Synopsis of Pediatric Emergency Care

Second Edition

Editors

Sunit Singhi, MBBS, MD, FIAP, FAMS
Professor
Head, Department of Pediatrics
Head, Emergency and Intensive Care Units
Advanced Pediatrics Centre
Postgraduate Institute of Medical Education and Research, Chandigarh (India)

Jagannath S. Surpure, MD, FAAP, FACEP
Clinical Professor of Pediatrics
University of Nevada, School of Medicine
Director, Pediatric Emergency Department
University Medical Center, Las Vegas, Nevada

Associate Editor
John J. Fraser, Jr., M.D., J.D., M.P.H.
Clinical Professor of Surgery
UTMB Division of Emergency Medicine
301 University Blvd.
Galveston, TX 77555-1173

PEEPEE
PUBLISHERS AND DISTRIBUTORS (P) LTD.

Synopsis of Pediatric Emergency Care

Published by
Pawaninder P. Vij

Peepee Publishers and Distributors (P) Ltd.
Head Office: 160, Shakti Vihar, Pitam Pura, Delhi-110 034 (India)

Correspondence Address:

7/31, First Floor, Ansari Road, Daryaganj,
New Delhi-110 002 (India)
Ph: 41512412, 9811156083
e-mail: peepee160@yahoo.co.in
e-mail: peepee160@gmail.com

www.peepeepub.com

Reprint 2024

ISBN: 9788184450767

Preface to the Second Edition

A good pediatric emergency care can have a profound impact on survival and quality of life of children with acute life threatening illnesses. Many common illnesses present in the emergency, and their timely and stepwise management, can be really rewarding. Over the past few decades emergency care has grown as a specialty all over the developed world. It has taken longer for this to happen in developing countries. It is time that pediatric emergency care is accepted as a specialty in developing countries. We are happy that the publication of this book coincides with the launching of India's first integrated specialty course in Pediatric Emergency and Intensive Care at PGIMER, Chandigarh.

This book has its genesis and foundation in years of experience of two senior editors from different worlds – developed and developing. We felt that there is a need for text which can form the framework for guiding pediatric residents and pediatric-practitioners all over the world. The book has contributions from two diverse geographical regions and amalgamates the knowledge and wisdom of both. The topics in this book cover emergency needs of children in a comprehensive manner, from resuscitation to evaluation, and diagnostic approach to specific management of disease. The distinguished contributors from USA have covered the subjects in which they have greater experience such as trauma, whereas diseases seen in tropics are covered by the Indian authors. We trust therefore that the book will have a global appeal

It had been our endeavor to include internationally acceptable management guidelines, along with a mention of recent advances and various treatment options. We have also tried to present the information in a concise and non-controversial manner. Wherever possible, flow charts have been used to simplify the information. A unique feature of the book is a symptom-wise approach to common problems that present to the emergency room where immediate diagnosis may not be forthcoming, such as airway obstruction, chest pain, headache, acute paralysis etc. The book also covers common neonatal emergencies and environmental emergencies. Two chapters detailing guidelines for organizational, administrative, structural and functional requirements for setting up pre-hospital emergency services and a pediatric emergency department in a large hospital have been specifically included. We think that these chapters will be particularly useful for those interested in pursuing emergency care as a specialty. We hope that the book will help pediatric trainees as well as pediatricians in developing a strong foundation for care of sick children and serve as a catalyst to initiate young pediatricians in developing subspecialty interest in Pediatric Emergency Care.

Sunit Singhi

Chandigarh **J. S. Surpure**

Preface to the First Edition

The growth of pediatric emergency medicine has been phenomenal; there has been an explosion of new knowledge in this area in the last decade. The numerous new courses (APLS, PALS), books, journals, and newsletters are the indicators of this parameter. The advancement of new knowledge, equipment, and life-support care has resulted in children now being resuscitated and cared for more efficiently. The establishment of specialized care centers and properly trained personnel and equipment at remote and small community hospitals will further improve the emergency care of ill and injured children. Obviously the ultimate goal is improved medical care for all children.

This book attempts to provide practical clinical information on the most important emergency children's problems that are seen in the emergency department on a daily basis. Hopefully this practical knowledge will assist the frontline clinicians in approaching precise diagnosis and management. This book is not an attempt to provide a comprehensive review of all children's emergencies. Rather it presents a quick practical approach to most common and frequent childhood emergency problems faced by the clinician in daily practice. Each chapter uniformly provides a brief review of pathophysiology followed by discussion and presentation of diagnostic and therapeutic modalities. In most chapters, the clinical decisionmaking is simplified by an algorithmic approach.

We sincerely hope that this synopsis format will be of practical benefit to all health professionals who care for critically ill and injured children.

J.S. Surpure

Acknowledgements to the Second Edition

Almost 15 years ago I prepared a draft-outline of a book on Pediatric Emergency Care that would cover common emergencies seen in India. This was after several years of experience in a standalone Pediatric Emergency unit at the Postgraduate Institute of Medical Education and Research, Chandigarh. Thanks to Dr J. S. Surpure, a very senior and experienced Pediatric Emergency specialist, in whose unit I had spent some time in 1989, for his offer of a joint venture to write a book with contributions from USA and India, that the draft outline materialised into a book that was envisioned long ago!

I am indebted to Professor BNS Walia, who plunged me into this unchartered area of Pediatrics and gave constant support and encouragement to develop Pediatric Emergency Services. It was his motivation that helped us to develop Pediatric Emergency Care as a sub-specialty in the newly founded Advanced Pediatrics Centre.

I am extremely grateful to all the distinguished authors from USA and India, some of whom are our past trainees, for their excellent contributions. They worked hard and submitted their work promptly to keep up with the publication deadline. I am also grateful to all my colleagues, and students who enriched my knowledge and experience throughout the years of work in the Pediatric Emergency unit.

I remain indebted to my wife, Professor Pratibha Singhi, for encouraging me to work on this book and for being a critique of the contents. I wish to thank my colleague Dr Jayashree M, for her help in coordinating with various authors and copy-editing some of the chapters, and several of our senior residents who helped in proof-reading as well as searching the internet and library for academic resources on various topics. My thanks are also due to Mrs Naresh Kumari for secretarial help with manuscripts. Finally, I wish to thank the publisher, Mr Pawaninder P Vij, Director, PeePee Publishers and Distributors (Pvt) Ltd., New Delhi, for his enthusiasm and co-operation to ensure timely publication of the book.

Sunit Singhi

Acknowledgements to the First Edition

I am indebted to the eminent clinical experts who generously contributed the chapters, and much credit is owed to them. It would not have been possible to publish this book without their help. Indeed, the book is a true synopsis of many dedicated individuals' experience, knowledge, expertise, and sensitivity toward children.

Very special thanks to Judith Gimple, Bywater Production Services, for her superb assistance in proof reading and editing the manuscript. It was a great pleasure to work with her as she kept me on my toes with frequent reminders and suggestions. Appreciation also goes to Ed Johnson for his excellent computer work, and Arlene Conrad for her assistance in editing.

Finally, I thank the readers, and hope that this book will be useful for them in daily clinical practice and will guide them in caring for ill and injured children.

Contributors

Arun Bansal, MBBS, MD, MRCPCH
Assistant Professor
Department of Pediatrics
Postgraduate Institute of Medical Education and Research, Chandigarh, India

Deepak Bansal, MBBS, MD, DNB
Associate Professor
Department of Pediatrics
Postgraduate Institute of Medical Education and Research, Chandigarh, India

Bhavneet Bharti, MBBS, MD,DNB(Ped,Mch,HAH)
Assistant Professor
Department of Pediatrics
Postgraduate Institute of Medical Education and Research, Chandigarh, India

Roger Barkin, MD
Health Sciences Center Hospitals
University of Colorado
Denver, Colorado, USA

Steven Barrett, MD
Maitland, Emergency Medicine Physician
Florida Hospital, Orlando, Florida, 32803, USA

Jerry Ray Baskerville, MD, FACEP
Associate Professor of Surgery
The University of Texas Medical Branch
Galveston, Texas, USA

Joseph H. Chang, MD, MBA
Assistant Professor of Surgery
Division of Emergency Medicine
The University of Texas Medical Branch
Galveston, Texas, USA

Marcella M. Donaruma-Kwoh, MD
Assistant Professor of Pediatrics
Child Protection
Section of Pediatric Emergency Medicine
Baylor College of Medicine
Texas Children's Hospital, Houston, Texas, USA

John J. Fraser, Jr., MD, JD, MPH
Visiting Professor
Department of Emergency Medicine
The University of Texas Medical School at Houston
6431 Fannin Street, Suite JJL 429
Houston, Texas, USA

Glenda H. Grawe, MD
Assistant Professor of Pediatrics
Attending Physician, Pediatric Emergency Medicine
Baylor College of Medicine
Texas Children's Hospital
Houston, Texas, USA

Angela Gardner, MD
Assistant Professor of Surgery
Division of Emergency Medicine
The University of Texas Medical Branch
Galveston, Texas, USA

Yuri Gilhotra, MBBS (Hons) (Syd), FRACP
Pediatric Emergency Physician
Mater Children's Hospital, Brisbane
Senior Lecturer, University of Queensland
Australia

Frederick S. Huang, MD
Assistant Professor of Pediatrics
Director, Pediatric Hematology/Oncology
Scholar, John P. McGovern Academy of Oslerian Medicine, The University of Texas Medical Branch
Galveston, Texas, USA

Herndon William MD
Orthopedic Surgeon
Edmond, Oklahoma,73013, USA

Isaac Reena, MD
Assistant Professor of Pediatrics
Child Protection
Section of Pediatric Emergency Medicine
Baylor College of Medicine, Texas Children's Hospital, Houston, Texas, USA

Puneet Jain, MBBS, MD
Senior Resident
Department of Pediatrics
Postgraduate Institute of Medical Education and Research
Chandigarh, India

Alka Khadwal, MBBS, MD
Assistant Professor
Department of Pediatrics
Postgraduate Institute of Medical Education and Research, Chandigarh, India

Shiva Kalidindi, MD, MS, DTMH
Assistant Professor
Pediatric Emergency Medicine
University of Western Ontario
London, ON, Canada

Koza Joseph M, MD
Assistant Professor of Surgery
Division of Emergency Medicine
The University of Texas Medical Branch
Galveston, Texas, USA

Praveen Kumar MBBS, MD, DM (Neonatology)
Additional Professor
Department of Pediatrics
Postgraduate Institute of Medical Education and Research, Chandigarh, India

Jayashree M, MBBS, MD, DNB
Additional Professor
Department of Pediatrics
Postgraduate Institute of Medical Education and Research, Chandigarh, India

Radheshyam Miryala, MD
Assistant Professor of Family Medicine
The University of Texas Medical Branch
Galveston, Texas, USA

Nishat Ahmed, MBBS, MD
Senior Resident
Department of Pediatrics
Postgraduate Institute of Medical Education and Research, Chandigarh, India

Banani Poddar, MBBS, MD
Associate Professor
Department of Critical Care Medicine
Sanjay Gandhi Postgraduate Institute
Lucknow, India

Wayne C Rutledge, Jr, MD
Assistant Professor of Surgery
Division of Emergency Medicine
The University of Texas Medical Branch
Galveston, Texas, USA

Rayne H Rouce, MD
Resident in Pediatrics
The University of Texas Medical Branch
Galveston, Texas, USA

Dipak P Sheth, MD
Associate Professor
Pediatric Emergency Medicine Physician
Children's National Medical Center - Main Hospital
111 Michigan Avenue, NW
Washington, DC, USA

Sunit Singhi, MBBS, MD, FIAP, FAMS
Professor and Head, Department of Pediatrics
Head, Emergency and Intensive Care Units
Postgraduate Institute of Medical Education and Research, Chandigarh, India

Pratibha Singhi, MD, FIAP
Professor
Head, Pediatric Neurology and Neurodevelopment
Department of Pediatrics
Postgraduate Institute of Medical Education and Research, Chandigarh, India

Shiv Sajan Saini, MBBS, MD, DM (Neonatology)
Senior Research Associate
Department of Pediatrics
Postgraduate Institute of Medical Education and Research, Chandigarh, India

Deepti Suri, MBBS, MD
Assistant Professor
Department of Pediatrics
Postgraduate Institute of Medical Education and Research, Chandigarh, India

Robert Schafermeyer, MD
Department of Emergency Medicine
Carolinas Medical Center
Charlotte, North Carolina, USA

Sonia Singh MD, MPH, MBA
Assistant Professor
University of Pittsburgh, School of Medicine
Children's Hospital of Pittsburgh
3705 Fifth Avenue
Pittsburgh, PA 15213, USA

Lokesh Tiwari, MBBS, DNB
Sr. Resident, Fellow PICU
Department of Pediatrics
Postgraduate Institute of Medical Education and Research, Chandigarh, India

William Tsai, MD
Division of Pediatric Critical Care
Levine Children's Hospital
Charlotte, North Carolina, USA

Monira Vakil, DO
Assistant Professor of Emergency Medicine
University of Mississippi
Jackson, Mississippi, USA

Mickey J Viator, MD, FAAP
Assistant Professor of Surgery
Division of Emergency Medicine
The University of Texas Medical Branch
Galveston, Texas, USA

Hee-Kwang Yoo, DO
Assistant Professor of Surgery
Division of Emergency Medicine
The University of Texas Medical Branch
Galveston, Texas, USA

Brian S Zachariah, MD,MBA, FACEP
Associate Professor of Surgery
Division of Emergency Medicine
The University of Texas Medical Branch
Galveston, Texas, USA

Contents

1 Pediatric Triage

Triage refers to assessment of a patient in emergency room with a view to define urgency of care and priorities in management

GOALS OF TRIAGE

1. To rapidly identify patients with urgent, life-threatening conditions
2. To determine the most appropriate treatment area for patients presenting to the emergency department
3. To decrease congestion in emergency treatment areas
4. To provide ongoing assessment of patients

Main focus of triage is to identify patients in greatest need and prioritize care.

Triage Assignment: is based on "usual presentation", and objective measures such as vital signs and pain scales, and experience of the provider. Since there are multiple changes in size, development, normal parameters, and significance of presenting symptom-complexes at different ages, each child must be triaged according to age, developmental stage, and acuity. Family dynamics, cultural, and social variables are also important considerations in triage decisions.

Time responses during triage are not established standard of care. Triage levels may require upgrading if the time response has not been met. The triage process needs to be flexible because patients' status may change while in the emergency department.

After triage assessments patients can be categorised in 5-levels of priority. These are discussed below (as per guidelines of Canadian Association of Emergency Physicians.)

LEVEL 1: RESUSCITATION

(Time to physician IMMEDIATE)

Definition:

- Conditions that are threats to life or limb (or imminent risk of deterioration) requiring immediate aggressive interventions

Usual Presentation:

- Respiratory failure, shock, coma, or cardiopulmonary arrest
- Requires continuous assessment and intervention to maintain physiological stability

Sentinel Diagnosis

These include coma, seizures, moderate to severe respiratory distress, major burns, trauma, significant bleeding, and cardio-pulmonary arrest

LEVEL 2: EMERGENT

(Time to physician: 15 min)

Definition:

- Conditions that are a potential threat to life, limb, or function, requiring rapid medical intervention or delegated acts

Usual Presentation

- Moderate to severe respiratory distress
- Altered level of consciousness (GCS < 13)
- Severe dehydration
- Requires comprehensive assessment and multiple interventions to prevent further deterioration
- Fever: age < 3 months and temperature > 38° C.

Sentinel Diagnosis

Included in this level are children with sepsis, altered consciousness, ingestion, asthma, seizure (postictal), DKA, child abuse, purpuric rash, fever, open fractures, violent patients, testicular pain, lacerations or orthopedic injuries with neurovascular compromise, dental injury with avulsed permanent tooth.

LEVEL 3: URGENT

(Time to physician: 30 min)

Definition

- Conditions that could potentially progress to a serious problem requiring emergency intervention
- May be associated with significant discomfort or affecting ability to function at work or activities of daily living

Usual Presentation

- Alert, oriented, well hydrated, minor alterations in vital signs
- Interventions include assessment and simple procedures
- Febrile child >3 months with temperature > 38.5°C
- Mild respiratory distress
- Infant < 1 month

Sentinel Diagnosis

Patients with simple burns, fractures, dental injuries, pneumonia without distress, history of seizure, suicidal ideation, ingestion requiring observation only, head trauma with GCS 14 or 15 and alert, vomitings, are included at this level.

LEVEL 4 SEMI-URGENT

(Time to physician: 1 hour)

- Conditions that relate to patient age, distress, or potential for deterioration or complications
- Would benefit from intervention or reassurance within 1-2 hours

Usual Presentation

- Vomiting/diarrhea and no dehydration age > 2 years
- Simple lacerations/ sprain/ strains
- Alert with fever and simple complaints such as ear pain, sore throat, or nasal congestion
- Head trauma: no symptoms

LEVEL 5: NON-URGENT

(Time to physician: 2 hours)

Definition

- Conditions that may be acute but non-urgent, may be part of a chronic problem ± evidence of deterioration. Investigation or interventions could be delayed and referred to other areas of the hospital or health care system

Usual Presentation

- Afebrile, alert, oriented, well hydrated with normal vital signs.
- Interventions not usually required other than assessment/discharge instruction.
- Vomiting alone or diarrhea alone with no symptoms or signs of dehydration.

FURTHER READING

1. Beveridge R, Clark B, Janes L, et al. Canadian emergency department triage and acuity scale: implementation guidelines. Can J Emeg. Med. 1999: 1(3 suppl).
2. Canadian Association of Emergency Physicians. Canadian pediatric triage and acuity scale: implementation guidelines for emergency departments. Can J Emerg. Med. 2001;3 (4 suppl): 1-40.

Lokesh Tiwari and Sunit Singhi

2 Cardiopulmonary Resuscitation

Cardiopulmonary arrests in children occur infrequently compared to adults. Of children who require resuscitation, however, the majority are young (45 to 70 percent are less than one year old and 21 to 30 percent are one to four years of age). Though early reports suggested children have a better outcome than adults, recent reviews demonstrate that children who suffer *cardiopulmonary* arrests have poor outcomes with only 5 to 21 percent surviving to hospital discharge. In contrast, children who have just respiratory arrests have a much higher survival rate.

PATHOPHYSIOLOGY

Cardiopulmonary arrests in children are caused by a wide range of problems. The most common causes include intravascular volume depletion due to illnesses such as gastroenteritis, infectious diseases such as meningitis, sepsis, pneumonia, croup, and bronchiolitis. Unlike adults, cardiac arrest in children is asphyxial arrest rather than sudden cardiac arrest as a result of primary cardiac problems like congenital heart disease, myocarditis, or dysrhythmias. Though pediatric arrests are due to a wide range of etiologies, the final common pathway is usually respiratory failure and/or circulatory collapse, resulting in endorgan anoxia. Cardiac arrest probably occurs within five minutes of complete anoxia. Because cardiac arrest in children is predominately caused by anoxia, most children present with bradycardia or asystole. Only about 10 percent of children with cardiac arrest present with ventricular fibrillation and commonly have ventricular rhythms with cardiac arrest.

CLINICAL PRESENTATION AND DIFFERENTIAL DIAGNOSES

Recognition of a cardiopulmonary arrest is not difficult. Clinical characteristics are cyanosis, a grayish hue, diaphoresis, mottling, unresponsiveness, and absence of respiration or pulse. Rapid recognition and institution of advanced life support is critical. Identifying the etiology of a cardiopulmonary arrest should follow the establishment of an airway, ventilation, and circulation.

More difficult is the recognition of the pre arrest state-a child who is still awake but agitated and subtly tachypneic from hypoxia, and who has normal blood pressure but is tachycardiac with poor capillary refill. Given the poor outcome of children who suffer cardiopulmonary arrests, early intervention in these children can be lifesaving.

HISTORY, PHYSICAL EXAMINATION, LABORATORY AND MANAGEMENT

In an arrest situation, the classical approach of taking a history, performing a complete examination, and performing initial laboratory tests before deciding on management is obviously not applicable. Instead these elements are interwoven.

Pediatric Assessment

Use "assess-categorize-decide-act" model to evaluate and treat a seriously ill or injured child. At any point you identify a life-threatening problem, start life saving interventions immediately and get help by activating the emergency response system. General assessment that is rapid visual and auditory assessment using pediatric assessment triangle (PAT) can be completed within the first few seconds of patient encounter. From the information gathered during assessment, *categorize* the clinical condition of the child, *decide* what needs to be done, and *act* to implement appropriate treatment. Then reassess and repeat the process. Primary assessment includes rapid hands-on cardiopulmonary and neurological evaluation using ABCDE approach, assessment of vital signs and pulse oximetry if available. A child in cardiac arrest can be identified in first few seconds of encounter so life saving interventions must be started immediately. Further assessment via focused medical history, physical examination and ancillary lab studies to detect and identify the presence and severity of respiratory and circulatory abnormalities can be performed as dictated by the clinical situation.

Setting Up a Team

The presentation of a young child in cardiopulmonary arrest is anxiety provoking and often results in a chaotic resuscitation. Optimal performance is derived from having a well-trained, experienced team with members having preassigned specific roles. The ideal size of team ranges between five and eight people. Too small a team makes it difficult to move rapidly through the resuscitation algorithm; too large a team causes unnecessary confusion. The team should include a leader and a scribe as well as individuals assigned to manage the airway, perform chest compressions, establish venous access, place and maintain monitors, assess vital signs, draw up medications, and apply cardiac defibrillation. As soon as possible, an experienced team member should meet and talk with any family members available to ascertain recent and past medical history.

ESTABLISHING AN AIRWAY AND ASSURING VENTILATION

If child is non-responsive, open the airway using head tilt-chin lift, evaluate the airway and check for breathing for 5 to 10 seconds by looking quickly at the chest and abdomen for signs of movement and listening over the mouth and nose for the movement of air. If there are no signs of respiration, check the oropharynx for foreign objects, then suction the airway of excess secretions. Place the child in a "sniffing" position and give rescue breaths. If intubation cannot be accomplished immediately, patients can be ventilated temporarily with 100 percent oxygen by use of a bag and mask (most commonly a self-inflating bag with a reservoir). If placing fingers behind the angle of the jaw while bagging the child is not sufficient to maintain an open airway, either place an oropharyngeal airway or have a second person bag while the other maintains a patent, sealed oral airway. If an oral airway is placed, choose one with a tip that reaches approximately to the angle of the jaw.

Intubation should be accomplished as soon as feasible since it maximizes ventilation and minimizes the risk of aspiration. In hospital settings cuffed tubes have been found to be as safe as uncuffed tubes for infants and children. Cuffed tubes may be preferable in certain circumstances such as poor lung compliance, high airway resistance or large glottic air leak. Keep cuff inflation pressure less than 20 cm H_2O. The size of endotracheal (ET) tube can best be estimated by matching the external diameter of the tube to the diameter of the child's little finger. See Table 1. for estimates of ET tube, laryngoscope blade, and suction catheter sizes based on age. The time required to intubate should be monitored, and prolonged efforts should be avoided by intermittent ventilation with 100 percent oxygen by mask.

Appropriate placement of the ET tube should be promptly confirmed by physical

Table 1: Size of ET tubes, laryngoscopes, and catheters, based on age

	Internal Diameter of Endotracheal tube (mm)	*Laryngoscope blade size*	*Suction Catheters (F)*
Age	Uncuffed (age in years/4) + 4 Cuffed (age in years/4) + 3		2 X ET size
Newborn	2.5, 3.0 Uncuffed	0-1	6F
6 months	3.5, 4.0 Uncuffed	1	8F
18 months	4.0 Uncuffed	2	8F
3 years	4.5 Uncuffed 4.0 Cuffed	2	8F
5 years	5.0, 5.5 Uncuffed 4.5 Cuffed	2	10 F
6 years	5.5 Uncuffed 5.0 Cuffed	2	10 F
8 years	6.0 Cuffed	2	12 F
12 years	6.5, 7.0 Cuffed	2	12 F
16 years	7.0, 8.0 Cuffed	3	12 F
Adult (F)	7.5-8.0 Cuffed	3	12F
Adult (M)	8.0-8.5 Cuffed	3	14 F

examination i.e. adequate and symmetrical chest rise, equal breath sounds over proximal and peripheral lung fields and condensation in the tube with exhalation. Conformational devices include exhaled CO_2 detection by capnometry/ capnography, improvement in SPO_2, esophageal detector device to demonstrate aspiration of air from trachea and chest-X-ray to confirm tube position. If there is any doubt about proper placement, the tube should be pulled and the patient reintubated. Ventilation rates based on age are listed in Table 2. Ventilation volume should be 10 to 15 ml/kg; practically this volume can be approximated by bagging sufficient to lift the chest wall visibly. Auscultate the chest in anterior and lateral fields bilaterally, and quickly check for asymmetry of the chest wall and deviation of the trachea. A naso- or orogastric tube should be placed after intubation to evacuate the stomach of air and of any other contents.

Cricothyroidotomy or tracheostomy are *rarely* required (PALS). Complications from these procedures are common, and ventilation can almost always be maintained with bag and mask until intubation can be accomplished.

Airway and ventilation should be repeatedly reassessed throughout resuscitation. In addition, the oxygen delivery system should be double-checked to assure that maximum oxygen is being delivered to the patient.

ASSESSMENT OF CIRCULATION/CHEST COMPRESSIONS

After delivery of 2 rescue breaths, attempt to feel carotid or brachial pulse in the unresponsive, non-breathing victim for 5 to 10 seconds. If pulse is not felt definitely within 10 seconds, high quality cardiopulmonary resuscitation (CPR) should be started. Place heel of one hand in the centre of chest between nipples and other hand on top of the first hand to start effective compression. In infants compression should be delivered just below the nipple line. Deliver chest compressions that depress the chest of the infant and child by one third to one half the depth of the chest. Remember to *push hard, push fast* (rate of 100 compressions per minute), allow complete chest recoil between compressions, and minimize interruptions in compressions. Use a 30:2 compression-ventilation ratio for all 1-rescuer and all adult CPR and use a 15:2 compression ventilation ratio for infant and child 2-rescuer CPR. Once an advanced airway is in place (eg, endotracheal tube, Combitube, LMA) during 2-rescuer CPR, provide 100 compressions per minute without pausing for ventilation, and deliver 8 to 10 breaths per minute. See Table 2 for a summary of technique and rates based on age. Compressions should ideally be interrupted only for ventilation (until an advance airway is placed), rhythm check (after 2 minutes) and actual shock delivery.

Establishing Venous Access

After oxygenation and ventilation, vascular access is the next management priority in an acutely ill or injured child. Venous access should be obtained rapidly to allow the provision of fluids and drugs. Rapid venous access is more important than site of access. Immediate intraosseous access is recommended if no other intravenous access is already in place. If neither a bone marrow nor a specifically designed intraosseous needle is available, a two-inch, 18 to 20 gauge spinal needle can be used. The preferred location is on the flat, medial surface of the proximal tibial shaft 1 to 2 cm below the tibial tuberosity. Alternately, especially in older children or adolescents, a needle can be placed in the medial surface of the tibia proximal to the medial malleolus. All resuscitation drugs and fluids can be delivered rapidly and safely via this route.

Table 2: Compression/ ventilation standards for pediatric resuscitation

Maneuver	*Adult* *Adolescent and older*	*Child* *1 year to adolescent*	*Infant* *< 1 year*
Pulse check	Carotid or femoral		Brachial or femoral
Compression landmarks	Centre of chest, between nipples		Just below nipple line
Compression method	2 hands	2 hands or 1 hand	1 rescuer: 2 fingers 2 rescuers: 2 thumbs encircling hands
Compression depth	1.5 to 2.0 inches	Approximately ? to ½ the depth of chest	
Compression rate	Approximately 100 per minute		
Compression-ventilation ratio	30:2 (1 or 2 rescuer)	30:2 (single rescuer) 15:2 (2 rescuer)	

Child CPR guidelines for *healthcare providers* apply to victims from about 1 year of age to the onset of dolescence or puberty (about 12 to 14 years of age) as defined by the presence of secondary sex characteristics.

During attempted resuscitation if an endotracheal tube is in place but vascular access is not yet available, lipid soluble resuscitation drugs namely lidocain, epinephrine, atropine and naloxone (LEAN) may be administered through ET tube although optimal endotracheal doses are unknown and drug level and effects are unpredictable. Flush with a minimum of 5 mL normal saline followed by 5 assisted manual ventilations.

Central venous access is obtained most reliably and rapidly by the Seldinger guide-wire technique via the femoral vein (PALS). The use of this route does not impinge on other aspects of resuscitation. Cannulation by the open or percutaneous cutdown technique *in unexperienced hands* is difficult and slow and generally should be avoided (Figure 1).

Assessment of Cardiac Rhythm

Management of any seriously ill or injured child requires assessment of heart rate and rhythm. Asystole and bradycardia with a wide QRS complex are most common in asphyxial cardiac arrest, VF and pulseless electrical activity (PEA) are less common and more likely to be observed in children with sudden arrest. By far the most common rhythm found in apneic, pulseless children will be asystole or bradycardia. Patients who survive with this rhythm will usually do so with the initiation of ventilation or with the first couple of doses of epinephrine (14). Determine the rhythm, it may be slow (bradyarrhythmia), fast (tachyarrhythmia), or arrest (pulseless arrest). In pulseless arrest rhythm may be shockable (VF / VT without pulse) or nonshockable (asystole / pulseless electrical activity).

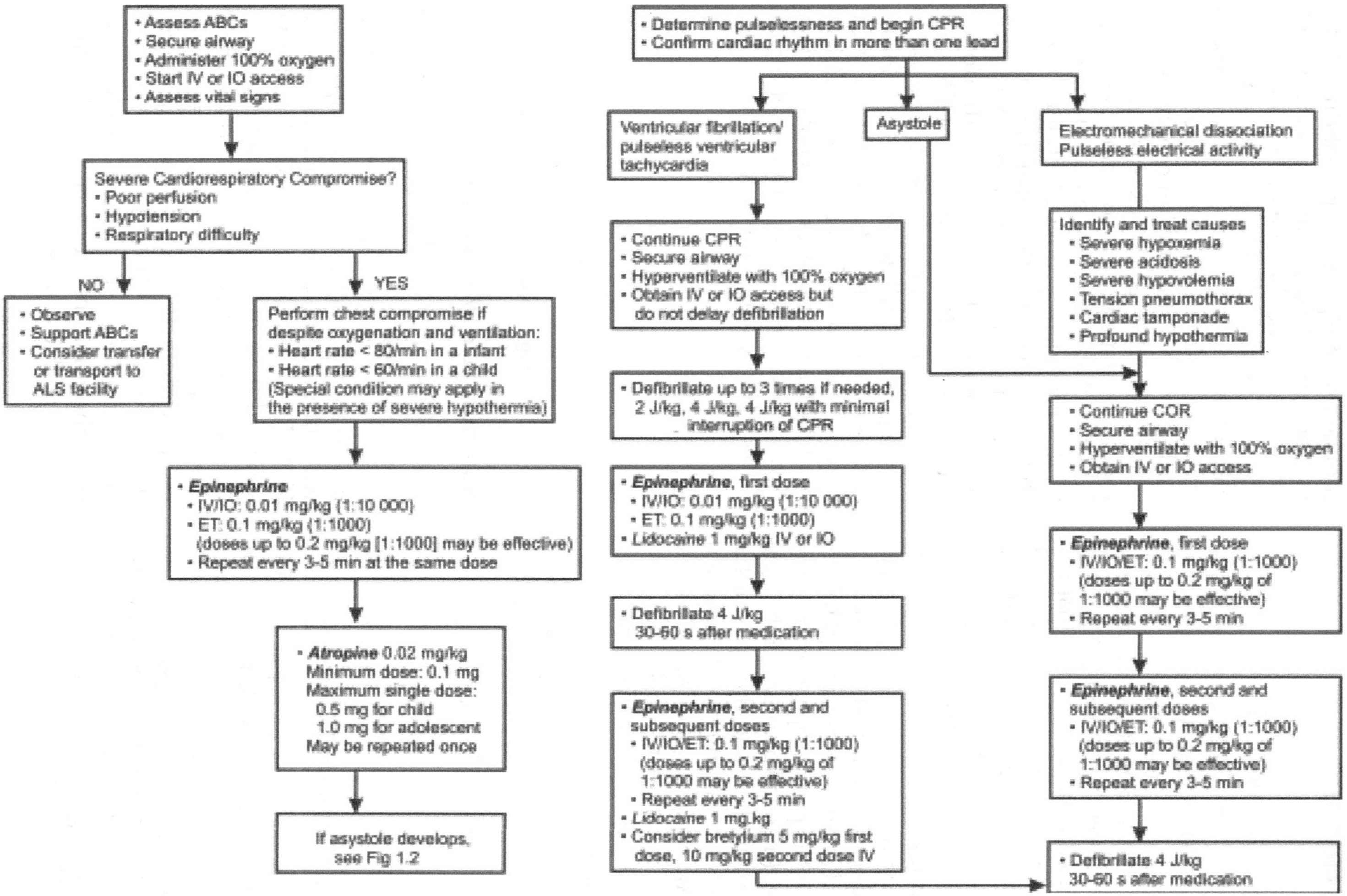

Fig. 1: Algorithm for pediatric cardiopulmonary resuscitation: (a) bradycardia decision tree (ABCs = airway, breating, circulation; ALS = advanced life support; IO = intraosseous; IV = intravenous) and (b) asystole and pulseless arrest decision tree (CPR = cardiopulmonary resuscitation). (Adapted from American heart Association. Guidelines for cardiopulmonary resuscitation and emergency cardiac care)

PULSELESS ARREST

Shockable Rhythm (VF / VT)

VF occurs in 5% to 15% of all pediatric victims of out-of hospital cardiac arrest and up to 20% of pediatric in-hospital arrests Defibrillation is the definitive treatment for shockable rhythms. When using a manual defibrillator use the largest paddles that will fit on the chest wall without touching each other. Use infant paddles for infanta weighing <10 kg and adult paddles (8 to 10 cm) for children >10 kg. Apply electrode–chest wall interface like conductive gel, electrode cream, paste, or self-adhesive monitoring-defibrillation pads. Do not use saline-soaked pads, ultrasound gel, bare paddles, or alcohol pads. Apply firm pressure on the paddles (manual) placed over the right side of the upper chest and the apex of the heart (to the left of the nipple over the left lower ribs). Alternatively place one electrode on the front of the chest just to the left of the sternum and the other over the upper back below the scapula.

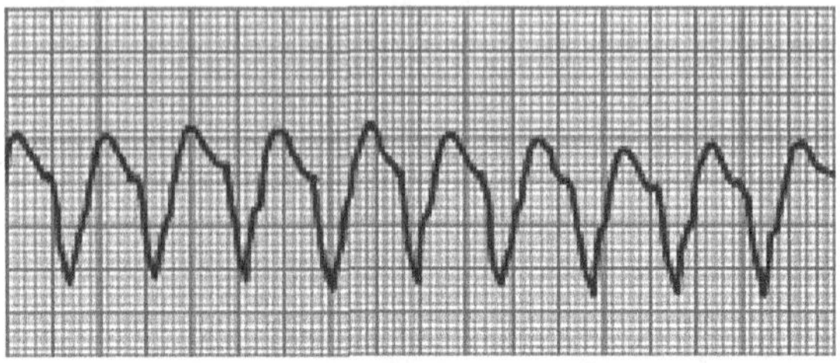

Fig. 2: Ventricular Tachycardia

Taking all precautions give 1 shock (2 J/kg) as quickly as possible and immediately resume CPR, beginning with chest compressions. Continue CPR for about 5 cycles (about 2 minutes) and again check the rhythm. If a shockable rhythm persists, give one shock (4 J/kg), resume compressions immediately and give a (standard) dose of epinephrine. There is no survival benefit from routine use of high-dose epinephrine, and it may be harmful, particularly in asphyxia (16). High-dose epinephrine may be considered in exceptional circumstances, such as beta-blocker overdose. Give the standard dose of epinephrine about every 3 to 5 minutes during cardiac arrest. If the rhythm continues to be "shockable," deliver a shock (4 J/kg), resume CPR immediately, and give amiodarone or lidocaine if amiodarone is not available while CPR is provided. Continue CPR for 5 cycles (about 2 minutes) before again checking the rhythm and attempting to defibrillate if needed with 4 J/kg. If defibrillation is successful but VF recurs, continue CPR while you give another bolus of amiodarone before you try to defibrillate with the previously successful shock dose. Search for and treat reversible causes. If there is an organized rhythm at any time, check for a pulse, if there is no pulse, treat it as pulseless electrical activity (PEA) and proceed accordingly.

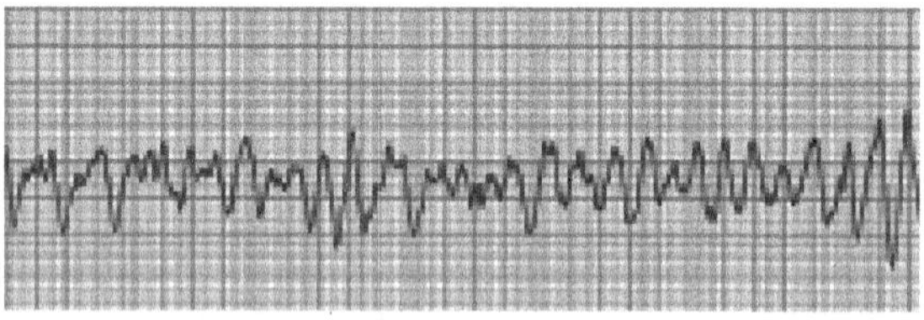

Fig. 3: Ventricular Fibrillation

Nonshockable Rhythm (Asystole / PEA)

The most common ECG findings in infants and children in cardiac arrest are asystole and PEA. PEA is organized electrical activity, most commonly slow, wide QRS complexes—without palpable pulses. For asystole and PEA: Resume high quality CPR and give standard dose of epinephrine after every 3 to 5 minutes. There is no survival benefit from routine high-dose epinephrine, use a standard dose for the first and subsequent doses except in circumstances such as beta-blocker overdose where high dose epinephrine may be beneficial. Search for and treat reversible causes.

Table 3: Possible contributing factors in arrhythmias

6 H's	*5 T's*
Hypovolemia	Toxins
Hypoxia	Temponade, cardiac
Hydrogen ion (Acidosis)	Tension pneumothorax
Hypo-/hyper-kalemia	Thrombosis (coronary or pulmonary)
Hypoglycaemia	Trauma (hypovolemia)
Hypothermia	

Tachycardia with Hemodynamic Instability

Because all arrhythmia therapies have the potential for serious adverse effects, consult an expert in pediatric arrhythmias before treating a hemodynamically stable child having tachycardia. If there are no palpable pulses, treat as pulseless arrest. If there is tachycardia on ECG monitor and pulses are palpable with patient having signs of hemodynamic compromise (poor perfusion, tachypnea, weak pulses), ensure ABC and assess QRS duration, determine if the QRS duration is =0.08 second (narrow-complex tachycardia) or >0.08 second (wide-complex tachycardia).

Narrow-Complex ($\leq$0.08 Second) Tachycardia

Differentiate between probable sinus tachycardia and probable supraventricular tachycardia on the basis of history and ECG findings (Table 4). If the rhythm is sinus tachycardia, search for and treat reversible causes. If it is probable supraventricular tachycardia attempt *vagal stimulation* (apply ice to the face without occluding the airway) while preparing for pharmacological or electrical cardioversion. Pharmacological cardioversion with adenosine (0.1 mg/kg) is very effective. If IV access is readily available administer adenosine using 2 syringes connected to a T-connector or stopcock; give adenosine rapidly with one syringe and immediately flush with >5 mL of normal saline with the other. If the patient is very unstable or IV access is not readily available, provide electrical (synchronized) cardioversion. Consider sedation if possible. Start with a dose of 0.5 to 1 J/kg.

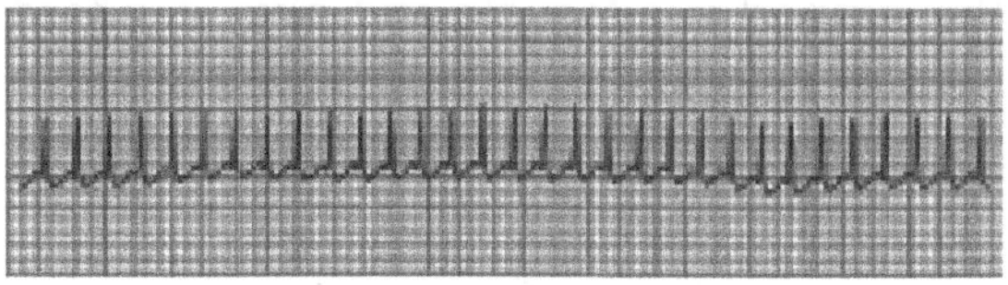

Fig. 4: Supra ventricular tachycardia

If unsuccessful, repeat using a dose of 2 J/kg. If a second shock is unsuccessful or the tachycardia recurs quickly, consider antiarrhythmic therapy (amiodarone or procainamide) before a third shock. Consider obtaining expert consultation.

Wide-Complex (>0.08 Second) Tachycardia

Wide-complex tachycardia with poor perfusion is probably ventricular in origin but may be supraventricular with aberrancy.

Table 4: Differentiating features between Sinus Tachycardia and Supraventricular Tachycardia

Probable sinus tachycardia	*Probable supraventricular tachycardia*
• Compatible history consistent with known causes	• Vague and non specific history, abrupt rate changes
• Normal P wave	• Abnormal or absent P wave
• Constant PR with variable RR	• Fixed heart rate
• Infants: rate usually <220	• Infants: rate usually $\geq$220
• Children: rate usually <180	• Children: rate usually $\geq$180

Treat with synchronized electrical cardioversion (0.5 J to 1 J/kg). If readily available, try a dose of adenosine first to determine if the rhythm is SVT with aberrant conduction. If a second shock (2 J/kg) is unsuccessful or tachycardia recurs quickly, consider antiarrhythmic therapy (amiodarone or procainamide) before a third shock.

OTHER RHYTHM ABNORMALITIES

Bradycardia

If pulses, perfusion, and respirations are normal, no emergency treatment is necessary. If heart rate is <60 beats per minute with poor perfusion despite effective ventilation with oxygen, start chest compressions. Verify that the support is adequate and give standard dose of epinephrin. If bradycardia persists or responds only transiently, consider a continuous infusion of epinephrine or isoproterenol. If bradycardia is due to vagal stimulation, give atropine. Emergency transcutaneous pacing may be lifesaving if the bradycardia is due to complete heart block or sinus node dysfunction unresponsive to ventilation, oxygenation, chest compressions, and medications, especially if it is associated with congenital or acquired heart disease. Pacing is not useful for asystole or bradycardia due to post-arrest hypoxic/ischemic myocardial insult or respiratory failure.

Torsades de Pointes (Figure 5)

This polymorphic VT is seen in patients with a long QT interval, which may be congenital or may result from toxicity with antiarrhythmics, tricyclic antidepressants, digitalis, or drug interactions. Regardless of the cause, treat torsades de pointes with a rapid (over several minutes) IV infusion of magnesium sulphate.

DRUG THERAPY

Recommendations for drug therapy during pediatric resuscitation have changed significantly over the last 10 years. Several issues remain unresolved and recommendations may continue to change. See Table 5 for current dosing recommendations.

Oxygen

Most arrests occur as a result of inadequate delivery of oxygen to the tissues. It is therefore imperative that 100 percent oxygen be used throughout the resuscitation to minimize tissue hypoxia.

Epinephrine. After oxygen, epinephrine is widely considered to be the most effective drug in resuscitation. It is indicated for asystole, bradycardia, EMD, and ventricular fibrillation. The mechanism of action appears to be largely due to its effects, which result in increased coronary perfusion pressure and cerebral blood flow. Low-dose infusions (<0.3 µg/kg per minute) generally produce β-adrenergic action (potent inotropy and decreased systemic vascular resistance), and higher-dose infusions (>0.3 µg/kg per minute) cause α-adrenergic vasoconstriction.

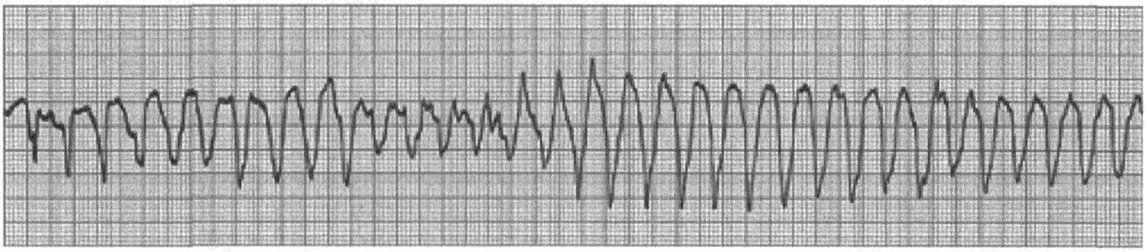

Fig. 5: Torsades de Pointes

Table 5: Common drugs used during resuscitation

Drug	Dose	Concentration	Comment
Atropine	0.02 mg/kg/dose	Range 0.1 mg to 1.2 mg/ml	Recommended minimum dose 0.1 mg, maximum dose 0.5 mg for a child
Adenosine	0.1 mg/kg IV/IO	3 mg/ml	Rapid bolus using two syringe technique
Calcium chloride	20 mg/kg/dose	100 mg/ml(10%)	Use with central venous access
Dopamine	2-20 μg/kg/min	40, 80 and 160 mg/ml	Titrate to desired effect
Epinephrine	0.01 mg/kg/dose	0.1 mg/ml (1:10,000)	High dose not recommended
Epinephrine (infusion)	0.1-1.0 μg/kg/min		Titrate to desired effect
Glucose	0.5 to 1 gm/kg/dose	D5W (0.05 gm/ml) D10W (0.1 gm/ml) D25W (0.25 gm/ml) D50W (0.5 gm/ml)	More important in neonates
Lidocaine	1 mg/kg/dose	10 & 20 mg/ml	Give bolus undiluted over 2-4 min
Lidocaine infusion	20-50 μg/kg/min	(1 &2%)	
Sodium bicarbonate	1 mEq/kg/dose	0.5-1 mEq/ml (4.2 & 8.4%)	Use only if ventilation is established
Amiodarone	5mg/kg over 20-mins		

Because there is great interpatient variability titrate the drug to the desired effect.

Adenosine

It is very short acting antiarrhythmic drug with half life < 10 seconds so given as rapid push using two syringe technique. It is used for pharmacological cardioversion in supraventricular tachycardia. It briefly blocks conduction through AV node and depresses sinus node automaticity. Recommended dose is 0.1 mg/kg IV/IO rapid push (maximum dose 6 mg) as first dose and double the dose for second dose.

Amiodarone

It is class III antiarrhythmic agent used in treatment of ventricular fibrillation and pulseless ventricular tachycardia. Other indication are ventricular tachycardia with pulse and supraventricular tachycardia non responsive to cardioversion. Recommended dose is 5 mg/kg IV/IO load over 20 to 60 minutes (maximum dose 300 mg), repeat to maximum total dose of 15 mg/kg.

Glucose

The myocardium uses glucose as its major

energy substrate, and infants, especially those who are chronically ill, have limited glycogen stores. Consequently early assessment of a child's serum glucose is essential. Blind or repeated administration of glucose is not warranted, however, as it may result in a hyperosmolar state.

Atropine

This is generally recommended for both asystole and bradycardia. Since bradycardia most commonly stems from hypoxia, however, attention should be directed toward adequacy of airway and ventilation before atropine is given.

Sodium Bicarbonate

Controversy surrounds the use of bicarbonate in an arrest situation. Evidence is accumulating that the administration of bicarbonate can cause a *lowering* of intracellular pH. To date, a consensus has formed that bicarbonate should not be given until adequate ventilation has been established, and arterial blood gases drawn subsequently demonstrate a residual metabolic acidosis.

Calcium

No longer recommended in an arrest situation unless hypocalcemia is demonstrated or there is a specific therapeutic indication such as hyperkalemia, hypermagnesemia, or calcium channel blocker overdose (PALS).

Lidocaine

Ventricular fibrillation or unstable tachycardia that does not respond to defibrillation is indications for the use of lidocaine. If one bolus dose is not effective, a repeat bolus dose may be given in 10 to 15 minutes. Start a continuous infusion immediately. A third bolus may be needed 10 to 15 minutes later while the infusion is reaching steady-state concentrations.

Dopamine

Titrate dopamine to treat shock that is unresponsive to fluid and when systemic vascular resistance is low. Typically a dose of 2 to 20 μg/kg per minute is used. At doses (>5 μg/kg per minute), dopamine stimulates cardiac beta-adrenergic receptors, but this effect may be reduced in infants and in chronic congestive heart failure.

Dobutamine Hydrochloride

Dobutamine has a selective effect on β_1 and β_2 adrenergic receptors; it increases myocardial contractility and usually decreases peripheral vascular resistance. Titrate an infusion to improve cardiac output and blood pressure, especially due to poor myocardial function.

Norepinephrine

Norepinephrine is a potent inotropic and peripheral vasoconstricting agent. Titrate an infusion to treat shock with low systemic vascular resistance (septic, anaphylactic, spinal, or vasodilatory) unresponsive to fluid.

Sodium Nitroprusside

Sodium nitroprusside increases cardiac output by decreasing vascular resistance (afterload). If hypotension is related to poor myocardial function, consider using a combination of sodium nitroprusside to reduce afterload and an inotrope to improve contractility.

Inodilators

Inodilators (inamrinone and milrinone) augment cardiac output with little effect on myocardial oxygen demand. Use an inodilator for treatment of myocardial dysfunction with increased systemic or pulmonary vascular resistance. Administration of fluids may be required because of the vasodilatory effects. Inodilators have a long half-life with a long delay in reaching a new steady-state hemodynamic effect after changing the infusion rate (18 hours with inamrinone and 4.5 hours with milrinone). In case of toxicity, if you stop the infusion the adverse effects may persist for several hours.

Guidelines for Stopping Resuscitation Efforts

There are no established standards for terminating resuscitative efforts in an emergency setting. Based on epidemiologic studies of cardiopulmonary resuscitation, however, some general statements and broad guidelines can be derived. Unwitnessed cardiopulmonary arrests or patients who have a delay of greater than 12 minutes before cardiopulmonary resuscitation (CPR) is initiated have a poor prognosis. Children presenting with asystole do much worse than do children presenting with other types of rhythm. Children who develop sinus rhythm and perfusion after more than two doses of epinephrine also have low long-term survival. The exception is children who are hypothermic, most commonly from cold-water drowning. Establishing brain death by strict criteria takes time, however, and is impossible to do in an emergency setting.

Based on this set of facts, it is reasonable to intubate, ventilate, and perform compressions on all children who present in cardiopulmonary arrest until their hypoxia and respiratory acidosis is reversed, their core temperature is raised to 35°C, and they have been given at least two doses of epinephrine and *as indicated* counter shocked or given drugs such as glucose. Resuscitative efforts should be continued on children who intermittently restore perfusion or demonstrate supraventricular tachycardia or a ventricular rhythm. Regardless of the duration of suspected anoxia, any child who restores perfusion should continue to be treated. Though the prognosis for some of these children will be poor, termination can only be medicolegally carried out in an intensive care setting and should not be terminated in the field. Resuscitation can be stopped, however, on children who remain unresponsive without pulse and rhythm after the resuscitative efforts outlined above have been completed.

CONCLUSIONS

Survival rates from cardiopulmonary resuscitation in children are low. Hence vigilant monitoring of children with potentially fatal diseases is essential. Early intervention prior to arrest will result in the highest possible rates of recovery. Since all cardiopulmonary arrests are not completely preventable, however, the highest survival rates will result from prompt, well-organized resuscitative efforts.

Last, the physiology and pharmacology of cardiopulmonary resuscitation are evolving sciences. Changes in approach and outcome can be expected to continue to occur over the next decade.

FURTHER READING

1. Ludwig S, Fleisher G. Pediatric cardiopulmonary resuscitation: a review and a proposal. Pediatr Emerg Care 1985;1:40.
2. Silverman BK. Advanced pediatric life support. Dallas: American Academy of Pediatrics & American College of Emergency Physicians, 1989;1-14.

3. Deakers TW, Reynolds G, Stretton M, Newth CJ. Cuffed endotracheal tubes in pediatric intensive care. *J Pediatr*. 1994;125:57– 62.
4. Parwani V HI-H, Hsu B, Hoffman RJ. Experienced emergency physicians cannot safely or accurately inflate endotracheal tube cuffs or estimate endotracheal tube cuff pressure using standard technique. *Acad Emerg Med*. 2004;11:490–491.
5. *Circulation* 2005;112;IV-12-IV-18;
6. PALS 2007
7. Garcia LA, Kerber RE. Transthoracic defibrillation: does electrode adhesive pad position alter transthoracic impedance? *Resuscitation*. 1998;37:139 –143.
8. Perondi M, Reis A, Paiva E, Nadkarni V, Berg RA. A comparison of high-dose and standard-dose epinephrine in children with cardiac arrest. *N Engl J Med*. 2004;350:1722–1730.

In the previous edition this chapter was written by David Johnson, MD Assistant Professor of Pediatrics Divisions of Emergency Medicine & Clinical Pharmacology, The Hospital for Sick Children Toronto, Ontario, Canada

Sai Sunil Kishor M and Praveen Kumar

3 Neonatal Resuscitation

Resuscitation of the newborn infant is a medical emergency. It is required for any neonate who, in the first few minutes of life, cannot establish adequate effective ventilation to meet the needs for oxygenation and carbon dioxide excretion or whose cardiovascular status is inadequate to perfuse the central nervous system (CNS), heart, and other vital organs. Ineffective oxygenation and inadequate perfusion in the newborn may start at a variable period before delivery secondary to conditions that interrupt the placenta's ability to remove carbon dioxide and hydrogen ions or to supply oxygen (fetal asphyxia). This may progress through the intrapartum and the immediate postpartum period. Conditions that reduce the neonate's ability to initiate and/or maintain breathing at birth, however, will also regularly result in asphyxia.

Transition from fetal to neonatal life requires many adjustments that the newborn must accomplish in order to function normally at birth. Some infants have difficulty making this transition and require resuscitation in the first few minutes after birth. An effective resuscitation requires, besides capable personnel and a smooth working team, an understanding of the physiology of progressive asphyxia, temperature regulation, and appropriate ventilatory and monitoring equipment, drugs, and fluids. In the emergency department, good communication should be maintained between obstetrics, pediatrics, anaesthesiology, and the nursing service. At least two persons are required to perform proper neonatal resuscitation. High-risk conditions that may result in an asphyxiated newborn infant are given in Table 1. If possible these conditions should be anticipated and preparation made well in advance.

PATHOPHYSIOLOGY OF ASPHYXIA

An understanding of the pathophysiology of asphyxia is a prerequisite to anyone performing neonatal resusitation. Much of the information about the physiological changes associated with asphyxia comes from experiments on animals. Although differences exist among the diverse species studied, the species that is most closely analogous to the human fetus when it is subjected to total asphyxia is the Rhesus monkey fetus. A Rhesus monkey fetus was delivered via caeserian section with catheters placed in the fetal vessels prior to delivery; it prevented from gasping with a saline-filled rubber bag

Table 1: Conditions of high risk for the newborn

Prenatal	*Natal*	*Postnatal*
Maternal age more than 3.5 years	Abnormal presentation	Birth asphyxia
Diabetes	Premature delivery	Respiratory distress
Hypertension	Multiple births	Hypothermia
Hemorrhage	Maternal hypertension	Meconium staining
Infection	Prolonged labor	Premature infant
Prolonged rupture of	Prolapse of the cord	Intrauterine growth
Membranes		Retardation (IUGR)
Drug therapy	Maternal anesthesia	
Drug dependency	Caesarean section	
Heroin	Abnormal fetal heart rate	
Methadone	Meconium-stained amniotic fluid	
Cocaine	Polyhydramnios	

placed over its head. The animal was observed over a period of several minutes and the physiological changes that occurred were recorded during this "total asphyxia." Rapid gasps occurred shortly after the onset of asphyxia accompanied by muscular efforts producing thrashing movements of the arms and legs. This ceased after little more than a minute and heralded the onset of *primary apnea.* During primary apnea, spontaneous respirations could still be induced by appropriate sensory stimuli. This apnea lasted for about a minute. The heart rate dropped but was still above 100 per minute. A series of spontaneous deep gasps then followed for the next four or five minutes, gradually becoming weaker and terminating at the last gasp followed by *secondary apnea.* This occurred after approximately eight minutes of total anoxia. During secondary apnea, respirations could not be induced by sensory stimuli, and death would occur if secondary apnea was not reversed within several minutes. The longer the delay in resuscitation after the last gasp, the longer the time to the first gasp after resuscitation.

When an asphyxiated newborn is encountered in the emergency department, it is extremely difficult to determine whether primary or secondary apnea is present. In all situations, secondary apnea must be assumed and resuscitative efforts should be initiated immediately.

Dramatic changes in the acid base parameters of the Rhesus monkey occurred during asphyxia. During 10 minutes of asphyxia pH dropped from 7.3 to 6.8, PC02 rose from 45 to 150 mmHg and P02 fell from 25 to almost 0 mmHg. Associated with this was an increase in the blood lactate level (anaerobic glycolysis), free fatty acid and glycerol (release of epinephrine and norepinephrine), and mobilization of hepatic glycogen. This mobilization of glycogen makes it an unusual event to find hypoglycemia in an asphyxiated newborn infant. Therefore infusion of hypertonic glucose solutions are not recommended during resuscitation.

During the course of asphyxia blood pressure fell gradually after an initial transient rise. The skin became blotchy and blue in response to circulatory failure. Blood was preferentially redistributed, however, to vital organs like the heart, the brain, and the adrenal glands at the expense of less vital organs like the kidneys, the spleen, and the lungs *(diving reflex).* This situation resulted in asphyxial damage to virtually every organ in the body like necrotizing enterocolitis in the gastrointestinal tract, postasphyxial icterus, shock lung, persistent pulmonary hypertension, renal failure, and sclerema of the skin secondary to asphyxial injury to the dermal capillaries.

The most common antecedent of persistent neurologic dysfunction in a newborn infant is perinatal asphyxia. This is true because, although the brain is less than 2 percent of the body weight, it accounts for almost 20 percent of the total oxygen consumption. Thus the brain is dependent on a continuous, uninterrupted supply of oxygen and glucose in order for it to function normally. Asphyxia also leads to a loss of the brain's ability to control its own blood supply *(auto regulation)*. Such a loss in the brain's ability to control circulation exposes the brain to fluctuations in systemic blood pressure. This could result in intracranial hemorrhage. A wide array of typical pathological lesions have been described in the brain of asphyxiated newborn infants. The asphyxiated neuronal cell membrane becomes vulnerable to cation and water flux since acidosis alters its intrinsic ion pumping mechanisms. Potassium leaks out and sodium enters the neuron. This is the biochemical basis for the brain swelling found in postasphyxia.

Newborn infants have some protective mechanisms to tolerate asphyxia such as a lower metabolic rate of any particular tissue than the adults do, availability of substrates for anaerobic degradation, and an intact circulation to redistribute lactate and hydrogen ion to tissues still being perfused. Severe sustained asphyxia, however, will overcome these protective mechanisms, and severe brain damage and death will occur if asphyxia is not reversed.

The description of asphyxia and its consequences described above generally refers to severe total asphyxia. In practice, various grades of asphyxia much milder than this will be encountered. Also modern obstetrical management with fetal monitoring and determination of fetal acid base status with scalp blood sampling can detect impending asphyxia *in utero*, and preventive measures can be undertaken before delivery.

CLINICAL PRESENTATION

In the emergency department, neonatal resuscitation should be an infrequent event. In the few situations that require resuscitation, however, both skill and quick response is required to prevent the damaging effects of prolonged asphyxia. Clinical presentation could vary from mild asphyxia, where an infant presents with slight disturbances in the stability of cardiorespiratory system, to complete cardiac and respiratory arrest associated with shock, severe hypothermia, and metabolic acidosis.

Therefore the worst situation should be anticipated, and preparation should be made in the emergency department. All the necessary equipment for performing neonatal resuscitation should be available at all times (Table 2). A radiant warmer should be ready with proper lighting. All resuscitative procedures should be performed with gloved hands, as the physician invariably has to respond to infants with very little knowledge of their prenatal history. All ancillary services should be informed of the arrival of the asphyxiated newborn infant.

EVALUATION OF THE NEWBORN INFANT

Immediately after arrival, infants should be placed under a radiant warmer and Apgar scores should be determined. The components of the Apgar scores are given in Table 3. These parameters can be assessed very easily at the bedside within a few seconds. Traditionally Apgar Scores are given in the delivery room at one and five minutes after birth. The evaluations and decisions regarding the resuscitation measures should be guided by assessment of respiration, heart rate and color. Apgar scores are

Table 2: Resuscitation equipment

Radiant Warmer	Laryngoscope blades, nos, 0 and 1
EKG/respiration monitor	Umbilical catheters 3.5 and 5 Fr
Suction with manometer	Three- way stopcock
Wall oxgen with flow meter	Sterile umblilcal catherizaiton tray
Suction catheters, sizes 5, 6, and 8 Fr	ET tube adaptior for meconium suctioning
Resuscitation bag with manometer	Gloves
Face masks-small, medium and large	Stethoscope
Oral airways	Warm towels
ET tube, sizes 2.5, 3 and 3.5mm	Cap to cover the scalp
ET tube stylette	Umbilical cord clamp
Laryngoscope	

Table 3: Apgar Scores

	Score		
Sing	0	1	2
Heart rate	Absent	Less than 100	More than 100
Respiratory effort	Absent	Weak, irregular	Good, crying
Muscle tone	Flaccid	Some flexion	Well flexed
Reflex irritability	No response	Grimace	Cry
Color	Pale	Blue	Pink

conventionally assigned after birth at 1 and 5 minutes. The decision to initiate resuscitation is taken much before assigning the Apgar score and does not depend on it. The 1 minute Apgar score generally correlates with umbilical cord blood pH and is an index of intrapartum hypoxia. The Apgar score at 5 minutes and beyond are reflective of the neonate's response to resuscitative efforts. If the five-minute Apgar score is less than seven, additional scores should be obtained every five minutes up to twenty minutes unless two successive scores are eight or greater. Apgar scores should be given by a person not directly involved in the resuscitation (for example, a nurse). Apgar scores, particularly when they indicate delay in return of tone, indentify neonates who have sustained significant CNS insults. Low Apgar scores at ten, fifteen, and twenty minutes are useful in predicting neonatal, and later, mortality and morbidity.

LABORATORY EVALVATION

Generally laboratory evaluation will not be of any benefit in the immediate management of the newborn infant. Besides obtaining the vital signs, the temperature, and the acid base status, no other laboratory evaluation will be necessary. As time becomes the limiting factor, quick clinical assessment and immediate action should be carried out. Biochemical markers of asphyxia other than acid base status have been described in the literature. These markers are generally not useful in the immediate management of the infant.

MANAGEMENT

Goals of Resuscitation

The major objectives of resuscitation of the newborn infant are to maintain neutral thermal environment, to provide adequate ventilatory support, to maintain adequate circulation that will provide adequate oxygen-carrying capacity and blood supply to the brain, to minimize fluid and electrolyte shifts within the brain, and to provide sufficient calories for optimal brain metabolism. The process of resuscitation is a continuum and the person involved in resuscitation should stop at every step of the process and reassess whether the objective has been achieved. If the objective has been achieved, resuscitative efforts should be stopped, the infant should be observed briefly, and efforts should be resumed as indicated. Overzealous attempts at resuscitation without close attention to the infant's condition will lead to complications. An algorithm for management is given in Figure 1. As can be seen, heart rate color and respiratory efforts should be the guide to the resuscitative process.

Thermal Environment

All infants should be maintained under neutral thermal environment where metabolic demands are minimal. Infants who are asphyxiated have a particularly unstable thermoregulatory system, and recovery from acidosis will be delayed if hypothermia is present. Immediately after its arrival in the emergency department or delivery, the infant should be placed under a radiant warmer and completely dried.

Skin temperature should be maintained

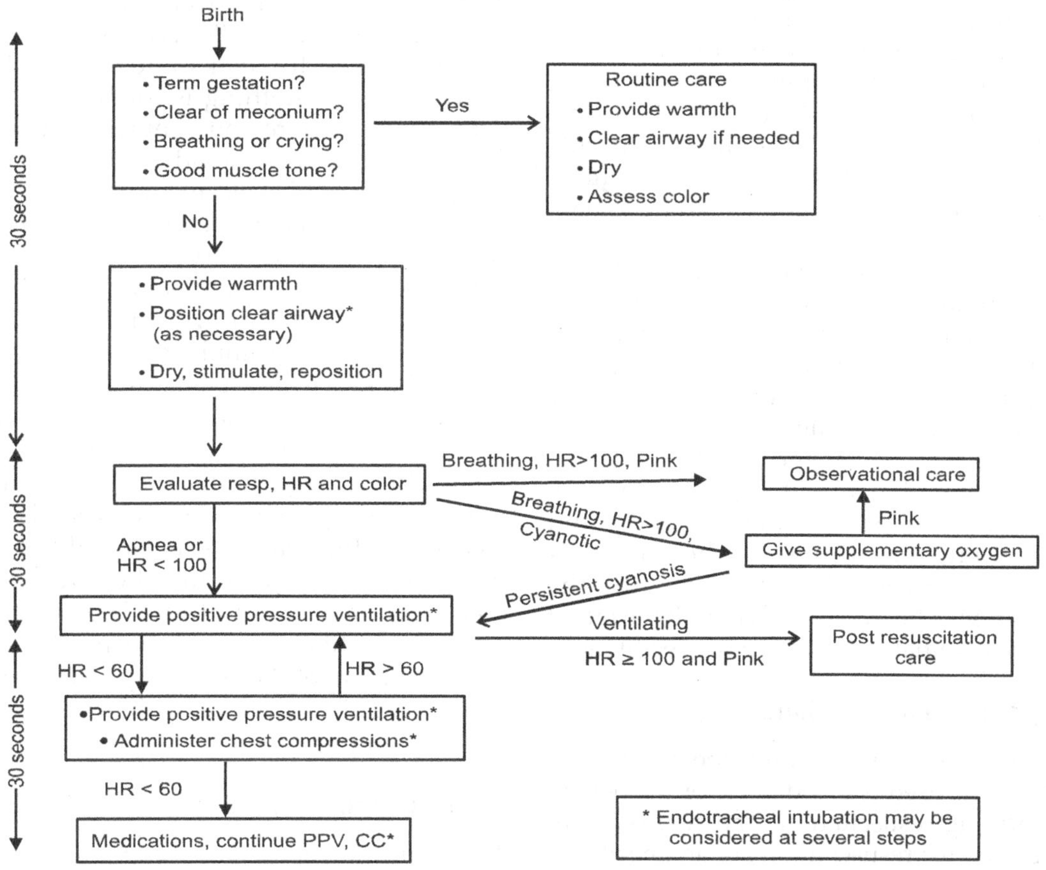

Fig. 1: Management of an asphyxiated newborn infant

between 36.2 and 36.8 C. Under the radiant warmer, heat losses are markedly reduced and the infant is readily accessible for resuscitative efforts.

Establishment of Adequate Ventilation and Circulation

After it has been dried, the infant should be placed in a slight Trendelenburg position with the neck slightly extended. Care should be taken to not hyper or underextend the neck as this may affect the entry of air. First the mouth is suctioned then the nose with either a bulb syringe, a DeLee suction catheter, or a mechanical suction catheter. Irrespective of the suction device used, the mouth should always be suctioned first in order to avoid aspirating the material from the mouth into the trachea. Special precautions to be followed when meconium is present in the amniotic fluid are described at the end of this chapter. This procedure itself will provide some stimulation. If the infant is breathing, evaluate the heart rate, and if it is above 100/min, evaluate color. If the infant is pink, continue to observe. If the heart rate is below 100/min, initiate bag and mask ventilation. If the infant has central cyanosis, administer supplementary oxygen, lowering the concentration as the infant gradually improves, or continue to administer it if cyanosis persists. If the infant is apneic, provide stimulation with a gentle slapping of the foot or by rubbing the back, and re-evaluate breathing. If the infant is breathing, proceed as before with the evaluation of heart rate and color. If the infant is apneic, initiate bag and mask vecitilation.

Bag and Mask Ventilation

A clear understanding of the operation of the type of bag used is mandatory for the person performing resuscitation. The two types of bags used for resuscitation are an anesthesia bag (flow-inflating bag) and a self-inflating bag. A pressure release valve set to release at 30 to 35 cm H2O is a common feature in most self-inflating bags. More pressure can be achieved when necessary by occlusion, bypassing the pressure release valve in some bags. Extreme caution should be used when this is used as excessive pressure may be transmitted to the lungs. A pressure manometer attached to bag may help to control the pressure in this situation.

When bag and mask ventilation becomes necessary, select the appropriate bag and mask, and check to make sure the connections and the pressure release mechanisms are working properly. Connect the bag to an oxygen source capable of delivering 90 percent to 100 percent. Then position the bag and mask on the infant and ventilate, observing chest wall movement. If there is a rise, ventilate for 15 to 30 seconds. If there is no rise, check for leaks and/or blocked airways, and if nothing is found, increase ventilation pressure and ventilate as before. The ventilation rate should be 40 to 60/min at a pressure of 15 to 20 cm for normal lungs. After this, evaluate the heart rate. If the heart rate is below 60/min, continue to ventilate and initiate chest compressions. If the heart rate is above 60/min, and increasing, continue to ventilate until it reaches 100/min. When the heart rate stabilizes above 100 / min, reduce the rate and pressure of assisted ventilation until effective spontaneous respirations are established. When color improves, supplemental oxygen can also be weaned. If the heart rate, color and tone do not improve, check for the effectiveness of bag and mask ventilation. The positive pressure ventilation may be ineffective due to one or more of these reasons: i) the seal is inadequate ii) the airway is blocked or iii) not enough pressure is being given.

Chest Compressions

The indication for chest compressions is a heart rate of < 60/min and one that does not increase after 30 seconds of effective bag and mask ventilation. During chest compressions, ventilation should continue as before except during heart rate checks. This maneuver is usually performed using two fingers in the lower one third of the sternum just above the xiphoid. The compressions are performed at a rate of 120/min. Chest compressions interposed with ventilation in a 3: 1 ratio may be more effective than simultaneous ventilation and compressions. The three compressions are followed by a pause to allow delivery of an effective breath. This will result in provision of 90 compressions and 30 breaths in each minute. After 30 seconds of the procedure, stop and count the heart rate. If it is increasing and is above 60/min, stop compression, and continue to ventilate until respiration is established. If it is still below 60/min, continue chest compressions and ventilation, and prepare for endotracheal intubation.

Endotracheal Intubation

The indications for intubation during resuscitation are: (a) When the positive pressure ventilation is ineffective (b) When prolonged bag and mask ventilation is required (c) when chest compressions are needed (d) When tracheal suction is required (meconium stained amniotic fluid) (e) To give epinephrine through endotracheal tube (f) Congenital diaphragmatic hernia. Intubation should be accomplished within a short period of time (20 seconds) with free flow of 100 percent oxygen provided close to the infants nostrils. The infant should be bagged, making certain that the rise in chest movement is equal, that breath sounds are equal on both sides, and that there is no gastric distention.

Medications During Resuscitation

Medications are rarely required during resuscitation. Epinephrine should be administered if the heart rate remains <60 / min after 30 seconds of effective positive pressure ventilation and another 30 seconds of coordinated chest compressions and ventilation. Epinephrine can be administered either intravenously or by endotracheal route. When given intravenously, flush with 0.5-1 ml of normal saline. Epinephrine can be repeated every 3-5 minutes if the heart rate continues to be <60/min. Resuscitation medications, route of administration, and indications for their use are given in Table 4. Quick access for intravenous medications can be achieved by insertion of an umbilical venous catheter.

Special circumstances include:

Meconium stained amniotic fluid. While resuscitating the newborns born through meconium stained amniotic fluid, the clearing of the airway during initial steps depend upon whether the neonate is 'vigorous' or not. 'Vigorous' baby is identified by presence of strong respiratory efforts, good muscle tone and heart rate > 100/min. If any of these parameters is abnormal, baby should be considered as non-vigorous. In case of non-vigorous neonates, endotracheal suction needs to be done. Repeat endotracheal suction can be done as necessary until little meconium is recovered or baby's heart rate indicates that resuscitation must proceed without delay. If the neonate is vigorous do suction of only mouth and nose using a 12-14 Fr suction catheter.

Asphyxial myocardiopathy. With severe and prolonged perinatal asphyxia, myocardial ischemia can occur with resulting congestive heart failure, systemic hypotension, and hypoperfusion. These babies present with hepatomegaly, the electrocardiogram (EKG) showing ischemic pattern and hypoglycemia. The specific treatment in this situation is to administer digitalis and a positive inotropic agent such as isoproterenol.

Table 4: Resuscitation Medications

Drug	*Indications*	*Dose*	*Route*
Epinephrine Available: 1:1,000 Administer: 1:10,000	HR <60 even after 30 sec. of coordinated chest compressions & ventilation	IV: 0.1-0.3 ml/kg ET: 0.3-1 ml/kg	IV or ET, give rapidly
Volume expanders Normal saline Ringer's Lactate O-ve blood	Shock with evidence of blood loss and baby is responding poorly to resuscitation	10 ml/kg	IV over 5-10 min.
Naloxane (0.4 mg/ml)	Respiratory depression even after restored HR & color and h/o narcotic administration in mother within past 4 hrs	0.1 mg/kg	IV

IV= intravenous, ET= endotracheal

Hydrops (etalis. Two skilled resuscitators are needed in this situation. One person manages the airway as before. The second person catheterizes the umbilical vein, performs abdominal paracentesis, and takes the steps to maintain adequate circulation. These infants have severe anasarca with very low serum protein levels. Rh negative blood, cross-matched against the mother's blood, is used to isovolumetrically exchange the blood volume to improve the hematocrit and oxygen carrying capacity.

FURTHER READING

1. Kattwinkel J, Text book on neonatal resuscitation, American academy of pediatrics. 5th ed. Ottawa; 2006.
2. American Heart Association; American academy of Pediatrics. 2005 American Heart Association (AHA) guidelines for cardiopulmonary resuscitation (CPR) and emergency cardiovascular care (ECC) of pediatric and neonatal patients: neonatal resuscitation guidelines. Pediatrics 2006;117(5):e1029-38.
3. Milner AD. Resuscitation of the newborn. Rinnie JM (editor) In: Roberton's Textbook of Neonatology. 4th Ed. Elsevier Churchill Livingstone; 2005. p.219-41.

In the previous edition this chapter was written by K.C. Sekar, MD Assistant Professor of Pediatrics/Neonatology Children's Hospital of Oklahoma Oklahoma City, Oklahoma

Shiv Sajan Saini and Praveen Kumar

4 Neonatal Seizures

Seizure is defined clinically as paroxysmal alteration in neurological function (i.e. behavioral, motor or autonomic function). Seizures are the most common neurological emergencies in newborns. These often point to the devastating form of brain injury.

CLASSIFICATION OF NEONATAL SEIZURES

Seizure type	*Manifestations*
Subtle (50%) Preterm > Term Most common form of seizures	Ocular movements (mc) - eye deviation, fixed stare, nystagmus. Others- oral bucco-lingual movements; rowing, swimming, bicycling, pedaling, and stepping limb movements; changes in heart rate and/or respiration; apnea (if associated with other seizure activity) and BP changes.
Clonic (25 – 30%) Term > Preterm	1-3 jerks /second, fast contraction and slow relaxation phase. Unifocal- Involves one side of body. Indicates underlying focal insult or metabolic cause. Multifocal-Migratory in nature. Usually metabolic. Common causes: (a) Unifocal - stroke, focal traumatic contusions, subarachnoid hemorrhage or metabolic disturbances; (b) Multi focal - metabolic.
Tonic (5%) Preterm > Term	Focal- Rigid posturing of one limb or asymmetrical posturing of the trunk or neck. Generalized- Sustained posturing resembling "decorticate", opisthotonic, or "decerebrate" rigidity. Common causes include diffuse neurological dysfunction and major Intraventricular hemorrhages.
Myoclonic (15-20 %)	Lightening fast contraction, non rhythmic character and the tendency to affect flexor muscle groups. Focal-Involve flexor muscles of the upper extremities. Multifocal-Asynchronous twitching of several body parts. Generalized- Bilateral jerks with flexion of upper and sometimes lower extremities. Common causes include serious brain dysfunction e.g. Perinatal asphyxia, IEM, cerebral dysgenesis or major brain trauma.

Etiology: Common causes responsible for neonatal seizures are as follows:

1. Hypoxic Ischemic Encephalopathy: Most common cause (60%). Characteristically seizures occur in first 24 hours.
2. Intracranial hemorrhage.
3. Intracranial infections- include bacterial meningitis as well as congenital viral infections.
4. Developmental defects.
5. Metabolic which include hypoglycemia, hypocalcemia, electrolyte disturbance and inborn errors of metabolism.
6. Epileptic syndromes.

Nonepileptic behaviors of newborns

Jitteriness: is tremors in quality and differentiated from seizures by tendency to stop with passive restraint and start with stimulation. Other features include lack of ocular phenomena and autonomic changes with jitteriness.

Benign neonatal sleep myoclonus: is bilateral or unilateral, synchronous or asynchronous myoclonus that occur during active sleep and is not stimulus-sensitive.

DIAGNOSIS

- *Maternal history*—TORCH infection, PIH, fetal distress, chorioamnionitis.
- *Antepartum history*—Type of delivery, use of local anaesthetics for the mother, which was ineffective. (Suggesting perhaps injected into baby), prolonged labour, instrumentation, apgar score and cord pH.
- *Postnatal history*—Age of onset, feeding history, sleep and activity prior to seizures. Tremulousness may suggest drug withdrawal or neonatal hypocalcemia. Lethargy and temperature instability may suggest an infection. Persistent hiccups may suggest nonketotic hyperglycinemia.
- *Family history of seizures*—genetic syndrome and IEM's.
- *Examination*- Detailed neurological examination, examination of scalp for in utero needle injuries, Inspection for skin lesions and assessment of fontanelle.

Laboratory Studies

- Serum glucose, ionized calcium (QoTc interval on ECG), magnesium, pH, Serum electrolytes, PCV and bilirubin (if baby icteric). Take BP in all cases.
- Lumbar puncture should be performed to determine the presence of infection.
- Neuroimaging: Perform ultrasound (USG) cranium to look for intracranial bleeds and malformations. In case of focal seizures computed tomography or magnetic resonance imaging is required to pick ischemic lesion which can be missed on USG.
- *Electroencephalography (EEG)*—A characteristic feature of neonatal seizures is the phenomenon of electroclinical dissociation (no motor symptoms in presence of electrical discharges). EEG correlation is not consistently seen with tonic, subtle and myoclonic seizures. The EEG should be analyzed for ictal activity as well as for background activity. EEG is useful in cases of repetitive motor activity to rule out seizures, to pick up electrical seizures in paralyzed neonate and for prognostication.
- Others (to be done in specific situations)
  - Thrombophilia evaluation if evidence of stroke or venous thrombosis.
  - Serum ammonia and lactate, Urine MR screening, Urine and serum amino acids and organic acids.
  - Investigation for congenital viral infections.
  - CSF studies: CSF:serum glycine ratio for Nonketotic hyperglycinemia; CSF lactate and pyruvate for mitochondrial cytopathies; CSF:serum glucose <0.5 in the presence of low CSF lactate levels suggests GLUT – 1 deficiency syndrome.
  - Assessment of other organ systems (eg, renal, hematologic, hepatic) may support a diagnosis of hypoxic ischemic encephalopathy or an inborn error of metabolism.

MANAGEMENT

Flowchart shows emergency room treatment of neonatal seizures.

Flowchart for acute management of neonatal seizures

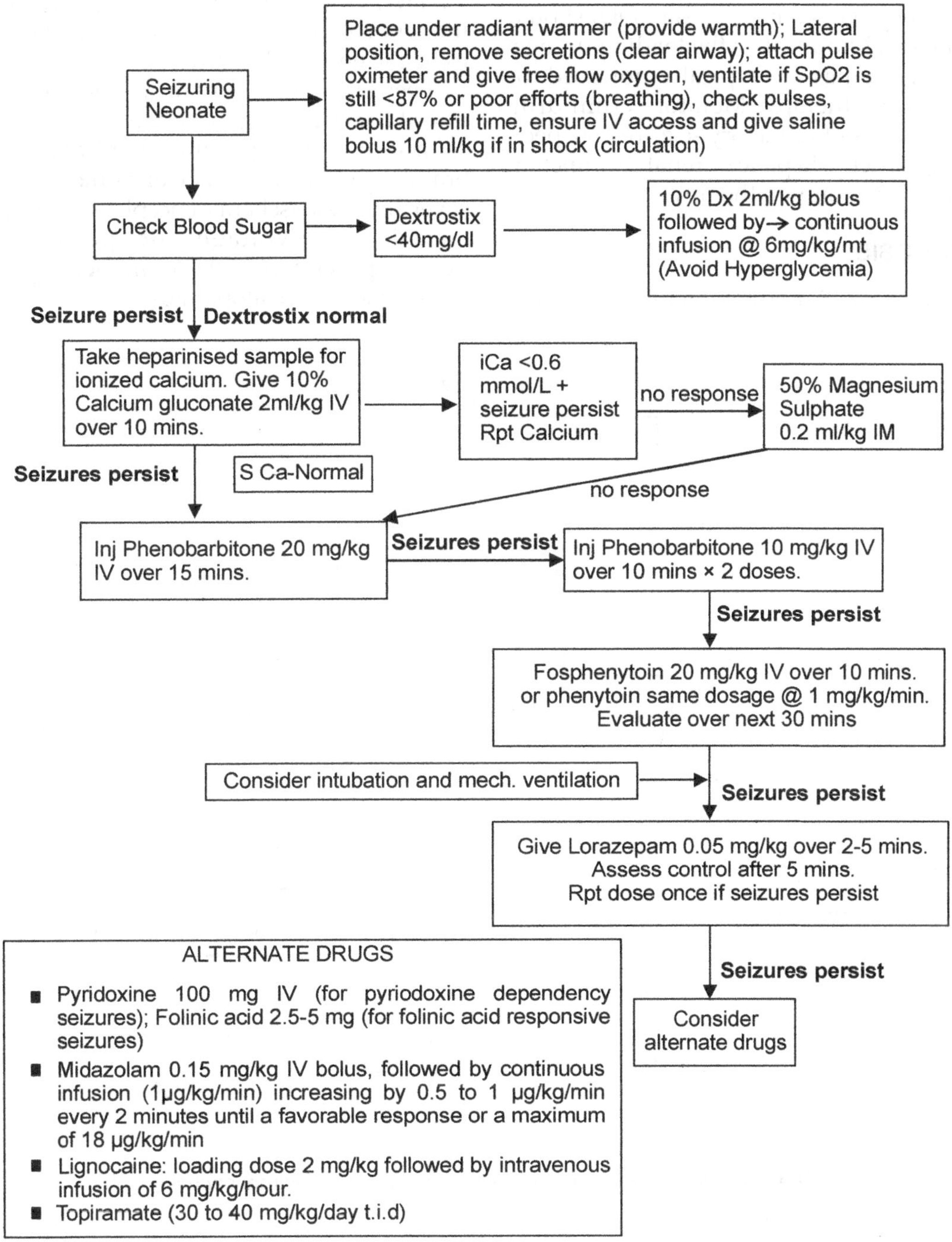

LONG TERM TREATMENT

Long-term treatment is directed against the specific cause of seizures. Maintenance dose of AED's (Phenobarbitone 3-4 mg/kg/day O.D; Phenytoin 4-8 mg/kg/day OD) should be started 12 hours after the loading dosage. Benzodiazepines are typically not used for maintenance therapy. Monitor serum drug levels in cases of refractory seizures, suspected drug toxicity, hepatic or renal dysfunction and if baby is on polytherapy.

PROGNOSIS

Good prognosis: A normal interictal EEG in a term newborn (not preterms), transient metabolic derangements, subarachnoid hemorrhage and hereditary neonatal convul -sions.

Variable prognosis: Symptomatic hypoglycemia, intracranial infection and moderate hypoxic-ischemic encephalopathy.

Poor prognosis: Early-onset seizures, frequent or prolonged seizures that are refractory to multiple anticonvulsants, cerebral dysgenesis, inborn error of metabolism, severe hypoxic-ischemic encephalopathy, isoelectric, low-voltage, or paroxysmal burst-suppression background activity and myoclonic encephalopathies.

Flow diagram on weaning and duration of AED

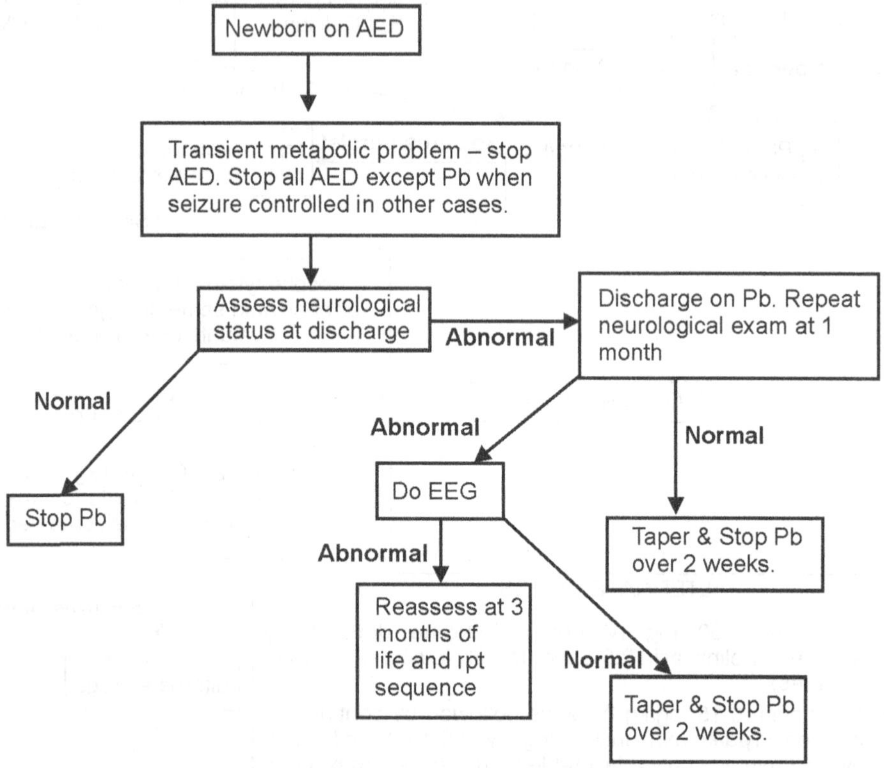

(Pb-Phenobarbitone, AED - antiepileptic drugs, EEG - Electroencephalography)

Anti-epileptic drug dose in the newborn

Drug	*Initial dose*	*Maintenance*	*Therapeutic level/ Remarks*
Phenobarbital	20 mg/kg IV	3-4 mg/kg O, IV	Therapeutic level 20 and 40 mg/L. Half-life varies from 100 to 270 hours, may be up to 400 hours in preterm infants.
Fosphenytoin	20mg/kg PE IV		PE = Phenytoin equivalents (1.5 mg fosphenytoin = 1 mg of Phenytoin)
Phenytoin	20mg/kg IV	3-4 mg/kg O,IV	Therapeutic level 6 to 15 mcg/ mL. Obtain initial trough level 48 hours after an IV loading dose. The half-life varies from 40 to 200 hours, with a mean of 100 hours.
Lorazepam	0.05mg/kg IV		May increase digoxin levels if given concurrently.
Midazolam	0.15 mg/kg	0.1-0.4mg/kg/hour	Monitor closely for CNS depression, hypotension, bradycardia, apnea, and/or respiratory depression.
Lignocaine	2 mg/kg	1-6 mg/kg/h	Therapeutic level 0.5-4 mg/L. levels of greater than 7.5 mg/L may actually induce seizure activity.

FURTHER READING

1. Volpe JJ. Neonatal seizures. Volpe JJ (editor). In: Neurology of the newborn. 5th Ed. Philadelphia: Saunders Elsevier; 2008. p. 203-44.
2. Barnette AR, Inder TE. Evaluation and Management of Stroke in the Neonate. Clinics Perinatol 2009; 36(1): 125-36.
3. Lombroso CT, Holmes GL. Value of the EEG in neonatal seizures. J Epilepsy 1993; 6(1): 39-70.

Sai Sunil Kishor M and Praveen Kumar

5 Neonate with Respiratory Distress

Respiratory distress is defined by presence of at least 2 of these features- tachypnea (RR > 60 per minute), retractions (intercostal and/ or sub costal) and grunt.

COMMON CAUSES

In preterm neonate	*In term neonate*
Hyaline membrane disease, pneumonia, delayed clearance of lung fluid, air leak.	Meconium aspiration syndrome, delayed clearance of lung fluid, air leaks, pneumonia,
Persistent hypertension	pulmonary (PPHN).

Common to Both

Surgical causes: Choanal atresia, tracheoesophageal fistula, diaphragmatic hernia.
Cardiac: Congestive cardiac failure and ductus dependant lesions.
Metabolic: Acidosis, hypoglycemia, polycythemia, anemia.

Intracranial bleed.

EVALUATION

History

A relevant antenatal and perinatal history should be taken based on common causes.

- Gestation.
- Antenatal steroids in a preterm baby.
- Premature or prolonged rupture of membranes, fever, unclean P/V examination, foul smelling liquor, chorioamnionitis.
- Fetal bradycardia, meconium stained liquor, perinatal asphyxia, traumatic delivery.
- Antepartum hemorrhage, diabetes mellitus.

Examination

- Hyperinflated chest, meconium staining of cord/nails-MAS
- Scaphoid abdomen, location of heart sounds- CDH
- Equality of air entry, transillumination (air leak)
- Evidence of CHF-hepatomegaly, tachycardia, murmur, cyanosis
- Preductal and postductal saturation difference- PPHN
- Evidence of IC bleed- bulging AF, pallor, hypotonia, pupillary size and reaction, encephalopathy

Assessment of severity of distress: Two important scoring systems available are the Downe's score and the Silverman-Anderson retraction score.

Table 1: Downe's score (total score of >6 indicates severe respiratory distress)

Parameter	0	1	2
RR(/min)	< 60	60-80	>80
Cyanosis	Absent	In room air	In 40% oxygen
Grunt	Absent	Audible with a stethoscope	Audible with a naked ear
Retractions	Absent	Mild	Moderate - severe
Air entry	Good	Diminished	Barely audible

Monitoring and workup

1. Vitals, SpO_2 monitoring, Downe's score
2. ABG, electrolytes, Blood glucose, PCV
3. Sepsis work up
4. Chest X-ray, shake test
5. Assessment of gas exchange: Alveolar-arterial oxygen gradient ($AaDO_2$), Oxgenation index (OI)

Supportive therapy

- Maintain thermo-neutral environment
- Maintain pH, fluid & electrolyte balance
- Correct hypotension
- Treat hypoglycemia, hypovolemia, anemia

INITIAL MANAGEMENT

For algorithm *See* next page figure.

Oxygen therapy

Indications: Clinical central cyanosis, Hypoxemia (O_2 saturation <87%* and / or PaO_2<50 mmHg in room air), Presence of respiratory distress irrespective of O_2 saturation.

Saturation targets: Preterm: 87-95%, Term: 90-100%, Bronhopulmonary dysplasia: 90-95%, PPHN: >95%.

Commonly used oxygen delivery systems in neonates:

Use pre-warmed and humidified oxygen. Low flow systems are commonly available

Type	Length of insertion (in cm)	RFR (l/min)*	FiO_2 (%) (at an average RFR)	Complications	Remarks/ precautions
Nasal cannula	Nares to the inner canthus	1 - 2	25 - 45	Crusting, septal trauma, erosion, the eyebrow inadvertent PEEP	Alternate between nares every 12 hours
Nasophary-ngeal cannula	Ala nasi to the tragus	1 - 2	45-60	Crusting, septal trauma, septal erosion, inadvertent PEEP	Alternate between nares every 12 hours
Nasal prongs	0.5-1 cm	1 - 2	25-45	Crusting, erosion	Short, binasal prongs are recommended
Oxygen hood	—	2 - 4	30-70%	—	Keep flow above 3 lit. to avoid rebreathing

*RFR – recommended flow rate, PEEP – positive end-expiratory pressure

The indications for CPAP and mechanical ventilation are mentioned in the management algorithm.

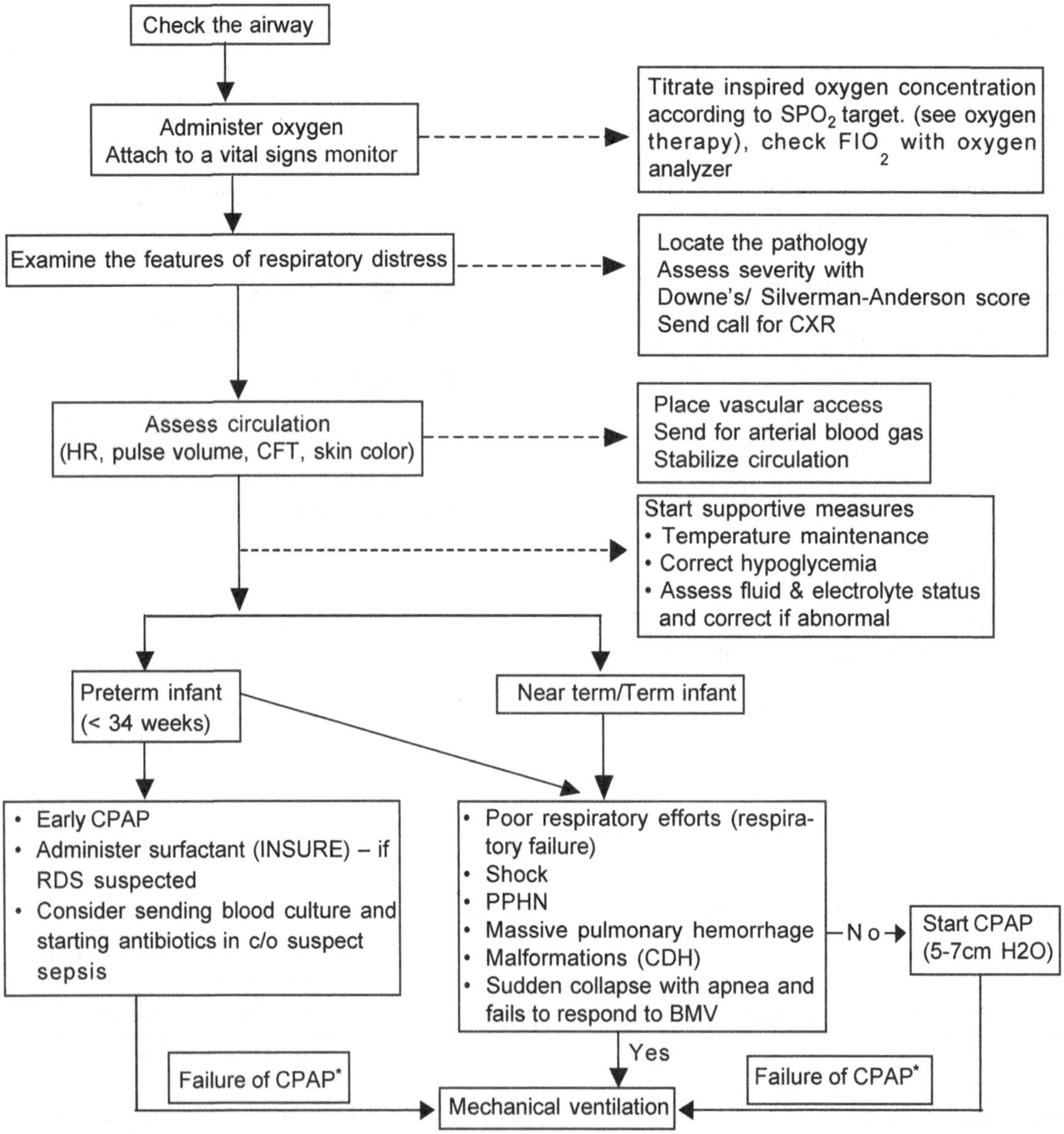

Fig. : Algorithm for initial management of a neonate with respiratory distress

(***Failure of CPAP:** Even on a CPAP of 7cmH_2O and 70% FiO_2 if the neonate has excessive work of breathing (or) PCO_2> 60mmHg with pH <7.2 (or) recurrent apnea or hypoxemia (PaO_2 <50 mmHg), this should be considered as failure of CPAP.)

and used in neonates. These systems provide a variable FiO_2 depending on the flow.

FURTHER READING

1. Greenough A, Milner AD. Pulmonary disease in the newborn: Acute respiratory disease. Rennie JM (editor). In: Roberton's Textbook of Neonatology. 4th Ed. Philadelphia: Elsevier Churchill Livingstone; 2005. p. 468-553.
2. Ambalavanan N, Schelonka RL, Carlo W. Ventilatory strategies. In: Goldsmith JP, Karotkin EH (editors) Assisted Ventilation of the Neonate. Philadelphia: Saunders; 2003. p.249-60.
3. Bhtutani VK, Sivieri EM, Abbasi S, Shaffer TH. Evaluation of neonatal pulmonary mechanics and energetics. Pediatr Pulmonol 1988;4:150-8.
4. Greenough A, Donn SM. Matching Ventilatory Support Strategies to Respiratory Pathophysiology . Clinics Perinatol 2007;34(1):35-53.

Shiv Sajan Saini and Praveen Kumar

6 Neonatal Jaundice

Jaundice is most common sign in neonatal medicine. Almost 2/3rd of term and virtually all preterm babies develop clinically visible jaundice in first week of life. Jaundice increases till 3rd to 5th day of life and then decreases. The following situations warrant evaluation of a jaundiced neonate and is termed as **pathologic** or **non-physiologic jaundice**.

a. Clinical jaundice in first 24 hours of life.
b. Any jaundice requiring phototherapy (>95th percentile for the postnatal age in hours).
c. TSB increasing by > 0.5 mg/dl/hour.
d. Conjugated hyperbilirubinemia (direct bilirubin level >1 mg/dl when the TSB is < 5 mg/dl or > 20% of the total, if the TSB is > 5 mg/dl).
e. Clinical jaundice persisting for more than 14 days of life in term and 21 days of life in preterm.

EVALUATION

The history and examination are directed towards assessing the severity, complication and the etiology of jaundice.

History in a Jaundiced Infant

1. Antenatal
   a. Maternal fever and rash during pregnancy- Intrauterine infections.
   b. Maternal drugs (sulfonamides, nitrofurantoin, antimalarials)- Hemolysis in a G6PD deficient infant.
2. Intrapartum
   a. Mother- Use of oxytocin, excess hypotonic fluids.
   b. Baby- Delayed cord clamping, asphyxia, birth trauma.
3. Family history
   a. Previous sibling with neonatal jaundice or family history of anemia, splenectomy- Blood group incompatibility (Rh, ABO), G6PD deficiency, spherocytosis, Crigler-Najjar syndrome.
   b. Liver disease in the family- Galactosemia, α-1 antitrypsin deficiency.
4. Neonatal course
   a. Prolonged parenteral nutrition- Cholestatic jaundice.

Examination- Key examination objectives include judging severity of jaundice and presence of complications like acute bilirubin encephalopathy apart from finding the cause of jaundice.

1. Severity of Jaundice

Jaundice in newborn progresses in a cephalocaudal direction. Clinical jaundice becomes apparent at TSB levels of 5-7 mg/dl. The severity can be assessed by blanching the skin in day light.[1] The interpretation may be wrong by inexperienced examiner, poor light and dark skin of the baby. Transcutaneous bilirubinometry can be useful noninvasive tool to screen the babies, which can overcome all these problems.

Dermal Zone	Mean ± SD (mg/dL)
1	5.9 ± 0.3
2	8.9 ± 1.7
3	11.8 ± 1.8
4	15.0 ±1.7
5	> 15.0

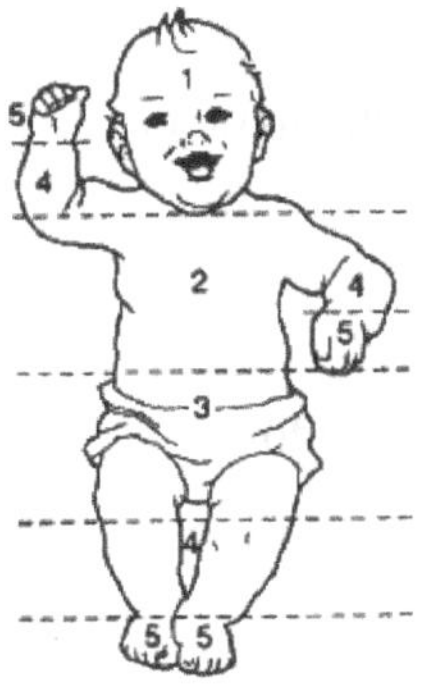

Fig 1: Dermal zones according to Kramer's rule.[1]

2. Complications

A complete neurological examination especially of the mental status, muscle tone and cry is required.

Acute bilirubin encephalopathy (ABE)[2]			
	Initial phase	*Intermediate phase*	*Advanced phase*
Mental status	Sleepy	Lethargy, irritability	Semicoma, seizures
Muscle tone	Slight hypotonia,	Hyper or hypotonia	Usually increased,
	Paucity of movement	depending on arousal state, mild arching	Retrocollis, opisthotonos
Cry	Slightly high-pitched	High-pitched	Shrill cry
Feeding	Poor feeding	Minimal feeding	No feeding

Preterm babies may differ from term babies in evolution of acute bilirubin encephalopathy.

3. Physical Examination

Physical examination		Relevance
Anthropometry	Weight loss since birth	Dehydration
	Microcephaly	Intrauterine infections
	Small for date	Polycythemia, intrauterine infections
General Physical Examination	Pallor	Hemolytic anemia, extravasation of blood
	Bruises, cephalhematoma	Increased bilirubin formation
	Petechiae	Intrauterine infections, sepsis, erythroblastosis
Systemic Examination	Hepatosplenomegaly	Hemolytic anemia, intrauterine infections, liver disease
Chorioretinitis		Intrauterine infections
Urine staining diapers and clay colored stool		Cholestasis

Lab Investigations

For Etiology of Jaundice (All Babies Receiving Phototherapy)

- Blood grouping and DCT (if mother group O or Rh negative).
- G6PD activity.
- Hemogram for evidence of hemolysis (↑ed retic count, fall in PCV and peripheral smear for spherocyte, nucleated RBC, anisopoikilocytosis and polychromasia).
- Serum sodium, serum osmolality as an objective measurement of dehydration.
- Conjugated bilirubin fraction when cholestasis is suspected.
- Sepsis work up, if presentation suggests so.

Severity of Jaundice

TSB should be done

1. At birth, if there is setting of Rh incompatibility.
2. If jaundice is apparent within first 24 hours of life.
3. When pathological jaundice is suspected based on Kramer's rule.
4. When there is a doubt in visual estimation of jaundice.

Once under phototherapy TSB should be repeated every 4-12 hrly depending on the severity of jaundice. More frequent assessment of jaundice is done when hemolysis is suspected or the TSB value was near exchange zone.

TREATMENT

Phototherapy and exchange transfusion are two main treatment modalities.

For Newborn Infant ≥ 35 Weeks of Gestation

Local modification of American Academy of Pediatrics (AAP) charts[2] should be used to take decisions for phototherapy (Figure 2) and exchange transfusion (Figure 3).

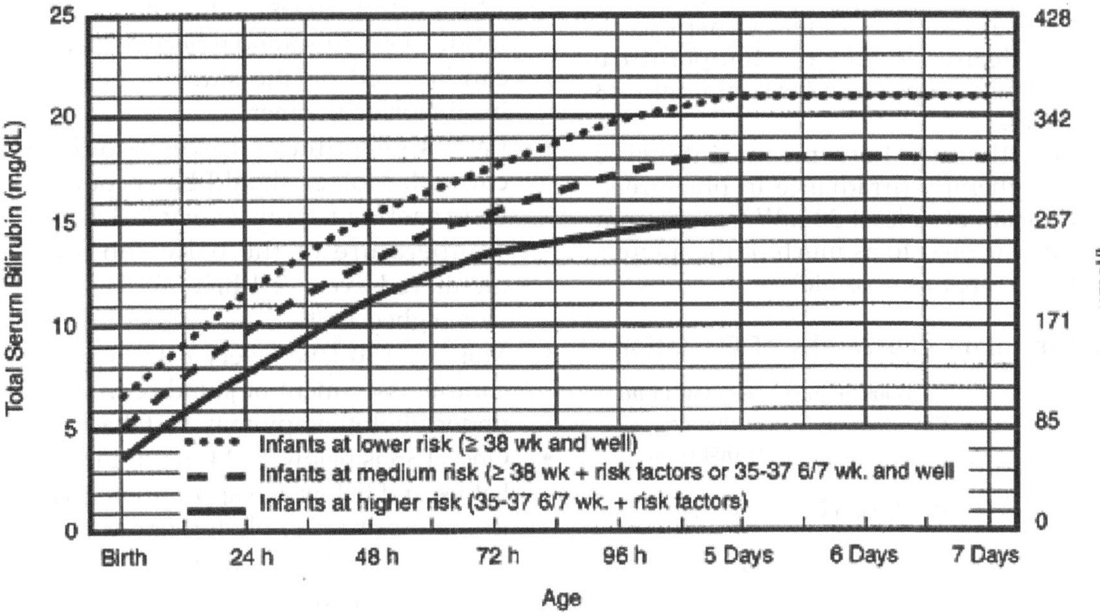

Fig 2: Guidelines for phototherapy in neonates of 35 or more weeks gestation[2].

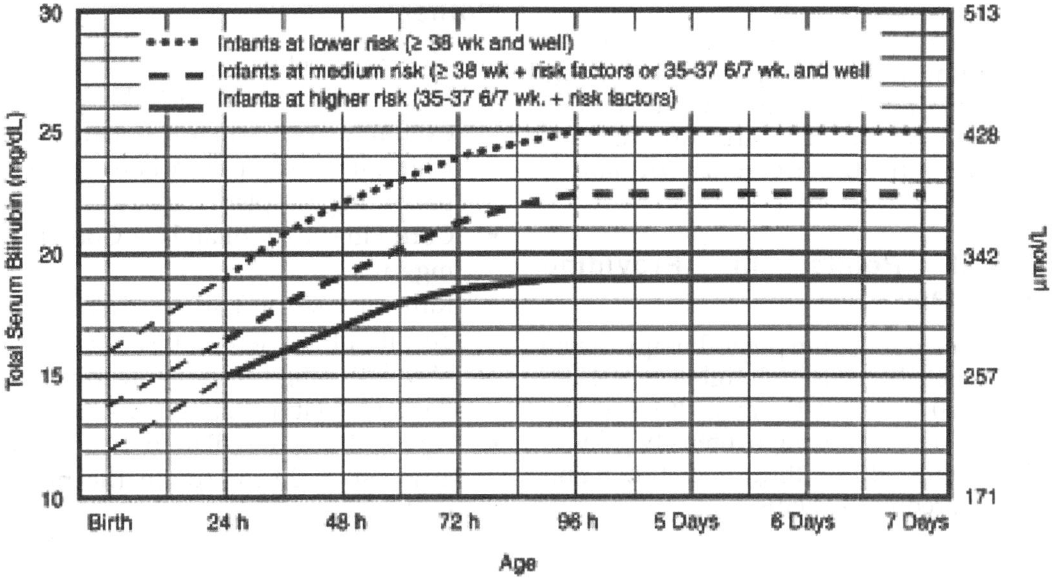

Fig 3: Guidelines for exchange transfusion in infants 35 or more weeks gestation[2].

- Medium risk line should be used for neonates ≥ 38 wk and no risk factors.
- High risk line ≥ 38 wk with risk factors, 35-37 6/7 with or without risk factors. Risk factors - isoimmune hemolytic disease, G6PD deficiency, asphyxia, significant lethargy, temperature instability, sepsis, acidosis, albumin <3 gm/dl.
  Phototherapy here means intensive phototherapy (irradiance in blue-green spectrum of at least 30 mW/cm^2 per nm and delivered to as much of the infant's surface area as possible).[2]

Preterm Infant <35 Weeks of Gestation

Birth Weight	Decision to start Phototherapy	Decision to do exchange transfusion
<1000 grams	Visible Jaundice	10-12 mg%
1000-1500 grams	7-9 mg%	12-15 mg%
1500-2000 grams	10-12 mg%	15-18 mg%
2000-2500 grams	13-15 mg%	18-20 mg%

Cockingtons charts[3] can be used alternatively for deciding phototherapy and exchange transfusion. If TSB is in the indefinite zone as per the Cockingtons charts, do exchange transfusion in the presence of above mentioned risk factors.

Practical Points in Providing Phototherapy

- Blue green spectrum phototherapy can be provided by blue tubelights (PHILIPS TL52, 20W), blue CFL lamps (OSRAM 18 W), halogen lamps, high intensity gallium nitric blue light emitting diode (LED) unit and fibreoptic systems.
- Dose: minimum of 10-15 µW/cm^2/nm. The higher the irradiance, the better is the effect. To increase the dose, use double surface photo-therapy, keep baby 10-15 cm from tubes, periodically monitor irradiance of tubes and reflective material can be used on the sides of bassinet, incubator or warmer.
- Baby's genetilia and eyes should be covered. Mother should be encouraged to breastfeed baby every 2-3 hours. Temperature of the baby should be monitored every 2-4 hrly. Baby should be weighed daily.
- Monitor TSB level every 8-12 hourly as clinical assessment of jaundice in babies under phototherapy may be fallacious.
- Once TSB is below 13-14 mg d/l in term babies and below age appropriate cut off in preterm babies, phototherapy can be stopped. Check for rebound rise in TSB after 12-24 hours.

Indications for ET at or Soon After Birth in a Baby Born to Rh Isoimmunized Mother

- Hydrops foetalis.
- History of previous sibs requiring exchange transfusion because of Rh isoimmunization, in a baby born with pallor, hepatosplenomegaly and + DCT.
- Cord Hb < 10 g/dl and/or Cord TSB > 5 mg/dl.
- Rate of rise of TSB > 1 mg/dl/hour despite phototherapy OR rate of rise of TSB > 0.5 mg/dl/hour despite photo-therapy if Hb is between 10-12 g/dl.
- Any TSB > 12 mg/dl in first 12 hours and any TSB > 20 mg/dl in the neonatal period.

Which Blood Group to Ask For?

Rh isoimmunization	Rh-negative blood of baby's ABO type or O-ve blood.
ABO incompatibility	O+ve cells suspended in AB plasma/ O+ve whole blood
For other babies	Baby's blood group is to be used

Post-exchange baby should receive vitamin K and all medications which the baby was receiving. Monitor RR, HR, Color and temperature ½ hourly for 2 hours. Check blood sugar, TSB & PCV at 2 hours following exchange. Baby can be fed after 1-2 hours of DVET, if baby is well.

Fluid Supplementation

Giving fluid supplementation to term neonates with severe nonhemolytic jaundice (TSB >18), decreases the need for exchange transfusion[4]. The fluid (N/5 in 5% Dextrose) is given I.V. over 8 hours (50 ml/kg + 20 ml/kg phototherapy allowance + ½ of 8 hour maintenance fluid requirement). One should consider giving fluid relaxation in all such cases and in the waiting phase before DVET.

Drugs

IV Immunoglobulins

IV immunoglobulin given in the dose of 0.5-1 g/kg over 2-4 hours can prevent repeated exchanges in jaundiced babies due to Rh isoimmunization or proven ABO incompatibility.

Phenobarbitone

It has been shown to be useful in reducing the need for ET and duration of phototherapy in VLBW babies if started on day 1 of life. However it takes 2-3 days to induce the enzymes and hence would have a limited role if jaundice is already at its peak. Though limited follow up data has shown its safety, still there are concerns about its effect on long term neurodevelopment.

Approach to jaundice in non-isoimmunized neonates

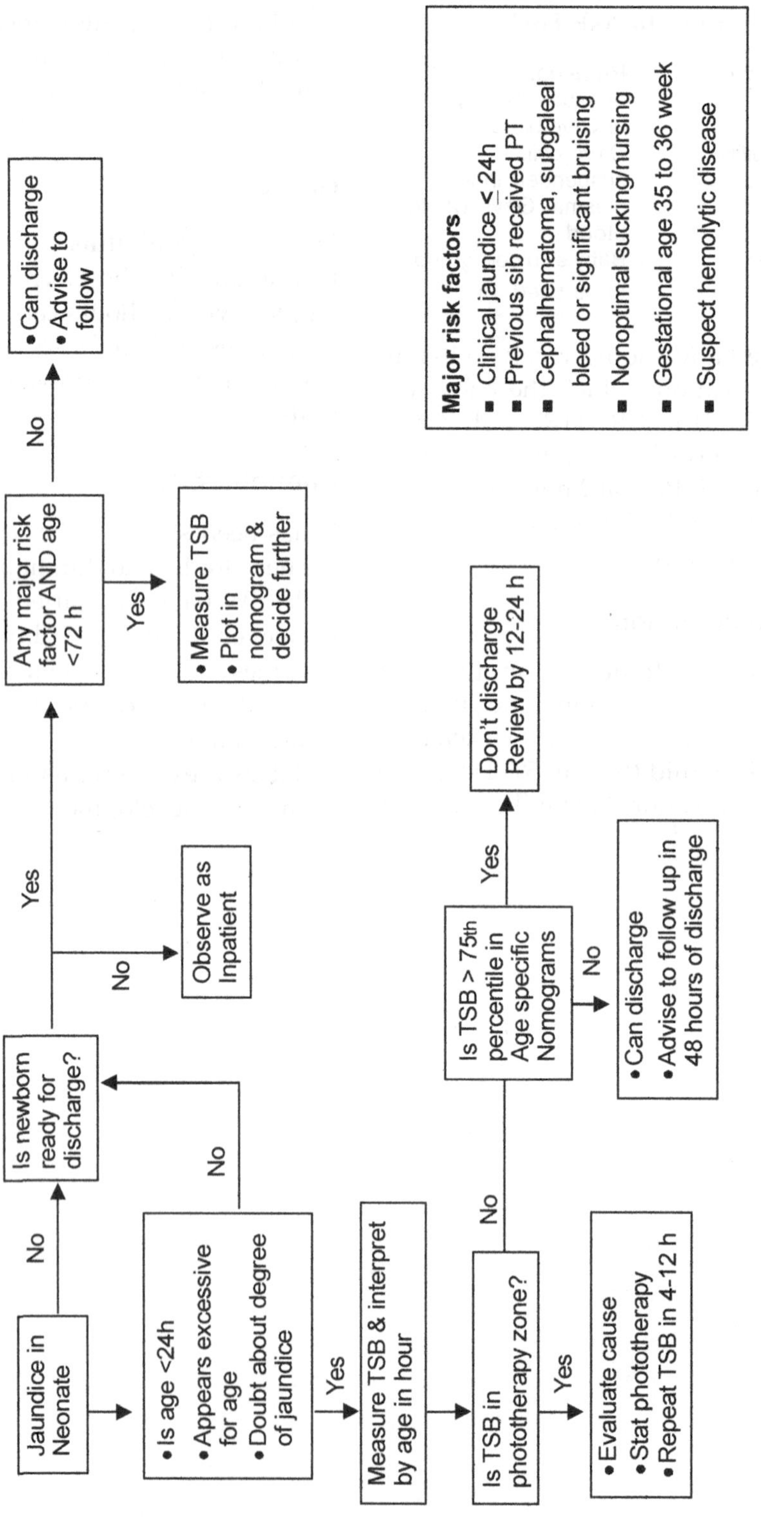

Approach in Rh isoimmunized mother

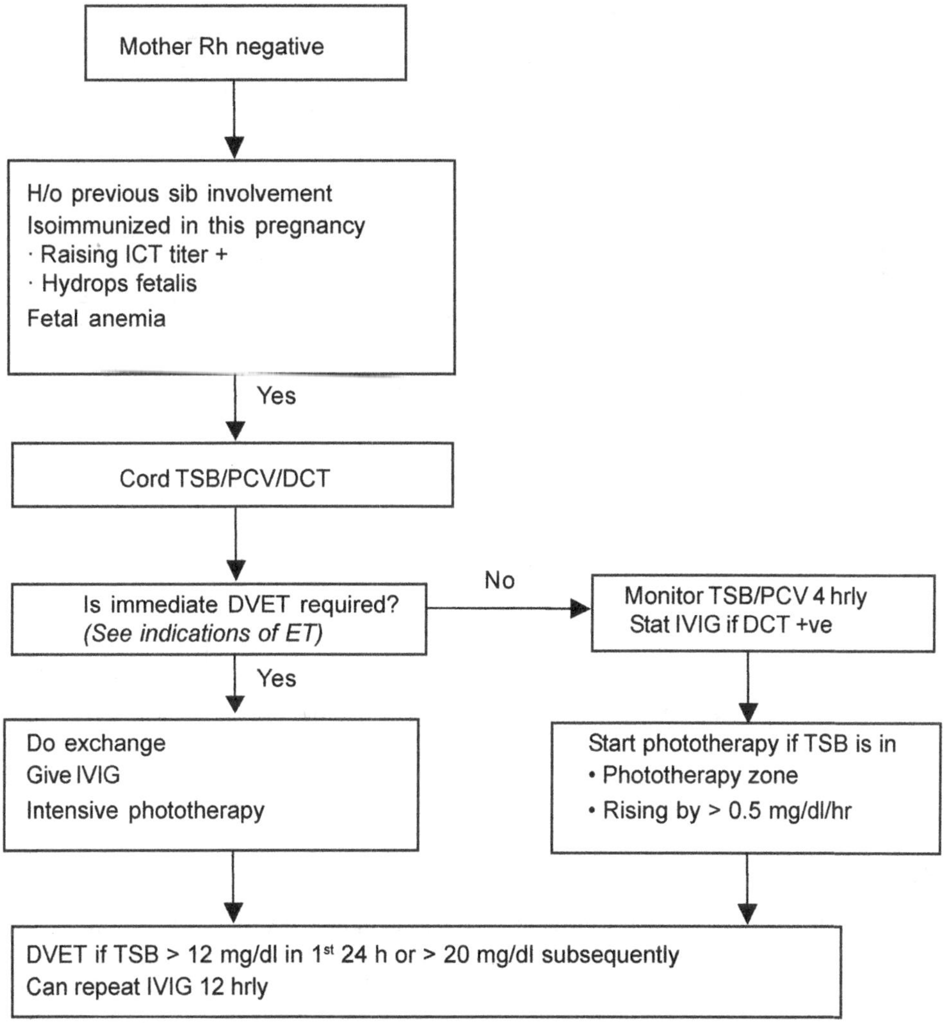

Approach to baby with Cholestasis

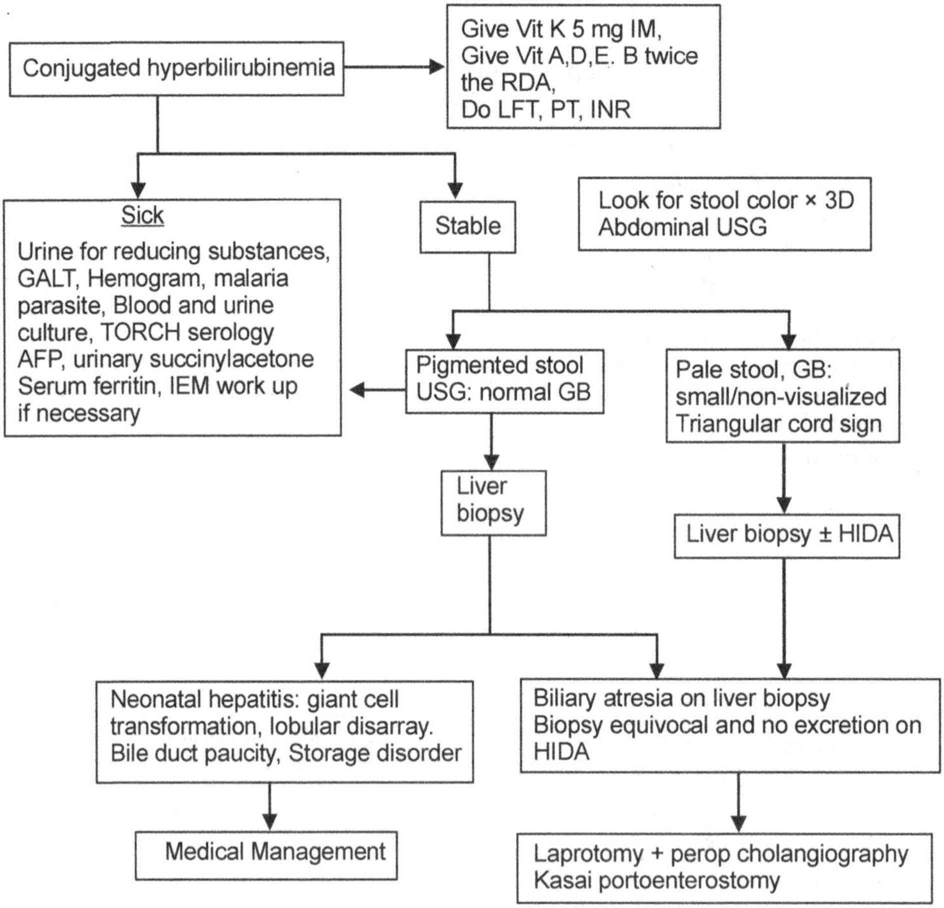

FURTHER READINGS

1. Kramer LI. Advancement of Dermal Icterus in the Jaundiced Newborn. Amer J Dis Child. 1969; 118: 454-458.
2. American Academy of Pediatrics Subcommittee on Hyperbilirubinemia. Management of hyperbilirubinemia in the newborn infant 35 or more weeks of gestation. Pediatrics. 2004; 114(1):297-316.
3. Cockington RA. A guide to the use of phototherapy in the management of neonatal hyperbilirubinemia. J Pediatr 1979;95:281-285.
4. Mehta S, Kumar P, Narang A. A randomized controlled trial of fluid supplementation in term neonates with severe hyperbilirubinemia. J Pediatr 2005;147(6):781-5.

Sai Sunil Kishor M and Praveen Kumar

7 Bleeding Neonate

Neonates, especially preterms, are at higher risk of bleeding due to decreased activity of certain coagulation factors and impaired platelet function. Bleeding is a common problem in sick neonates and can be life threatening.

HOW TO APPROACH?

1. Is the baby is sick or well at the onset of bleeding- see in the differential diagnosis below.
2. Was Vit K given to the baby at birth?
3. Is the bleeding generalized or localized?- Generalized bleed almost always due to coagulopathy or thrombocytopenia or both.
4. Family history of bleeding- is more relevant in well baby with bleeding.
5. History of maternal illness [those causing immune thrombocytopenia like ITP & connective tissue disease, PIH and drug intake (barbiturates, phenytoin, aspirin, rifampin, INH and warfarin)]
6. Age of onset of bleeding- immune thrombocytopenia presents usually in first 24 hrs, classic Vit K deficiency bleeding between 2nd to 4th day of life.
7. Presence of petechiae, small mucosal hemorrhages generally indicate thrombocytopenia and large bleeds indicate coagulopathy.
8. Coexisting signs like jaundice, organomegaly point to infection, liver disease and erythroblastosis.

INVESTIGATIONS & INTERPRETATION

Investigations

Required in all cases

1. Platelet count
2. Coagulogram
3. Peripheral smear

Required on case to case basis

1. Apt test
2. D-dimer
3. PIVKA
4. Anti-platelet antibodies
5. Maternal platelet count
6. Neuroimaging for CNS bleed

Normal & Abnormal Values

- **Platelet count:**

  Thrombocytopenia if < 1.5 lakh/ mm^3

  Severe thrombocytopenia < 50,000/ mm^3.

- **Coagulogram:**

  PT of ≥ 17 sec is abnormal in term and preterm.

  APTT of > 45 sec in term

  >55 sec in preterm are abnormal

Practical tips

**Coagulogram:* Normal ratio of blood: anticoagulant should be 9:1 in the vial. If there is polycythemia, it should be 19:1. If the sample gets clotted, it should not be assumed that neonate's coagulation profile is normal, but send another coagulogram.

Apt test-

1. It is used to rule out ingested maternal blood which presents in first 3 days of life.
2. This should be done in a well baby with isolated gastro-intestinal bleed
3. Mix 1 part of gastric aspirate / stool/ vomitus with 5 parts of distilled water. Centrifuge it and separate the clear pink supernatant. Add 1 ml of 1%NaOH to 4 ml of hemolysate. Sample containing maternal blood will turn brown while fetal blood remains pink.

PIVKA (Protein Induced in Vitamin K Deficiency)- for confirmation of vitamin K deficiency. This can be done even up to 72 hrs after Vit K administration.

Table 1: Differential diagnosis

Clinical condition	*Platelets*	*PT*	*APTT*	*Diagnosis*
Sick neonate	↓	↑	↑	DIC
	↓	N	N	Sepsis, NEC
	N	↑	↑	Liver disease
	N	N	N	Stress bleed
Well neonate	↓	N	N	Immune thrombocytopenia, kasabach-meritt syndrome Bone marrow hypoplasia
	N	↑	↑	Vit K deficiency bleeding
	N	N	↑	Heriditory clotting factor def.,
	N	N	N	Swallowed blood, trauma, qualitative platelet defects, Factor XIII def.

TREATMENT

General Principles

1. If there is hypovolemic shock/ blood loss >10% of blood volume due to acute blood loss, give whole blood or volume expander.
2. Give Vit K_1 1 mg IV.

3. Keep cross matched blood ready for emergency transfusion and for further transfusions.
4. Look for the underlying cause and treat it.

Platelet Transfusion

- **Indication:** (modified from Cassandra and Strauss 2006)
  1. Count is <50,000 with in a sick neonate (or) minor bleeding (puncture site, skin & mucosal) (or) undergoing invasive procedure (or) <100, 000 with major bleed
  2. <20,000 even without bleed.
  3. Qualitative platelet defect with bleeding with any platelet count.
- How much? – Chart 10 ml/kg of platelet concentrate over 1 hour.
- The platelet concentrates to be kept in room temperature only.
- Start transfusion as early as possible after issuing because of the risk of aggregation.
- Avoid transfusion through the central line, due to the risk of thrombosis.

Fresh Frozen Plasma/Single Donor Plasma

- **Indications:**
  1. Coagulopathy with bleeding/or under-going invasive procedure
  2. Factor replacement when concentrates are not available (factor II, V, X and XI).
  3. At the initiation of heparin therapy
- **How much?**- 10 ml/kg over 2-3 hours. Sometimes with active bleeding one need to raise the concentration of the clotting factors to 20% of the normal. This can be done by repeating 10 ml/kg.
- FFP/SDP can be stored temporarily in the freezer compartment for less than 12 hours. Once thawed transfuse immediately and do not refreeze.

Treatment of Vit. K Deficiency Bleeding (Table 2)

Give Inj. Vit K_1 1–5 mg slowly. Infants with late VKDB may need higher dose up to 5 mg. Coagulation parameters will normalize and there will be cessation of bleeding within a few hours. Serious bleeding, particularly in premature infants or those with liver disease, may require a transfusion of fresh frozen plasma or whole blood.

DIC:

- Treat the underlying cause
- Give Vitamin K_1- 1 mg IV
- Platelets and fresh frozen plasma @ 10 ml/kg each
- Consider exchange transfusion, if bleeding persists.
- In case of thrombotic DIC give unfractionated heparin or LMW.

Table 2: Vitamin K Deficiency Bleeding (VKDB)

Type	*Age*	*Site of bleed*	*Cause*
Early	<24 hrs	Intracranial, Gastro-intestinal, Intra-abdominal	Maternal drugs, Inherited coagulopathy
Classic	2-7 d	GIT, mucosal, umbilical stump, injection sites	Missing the dose of Vit K at the birth
Late	1-3 months	Intracranial, GIT, skin	Cholestasis, diarrhea, idiopathic

FURTHER READING

1. Monagle P, Andrew M. Developmental Hemostasis: Relevance to newborn and Infants. Nathan DG, Ginsburg D, Orkin SH, Look AT (editors). In: Nathan and Oski's Hematology of Infancy and Childhood. 6th ed. Philadelphia: WB Saunders Company; 2003. p. 121-68.
2. Lusher JM. Clinical and Laboratory approach to the patient with bleeding. Nathan DG, Ginsburg D, Orkin SH, Look AT (editors). In: Nathan and Oski's Hematology of Infancy and Childhood. 6th ed. Philadelphia: WB Saunder's Company; 2003. p.1515-26.
3. Wu YY, Stack G. Blood Product Replacement in the Perinatal Period. Semis Perinatol 2007; 31: 262-271.
4. Manco-Johmson MJ. Bleeding disorders in the neonate. Neoreviews 2008; 9:e 162-169.
5. Thornburg C, Pipe S. Neonatal thromboembolic, emergencies. Archives fetal neonatal Med 2006; 11: 198-206.
6. Pramanik AK. Bleeding disorders in neonates. Pediatr Rev 1992; 13: 163-173.

8

Sunit Singhi

Acute Upper Airway Obstruction

Acute airway obstruction in children is one of the most common life-threatening emergencies in pediatric practice. It usually generates a great deal of anxiety since there is little time for deliberation, and it may lead to significant morbidity and indeed mortality. Protocols outlining the management of airway obstruction are useful in facilitating the care of these patients and should be readily available.

Stridor is a harsh crowing sound usually heard during inspiration. It indicates upper airway obstruction (pharynx to trachea). Inspiratory stridor is usually supraglottic, while expiratory stridor emanates from the trachea. Any patient with a persistent stridor of acute onset must be hospitalized for treatment and observation.

PATHOPHYSIOLOGY

The anatomy of the upper airway renders the child at a considerable disadvantage when compared to the adult and predisposes children to upper airway obstruction. For example, the larger occiput in the infant is more likely to compromise the airway by flexion of the cervical spine while the relatively large tongue with less muscle tone increases the likelihood of posterior displacement and obstruction of the airway. Epiglottic enlargement is also more hazardous in children since the epiglottis is relatively longer and stiffer and projects more posteriorly as compared to adults. In addition, the submucosa in the subglottic area is more loosely attached; facilitating accumulation of fluid and development of edema, while the soft, cartilaginous airway in infants may collapse during inspiration.

Since resistance to airflow is related to the fourth power of the radius (Poisslle's Law), small changes in the airway diameter can have profound effects on airway resistance in the pediatric patient. Flow of air into the airway during inspiration results from the generation of a negative intrathoracic pressure (that is, a drop in intrathoracic and intratracheal [IT] pressure below extrathoracic pressure) (Figure 1). Since the difference in intrathoracic and extrathoracic pressures necessary to maintain flow is proportional to the fourth power of the airway radius, a 50 percent decrease in radius may increase the pressure by a factor of 32. Attempts to generate this high negative intrathoracic pressure result in the typical physical findings of retraction of the chest wall and pulsus paradoxus. The high negative pressure also results in collapse of

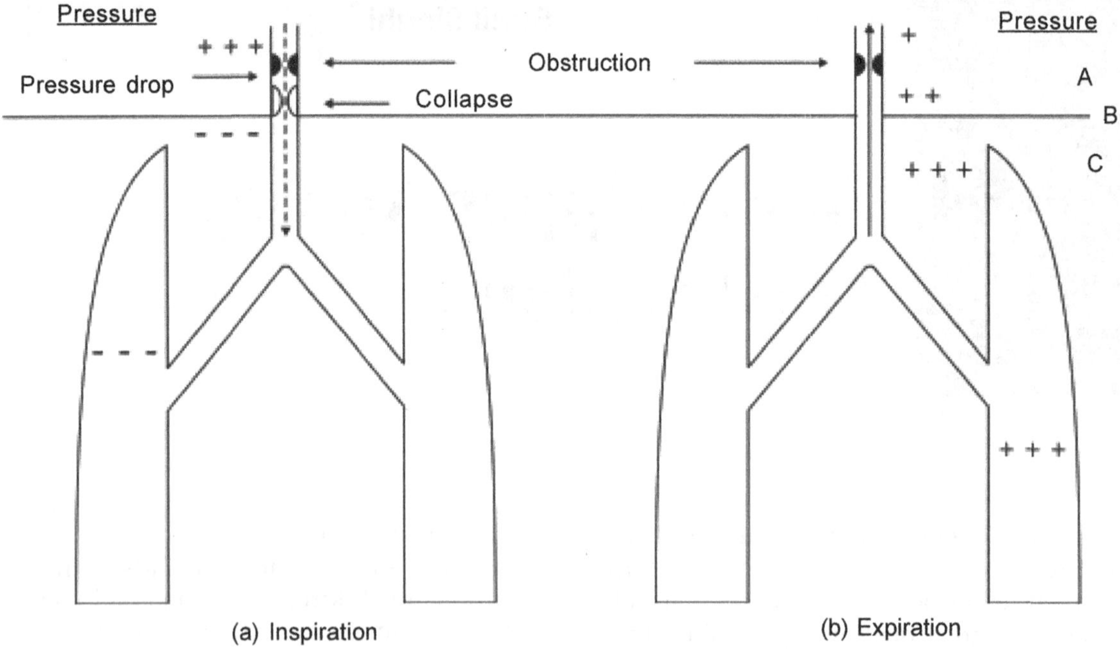

Fig. 1: A = extrathoracic airway; B = intrathoracic structures including the lung; C = thoracic inlet. During inspiration, there is greater negative intrathoracic pressure conducted to the lungs and major intrathoracic airways. There is airflow from the upper airway, which is at atmospheric pressure, causing a net pressure differential (pressure drop) to further collapse the extrathoracic airway and hence causing further airway narrowing. During expiration, the positive pressure in the airway exceeds atmospheric pressure, and hence the airway is held open.

the soft extrathoracic airway and worsening of the obstruction.

CAUSES OF UPPER AIRWAY OBSTRUCTION IN CHILDREN

Obstructions of the upper airway can be divided into those that involve the supraglottic structures and those involving the subglottic structures. Supraglottic obstruction may be associated with muffled voice and dysphagia while subglottic obstruction is accompanied by hoarseness of voice or cry and barking cough. In addition to the anatomic classification, airway obstruction may also be categorized etiologically as either infectious or noninfectious.

The common infectious causes of upper airway obstruction are acute laryngotracheitis (viral croup), acute epiglottitis, diphtheria, bacterial tracheitis, retropharyngeal abscess and acute severe tonsillitis with superimposed tonsillar and adenoidal hypertrophy. Foreign body in trachea/larynx is the most common noninfectious cause of airway obstruction in children. Less common causes of acute stridor are hypocalcemic laryngeal tetany and angioneurotic edema. Chronic stridor is seen with congenital malformations such as laryngomalacia, tracheomalacia, laryngeal web, and vascular rings.

EVALUATION

In a child with stridor check other symptoms, such as voice change and fever, history of trauma to head or neck, and history of choking, which could lead to foreign body aspiration.

- Throat should be examined for evidence of acute inflammation, exudates and membrane.
- In the neck look for any extrinsic mass, evidence of trauma and tracheal position.
- If the patient's condition permits, consider a laryngoscopic examination and obtain a lateral X-ray of neck in children with severe distress. Laryngoscopy or any procedure that may agitate the patient is postponed till an emergency airway is established. Visualization of epiglottis in a suspected case of epiglottitis should be attempted only after making preparations for immediate intubation or tracheostomy.
- Few investigations are required to support the clinical impression. Hematologic and radiologic evaluations are often unnecessary and may exacerbate the anxiety and delay appropriate treatment. Sending an acutely ill patient to the X-ray department delays treatment and increases the likelihood of airway obstruction with supine positioning especially in patients with epiglottitis. A physician who is competent in providing airway support may accompany stable patients to the X-ray department.

SPECIFIC CAUSES

Acute Laryngotracheitis (Viral Croup)

The attack rate of viral croup is between three and fifteen per thousand children per year between six months and five years of age with the highest incidence being in children between six and eighteen months of age. Of these, approximately one percent requires hospitalization, and a significantly lower number require airway intervention. Parainfluenza virus type 1 accounts for most cases of viral croup followed by Type 2, Type 3, influenza A and B, and respiratory syncytial viruses. Parainfluenza primarily infects the ciliated respiratory epithelium thus the ventricular and subglottic regions are the chief sites involved in viral croup. In addition to edema, laryngeal muscle spasm as a result of Type 1 hypersensitivity response to parainfluenza virus with the release of spasmogenic mediators may also contribute to airway obstruction.

The child with viral croup often has an antecedent viral upper respiratory tract infection and may be mildly febrile. After a few days, the child develops a barky or seal-like cough that is accompanied by an inspiratory stridor that is worse at night and is more pronounced during agitation. The course tends to be insidious peaking at three to four days and resolving over a one-week period. Most patients will follow this typical course without significant respiratory difficulty. Severe disease is usually indicated by marked tachypnea, the use of accessory muscles and supraclavicular, intercostal and subcostal indrawing. In severe disease, stridor may be marked; however, a decrease in stridor may be an ominous sign of critical airway obstruction or impending respiratory failure.

Acute Epiglottitis

Epiglottitis accounts for one in every thousand pediatric admissions to a hospital with the peak incidence occurring in children between two and six years of age. It is usually of bacterial etiology. H. influenzae Type B is responsible for almost all cases of epiglottitis in otherwise healthy children. H. influenzae is carried in the nasopharynx of five percent of asymptomatic children. Invasive disease occurs, however, in one percent of these carriers. The organism is believed to spread hematogenously to the epiglottis, resulting in local inflammation and the typical cherry red edematous epiglottis. Less commonly S. pneumoniae may be the causative organism; a variety of other agents, however, may be responsible in the immunocompromised patients.

Epiglottitis, unlike croup, is sudden in onset and rapidly progressive in symptomatology. The preceding illness, unlike viral croup, may only be a few hours in duration. The initial symptoms are sore throat, fever, and cough followed by dysphagia, drooling, and respiratory distress. On examination the child is drooling, anxious, looks acutely ill, and is typically sitting forward with the neck hyper extended, occasionally in a tripod position. Attempts at direct visualization of the pharynx and epiglottis in this situation may induce complete obstruction and is therefore not recommended. Febrile dysphagia in children should always be considered to be epiglottitis until proven otherwise. The two classical X-ray findings of epiglottitis are enlargement of the epiglottis and distention of the hypo pharynx (Figure 2).

In most cases, the clinical presentation of viral croup and epiglottitis are quite classical with distinctive differences making them often relatively easy to differentiate (Table 1).

Diphtheria

Diphtheria is an acute, contagious bacterial disease caused by the bacterium *Corynebacterium diphtheriae*. This is not an invasive organism and ordinarily remains in the superficial layers of the respiratory mucosa or skin lesions, where it can induce an inflammatory reaction in the local tissues. Toxigenic strains produce a potent exotoxin,

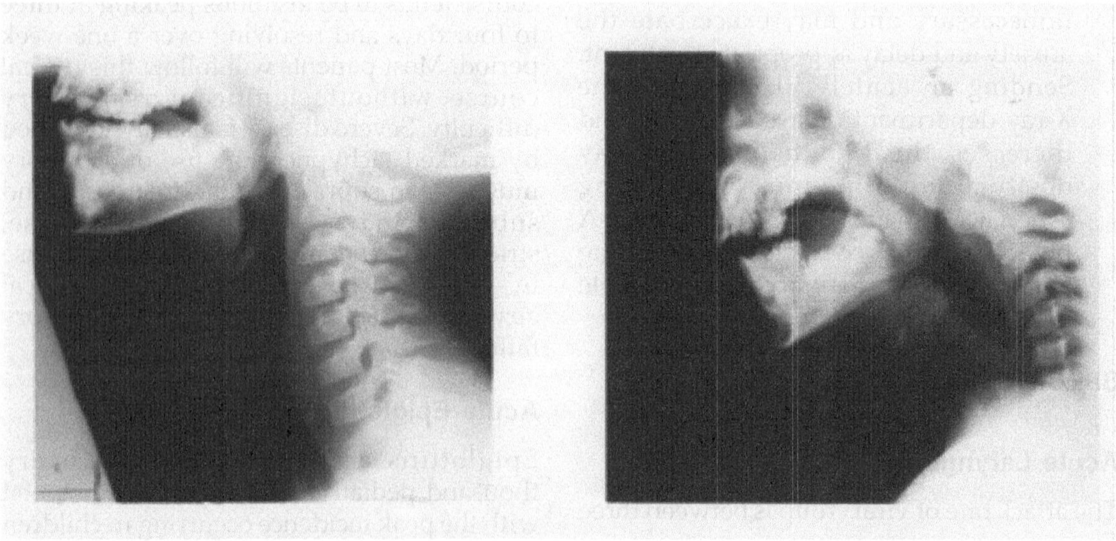

Fig. 2: The normal radiograph of the upper airway is demonstrated on the left with the well-defined epiglottis. On the right radiograph, the epiglottis is swollen and thumb-like in appearance

Table 1: Differentiating features between croup and epiglottitis

	Croup	*Epiglottitis*
Incidence	More common	Less common
Etiology	Viral	H. influenza Type B
Site of obstruction	Subglottic	Supraglottic
Age	6 months to 3 years	2 to 6 years
Recurrence	5%	Rare
Clinical features		
Symptoms		
Onset	Gradual (days)	Sudden (hours)
Fever	Low grade	High
Cough	Barky	Minimal
Dysphagia	None	Severe
Drooling	None	Present
Voice	Hoarse	Clear or muffled
Sore throat	Common	Common
Signs		
Posture	Recumbent	Sitting (Tripod)
Toxic	Absent	Present
Temperature	Normal/Low grade	High
RR	Rapid	Initially normal
Retractions	Present	Absent early
Cyanosis	Absent early	Absent early
Investigations		
CBC (Total WBC)	12,000	24,000
(differential count)	60% PMN	85% PMN
X-ray*		
LAT	Subglottic narrowing (1 cm below the glottis)	Enlarged epiglottis Distended hypopharynx
PA	Distention of hypopharynx Tapering of trachea (Steeple sign)	

* X-rays should not be attempted when the diagnosis of epiglottitis is strongly suspected on clinical grounds.

CBC = complete blood count
WBC = white blood cell
LAT = lateral
PA = postanterior
PMN = polymorphonuclear neutrophil leukocytes

which inhibits protein synthesis in mammalian cells. Infection due to toxigenic strains initially causes oedema followed by epithelial necrosis and acute inflammation. Coagulation of the fibrinopurulent exudate produces a pseudomembrane, which contains large amounts of the bacteria. The exotoxin produced acts locally, causing necrosis and contributing to the formation of the pseudomembrane.

Clinical Features

The disease typically has a short incubation period of 2 to 5 days followed by a prodromal period of between 12 to 24 hours. Its clinical course can vary from several days to several months if complications occur. The pharynx or tonsils are most commonly infected (50–67% of cases), but laryngeal or nasal mucosa may also be affected, often secondary to spread from the pharynx.

Pharyngeal diphtheria: Early symptoms include malaise, sore throat, anorexia, and a low-grade fever (37.8–38.9°C). After 2–3 days a bluish-white sharply demarcated pseudomembrane may form, often starting as spots on the tonsils that extend and coalesce. The membrane can spread beyond the margins of the tonsils onto the soft palate; it may turn a grayish-green colour and on occasion, can be black if there has been bleeding. The membrane is tough and fibrinous and may adhere firmly to surrounding tissue. Extensive membrane formation can result in respiratory obstruction. Infection at these sites is usually associated with substantial systemic absorption of toxin. Those patients without toxicity exhibit discomfort and malaise associated with local infection, whereas those with severe toxicity develop severe prostration, pallor, tachycardia, stupor, and coma and may die within 6 to 10 days. A proportion of patients with severe disease develops cervical lymphadenopathy and associated neck oedema, resulting in the classical 'bull-neck' appearance.

Laryngeal diphtheria: The larynx is the infection site in 25% of cases. Because the illness can have an insidious onset (increasing hoarseness, cough and mild fever), the diagnosis is often missed, unless accompanied by pharyngeal diphtheria. It may lead to airway obstruction, coma and death.

Anterior nasal diphtheria: Onset of nasal infection with toxigenic *C. diphtheriae* is often indistinguishable from the common cold. Patients may subsequently present with a unilateral or bilateral mucopurulent nasal discharge, which may be irritant to the nose or upper lip. A white membrane usually forms on the nasal septum. In general, it tends to cause a fairly mild disease due to poor systemic absorption of the toxin from the nares.

Complications: Most complications of diphtheria are attributable to the toxin. Disease severity and the development of complications are generally related to the extent of local disease. These include asphyxiation due to extensive pseudo membrane formation, myocarditis and neuropathy. The majority of deaths occur in the first week of illness, usually from asphyxia or myocarditis. In general, the likelihood of complications and mortality from diphtheria is directly related to the severity of the local disease, and inversely related to the speed of diagnosis and treatment with antitoxin.

Bacterial Tracheitis

It should be suspected when a clinical picture similar to that of viral croup is complicated by high grade fever, toxicity and copious purulent tracheal secretions. *Staphylococcus aureus*, Streptococci and *H. influenzae* are common etiologic agents.

Retropharyngeal Abscess

It is an uncommon cause of stridor. It occurs in infants and young children because of secondary infection of retropharyngeal space and lymph nodes following an upper respiratory infection. The infection is most often a mixed one caused by Streptococci, *Staphylococcus aureus* and anaerobic organisms. Typically, there is high fever, sore throat, inspiratory stridor and difficulty in swallowing. The neck is generally hyperextended so as to achieve maximum airway. A lateral X-ray of neck is diagnostic. It shows airway narrowing and widening of retropharyngeal space. Presence of air leucencies indicates perforation.

Tonsillar and adenoidal hypertrophy superimposed on acute severe tonsillitis is an important cause of severe upper airway obstruction. Inflammatory edema extending down to larynx may further aggravate obstruction of airway.

Foreign Body in Trachea/Larynx

An acute episode of coughing, choking or gagging followed by stridor in infants and toddlers while eating nuts or playing with small objects is typical of a foreign body aspiration. In 30% of patients below 3 years of age, however, such a history may not be available. Besides stridor, aphonia, dysphagia and severe air hunger are the predominant signs of laryngeal and tracheal foreign bodies.

MANAGEMENT

General Management

Assess the child for severity of respiratory distress and give resuscitative or supportive therapy accordingly.

Acute Laryngotracheitis (Croup)

In the assessment of the child with croup, determination of the severity and the anticipated progression needs to be made in order to determine further management. The croup score (Table 2) has been recommended as a tool to aid in the decision making process but should not be used to replace good clinical judgement. In making decisions regarding triage of patients with croup, emphasis should be placed on the age of the child and on the ability of the parents to assess and respond appropriately if the child's condition deteriorates. The younger the child, the lower should be the threshold for hospitalization. Radiologic evaluation of the patient with classical signs and symptoms of croup is unnecessary. If, however, the symptoms are causes of obstruction, the lateral view of the neck often demonstrate subglottic narrowing, usually extending one

Table 2: Clinical croup score

Parameter	*0*	*1*	*2*
Inspiratory breath sounds	Normal	Harsh with rhonchi	Delayed
Stridor	None	Inspiratory	Inspiratory and expiratory
Cough	None	Hoarse cry	Bark
Retractions flaring	None	Flaring and suprasternal retractions	Flaring, suprasternal intercostal retractions
Cyanosis	None	In air	In 40% oxygen

Reprinted with permission from Downes JJ, Raphaely RC. Anaesthesiology. Pediatric Intensive Care 1975; 43; 238-250.

cm below the demonstrated narrowing of the subglottic region, the Steeple sign (Figure 3).

Management of the various levels of severity in croup is illustrated in Figure 4 and discussed in more detail in the following subsections.

Mild Croup

Children with mild disease usually do not have stridor at rest; they often have a barky cough, however, and may develop stridor with agitation. These children have a croup score of less than two. If the parents are reliable and will react appropriately to increasing distress, the child may be discharged home with the recommendation to use a cool mist vaporizer.

Mild to Moderate Croup

These children have very mild stridor at rest; this may become more pronounced, however, with agitation (croup score 2 to 4). These children may be observed in the emergency department in a humidified tent. Nebulized budesonide (1,000 µg given 30 minutes apart) or oral dexamethasone provides prompt and significant clinical improvement in children with mild to moderate croup and reduces the need for hospitalization. If in the physician's judgement the parents are reliable and will return to the hospital if deterioration occurs, the child can be discharged. In that event, the parents would be advised to continue cold mist therapy. These children may also benefit from a stroll outside in cold weather.

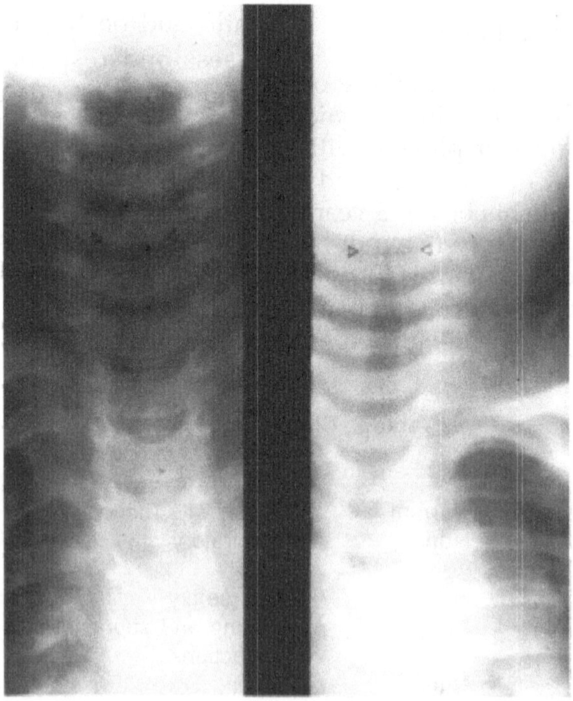

Fig. 3: The radiograph on the left demonstrates the normal anatomy of the upper airway with normal tapering in the subglottic region. On the right is the radiograph of a child with croup. This demonstrates the manifested narrowing in the subglottic region, the Steeple sign

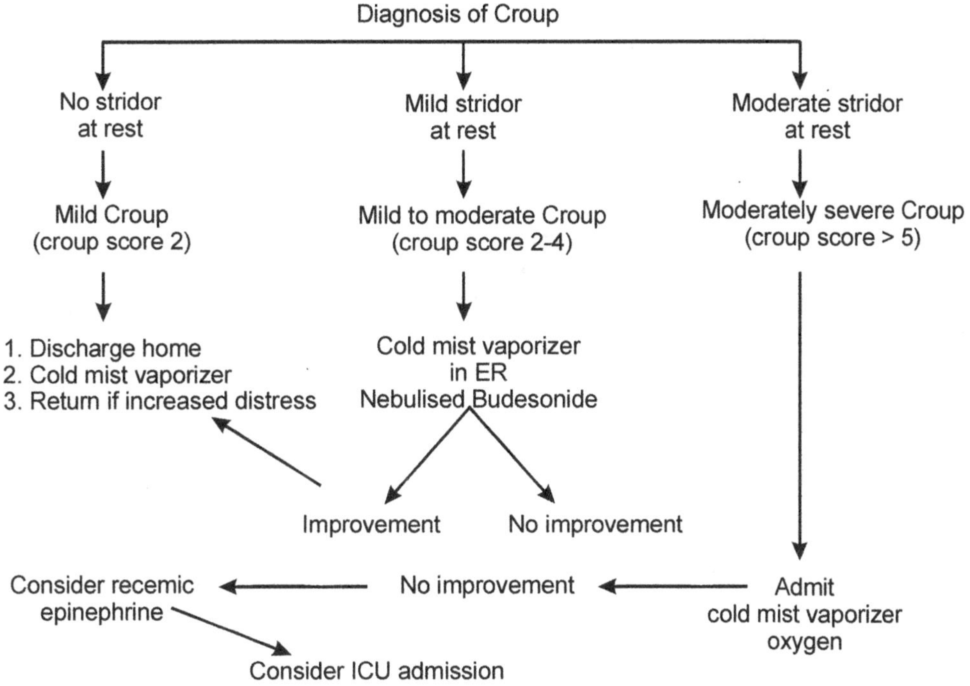

Fig. 4: Algorithm for the treatment of mild to moderately severe croup

Moderately Severe Croup

Children with easily audible stridor at rest without the use of a stethoscope (croup score greater than 5) should be admitted to the hospital. These children should be placed in a humidified tent with oxygen. Further deterioration of the child's condition may require the use of racemic epinephrine. Nebulized racemic epinephrine (0.25 to 0.5 cc in 2 cc normal saline) can be given as often as is required clinically; after repeated doses, however, the child should be considered for intensive care monitoring and an ear, nose, and throat (ENT) and anesthesia evaluation. Steroids have been demonstrated to be beneficial in alleviating the signs and symptoms and may be used with this group of patients.

Severe Croup

These patients are in significant distress and clinically there is decreased air entry, use of accessory muscles, subcostal and intercostal indrawing, and possibly cyanosis (Figure 5). These patients are considered in the same context as are acute epiglottitis and constitute medical emergencies. Any maneuvers that would agitate the child should be avoided. Oxygen is provided in a non-threatening manner with the child in the parent's arms. Racemic epinephrine should be attempted to provide relief of the obstruction. Severe cases should receive hydrocortisone 10 mg/kg or dexamethasone 0.3-0.6 mg/kg/dose IV 6 hrly for four doses. If there is a favorable response, the child should be transferred to the critical care unit for further management (NPO [nil per oral-nothing by mouth], humidity and oxygen) and close monitoring. Children who do not respond to racemic epinephrine and are becoming exhausted and obtunded should be considered for emergency

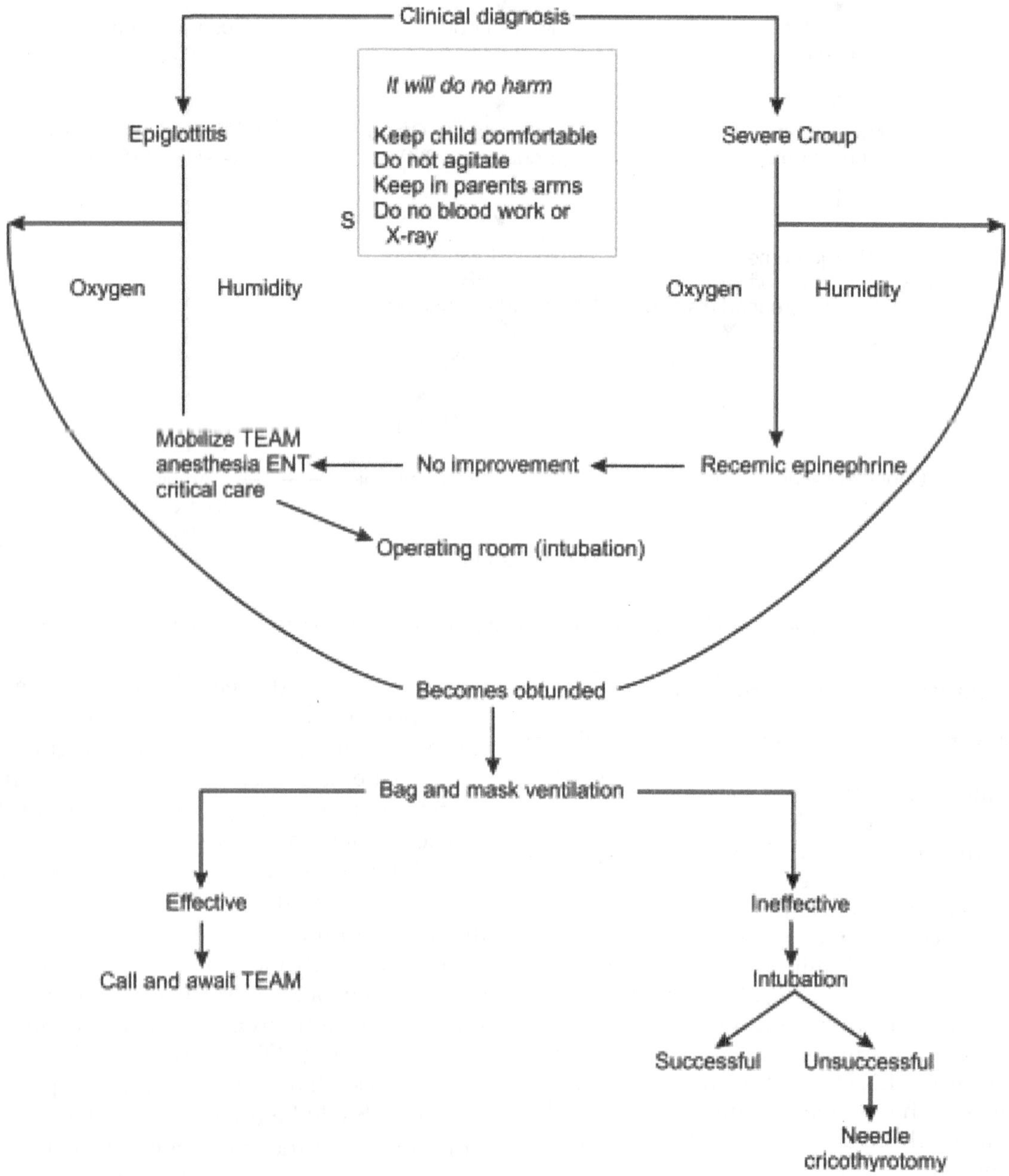

Fig. 5: Algorithm for the management of epiglottitis and severe croup

intubation. It is preferable to intubate the child electively in a controlled fashion rather than to perform a crisis intubation at the time of cardiopulmonary collapse. Intubation is best conducted in the operating room, following inhalation anesthesia with ENT and with anesthesia present.

If the child with severe croup becomes obtunded or is unable to ventilate adequately, bag and mask ventilation should be initiated. In spite of the degree of obstruction, many of these patients can be effectively bag and mask ventilated. If this is effective, then awaiting more experienced personnel is advisable since inexperienced manipulation of the airway may cause further trauma and increase the degree of obstruction. If bag and mask ventilation is ineffective, the physician who is most skilled in the procedure should attempt intubation. If this fails, a needle cricothyrotomy should be performed.

Epiglottitis

The management of the child who presents with epiglottitis (see Figure 5) is anxiety provoking, and therefore all emergency departments involved with the care of children should have a management protocol with which their medical staff is familiar. Once the diagnosis is strongly suspected depending on the institution, a combination of otolaryngology, anesthesia, and critical care should be notified. Oxygen is provided to the child in a nonthreatening manner. Aggressive examination of the patient, especially oral examination, as well as hematological and radiological investigations should be avoided. The child should be transported to the operating room accompanied by the parent as well as by the appropriate personnel and equipment necessary to secure an emergency airway if necessary.

In the operating room, following an inhalation anesthetic, nasotracheal intubation should be performed and antibiotics administered (ceftriaxone). Blood and supraglottic specimens are sent for culture. After securing the endotracheal (ET) tube and proper restraints and sedation, the child will be transported to the pediatric critical care unit for further therapy. Close monitoring for complications (pulmonary edema, pneumonia, metabolic abnormalities, and infection) is required. The child is usually extubated in 24 to 48 hours. Prophylactic rifampin (20 mg/kg/dose [max 600 mg]) orally once daily for four days) is recommended for all contacts in households with at least one contact younger than 48 months. The patient with epiglottitis should also be given a course of rifampin.

Diphtheria

Because prompt treatment is crucial, diagnosis is usually made on the basis of clinical findings with microbial culture later confirming the diagnosis. As soon as respiratory diphtheria is suspected, patients should be given diphtheria antitoxin followed by antibiotic treatment with either erythromycin or penicillin. Although antibiotic therapy eradicates the bacteria, it has no apparent effect on the clinical course of the disease. Respiratory support and airway maintenance should also be administered as needed.

(i) Send throat swab for bacteriological studies (Albert's stain and culture) to confirm the diagnosis.

(ii) If severe obstruction (stridor, severe distress and cyanosis) is present, establish emergency airway and *consider an early tracheostomy. It is often needed.*

(iii) Give diphtheria antitoxin 80,000-120,000 units preferably IV or IM.

(iv) Give procaine penicillin 50,000 U/kg/day IM for 7 days.

Prevention

To prevent the spread of the disease,

isolation of cases is essential and individuals in close contact with infected persons should receive prophylactic antibiotics and be immunized with an appropriate dose of diphtheria toxoid. If previously immunized, a booster dose is recommended, but if the immunization status is uncertain close contacts should receive a primary immunization series appropriate for their age. Convalescing patients should also be immunized, since the infection does not always induce adequate levels of antitoxin.

Bacterial Tracheitis

When it is suspected, antimicrobial agents to cover *S. aureus*, *Streptococci*, and *H. influenzae* are required. It is recommended to use a combination of cloxacillin (100-200 mg/kg in 4 divided doses per day) and gentamicin (5 mg/kg/day in 3 divided doses). Early intubation is necessary for effective clearing of the airways.

Retropharyngeal Abscess

The following steps of management are followed:

(i) Antibiotics: Cloxacillin (100-200 mg/kg/day q 6h) and gentamicin (5 mg/kg/day q 8h) IV.

(ii) Active management of airways. Endotracheal intubation should be done in any child with a significant degree of obstruction even if air exchange appears adequate initially. Orotracheal intubation is preferred because of the risk of rupture of the abscess.

(iii) Surgical drainage.

Foreign Body in Trachea/Larynx

(i) Establish the location of the foreign body by taking X-ray chest PA and lateral views, and both inspiratory and expiratory films.

(ii) If it is suspected in upper airway, remove it as early as possible. Place the child face downward across your knees and give 3 to 4 blows to the back. If this fails, proceed with rapid compressions of chest four times as if performing external cardiac massage to raise intrathoracic pressure. In children over one year of age, Heimlich maneuver may also be perfor-med. It is most easily performed from behind the patient, by placing one's hands on the upper abdomen and rapidly squeezing it towards epigastrium. Sudden compression of upper abdomen forces the diaphragm up and propels the object out of the airway.

(iii) If these procedures fail, it may be possible to remove the foreign body by visualization under direct laryngoscopy and use of a Magill's forceps. An emergency airway with wide bore cannula inserted through cricothyroid membrane in trachea must be established before the procedure.

(iv) If this fails urgent bronchoscopic removal is indicated.

(v) If the child is breathing and able to cough, give oxygen and leave in position of comfort. Arrange for bronchoscopy as soon as possible, even if there is complete relief of symptoms. It is especially true of peanut aspiration. This is one situation where a negative endoscopy is preferable to missing the foreign body.

Angioneurotic Edema

The condition is treated by administration of adrenaline (1:1000), subcutaneously 0.01 ml/kg (maximum 0.3 ml); hydrocortisone 10 mg/kg IV and antihistamines like chlorpheniramine.

Table 3: Specific treatment priorities with respect to cause of upper airway obstruction

Diagnosis	*Therapy*
Mild laryngotracheitis	Observation at home, mist or steam
Moderate laryngotracheitis	Admission to hospital, observation, inhaled budesonide and mist
Severe laryngotracheitis	Close observation, oxygen, intravenous dexamethasone and nebulized adrenaline; may require intubation
Spasmodic croup	Usually nebulized budesonide, may need adrenaline nebulization
Diphtheria	Antitoxin and penicillin Usually require tracheostomy
Retropharyngeal abscess	Surgical drainage, and antibiotics
Tonsillar obstruction	Antibiotics if bacterial cause, steroids unproven in EBV infection Occasionally require nasopharyngeal airway, or endotracheal intubation
Acute angioneurotic edema	Adrenaline SC or IM

In recent years, mortality and morbidity as a result of upper airway obstruction, especially due to severe croup and epiglottitis has significantly decreased. Much of this is attributed to a better understanding of the pathophysiology of the disease and to an appreciation of the rapidity with which patients can deteriorate. The major impact is as a result of medical personnel being familiar with appropriate protocols for the management of these children and because of subsequent skilled airway management.

FURTHER READING

1. Backofen JE, Rogers NC. Upper airway disease. In Rogers MC, ed. Textbook of pediatrica Intensive care. Baltimore: Williams & Wilkins 1987; 171-197.
2. Committee on Infectious Disease, Report of the committee on infectious disease, 22nd ed. Elk Grove Village, Ill: American Academy of Pediatrics 1991; 222-223.
3. Grad R, Taussig LN. Acute infections producing upper airway obstruction. In Chernick V, ed. Kendig's disorders of the respiratory tract in children, 4th ed. Philadelphia: Saunders 1989; 336-348.
4. Kairys SW, Obnstead EM, O'Connor GT. Steroid treatment of laryngotracheitis. A metaanalysis of the evidence from randomized trials. Pediatrics 1989; 83: 683-693.
5. Mauro RD, Poole SR, Lockhard CH. Differentiation of epiglottis from laryngotracheitis in the child with stridor. Arch Dis Child 1988; 142: 679-682.
6. Rapkin RH. Epiglottitis and Severe Croup. In Dickerman D, ed. The critically ill child, diagnosis and medical management, 3d ed. Philadelphia: Saunders 1985; 1-17.
7. Travis KW, Todres ID, Shannon DC. Pulmonary edema associated with croup and epiglottitis. Pediatrics 1977; 59: 695-698.

In the previous edition this chapter was written by Niranjan Kissoon, MB, BSc, FRCP(C), FAAP Associate Professor Pediatrics, Department of Pediatrics University of Florida—Health Sciences Center Jacksonville, Florida

Steven M. Barrett

9 Respiratory Failure

Disorders of the respiratory system are the most common childhood emergencies. Deaths from respiratory disorders account for one third of all mortality in children under fifteen years of age and for almost one half of all deaths under one year of age. Most pediatric cardiac arrests are secondary to a respiratory etiology.

PATHOPHYSIOLOGY

Respiratory failure is defined as an impairment of adequate oxygen absorption for the body's metabolic requirements or of adequate carbon dioxide excretion. Hypercapnia, hypoxemia, or both result from one or more of three mechanisms: (1) inadequate alveolar ventilation, (2) mismatching of alveolar ventilation and pulmonary perfusion, or (3) abnormal diffusion of gases across the alveolar capillary interface. Respiratory distress is the clinical state characterized by an abnormal respiratory rate or by increased work of breathing. Respiratory distress may progress to respiratory failure. Some patients in respiratory failure, however (for example, from certain neuromuscular disorders or respiratory muscle exhaustion) may have little or no evidence of respiratory distress such as tachypnea or other clues of increased respiratory effort.

Alveolar ventilation depends on input from the central nervous system (CNS) and the function of the thoracic pump (peripheral nerves, intercostal and accessory muscles, diaphragm and rib cage) and the lungs. The lung can be divided into conducting airways (the trachea and bronchi) and the alveoli. The conducting airways constitute anatomic dead space since the air in these airways does not participate in gas exchange. Anatomic dead space differs from physiologic dead space, which is defined as those areas of abnormal lung in which ventilation-perfusion *(V/Q)* mismatch prevents normal gas exchange. *Tidal volume* is the amount of air inspired in a single breath and includes both the anatomic dead space volume and the alveolar volume. Tidal volume is a function of respiratory effort, airways resistance, alveolar compliance, and chest wall elasticity. The product of tidal volume and respiratory rate is the minute ventilation. The product of dead space volume and respiratory rate is the dead space ventilation. Subtracting dead space ventilation from minute ventilation yields alveolar ventilation. In a normal subject deal space ventilation (V_D) accounts for 20%-30% of ventilation. A reduction in alveolar ventilation results in hypercapnic respiratory failure ($PaCO_2 > 50$ mmHg).

The normal tidal volume in most children is 5 to 7 ml/kg. In the young patient, the thoracic cage is pliable and may fail to support the lung adequately during respiratory distress. The clinical manifestation of this compromised lung expansion is paradoxical chest wall movement (sternal and intercostal retractions) during inspiration. Furthermore, air movement in the pediatric patient is more dependent on diaphragmatic motion than it is in the adult. When diaphragmatic movement is impeded by pressure from above (for example, air trapping in obstructive airways disease) or from below (for example, abdominal distention), effective respiration is threatened because the pliable chest wall may not be able to compensate.

The upper airways in infants and children are small and more easily obstructed by foreign bodies, local swelling, or the tongue than is the case in adults. In addition, an upper respiratory infection or rhinitis may cause significant respiratory compromise in the infant less than 4 months old who is an obligate nose breather. The lower airways in children are also smaller and have incompletely developed supporting cartilage. Therefore alveolar ventilation may also be easily compromised at this level if the lower airways become obstructed by mucus, blood, pus, edema, or bronchoconstriction.

The adequacy of V/Q matching is determined by the composition of alveolar gas (oxygen and carbon dioxide) and the degree to which alveolar ventilation and pulmonary perfusion are balanced. A difference exists between the alveolar and arterial oxygen levels ($A\text{-}aDO_2$); this value is 10 to 20 mmHg and is due to venous admixture from anatomic shunts through the bronchial and the besian circulation.

Abnormalities in gas exchange that occur as a result of changes in the composition of alveolar gas include a reduced inspired oxygen fraction (FjO_2) (for example, high altitude), an increased arterial carbon dioxide tension ($PaCO_2$) (for example, hypoventilation), and alterations in the respiratory exchange ratio (for example, increased CO_2 production from excessive glucose metabolism). These causes of respiratory failure are characterized by hypoxemia (PaO_2 <60 mmHg) with a normal $A\text{-}aDO_2$ and generally with hypercapnia ($PaCO_2 > 50$ mmHg).

In addition to the composition of alveolar gas, the adequacy of gas exchange is determined by the balance of alveolar ventilation and pulmonary perfusion. The ideal V/Q match is altered by a reduction in alveolar ventilation (for example, pulmonary edema or atelectasis) or by a reduction in pulmonary blood flow (for example, pulmonary embolism). The extreme example of reduced ventilation (V/Q = 0) is defined as intrapulmonary shunting; the extreme of reduced perfusion is dead space ventilation (V/Q = 00). The shunt refers to that fraction of blood that passes through the lungs and is not oxygenated. A low V/Q is greater than zero but less than the ideal. In most clinical disorders of V/Q balance, the V/Q ratios are between the extreme values along a spectrum. Most of these patients will have a mixture of both V/Q mismatch and absolute shunt. The actual V/Q ratio is influenced by protective reflexes, such as hypoxic vasoconstriction in areas of reduced ventilation.

Respiratory failure as a result of V/Q mismatch is manifested by hypoxemia with an increased $A\text{-}aDO_2$ (that is, > 20 mmHg). Increasing the FiO_2 will usually improve hypoxemia caused mainly by V/Q mismatch but will not significantly raise the PaO_2 when hypoxemia is caused mainly by an absolute shunt. Any condition that reduces the mixed venous oxygen tension (for example, reduced cardiac output) or that increases oxygen consumption (for example, increased metabolic rate) will worsen hypoxemia in the presence of V/Q imbalance. Hypoxemia is a stimulus to increase minute ventilation; thus the patient with hypoxemic respiratory failure from low or zero V/Q balance will usually present with hypocapnia ($PaCO_2 < 35$ mmHg) as long as the respiratory muscles can sustain the hyperventilation.

Increased dead space ventilation occurs when pulmonary perfusion is reduced relative to alveolar ventilation. This situation may be present as the result of pulmonary vasoconstriction (for example, pulmonary hypertension in the newborn), obliteration of small vessels in the pulmonary arterial bed (for example, acquired respiratory distress syndrome), or multiple pulmonary emboli (for example, secondary to endocarditis).

The third influence on gas exchange is the ability of oxygen and carbon dioxide to diffuse across the alveolar-capillary membrane. In general, a blood-gas tension abnormality results from abnormal diffusion of gases only when at least two of the following three factors are present: (1) decreased PaO_2 which reduces the driving pressure of O_2; (2) increased thickness of the alveolar-capillary membrane, which increases the resistance to gas diffusion (for example, interstitial edema or fibrosis); (3) either a reduction in the cross-sectional area of the pulmonary capillary bed (for example, adult respiratory distress syndrome) or a reduction in the time for red blood cell oxygen loading in the capillary bed (for example, high cardiac output states).

Pediatric patients are also at greater risk than are adults for respiratory compromise because of their generally higher metabolic rate and, therefore, their increased oxygen consumption and carbon dioxide elimination. Respiratory distress adds to this metabolic demand on the ventilatory system by increasing the work of breathing, thus exacerbating the disparity between demand and supply. Causes of respiratory failure are categorized in Table 1.

CLINICAL PRESENTATION

During the initial history and physical examination, certain symptoms and signs may suggest the presence of hypercapnia (Table 2) or hypoxemia (Table 3). Patients with primary hypercapnic respiratory failure will generally be hypoxemic, and those with primary hypoxemic respiratory failure will usually have normal or decreased values of $PaCO_2$. Immediate evidence for the presence of respiratory failure includes severe respiratory distress in an agitated or anxious patient or inadequate air exchange in an obtunded patient.

The child who is not critically ill should be allowed to remain in the parent's lap or arms in a comfortable position. The respiratory rate, rhythm, and effort should be observed. Normal respiratory rates are age-related. In general, rates above 50 per minute are abnormal for an infant, and rates above 40 per minut are abnormal for a child. Other signs of increased work of breathing include the use of accessory neck muscles (sternocleidomastoid and scalene muscles), retractions (intercostal, subcostal, lower sternum, or supraclavicular), nasal flaring, and paradoxical chest or abdominal wall motion. Chest retractions and nasal flaring are more specific for respiratory tract disorders than is tachypnea. Retractions of different parts of the thorax are often striking in infants and young children with respiratory distress because of the highly compliant chest wall.

Dysphagia and drooling suggest upper airway obstruction. Stridor is an inspiratory crowing sound that is present in upper respiratory tract obstruction. Stridor has a high-pitched quality with croup and laryngeal foreign body aspiration and a low-pitched muffled quality with epiglottitis. A harsh, brassy cough, particularly when it is associated with inspiratory stridor, likewise suggests the presence of laryngeal or subglottic obstruction (for example, foreign body or croup). Grunting is caused by early

Table 1: Causes of respiratory failure

Hypercapnic ($PaCO_2$ > 50 mmHg)

1. Decreased alveolar ventilation
   a. CNS depression from head injury, coma, status epilepticus, drug overdose
   b. Peripheral nervous system dysfunction from spinal cord trauma, Guillain-Barre syndrome, botulism, myasthenia gravis
   c. Upper airway obstruction from foreign bodies, diphteria, vocal cord palsy, epiglottitis, croup, aspiration, thermal injury, tracheomalacia
   d. Increased airway resistance from asthma, bronchiolitis, cystic fibrosis, organophosphate poisoning
   e. Decreased lung compliance from pulmonary edema, interstitial fibrosis
   f. Increased chest wall compliance from flail chest
   g. Pleural space dysfunction from pneumothorax, hemothorax, pleural effusion
   h. Respiratory muscle fatigue from excessive work of breathing, shock states
   i. Respiratory muscle failure from muscular dystrophies
2. Increased dead space ventilation
   a. Decreased pulmonary blood flow from multiple pulmonary emboli, pulmonary hypertension syndromes, decreased cardiac output states
   b. Air trapping and alveolar overdistention from asthma, bronchopulmonary dysplasia (BPD)
3. Increased production of CO_2
   a. Increased metabolic rate with major burns
   b. Altered respiratory quotient from excessive glucose administration

Hypoxemic (PaO_2 <60 mmHg)

1. Decreased FiO_2
   Alveolar hypoxia, for example, from altitude illness
2. Intrapulmonary shunting with increased pulmonary vascular resistance
   Diffuse alveolar flooding with pulmonary vascular obliteration from adult respiratory distress syndrome (for example, due to shock states, sepsis, disseminated intravascular coagulation, fat embolism)
3. Intrapulmonary shunting without increased pulmonary vascular resistance
   Local alveolar flooding from pneumonia, lung contusion
4. Low V/Q match with increased pulmonary vascular resistance
   Bronchospasm with increased pulmonary artery tone from meconium aspiration syndrome
5. Low V/Q match without increased pulmonary vascular resistance
   Alveolar flooding from cardiogenic or noncardiogenic pulmonary edema (for example, due to smoke inhalation, toxic gas inhalation, near-drowning, salicylate or opiate toxicity, gastric juice aspiration)
6. Intracardiac shunting with increased pulmonary vascular resistance
   Right-to-left shunting with increased pulmonary artery tone from endocardial cushion defect
7. Intracardiac shunting without increased pulmonary vascular resistance
   Right-to-left shunting without pulmonary vascular disease from pulmonic stenosis with a ventricular septal defect
8. Hypoventilation
   Decreased alveolar ventilation from upper airway obstruction, congenital lobar emphysema, diaphragmatic hernia, gastric distention, abdominal distention
9. Diffusion impairment
   Interstitial space dysfunction from pulmonary fibrosis
10. Decreased mixed venous oxygen tension
    Increased oxygen extraction by tissues in cardiogenic shock

Table 2: Evidence for hypercapnia

Headache	Wheezing
Drowsiness, coma	Decreased air entry by auscultation
Sweating	Asymmetric air entry by auscultation
Tachycardia	Excessive work of breathing
Hypertension	Paradoxical chest wall motion
Peripheral vasodilation	Paradoxical abdominal wall motion
Stridor	Apneic episodes

Table 3: Evidence for hypoxemia

Dyspnea	Tachycardia
Confusion	Hypertension
Agitation	Peripheral vasoconstriction
Restlessness	Rales by auscultation
Tachypnea	Murmur by auscultation
Retractions	Dysrhythmias
Nasal flaring	Bradycardia
Grunting	Hypotension
Sweating	Cyanosis

closure of the glottis during exhalation. Grunting increases expiratory airway pressure, thus preventing airway collapse in a manner similar to the mechanism of positive end expiratory pressure (PEEP). Grunting may occur in patients with lower respiratory tract diseases (for example, pneumonia, asthma, or bronchiolitis), especially if diminished lung compliance is present (for example, pulmonary edema). Children suffering pain from any illness or injury, however, may also have grunting.

The adequacy of tidal volume can be assessed by inspection of abdominal excursions in the infant and chest filling in the child and by auscultation of breath sounds bilaterally. Wheezing bilaterally suggests asthma or bronchiolitis (or occasionally congestive heart failure); foreign body aspiration may induce unilateral wheezing. Restlessness and irritability in an infant may be due to hypoxemia, hypercapnia, shock, or pain. Bradycardia is ominous in patients with respiratory failure and can occur in infants in response to hypoxemia. The presence of cyanosis in central tissues such as the tongue and the face should be noted. Peripheral cyanosis without central cyanosis can result from peripheral vasoconstriction in shock states or hypothermia or as a normal physiologic response in infants. The absence of cyanosis does not imply that oxygenation is adequate.

Disorders that lead to respiratory distress or failure may be progressive, sometimes acutely progressive. Patients may present with impending respiratory failure, or they may be at risk for respiratory compromise. These patients must be examined repeatedly for evidence of developing respiratory distress so that respiratory failure can be anticipated and possibly prevented with timely medical management decisions.

LABORATORY EVALUATION

Respiratory distress with tachypnea may be present in patients with disorders that are not primarily related to the respiratory system such as sepsis, congenital heart disease, or metabolic acidosis (due to salicylate toxicity, diabetic ketoacidosis, or gastroenteritis with dehydration). Therefore confirmation of the clinical diagnosis of respiratory failure or impending failure generally requires arterial blood-gas and pH measurements. Respiratory failure is present if the $PaCO_2$ is greater than 50 mmHg (assuming no preexisting lung disease with chronic CO_2 elevation) in the presence of acidosis or if the PaO_2 is less than 60 mmHg (assuming no cyanotic congenital heart disease) in a patient breathing room air.

The alveolar-arterial oxygen difference ($A\text{-}aDO_2$) can be estimated in a patient with normal cardiac output who is breathing room air (ideally at sea level). In this situation, the alveolar O_2 tension added to the alveolar CO_2 tension equals approximately 145 mmHg. Assuming intact diffusion of blood gases at the alveolar-capillary interface, the alveolar CO_2 tension is essentially the same as the measured arterial CO_2 tension. Therefore the alveolar O_2 tension is approximately equal to 145 minus the measured $PaCO_2$. The measured PaO_2 is now subtracted from the calculated alveolar O_2 tension to yield A-aDO_2. An A-aDO_2 value of less than 20 mmHg is normal, 20 to 30 mmHg represents mild pulmonary dysfunction, 30 to 50 mmHg moderate dysfunction, and greater than 50 implies severe respiratory decompensation. Hypoxemia with a normal A-aDO_2 results from hypo ventilation. Hypoxemia with an increased A-aDO_2 suggests either an intrapulmonary shunt, a low V/Q match, or a diffusion impairment.

If the patient is breathing oxygen, the PaO_2/FiO_2 ratio can be calculated. The normal value for this ratio is about 500 to 600, and a ratio of 200 (for example, PaO_2 of 80 mmHg with FiO_2 of 40 percent or 80/0.4) corresponds to an intrapulmonary shunt of about 20 percent, which generally indicates a need for ventilatory support. Further information may be gained by administering 100 percent O_2 to the hypoxemic patient. If the PaO_2 value increases to over 100 mmHg, either a low V/Q match or a diffusion impairment is present; if the PaO_2 value remains below 100 mmHg, an intrapulmonary shunt is the cause of hypoxemia. Even temporary administration of 100 percent O_2, however, is not completely innocuous; it can induce absorption atelectasis resulting in the measurement of a falsely elevated shunt fraction.

Pulse oximetry is useful for continuous measurement of O_2 saturation of hemoglobin. The relationship between PaO_2 and oxygen saturation of hemoglobin is expressed by the sigmoid-shaped oxygen-hemoglobindissociation curves. When the $PaCO_2$" pH, and body temperature are normal, an oxyhemoglobin saturation of 90 percent correlates with a PaO_2 of about 60 mmHg. Hypercarbia, acidosis, or hyperthermia will shift the dissociation curve to the right so that an oxyhemoglobin saturation of 90 percent then correlates with a PaO_2 greater than 60 mmHg.

A chest roentgenogram is indicated and may reveal abnormalities that require intervention such as a pneumothorax or a malpositioned endotracheal tube. Furthermore the chest film can help with diagnosis of certain causes of respiratory failure. Other evaluations that may be indicated include a soft tissue lateral neck roentgenogram, electrocardiogram (EKG), complete blood count, electrolytes, glucose and toxicology screen. A lateral decubitus chest roentgenogram is useful for evaluation of the dependent side for free pleural fluid or evidence of air trapping and the nondependent side for pneumothorax, air-fluid levels or basilar infiltrates hidden behind the diaphragm, or behind pleural effusion. Air trapping on the dependent side suggests that an ipsilateral endobronchial foreign body is not allowing the dependent lung to deflate as expected.

MANAGEMENT

Respiratory failure must be anticipated and prevented, if possible, with appropriate therapy. The goals of management of the patient with impending or fully developed respiratory failure include reestablishing adequate gas exchange in the lung and oxygen delivery to tissues. The etiology of failure should be identified, and the patient should be monitored so that the course of the disease process and the adequacy of therapy can be followed.

The patient's upper airway patency, respiratory rate and effort, vital signs, level of consciousness, color and status of peripheral perfusion (skin temperature and capillary refill time) should be initially assessed and repeatedly monitored. Available monitoring devices include continuous pulse oximetry, indwelling arterial catheters, and end-tidal CO_2 samples (capnography). Serial measurements of arterial blood gases and pH may be indicated. The patient should be reassessed repeatedly and after any therapeutic maneuver.

Sufficient oxygen should be administered to produce a hemoglobin-saturating PaO_2, that is, about 70 mmHg. In the patient with shock, an even higher PaO_2 should be attained if possible so that distal tissue watershed areas can be protected from hypoxia. A PaO_2 of less than 40 mmHg is a profound stimulus to the development of pulmonary hypertension and right heart failure. A continually high FiO_2 can eventually cause oxygen toxicity in the lung, but the duration of this exposure necessary to produce toxicity is uncertain, and patients vary in susceptibility. Furthermore the use of positive pressure ventilation itself may play a role in the production of lung damage. Concerns about oxygen toxicity should not prevent adequate oxygenation of the patient, and a high FiO_2 is occasionally necessary for temporary periods. The overall management protocol, however, should allow reduction of the FiO_2 to 60 percent or lower as soon as this is practical.

If a hemoglobin-saturating PaO_2 cannot be achieved in a patient who is spontaneously breathing oxygen by mask, more advanced airway support may be required. Most children in respiratory distress or failure can be managed initially with bag-valve-mask ventilation and oxygenation. If early respiratory support efforts prove inadequate, endotracheal (ET) intubation and mechanically assisted ventilation may be indicated to reduce a possible low V/Q match or intrapulmonary shunt. The amount of assisted ventilation required is that which produces adequate chest wall expansion, usually a tidal volume of 10 to 15 mVkg.

Other therapeutic options depend on the type of respiratory failure identified and the specific etiology of failure (Tables 4 and 5). For example, bronchodilator therapy is

Table 4: Examples of management options for hypercapnic respiratory failure

Disorder	*Goal*	*Treatment*
CNS or peripheral nervous system hypoventilation	Increase alveolar ventilation	Assisted ventilation
Upper airway obstruction	Relieve or bypass obstruction	Endotracheal intubation, laryngoscopy, bronchoscopy
Increased airways resistance	Bronchodilation	Beta-adrenergic agonists, theophylline, steroids
Decreased lung compliance	Correct lung volume	Assisted lung ventilation, PEEP, diuretics
Respiratory muscle fatigue	Muscle rest Improve muscle function	Assisted ventilation Beta-adrenergic agonists, theophylline
Increased dead space ventilation	Improve pulmonary blood flow	Vasodilators, reduced PEEP, inotropes, heparin

Reprinted with permission from Anas NG. Respiratory failure. In Leven DL, Morriss FC, eds. Essentials of pediatric emergency care. St. Louis: Quality Medical Publishing, 1990;64-71.

Table 5: Examples of management options for hypoxemic respiratory failure

Disorder	*Goal*	*Treatment*
Intrapulmonary shunt	Convert shunt to low or normal V/Q	Bronchodilators, diuretics, PEEP
Low V/Q	Correct hypoxemia	Increase FiO_2
	Correct lung volume	Bronchodilators, diuretics, PEEP, surfactant replacement
Intracardiac shunt		
Ductus arteriosus-dependent lesions	Maintain patency of ductus	PGE_1 infusion
Tetralogy of Fallot	Relax pulmonary infundibulum	Morphine sulfate, propranolol
Hypoventilation	Increase alveolar ventilation	Assisted ventilation, racemic epinephrine
Diffusion impairment	Increased alveolar O_2	Increase FiO_2
	Reduce resistance to diffusion	Diruetics, steroids

Reprinted with permission from Anas NG. Respiratory failure. In Leven DL, Morriss FC, eds. Essentials of pediatric emergency care. St. Louis: Quality Medical Publishing 1990;64-71.

indicated when hypercapnic respiratory failure from increased airways resistance is diagnosed. Response to bronchodilators is poor in most patients under 18 months of age, even in those patients later diagnosed with asthma, so that a bronchodilator therapeutic trial may be an unreliable test to differentiate asthma from bronchiolitis. Especially in patients with hypoxemic respiratory failure, careful fluid balance is important so that crystalloid overload can be avoided.

CONCLUSIONS

An understanding of the pathophysiology and appropriate initial assessment and management of infants and children with acute respiratory distress and failure will enable optimal care for these patients. Some causes of distress and failure are rapidly reversible with prompt recognition and proper therapy. Other disorders will follow a prolonged course to eventual improvement and recovery or to progressive deterioration and mortality despite optimal management decisions. Decompensation in these patients can occur rapidly, thus continual reevaluation and continuous monitoring are critical.

FURTHER READING

1. Benditt JO. Initiating noninvasive management of respiratory insufficiency in neuromuscular disease. Pediatrics. 2009 May;123 Suppl 4:S236-8.
2. Panitch HB. The pathophysiology of respiratory impairment in pediatric neuromuscular diseases. Pediatrics. 2009 May;123 Suppl 4:S215-8.
3. Kissoon N, Skippen P. Adjunct pharmacotherapy in acute lung disease in children. Minerva Pediatr. 2007 Aug;59(4):379-88.
4. Bansal A, Singhi SC, Jayashree M. Penicillin and gentamicin therapy vs amoxicillin/clavulanate in severe hypoxemic pneumonia. Indian J Pediatr. 2006 Apr;73(4):305-9.
5. Kennedy JD, Martin AJ. Chronic respiratory failure and neuromuscular disease. Pediatr Clin North Am. 2009 Feb;56(1):261-73, xii.
6. Lecky F, Bryden D, Little R, Tong N, Moulton C. Emergency intubation for acutely ill and injured patients. Cochrane Database Syst Rev. 2008 Apr 16;(2):CD001429

Sunit Singhi and Nishat Ahmed

10 Asthma/Bronchiolitis

ASTHMA

Asthma afflicts upto 10 percent of all children. Epidemiologic evidence indicates that this disease is becoming more frequent and more severe with a marked increase in emergency visits, hospital admissions and deaths. Evidence also suggests that under diagnosis and under treatment contributes to asthma's morbidity and mortality. Children come to the emergency department for exacerbations of asthma that range from chronic, aggravating cough to respiratory failure. The clinician must recognize and manage this wide spectrum of disease with the goal of relieving symptoms and averting disaster.

Pathophysiology

The clinical pathology of asthma results from a reversible obstruction of the large and small airways that impedes the egress of gas on exhalation. The trapping of intrapulmonary air causes areas both of hyperexpansion and postobstructive atelectasis, resulting in ventilation-perfusion mismatch. Airway obstruction appears to arise from two separate but interrelated processes:

1. Muscular constriction of the tracheobronchial tree.
2. Obstruction of the lumen of the airways with mucosal edema, secretions, and other products of inflammation.

Tracheobronchial muscle tone is controlled by the competing activity of acetylcholine and endogenous sympathomimetic agents. Drugs that stimulate sympathomimetic beta-receptors or inhibit acetylcholine can reverse tracheobronchial constriction and obstruction of airflow. This phenomenon forms the basis of the treatment of asthma with beta-agonist and anticholinergic agents.

Airway inflammation is a complex process controlled by a multitude of mediators, many of which are potent bronchoconstrictors. If it is allowed to proceed unchecked, inflammation ultimately leads to intraluminal airway obstruction from mucosal edema and thick, tenacious secretions. Because they have relatively narrow peripheral airways, and underdeveloped alveolar capacity, infants and young children are especially vulnerable to the effect of airway obstruction. Autopsies of children dying from asthma show greatly over distended lungs with severe mucus plugging of larger and smaller airways.

Clinical Presentation

The most common clinical manifestation of asthma is expiratory wheezing. Most children will have a history of reactive airway disease and will be receiving outpatient treatment. The diagnosis can be difficult in the "first-time wheezer" or in a child with atypical symptoms. In infants, bronchiolitis is the most common cause of wheezing. Congenital anomalies also tend to present in younger patients, and it is in this group that the greatest danger of a tracheal or esophageal foreign body exists. While on an emergent basis there is no diagnostic test for asthma, a family history of reactive airway disease, a history of recurrent symptoms, and a good response to therapy all support the diagnosis. While it has been said that "all that wheezes is not asthma," most that wheezes is indeed reactive airway disease. Indeed, asthma tends to suffer more from underdiagnosis than it does from overdiagnosis.

Asthma can cause vague complaints such as decreased exercise tolerance or atypical chest pain, but the most common clinical manifestation other than wheezing is cough. Patients or parents often describe the cough as harsh, chronic and worse at night. Small children often suffer posttussive regurgitation from gagging on thick, tenacious secretions. These patients are often misdiagnosed as having pneumonia, especially when small areas of atelectasis that are seen on a chest X-ray are interpreted as infectious infiltrates. Children with "cough equivalent asthma" are often unnecessarily treated with multiple courses of antibiotics.

Any child diagnosed as having more than one episode of pneumonia or labelled as suffering from "chronic bronchitis" must be strongly suspected of having an underlying problem. Most commonly these patients suffer from asthma (Table 1).

- Principles of management
- Assessment.
- Correction of hypoxemia with oxygen.
- Rapid reversal of airflow obstruction using inhaled β_2-agonists.
- Early addition of corticosteroids to speed the rate of improvement.
- Close monitoring of response with help of clinical signs and PFER, FEV1.

Table 1: Different diagnosis of wheezing

Infancy	Bronchiolitis, viral upper respiratory tract infection, pertussis, cystic fibrosis, bronchopulmonary dysplasia, congenital malformation (vascular ring, choanal atresia, tracheoesophageal fistula, web), gastroesophageal reflux, laryngotracheomalacia, immunodeficiency syndromes, congenital heart disease.
Childhood	Aspiration (foreign body or incompetent lower esophageal sphincter), croup, gastro-esophageal reflux, cystic fibrosis, hypersensitivity pneumonitis, tuberculosis, tumor, allergic bronchopulmonary aspergillosis, ciliary defects, parasitic pneumonitis, immunodeficiency syn-dromes, habit or imitation cough.
Adolescence	Aspiration (particularly with neurologic disorder), cystic fibrosis, gastroesophageal reflux, α_1-anti-trypsin deficiency, ciliary defects, immunodeficiency or autoimmune collagen disorders, tuberculosis, tumor, allergic broncho-pulmonary pneumonitis, cardiac disease, hyperventilation syndrome, sighing dyspnea, vocal cord dysfunction.

Evaluation

The evaluation of a child with an acute exacerbation of asthma begins with an assessment of the severity of the respiratory distress. Several factors are important in determining the degree of airway obstruction:

Mental status: The patient's mental status should be noted—a happy or calm patient usually denotes, at the most, mild distress, while an anxious asthmatic indicates severe airway obstruction and probably hypoxia. Increasing lethargy or obtundation signals imminent respiratory arrest.

Accessory muscle use: After assessment of mental status, the patient should be observed for the presence or absence of chest wall retractions and for nasal flaring. The use of accessory muscles of respiration implies moderate to severe airway obstruction. The more pronounced the retractions the more severe the respiratory distress.

Respiratory rate: Tachypnea is an important part of the response to airway obstruction and is virtually always present in acute asthma. Especially in infants and young children, careful attention must be given to the respiratory rate since their limited alveolar capacity demands that they increase minute ventilation mainly through breathing faster.

Auscultation: Auscultation of the chest can be helpful in determining the effectiveness of air exchange. In most patients, airway obstruction results in prolonged expiration. The loudness of wheezing should be noted but must be evaluated in the context of air exchange. The absence of wheezing implies inadequate air exchange and indicates severe airway obstruction—the "silent chest" demands urgent attention. Symmetry of breath sounds should also be noted. Unilateral diminished breath sounds can indicate severe postobstructive atelectasis or can be a manifestation of a pneumothorax.

Peak flow and spirometry: In older children, peak flow and spirometry provide useful information regarding the degrees of airway obstruction. This is especially true if the patient's baseline is known. These physiologic measurements often indicate a higher degree of airway obstruction than is predicted by the physical examination and thus may help to avoid underestimating a patient's illness. Peak flow predominantly measures obstruction in larger airways, while spirometry is useful in assessing the more peripheral airways.

Oxygen saturation: Another useful adjunct in determining the degree of illness is oxygen saturation, which can now be measured transcutaneously. While some degree of hypoxia occurs in virtually all acute asthma, a decrease in oxygen saturation (probably below 93 percent) implies significant ventilation-perfusion mismatch.

Chest X-ray: The chest X-ray is usually not helpful in an acute asthma episode. It commonly shows small areas of atelectasis that are easily confused with pneumonia. In some cases, however, an X-ray may be useful in excluding a foreign body, pneumothorax, or severe atelectasis.

History

Concomitant with the physical exam, a history should be obtained regarding the potential trigger of the acute attack, the duration of symptoms, the use of medications and the time of administrations. Short episodes provoked by known irritants are often easily reversed, while a patient with prolonged symptoms often has more resistant airway obstruction. This is especially true in patients who have either been compliant with, or have increased the frequency of, therapy with inhalational beta-agonists. A crescendo pattern of inhaler use implies a relatively severe and potentially resistant attack with a significant inflammatory component. The dose and timing of administration of asthma drugs should be ascer- tained. Some patients inappropriately increase their dosage during an acute attack and are therefore at risk of toxicity. A history regarding past or present use of steroids must be obtained. An asthmatic who deteriorates while on steroid therapy has a particularly refractory attack and is at risk for respiratory failure. Presence of precipitating factors such as infection, allergens, drugs, exercise and course of previous episode and outcome should also be taken into consideration.

Risk Factors

It is vital to identify those patients most likely to progress to a life-threatening episode (Table 2). These patients represent a population that can be considered as "high risk" collectively and mandate a cautious approach to management and disposition. Patients who are steroid dependent or require frequent steroid therapy fall into this category as do patients requiring frequent emergency department visits or hospitalization. Especially ominous is a history of admission to an intensive care unit (ICU), or a history of mechanical ventilation. While any episode of acute asthma can progress to respiratory failure, patients with a history of frequent or severe attacks are at relatively greater risk for deterioration than are patients with infrequent, mild attacks.

Table 2: Risk factors for life-threatening asthma

1. Early onset of severe asthma, particularly less than one year of age
2. Frequent need for hospitalization to control asthma
3. Dependence on corticosteroids, either oral or inhaled
4. Noncompliance or abuse of medication
5. Labile asthma with pronounced "morning dipping" diurnal airway obstruction
6. Britrle asthma with unexpected rapid deterioration of pulmonary function
7. Teenager with long-standing asthma of early onset
8. Depressive symptoms with chronic asthma

The patients at greatest risk for fatal asthma in USA appear to be urban adolescents of African-American descent who have a long history of severe disease. These patients may suffer from lack of access to health care as well as from the non-compliance common to adolescence. Both they and their physicians, however, often tend to underestimate the potential severity of their acute asthma attacks and therefore undermanage the illness with potentially catastrophic results.

Clinical manifestations of acute severe asthma and life-threatening attack are enumerated in the Tables 3 and 4. Marked tachypnea, chest wall retractions, use of accessory respiratory muscles, diminished or absent breath sounds, cyanosis, pulsus paradoxus above 15-20 mm Hg indicate severe life-threatening attack of asthma. Fatigue somnolence, disorientation and air hunger indicate impending respiratory failure.

Table 3: Clinical manifestations: Severe acute asthma

- PEFR < 40% of predicted.
- Tachycardia > 120 beats/min.
- Tachypnoea > 40 breaths/min.
- Dyspnoea. Inability to speak.
- Accessory muscle use.
- Pulsus paradoxus > 15 mmHg.
- SaO_2 90%-94%.

Table 4: Signs of a life-threatening attack

- Too dyspneic to speak
- PEFR < 25% of predicted or patient's best.
- Cyanosis.
- Respiratory muscle fatigue (e.g. Abdominal paradox).
- Altered consciousness—confusion, coma.
- A silent chest on auscultation.
- Pneumothorax.
- Bradycardia, hypotension.
- SaO_2 <90-92%, PO_2 <60 mmHg $PaCO_2$ 45 mmHg.

Why do patients die from asthma?

- Inadequate assessment of asthma severity.
- Delay in referral to hospital.
- Over-reliance on bronchodilators.
- Underuse of systemic steroids, prophylactic agents.
- Inadequate supervision, lung function not monitored.
- Socio-economic deprivation–poor access to health care.
- Psychosocial problems–non compliance.
- Drug toxicity.

Management

FEV1 or PEF values provide important information about the level of airflow obstruction both initially and in response to treatment. Because low PEF values cannot distinguish between poor effort, restrictive ventilatory disorders (e.g. neuromuscular weakness, pneumonia), and obstructive ventilatory disorders (e.g., asthma), FEV1 measurements are preferable if they are readily available. In the initial assessment of a life-threatening asthma exacerbation, FEV1 or PEF are not indicated. Very severe exacerbations may preclude performance of a maximal expiratory maneuver and, in such cases, the clinical presentation should suffice for clinical assessment and prompt initiation of therapy. In less severe exacerbations, in the office or ED, FEV1 or PEF should be obtained on arrival and 30-60 minutes after initial treatment. In the hospital, FEV1 or PEF should be measured on admission and 15-20 minutes after bronchodilator therapy during the acute phase and at least daily thereafter until discharge. Any FEV1 or PEF value <25 percent of predicted that improves by <10 percent after treatment or values that fluctuate widely are potential indications for ICU admission and close monitoring for respiratory failure.

Drugs

Humidified oxygen should be given by face mask or nasal catheter

Bronchodilators: The most important drugs used to reverse the acute bronchospastic component of airway obstruction are beta-receptor agonists. For many years, the most commonly used drug for acute asthma was epinephrine, which is a potent bronchodilator that is usually administered subcutaneously. Because it stimulates both pulmonary and cardiac betareceptors, epinephrine often causes tachycardia, and its use has been supplanted by inhaled beta-agonists with a high degree of specificity for pulmonary tissue. During nebulization, little systemic absorption occurs; thus systemic side-effects are minimized. Recent studies have focused on increasing the frequency and the dosage at which nebulized beta-agonists can be safely administered; these studies have demonstrated that cardiac toxicity is not a limiting factor. The onset of action for SABAs (short acting beta-agonist) is less than 5 minutes; repetitive administration produces incremental bronchodilation. In about 60–70 percent of patients, response to the initial three doses in the ED will be sufficient to discharge them, and most patients will have a significant response after the first dose. Nebulized salbutamol is the most commonly used bronchodilator. Some institutions also use nebulized terbutaline. These drugs are available in metered dose inhalers for home use, and for young children, they can be given as an oral suspension (Table 5).

Anticholinergic drugs also function as bronchodilators, with their primary effect probably being on larger airways. Some studies have found these agents useful in acute asthma and recommend they be used concomitantly with beta-agonists. Ipratropium bromide is available for use as nebulized agents and in metered dose inhalers. Adding multiple high doses of ipratropium bromide (0.5 mg nebulizer

Table 5: Drugs for treatment of acute attack

Drug	Administration	Dosage		Frequency
		Child	Adult	
Terbutaline	Subcutaneuos	0.01 mg/kg	0.25 ml	20 min (×2)
Epinephrine aqueous 1:1000 sol (1 mg/ml)*	Subcutaneuos	0.01 mg/kg	0.3 ml	20 min (×3)
Salbutamol 1:200 (5 mg/ml)	Nebulized aerosol	0.02 ml/kg up to 0.5 ml (100 ug/kg)	0.5 to 1.0 ml in 2.0 ml saline	30 min (×3)
Terbutaline 1:1000 (1 mg/ml)	Nebulized aerosol	1 ml in 1 ml saline	0.2 ml in 1.0 ml saline	30 min (×3)
Ipratropium bromide (0.25 mg/mL)	Nebulizer solution	0.25–0.5 mg	0.5 mg	20 min (×3)

In moderately severe or severe attack, it is best to administer drug via, or concomitant with, oxygen.
*. for use in life-threatening attack.

solution or 8 puffs by MDI in adults; 0.25–0.5 mg nebulizer solution or 4–8 puffs by MDI in children) to a selective SABA produces additional bronchodilation, resulting in fewer hospital admissions, particularly in patients who have severe airflow obstruction.

Theophylline, a methylxanthine derivative that functions at least in part as a bronchodilator, has been used for many years in the treatment of acute asthma. Recent evaluation of this drug has cast doubt on its efficacy in acute asthma, suggesting that the potential for toxicity outweighs the therapeutic benefits. However, many would consider it worth trying in a severe attack. Side effects of theophylline include vomiting and tremulousness. Higher levels can cause tachydysrythmias and, in severe cases, seizures. The metabolism of theophylline is notoriously erratic. It is wise to obtain a serum level on a patient taking theophylline prior to giving a "loading dose". Levels must be monitored closely on patients who are placed on theophylline infusions.

Corticosteroids: Systemic corticosteroids are the mainstay of therapy for the inflammatory component of airway obstruction. Their early use in an acute attack can prevent the need for hospital admission, and their use as outpatient therapy can reduce symptoms and prevent the need for a return visit to the emergency department. More importantly, by suppressing the inflamma-tion that produces the mucus plugging, atelectasis, and ventilation-perfusion mismatch characteristic of a severe attack, steroids can prevent an episode of asthma from progressing to respiratory failure. Steroids can be admini-stered intravenously, intramuscularly, or orally. While no definite guidelines have been derived regarding the dose, duration, or method of delivery of steroids during an acute asthma attack, most patients are treated with short, intensive bursts. Children appear to tolerate up to four one-week courses of steroid therapy during the course of a year with minimal risk of adrenal suppression. Oral administration of prednisone has been shown to have effects equivalent to those of intravenous methylprednisolone. A 5 days course following discharge is given to prevent early relapse. A common practice is to administer methylprednisolone 1-2 mg/ kg IV (intravenous) every six hours to an ill asthmatic. A patient discharged from the emergency department can be treated with prednisone 1mg/kg/day for five to seven days.

Corticosteroids should be administered immediately to any asthmatic in moderate or severe distress and should be strongly considered in any acutely ill patient with a history of severe attacks, frequent hospitalizations, or multiple courses of steroid use in the past. Patients with a history of prolonged, debilitating symptoms, especially those who have been resistant to aggressive inhalational therapy, are also candidates for steroids. A decrease in oxygen saturation implies significant ventilation perfusion mismatch and is an indication for administering steroids. Certainly not every child suffering from acute asthma needs treatment with steroids. However, failure to treat those patients aggressively, with a significant inflammatory component to their illness can result in unnecessary morbidity.

Management of the Severe Attack

Most children with mild, episodic asthma with acute symptoms will respond well to one or two nebulized treatments. Patients with more severe respiratory distress must receive very aggressive management. If nebulizer therapy is not immediately available, subcutaneous epinephrine should be administered. Steroids should be given at once. Patients in moderate to severe distress should receive nebulizer therapy at least every 20 to 30 minutes until improvement is noted. Oxygen should be administered continuously.

The asthmatic in severe respiratory distress who does not respond to treatment with frequent nebulized beta-agonists presents a management challenge. In such patients, IV beta-agonists have been used successfully to reverse bronchospasm and avert the need for mechanical ventilation. Salbutamol and terbutaline are used intravenously at some centers. These drugs are less active on the myocardium than isoproterenol is and to date have not been reported to cause myocardial ischemia in children. Beta-agonists can also be administered as continuous nebulized treatment on a milligram per hour basis, avoiding the potential complications of IV therapy. Further studies are needed before definite recommendations can be made regarding IV or continuous nebulized beta-agonist therapy. Both modalities are in use at many pediatric centers, however, where they play an important role in the treatment of critically ill asthmatics.

Consider intravenous magnesium sulfate (50 mg/kg/dose IV infusion in 30 ml normal saline) in patients who have life-threatening exacerbations and in those whose exacerbations remain in the severe category after 1 hour of intensive conventional therapy. Fluids and electrolytes should be corrected gradually over 24 hours, as children are mildly dehydrated with N/5 saline 5% D and potassium 40 meq/l as loss is increased by the use of steroids and theophylline induced dieresis. Hydration should be monitored and overhydration avoided as renal water excretion capacity is impaired in them.

Occasionally an asthmatic will not respond to the most aggressive therapy and will require mechanical ventilation. Intubation should be considered in the patient who develops a deteriorating mental status or progressive muscle fatigue. No absolute blood gas value mandates mechanical ventilation, but it must be considered in the setting of a rising pCO_2 or of refractory hypoxia. Most pediatric asthmatics tolerate moderate hypercarbia, but hypoxia can become lethal rapidly and must not be allowed to persist.

Most patients will need sedation prior to and following intubation. Benzodiazapines have hypnotic and anxiolytic properties and are often used to initiate sedation, but may not allow sufficient relaxation. Ketamine, a dissociative anesthetic agent, has been advocated as an induction agent in the intubation of children in status asthmaticus. In addition to sedation, ketamine causes bronchodilation and thus has some potential therapeutic benefit. Since it does not cause muscle paralysis, ketamine allows the patient to maintain some respiratory effort in the event that endotracheal tube placement is difficult. Ketamine can cause increased secretions, which can be reduced by prior treatment with an anticholinergic such as atropine or glycopyrrolate. Occasionally hallucinations can occur, and ketamine has infrequently been associated with laryngospasm. The recommended dose of ketamine is 0.5 to 2 mg/kg IV. Heliox-driven albuterol nebulization has been tried for patients who have life-threatening exacerbations and for those patients whose exacerbations remain in the severe category after 1 hour of intensive conventional therapy. Because of helium's low density, a mixture of helium and oxygen (heliox) could improve gas exchange in patients who have airway obstruction.

Protocol for Acute moderate and Severe Asthma

Immediate Treatment

If the patient is cyanosed and is having

Table 6:

Bronchiolitis	*Bronchial asthma*
No family history	Family history of asthma
Usually begins with URI	Sudden onset without preceding infection
Recurrent attacks may occur but < 5% will have viral infection as cause	Repeated episodes in the same infant
Normal WBC profile	Eosinophilia
Usually no response to aerosolised salbutamol.	Immediate response to a single dose of aerosolised salbutamol
Bacterial infection	*Viral LRTI*
Fever > 38.5°C	Fever < 38.5 °C
RR > 50/min	RR increase or normal
Chest recession	Hyperinflation
Clinical and radiological signs indicate consolidation rather than collapse	CXR – hyperinflation, 25% collapse
Wheeze not an early sign of primary bacterial LRTI	Cough, wheeze 50% of mycoplasma

altered sensorium immediately start oxygen, if necessary by bag and mask and give Inj. adrenaline 0.01 ml/kg (1:1000) subcutaneously.

Phase I: One to one and half hour

- O_2 by mask to keep O_2 saturation (SaO_2) > 90%.
- Start nebulisation with: Salbutamol 0.15-0.3 mg/kg/dose (max. 5 mg) and Budesonide (0.8 mg)/per dose, upto 3 doses of at 20-30 mins interval.
- Ipratropium 250 microgram every 30 minutes, up to 3 doses.
- Assess-Improved: Prepare for discharge
- No/inadequate improvement: Follow phase II.

Phase II:

1. Continue oxygen.
2. Continue nebulised salbutamol— 0-15 - 0.3 mg kg/dose hrly or 0.3 mg/kg/hr continuous nebulization till response.
3. Set up IV line.
4. Systemic steroid-*If conscious can accept orally—prednisolone 2 mg/kg/dose

* If cannot take orally—IV Hydrocortisone 10 mg/kg stat then 5 mg/kg 6 hrly or methyl prednisolone 1-2 mg/kg, 6 hrly.

5. IV $mgSO_4$ (50%), 50 mg/kg/dose IV infusion in 30 ml normal saline over 30 minutes.
6. Theophylline – After a bolus 5 mg/kg, 1mg/kg/hour by infusion
   It has beneficial therapeutic effect in children when given in combination with nebulized beta-agonists and systemic steroids.
7. Obtain blood counts, ABG's, Chest x-ray, electrolytes.
8. Treat infection if present with suitable antibiotics.
   Reassessment—At end of 4 hours.
   * Improved—Prepare for discharge.
   * Inadequate/No response : Hospitalise, *Follow phase III.*

Phase III

- Continue oxygen, and nebulised salbutamol continuous or intermittent.
- Continue Mg SO_4 (50%) infusion - 6 hrly.
- Intravenous beta-agonists intravenous terbutaline/salbutamol trial warranted in children with asthma who have failed to respond to nebulized bronchodilators and intravenous steroids.
- Intravenous salbutamol affects a rapid drop in $PaCO_2$ levels and averts need for ventilation in over two-thirds.

Dose:

- 0.5 μg/kg/min, increasing by 1 μg/kg every 15 min until the patient clinically improves and $PaCO_2$ falls or intubation and ventilation become necessary. The maximum infusion rate - 20 μg/kg/min, usually respond to 4 μg/kg/min.
- Assisted ventilation: Indicated if PaO_2 <50 on 50% O_2, PCO_2 >50, cyanosis on 50% O_2.
- Serial oxygen saturation, ABG's, cardiac and respiratory monitoring.

Discharge Preparation after Phase I

- Start salbutamol—by inhaler, in infants with spacer and mask, in small children with spacer.
- If already on steroid before exacerbation increase the dose of inhaled steroid for next two weeks.
- Review in OPD/ Clinic after - 1 week.

Discharge Advise-After phase II/III

- Salbutamol as above.
- Oral Steroid: Prednisolone 2 mg/kg/day x 5 days single morning dose.
- If severe exacerbation and/or history of >1 attack/per month uncontrolled on steroid - follow appropriate protocol.
- Send home after 12-24 hrs. With Clinic appointment / Review in OPD after - 2 days.

Disposition

No clinical scoring system predicts perfectly those patients who absolutely require admission. Even patients who have a resolution of wheezing and feel better after treatment can have significant residual airway obstruction and can relapse after responding well to initial therapy. A clinical improvement in air-exchange should be noted, and in infants, an improvement in respiratory rate and in the ability to feed well should be documented. Peak expiratory flow rate, which reflects obstruction in larger airways, can provide useful information but has been unreliable in predicting relapse. A decrease in oxygen saturation has been correlated with a need for hospital admission. Values between 91 to 93 percent have been associated with relapse, even in patients who appeared to improve with treatment. Oxygen saturation may reflect abnormalities in the smaller airways that result in ventilation-perfusion mismatch and that are not as quickly reversed as obstruction in larger airways. In at least one study, oxygen saturation was more sensitive than peak flow in predicting relapse.

Historical factors play an important role in determining disposition. Any patient with severe disease or a history of noncompliance should be discharged only with extreme caution. Patients or their parents must demonstrate an understanding of the illness and medical regimen, including how to use metered dose inhalers, and must have transportation to the hospital in the event of a relapse.

Summary

Fortunately the vast majority of asthmatics will not progress to respiratory failure, but by treating each episode of acute bronchospasm as a potentially life-threatening event, the emergency physician can avoid the pitfall of undermanagement. Recognition of the high-risk patient, aggressive management of patients with significant respiratory distress, and the judicious use of steroids are the current cornerstones of management.

BRONCHIOLITIS

Bronchiolitis is an extremely common cause of emergency department visits and hospital admissions. It is the most common cause of wheezing in infants less than one year of age. Pathologically the term bronchiolitis refers to inflammation in the peripheral airways. Clinically the term applies to a syndrome most often seen in young infants that is characterized by rhinorrhea, cough, retractions and wheezing. Bronchiolitis is most often caused by respiratory syncytial virus (RSV), the most common infectious cause of lower airway disease in infants and young children. Less commonly, bronchiolitis is caused by influenza, parainfluenza, or adenoviruses.

Epidemiology and Pathology

Bronchiolitis most commonly affects infants between two and six months of age.

The disease appears during the yearly epidemics of RSV infections that occur between October and June. By the time they reach the age of two, the vast majority of children show evidence of having been infected by RSV. Manifestations of infection range from mild lower airway disease to fulminant pneumonia with diffuse parenchymal involvement. Only a minority of children infected with RSV develop bronchiolitis. Why some children develop the characteristic bronchiolar inflammation and others do not is not fully understood.

In infants who develop bronchiolitis, RSV infection results in necrosis of respiratory epithelium and destruction of ciliated epithelial cells in the lower airways. The airway lumen becomes obstructed with cellular debris and edema in an uneven fashion, producing areas of air trapping and atelectasis. The diffuse inflammatory response may also produce bronchospasm, especially in infants with a tendency toward reactive airway disease. While the role of bronchospasm in bronchiolitis is not yet clear, upto 30 percent of children who wheeze in association with RSV infection go on to develop reactive airway disease. Thus bronchiolitis can be thought of as a virus induced pneumonia with asthmalike features. The diffuse airway obstruction produces ventilation-perfusion mismatch and can cause significant hypoxemia. Less commonly, air trapping can result in hypercarbia and respiratory failure. Most of the morbidity and mortality in bronchiolitis occurs in infants who are less than six months of age, where underdeveloped alveolar capacity and relatively narrow airways enhance the effect of any intraluminal obstruction. This illness tends to be especially severe in infants with underlying cardiopulmonary disease. Infants with congestive heart failure, cystic fibrosis, or immunosuppression are especially likely to develop respiratory compromise. However, patients at greatest risk for respiratory failure during the course of bronchiolitis are those infants with a 'history of prematurity who suffer from bronchopulmonary dysplasia (BPD), a condition that often results in chronic hypoxemia, hypercarbia, and brittle reactive airway disease. In these patients bronchiolitis can lead to respiratory failure quickly.

Clinical Presentation and Diagnosis

Early findings in bronchiolitis include an upper respiratory prodrome with copious nasal discharge, restlessness, cough and fever. The onset of lower airway involvement is characterized by tachypnea, tachycardia, and chest retractions. Auscultation of the lungs reveals wheezing with occasional fine rales. Lower airway obstruction results in prolonged expiration. Occasionally depression of the diaphragm can result in abdominal distension and the illusion of hepatosplenomegaly. Some infants develop conjunctivitis and pharyngitis.

Bronchiolitis must be distinguished from other causes of lower airway disease. These include bacterial pneumonia, chlamydia pneumonitis, anatomic anomalies such as vascular rings, and airway or esophagel foreign bodies. Congestive heart failure often presents with respiratory distress and wheezing in young infants and can easily be confused with bronchiolitis. Asthma can be difficult to distinguish from bronchiolitis, especially in the first-time wheezer; however, careful questioning often reveals prior pulmonary complaints. Although no bedside test accurately distinguishes between the two diseases, it is common clinical practice to administer a trial of beta-agonist therapy and to label patients with an unequivocal response as having *asthma* while those that do not seem to respond are considered to have *bronchiolitis.*

A definitive diagnosis of bronchiolitis can be made by culturing RSV from nasopharyngeal secretions or more rapidly by demonstrating the presence of RSV by immunofluorescent techniques. The chest X-ray is nondiagnostic. It can demonstrate diffuse hyperexpansion of the lungs, or it may show areas of patchy infiltrate that result from atelectasis.

Assessment

In the average healthy infant significant respiratory distress is indicated by pronounced tachypnea (respiratory rate of

60 to 80), poor retractions, air entry, anxiety or restlessness, and refusal to feed. Inability to feed is a manifestation of exertional dyspnea and an important clue to clinically significant respiratory insufficiency in an infant. Cyanosis is uncommon, but hypoxia is often present. Transcutaneous measurement is useful in revealing oxygen saturation. In severe cases, bronchiolitis can result in hypercarbia and respiratory failure. In patients who have significant respiratory distress or underlying cardiopulmonary disease, a blood gas should be obtained to assess respiratory status definitively.

The definitive mainstays of treatment for bronchiolitis are the maintenance of adequate hydration and oxygenation. Humidified oxygen 30-40%, may be given by placing the baby in a oxygen tent or through a headbox. As oral fluid intake cannot be maintained in a seriously ill infant IV hydration is necessary. Because of the asthma-like qualities of bronchiolitis and because it is thought that bronchoconstriction may play some role in the illness, common clinical practice also includes the use of beta-agonist therapy. Patients often receive nebulized treatment in the emergency department. Despite their wide use in the treatment of bronchiolitis, the efficacy of beta-agonists is controversial. This is especially true in young infants in whom improvement in pulmonary function is difficult to measure. Nebulised epirephrine is helpful in immidiate releif of distress and hypoxemia.

Indications for Hospitalization

- Age less than 3 months.
- Gestational age at birth of < 34 weeks
- Cardiopulmonary disease or immunodeficiencies.
- Respiratory rate > 70/ min.
- Lethargic appearance.
- Wheezing and respiratory distress associated with SpO2 < 92% on room air
- Hypercarbia.
- Atelectasis or consolidation on chest radiography.

In seriously ill patients, the antiviral agent ribavirin at dose of 50 mg/kg every 12 hourly for 3 to 6 days has been found to shorten the course of bronchiolitis and to reduce the time that mechanical ventilation is required in those patients who suffer respiratory failure. Currently ribavirin therapy is reserved for patients with underlying cardiopulmonary disease or for those who develop severe disease.

Apnea and Bronchiolitis

A common complication of RSV infection is apnea, which is especially likely to occur in very young infants or in those with a history of prematurity. The etiology of RSV-associated apnea is not known but it is felt to require assisted ventilation more often than is respiratory failure resulting from severe bronchiolitis. Any infant with a history of apnea requires hospital admission and close monitoring even if their bronchiolitis appears mild. Other viral infections can also cause apnea, but bacterial sepsis must be ruled out.

Summary

Bronchiolitis is a self-limited illness that, in the majority of healthy infants, can be managed safely at home. Patients who are unable to tolerate feeding require hospital admission and IV fluids to maintain hydration. Patients with hypoxemia require hospital admission for supplemental oxygen therapy. Any patient with significant hypercarbia is at risk for respiratory failure and should be considered a candidate for admission to a pediatric ICU.

Hospitalization should be strongly considered in patients with underlying cardiopulmonary disease, especially infants with bronchopulmonary dysplasia. Bronchiolitis is especially dangerous in infants with these risk factors. Infants less than two to three months of age with bronchiolitis should be discharged from the emergency department with extreme caution and only in the hands of an adequate caretaker. A next day follow-up visit is a good idea in these patients.

FURTHER READING

1. Schramm CM, Carroll CL. Advances in treating acute asthma exacerba-tions in children. Curr Opin Pediatr. 2009 Jun;21(3):326-32.
2. Rodrigo GJ. Rapid effects of inhaled corticosteroids in acute asthma: an evidence-based evaluation. Chest. 2006 Nov;130(5):1301-11.
3. Devidayal, Singhi S, Kumar L, Jayshree M. Efficacy of nebulized budesonide compared to oral prednisolone in acute bronchial asthma. Acta Paediatr. 1999 Aug; 88 (8):835-40.
4. Boyd M, Lasserson TJ, McKean MC, Gibson PG, Ducharme FM, Haby M. Interventions for educating children who are at risk of asthma-related emergency department attendance. Cochrane Database Syst Rev. 2009 Apr 15;(2):CD001290.
5. Mohammed S, Goodacre S. Intravenous and nebulised magnesium sulphate for acute asthma: systematic review and meta-analysis. Emerg Med J. 2007 Dec;24(12):823-30.
6. Yanney M, Vyas H. The treatment of bronchiolitis. Arch Dis Child. 2008 Sep; 93(9): 793-8.
7. Zhang L, Mendoza-Sassi RA, Wainwright C, Klassen TP. Nebulized hypertonic saline solution for acute bronchiolitis in infants. Cochrane Database Syst Rev. 2008 Oct 8;(4):CD006458.
8. Walsh P, Caldwell J, McQuillan KK, et al. Comparison of nebulized epinephrine to albuterol in bronchiolitis. Acad Emerg Med. 2008 Apr;15(4):305-13.
9. Corneli HM, Zorc JJ, Mahajan P, et al. A multicenter, randomized, controlled trial of dexamethasone for bronchiolitis. N Engl J Med. 2007 Jul 26;357(4):331-9.
10. Martinón-Torres F, Rodríguez-Núñez A, Martinón-Sánchez JM. Nasal continuous positive airway pressure with heliox versus air oxygen in infants with acute bronchiolitis: a crossover study. Pediatrics. 2008 May;121(5):e1190-5.

In the previous edition this chapter was written by William Ahrens, MD
Assistant Professor Emergency Medicine University of Illinois—Chicago
Chicago, Illinois

and

Gary Strange, MD
Associate Professor of Emergency Medicine Residency Program Director
University of Chicago, Chicago, Illinois

11 Foreign Body Aspiration

Foreign body aspiration most commonly occurs in children six months to six years of age with the majority less than 3 years of age. Aspiration occurs approximately twice as often in boys as it does in girls. In India, peanuts and food items are most common cause as also in USA. Food objects such as hot dogs, candies, nuts, and grapes are more commonly aspirated than nonfood objects (Table 1). Young children do not have molars and cannot adequately chew these foods. In addition, they do not have a perfectly coordinated swallowing mechanism, leaving ingested foods at the laryngeal inlet when the child inspires. Combining this with the facts that children put objects in their mouths out of curiosity, habit, or carelessness and that children often eat while playing and talking explains the etiology of foreign body aspiration. Approximately 300 to 400 deaths occur each year in the United States secondary to aspiration. This is half the mortality rate prior to the Consumer Products Safety Act of 1979. This act mandated that toys and toy pieces designated for children up to 3 years of age must be at least 1¼ inches in diameter and 2¼ inches in depth. Despite this, recent cases illustrate the variety of nonfood objects aspirated. These include balloons, earrings, straight pin during an attempt to blow the pin through a straw, aluminum foil tab from a juice container, Barbie™ doll curler and plastic sales tag holder. Balloons are now the leading cause of pediatric choking deaths from children's products.

PATHOPHYSIOLOGY

The pathophysiology of foreign body aspiration is related to the degree of airway obstruction. Factors determining the degree of obstruction include age of patient, size of foreign body, organic versus nonorganic, duration, and location of foreign body. Most reviews have found the right mainstem bronchus to be the most common location, probably because its angle with the trachea is less than the left mainstem. The remaining foreign bodies are lodged in the trachea or larynx, the later being the least common location (see Table 1).

Degrees of bronchial obstruction include partial obstruction on both inspiration and expiration and partial obstruction on inspiration but total obstruction on expiration and on inspiration and expiration. Total obstruction on expiration and not inspiration occurs secondary to intrathoracic negative pressure. This degree of obstruction results in air trapping and obstructive emphysema.

Table 1: Foreign body aspiration

	Number	Age Less Than 3 Years	M:F	Nature* Organic	Inorganic	Location† Bronchus	Right	Left	Laryngotracheal
Laks, Barzilay (1)	149	90	94:55	141	8		73	52	24
Kim, Brummitt, Humphry, et al. (2)	202	131	135:67	156	46		99	63	19
Moazam, Talbert, Rodgers (3)	40	33	26:14	27	13				
Daniilidis, Symeonidis, Triaridis, et al. (4)	79		48:31				22	39	18
Harboyan, Nassif (5)	213			197	16		121	55	36
Aytac, Yurdakul, Ikizler, et al. (6)	462	329	351:111	358	94		327	86	45
Merchant, Kirtane, Shah, et al. (7)	132	91	81:51	108	24		68	61	
Puhakka, Svedstrom, Kero, et al. (8)	83	46	56:27	49	34		41	25	13
Losek (9)	42		26:16	32	10		24	15	3
Blazer, Naveh, Friedman (10)	200	170	133:67	187	8		83	69	35
Abdulmajid, Ebeid, Motaweh, et al. (11)	250		110:140	212	38		175	32	43
Pyman (12)	230		150:80	155	75		117	74	33
TOTAL	2082	890/1268 (70%)	1210:659 (1.8:1)	1622 (82%)	366 (18%)	1721 (86%)	1150 (67%)	571 (33%)	269 (14%)

* The nature of some foreign bodies was unknown.

† Some patients had multiple foreign bodies in more than one location.

Note: Blanks indicate no report.

Total obstruction causes atelectasis. Organic versus non organic foreign bodies more commonly cause a local inflammatory reaction. Thus with time, a partial obstruction can progress to a total obstruction. If total obstruction is not corrected, trapped secretions dilate the bronchioles and result in bronchiectasis and fibrosis.

CLINICAL MANIFESTATIONS

The factors that determined the pathophysiology (the degree of airway obstruction) also determine the clinical manifestations. Initially the child may have cough, gagging, choking, stridor, wheezing, hoarseness, dysphonia, drooling, or cyanosis. The caretaker may not witness these initial symptoms, and if the child is too young to verbally report the aspiration, there will be no history of foreign body aspiration. This is not uncommon, as great as 62 percent of children in one review had no history of foreign body aspiration. Combining the studies referred to in Table 1, 81 percent of the children gave a history of foreign body aspiration.

Initial symptoms may resolve, and if so, a symptomless interval occurs. This interval may last hours, days, or months. In a review by Laks and Barzilay of 149 patients, 41 (27 percent) were asymptomatic at presentation. When a foreign body becomes lodged in a fixed position, the surface sensory receptors of the respiratory tract adapt to the constant pressure. The defense cough reflex stops with this adaptation of the surface receptors. Combining studies, cough was the most common symptom but still occurred in only 76 percent of the patients. Unless the foreign body moves or secretions stimulate new surface receptors, cough will not occur. The production of secretions is dependent on the inflammatory nature of the foreign body and on the length of time it has been lodged. This adaptive quality of the airway surface receptors accounts for the symptomless interval and is one of the factors that can lead to a subsequent delay in diagnosis.

Manifested symptoms are determined by the location of the foreign body in the respiratory tract and the degree of obstruction. Total obstruction at the level of the trachea or larynx will rapidly produce respiratory failure and an inability to ventilate with resuscitative breathing. Partial obstruction at the larynx may cause inspiratory stridor, drooling, gagging, and voice change. Whereas partial obstruction at the trachea may manifest as inspiratory stridor, choking, and cough. If obstruction is nearly complete at the trachea, expiratory wheeze may also occur. Partial obstruction of the bronchus results in wheezing and cough. The degree of obstruction will determine the degree of respiratory distress. For these reasons, symptoms can be quite variable. Combining studies, symptoms of foreign body aspiration include cough (76 percent), wheezing (50 percent), respiratory difficulty (36 percent), history of cyanosis (30 percent), and choking (30 percent). Eleven percent of the patients were asymptomatic. Location, duration, and nature of the foreign body also determine the signs of foreign body aspiration. Fever and rales support pneumonia and are more commonly found when patients present more than 24 hours postaspiration. Patients with laryngotracheal foreign bodies have significantly less wheezing, unilateral decreased air entry, and fever compared to patients with bronchial foreign bodies. Laryngotracheal foreign body patients, however, are more likely to have stridor and hoarseness. The classical physical finding of bronchial foreign body aspiration is unilateral decrease of air entry on the affected side. Combining studies, 61 percent of patients had unequal air entry: Other signs include wheezing (34 percent), tachypnea (30 percent), and rales (18 percent). Seven percent of the patients had normal examinations.

The initial roentgenograms for suspected foreign body aspiration are inspiratory/expiratory chest X-rays (Figures 1a and b). The affected side will be hyperinflated on the expiratory X-ray. The degree of

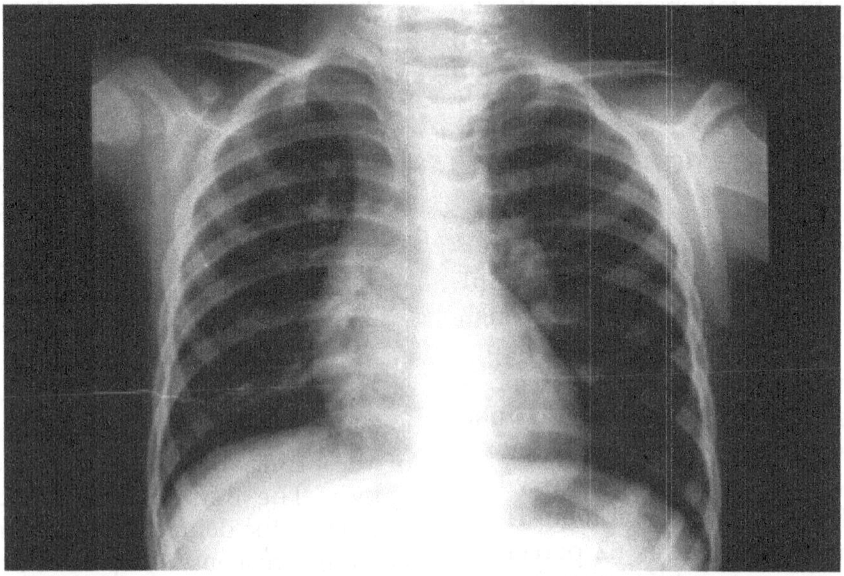

(a)

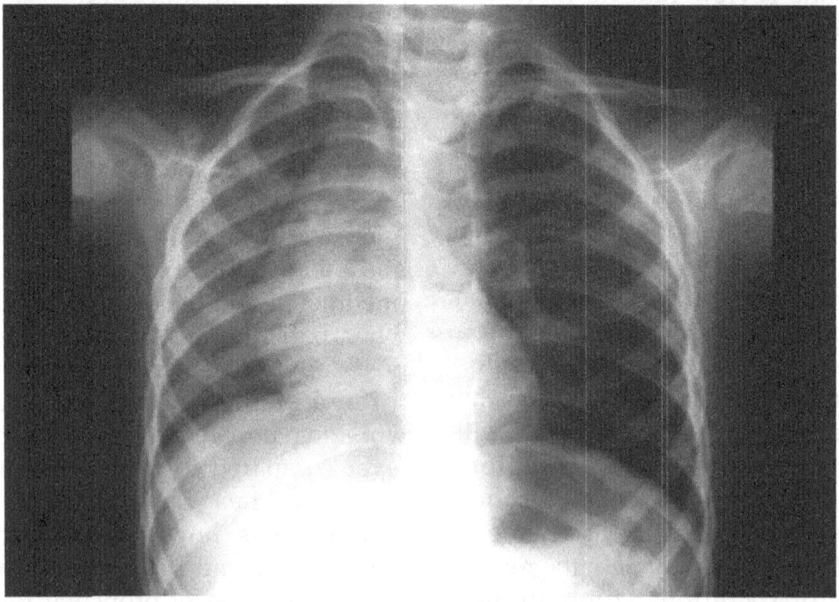

(b)

Fig. 1: Left mainstem bronchus foreign body causes the ball-valve effects illustrated in the inspiratory (a) and expiratory (b) chest X-rays. The expiratory film shows the depression of the diaphragm and hyperinflation of the involved left side, and the shift of the mediastinum and heart to the uninvolved right side.

hyperinflation is dependent on the degree of obstruction. Obstructive emphysema was the most common abnormal finding of previous reviews, occurring in 35 percent of the patients with foreign body aspiration. Since the majority of foreign bodies are organic, and thus radiolucent, only 8 percent of the foreign bodies were seen on chest X-rays. Other findings include infiltrate (15 percent) and atelectasis (11 percent). These findings, particularly infiltrate were more commonly found when the diagnosis of foreign body aspiration was delayed. In addition, discovering an infiltrate may further delay the correct diagnosis. Overall 31 percent of the chest X-rays were normal (1-12). For laryngotracheal foreign body, chest X-rays were normal in 60 percent of the patients reported by Blazer.

These limitations of plain chest roentgenograms in the diagnosis of foreign body aspiration are disturbing. An additional diagnostic procedure is fluoroscopy. The behavior of the mediastinal shadow is examined during the respiratory cycle. Widening of the mediastinal shadow during inspiration is a diagnostic sign of laryngeal, tracheal, or both main bronchi obstruction. This widening, however, can also occur during forced inspiration as happens with crying. Shift of the mediastinal shadow with inspiration indicates an unilateral bronchial obstruction. Combining previous reports, fluoroscopy was performed in 429 children and 317 of them (74 percent) were supportive of a foreign body aspiration. 'Fluoroscopy, lung scan, or CT (computerized tomography), however, do not improve diagnostic accuracy compared to history, physical examination, and chest X-rays.

MANAGEMENT

The diagnosis of foreign body aspiration is often delayed. Combining studies, 169 (18 percent) patients had a diagnostic delay of greater than 30 days (1-12). Delay is often caused by the physician attributing the patient's signs and symptoms to other, more common pediatric respiratory tract disorders. Pneumonia or asthma is often the initial misdiagnosis for foreign body aspiration. Antibiotic or bronchodilator treatment can result in improvement, therefore, a high suspicion for foreign body aspiration should be present in cases of recurrent pneumonia and prolonged bronchospasm. In addition, an esophageal foreign body may result in cough, respiratory distress, and stridor similar to the symptoms caused by a laryngotracheal foreign body.

Bronchoscopy is the treatment of choice. Combining studies, 2032 (98 percent) children with foreign body aspiration, had the foreign body removed via bronchoscopy, 10 (0.5 percent) spontaneously coughed the foreign body out, and 34 (1.6 percent) required thoracotomy. Complications from bronchoscopy include laryngeal edema needing tracheostomy (1.4 percent to 17 percent), pneumomediastinum-pneumo-thorax (1 percent to 2.3 percent) and cardiac arrest (1 percent to 2.3 percent). Prednisolone (1 to 2 mg/kg) is given prior to bronchoscopy to prevent laryngeal edema and subsequent need for possible tracheostomy. Cardiac arrest may be caused by the combination of hypoxia and reflex vagal stimulation, therefore, pre bronchoscopy atropine treatment is routine.

Bronchoscopy should be performed without delay for children with foreign body aspiration. A 24-hour trial of bronchodilator therapy, postural drainage, and chest physiotherapy in hopes of the patient spontaneously coughing up the foreign body are not recommended. Movement of the foreign body may convert a partial obstruction or one bronchus obstruction to a total tracheal obstruction. Deaths secondary to foreign body airway obstruction have occurred in children with asymptomatic intervals (25,26). Blazer found that a second or a third bronchoscopy was needed in 15 percent of the children with foreign body aspiration, either because the foreign body was not found in a previous procedure (9 percent) or because an incomplete removal was made (6 percent). A second, third, or fourth bronchoscopy was needed in 16 percent of the patients reported by Merchant. A negative bronchoscopy may also occur with an unsuspected esophageal foreign body.

In the emergent situation of respiratory failure secondary to foreign body aspiration, near-total or total obstruction at the level of the larynx or trachea is the most likely cause. Basic life-support therapy, including abdominal thrusts for the child one year of age and older or back blows and chest compressions for the child less than one year of age, can be initially attempted. In an emergency department, however, direct visualization with a laryngoscope and removal with McGill's forceps is recommended. If a foreign body is not visualized, a tracheal foreign body can be assumed. Endotracheal intubation is suggested with the intention of pushing the foreign body into one of the bronchi, thus permitting ventilation and oxygenation of at least one lung. Emergency tracheostomy or cricothyrotomy are final alternatives if endotracheal intubation is unsuccessful.

CONCLUSION

Foreign body aspiration occurs most commonly in children less than six years of age with the majority less than three years. Organic food materials are the most commonly aspirated foreign bodies. Prevention of the majority of cases is possible if young children are not permitted to eat peanuts, grapes, hot dogs, and other foods that require complete chewing. The presenting signs and symptoms of foreign body aspiration are variable, ranging from none to respiratory failure. Delay in diagnosis is not uncommon because the aspiration may be unwitnessed, airway adaption to the foreign body can result in an asymptomatic interval, 30 percent of chest roentgenograms are normal, and a more common pediatric respiratory disorder (asthma or pneumonia) is often diagnosed. Bronchoscopy without delay is the treatment of choice.

FURTHER READING

1. Digoy GP. Diagnosis and management of upper aerodigestive tract foreign bodies. Otolaryngol Clin North Am 2008;41:485-96.
2. Soodan A, Pawar D, Subramanium R. Anesthesia for removal of inhaled foreign bodies in children. Paediatr Anaesth 2004;14:947-52.
3. Hammer J. Acquired upper airway obstruction. Paediatr Respir Rev 2004;5:25-33.
4. Kumar P, Athanasiou T, Sarkar PK. Inhaled foreign bodies in children: diagnosis and treatment. Hosp Med 2003;64:218-22.
5. Pak MW, van Hasselt CA. Foreign bodies in children's airways: a challenge to clinicians and regulators. Hong Kong Med J 2009;15:4-5.

In the previous edition this chapter was written by Joseph D. Losek, MD, FAAP, FACEP Associate Professor of Pediatrics Medical College of Wisconsin Children's Hospital of Wisconsin Milwaukee, Wisconsin

Sunit Singhi

12 Sore Throat

Sore throat refers to any painful sensation in the pharynx or surrounding tissues and is a common complaint in childhood.

COMMON CAUSES

1. Infections
   1. Pharyngitis/tonsillitis
      1. Viral
      2. Bacterial
         1. Group A Streptococcus
         2. Other bacteria
   2. Peritonsillar, retropharyngeal and lateral pharyngeal abscesses
2. Irritants
   1. Excessive dryness
   2. Dust
   3. Smoke
   4. Postnasal drip secondary to allergic rhinitis or sinusitis
3. Trauma
   1. Vocal abuse
   2. Thermal injury
4. Foreign body
5. Caustic substances
6. Psychogenic

DIAGNOSTIC APPROACH

History and physical examination provide important clues for proper diagnosis of sore throat.

Most common clinical dilemma in child with pharyngitis is whether pathogen is virus or group A Streptococcus. Presence of conjunctivitis, cough, rhinitis, and hoarseness suggests viral etiology. Infectious mononucleosis is also a consideration, especially in older children and adolescents.

Tests to detect streptococcal antigen may be diagnostic, but if results of such tests are negative, throat culture should be performed.

Because many cases of pharyngitis are due to viruses, antibiotic use should be guided by antigen detection tests or culture. Neck radiography, flexible laryngoscopy and CT are useful for suspected foreign body or retropharyngeal/lateral pharyngeal abscess.

DIFFERENTIAL DIAGNOSIS

Acute Pharyngitis/Tonsillitis

Acute pharyngitis is an infection of the tonsils and or the pharynx. Pharyngitis, tonsillitis, and pharyngotonsillitis are interchangeable terms and are often used to describe the clinical diagnosis in patients with sore throats regardless of the etiology.

The exact incidence of pharyngitis is not known. However, pharyngitis is the second most common diagnosis in children 1-15 years of age in the ambulatory setting. Viral agents account for most cases of pharyngitis seen in children. Many viruses are known to cause pharyngitis/tonsillitis, including parainfluenza viruses, influenza A & B viruses, rhinoviruses, enterovirus, Herpes simplex type 1 and 2, Epstein Barr virus and respiratory syncytial virus.

In viral pharyngitis, coryza and cough predominate, whereas fever is a variable finding.

Some viral infections have typical clinical signs, which help in specific diagnosis. Herpangina is characterized by fever and painful vesicular lesions on pharynx and tonsils. Coxsackie A16 is characterized by vesicular lesions in the mouth and on hands and feet. Herpes simplex virus produces acute gingivostomatitis with fever and painful vesicles usually confined to anterior mouth, which may extend to anterior tonsillar pillars. Epstein-Barr virus is common cause of sore throat in adolescents. Other characteristic findings of infectious mononucleosis include fever, malaise, fatigue, cervical or generalized lymphadenopathy and hepatosplenomegaly. Adenovirus may cause pharyngoconjunctival fever. Follicular hyperplasia of tonsils and exudate may be seen.

Bacterial pharyngitis/tonsillitis is most commonly caused by group A beta Streptococcus(GABHS). It is implicated in 20-30% of all cases of pharyngitis. Classic clinical presentation is school-aged child with acute onset of fever and sore throat. Headache, abdominal pain, and vomiting also may occur. Rhinorrhea, cough, conjunctivitis, hoarseness and diarrhea are unusual. Tonsils are enlarged and inflamed with patches of exudate. Petechiae may sometimes be seen on palate. Anterior cervical lymph nodes may be enlarged on one or both sides and are often tender. Pharyngitis caused by group C or G Streptococcus is indistinguishable from that caused by group A Streptococcus.

Usual clinical dilemma is to distinguish between viral infection or group A streptococcal infection. It is difficult to distinguish them clinically. Throat culture is considered the gold standard for diagnosing GABHS pharyngitis, though it has limitations, including a relatively high incidence of false-negatives (10-20%). Also, positive throat culture for GABHS, without serologic evidence, does not distinguish between a carriage state and an acute infection. Rapid techniques are now available for detection of streptococcal antigen. Either rapid antigen test (sensitivity=95%) or throat culture (sensitivity>95%) should be performed if streptococcal pharyngitis is suspected.

C. diphtheriae is still an important cause of pharyngitis in our set-up. With this infection, acute onset of fever and sore throat is followed in 1–2 days by grayish membrane over pharynx and tonsils, which may extend into larynx and trachea. Positive throat culture confirms diagnosis of these pathogens.

GABHS may cause suppurative complications from local spread of infection. It includes peritonsillar cellulitis or abscess (quinsy), retropharyngeal abscess, cervical adenitis, otitis media, and sinusitis. Other important complications of GABHS include post-streptococcal glomerulonephritis (GN) and toxin-mediated disease such as scarlet fever and toxic shock syndrome. Treating streptococcal sore throat infection does not prevent post-streptococcal GN.

Peritonsillar abscess (PTA)

PTA are most commonly seen in older children and adolescents, but have been rarely reported in young infants. Patients often present with sorethroat, pain on swallowing a muffled voice, trismus, and drooling. Other complaints may include fever, ear pain, and neck pain. The abscess pushes the uvula away to the contralateral side of the oropharynx. The tonsils and pharynx are erythematous and there may be exudates on the tonsils.

It is often difficult to differentiate a peritionsillar cellulitis from an abscess. The significant asymmetry of tonsil size and the presence of uvular deviation and palatine fullness are more consistent with a PTA.

Streptococcus pyogenes is the most common pathogen. *Staphylococcus aureus* and H. *influenzae* or anaerobes (Peptostreptococcus, Fusobacterium species) are common pathogens as well. Many infections are polymicrobial.

Retropharyngeal abscess

Retropharyngeal abscess/cellulitis is an uncommon cause of sore throat. It occurs in children <4 years. Commonly, there is a recent history of an upper respiratory infection. Patients are often toxic and have fever. They may be drooling and have a stiff neck and tender cervical adenopathy. Respiratory symptoms of stridor or dyspnea are usually late findings. A midline mass can sometimes be seen in the posterior pharynx.

Usually, bacteria in the pharynx spread via lymphatic channels to the nodes of Rouvier, where they multiply and suppurate. Other possible mechanisms include trauma (causing a mucosal tear), hematogenous spread during bacteremia, or rarely, extension from vertebral osteomyelitis. The abscess can rupture into the prevertebral space or "danger space", which communicates with the mediastinum and descends as far the psoas muscles.A large RPA may obstruct the airway at the pharyngeal, laryngeal, or tracheal level.

RPA is usually a polymicrobial infection and may include Streptococcus species, Staphylococcus aureus, and anaerobes. Haemophilus influenzae type b has become a less common pathogen since the introduction of the vaccine.

Lateral neck X-ray may show bulging posterior pharyngeal wall. Prevertebral soft tissues at the level of C3 should measure less than two-thirds of the anterior-posterior width of the body of the third cervical vertebrae. The retropharyngeal space looks widened on a lateral radiograph in RPA. Crying can also lead to a widened appearance. If diagnosis is uncertain, a CT scan can be performed. CT with contrast is the most reliable test for evaluating an RPA. A hypodense region with rim enhancement is virtually diagnostic for an abscess, while a more heterogeneous mass without rim enhancement suggests retropharyngeal cellulitis.

Irritants

Sore throat may occur due to dryness of pharynx and frequently occurs with rhinitis, especially during winter months when humidity is low and mouth breathing is likely because of nasal congestion.

Exposure to dust or smoke also may cause irritation of pharynx.

Postnasal drip secondary to allergic rhinitis or sinusitis also may cause pharyngeal irritation and mild sore throat.

Excessive use of voice due to prolonged shouting or singing may cause sore throat.

Burn secondary to exposure of hot gases or liquid also may cause pharyngeal pain.

Psychogenic

Sometimes there does not seem to be an explanation for sore throat after history, physical exam, negative throat culture, and normal neck radiographs. In this case, psychosocial history is most valuable clinical tool.

MANAGENENT

Management is supportive and symptomatic as most are viral infections and self limiting.

Whenever in doubt, diagnosis should be confirmed by culture or rapid diagnostic methods. Specific causes of sore throat (like post nasal drip, voice abuse etc) when detected should be treated appropriately.

Bacterial (group A streptococcus) pharyngitis should be treated as has been known to be associated with acute rheumatic fever. Antibiotic options available are..

a. Oral Penicillin V for 10 days
b. Single dose of IM Benzathene penicillin
c. Oral erythromycin for 10 days in children allergic to penicillin
d. Amoxicillin for 10 days is also shown to be equally effective
e. Narrow spectrum cephalosporins for 10 days

A peritionsillar abscess should be aspirated by an ENT specialist. Aspiration of pus confirms the diagnosis and often gives the patient immediate symptomatic relief. Once drained, PTA is treated just like acute tonsillitis: antibiotics, hydration, and analgesics. Repeat aspirations are occasionally necessary. For patients who are allergic or have no response to penicillin, clindamycin provides excellent coverage.

A true retropharyngeal abscess requires incision and drainage, while cellulitis should be treated with antibiotics.

FURTHER READING

1. Worrall GJ. Acute sore throat. Can Fam Physician 2007;53:1961-2.
2. Del Mar CB, Glasziou PP, Spinks AB. Antibiotics for sore throat. Cochrane Database Syst Rev 2006;(4):CD000023.
3. Hayward G, Thompson M, Heneghan C, et al. Corticosteroids for pain relief in sore throat: systematic review and meta-analysis. BMJ. 2009 Aug 6;339:b2976. doi: 10.1136/bmj.b2976.
4. Altamimi S, Khalil A, Khalaiwi KA, et al. Short versus standard duration antibiotic therapy for acute streptococcal pharyngitis in children. Cochrane Database Syst Rev 2009;(1):CD004872.
5. Unuvar E, Yildiz I, Kilic A, et al. Is acetaminophen as effective as an antihistamine-decongestant-acetaminophen combination in relieving symptoms of acute nasopharyngitis in children? A randomised, controlled trial. Int J Pediatr Otorhinolaryngol 2007;71:1277-85.

Sunit Singhi

13 Chest Pain

Chest pain is a common pediatric complaint. It is perhaps the third leading pain syndrome in children. Chest pain has been reported to occur in 6/10000 children who visit an urban pediatric emergency department. It affects children of all ages and half of children with chest pain are less than 12 year old.

CAUSES

Among children presenting to emergency department up to 45% of children with chest pain are labeled" idiopathic". When a diagnosis can be found, **musculoskeletal injury** is the most common. Unlike adults children are far less likely to have a cardiac etiology for their pain. Most children with chest pain have a self-limited "benign" etiology. A list of common causes of chest pain is given in Table 1.

Table 1: Common Causes of Acute Chest Pain in Children

1. **Idiopathic:** most common; includes Texidor's twings
2. **Musculoskeletal:** chest wall muscle strain, costochondritis, slipping rib syndrome, Tietze's syndrome.
3. **Respiratory:** Violent cough, pneumothorax, asthma, pneumonia, pleuritis, pleurodynia
4. **Cardiac:** Arrhythmia (supraventricular tachycardia, ventricular tachycardia), infections (myocarditis, pericarditis), structural abnormalities (aortic stenosis, hypertrophic cardiomyopathy, anomalous coronary arteries), coronary artery disease (Kawasaki disease, familial hypercholestrolemia or lipidemia)
5. **Esophagel:** Gastroesophagel reflux, achlasia, hiatus hernia, foreign body.
6. **Dermal, neurogenic:** Herpes zoster, spinal nerve root compression.
7. **Vascular:** Vasoocclusive disease, Crises of sickle cell disease, Takayasu arteritis
8. **Abdominal causes (Rare):** Hepatitis, gall bladder diseases, peritonitis, hemoperitoneum, spleen rupture.

Young children are more likely to have chest pain related to a cardio-respiratory condition (cough, asthma, pneumonia, or heart disease). Children over the age of 12 years are more likely to have a psychogenic disturbance as the cause of their pain.

EVALUATION

It is important to ask the child to point to the location of the pain, since secondhand information from the parent may be misleading. The child may point to his epigastrium and call it his chest.

Significant points in the history should be: **Past history:** Has there been any prior surgery to the chest? Does the patient have asthma or sickle cell disease? **Family history:** Is there a family member who also has chest pain? Is there heart disease in the family? **Location:** Exactly where is the pain located? Can the child point to the area with one finger? **Character:** Exactly what does the pain feel like? Is it made worse by movement? Is it made worse by deep inspiration? **Time:** When does it occur? What does it keep the patient from doing?

Events preceding the pain, information on onset of pain, nature (sharp, cutting, dull), relationship with breathing, exercise, may help in establishing the origin of pain.

Examination of the heart and lungs is essential to look for any evidence of cardiovascular or pulmonary pathology. Chest wall inspection and palpation may yield clues to a musculoskeletal etiology. Signs of abuse must be looked for by the examiner. Examination of the abdomen may show that the pains referred to the chest are from intra-abdominal pathology.

Palpitation may be associated with mitral valve prolapse, paroxysmal supraventricular tachycardia, hyperventilation syndrome and anxiety (psychogenic chest pain).

Some children with chest pain may need further evaluation using X-ray, ECG and echocardiography (Table 2).

Table 2: Children with chest pain who need ECG and /or chest radiography

1. Presence of worrisome historical features such as acute onset of pain, pain associated with exercise, associated syncope, dizziness, palpitations, history of heart disease or a condition that can affect the heart or lungs, such as Kawasaki disease, Marfan's syndrome, asthma, anemia, sickle cell disease
2. Trauma
3. Foreign body ingestion
4. Fever
5. Those with an abnormal physical findings such as decreased or abnormal breath sounds, cardiac findings (murmur, rub, muffled heart sound, gallop, arrhythmia), subcutaneous emphysema.

DIFFERENTIAL DIAGNOSIS

Musculoskeletal pain

The onset is sudden or acute. Point pain is more frequent. It frequently occurs from strained chest wall muscles while carrying heavy books or exercising or from a direct blow to the chest that results in a mild contusion or in rarely a rib fracture.

Costochondritis accounts for about 10-20% of cases of chest pain. This musculoskeletal disorder usually involves 4th to 6th costocondral junction and produces, localized tenderness. The pain is exaggerated by physical activity or breathing. Musculoskeletal pain is often reproducible by palpation of the chest wall or moving the arms and chest through a variety of positions.

Texidor's twing or precordial catch "or" stitch in the side".

It is a syndrome of left-sided chest pain that is of less than 5 minute duration and sporadic. This pain may recur frequently in some and may remain absent for several months. The pain seems to be associated with a slouched posture or bending and is not related to exercise. It is usually relieved when the individual takes a few shallow breaths or sometimes one deep breath and assumes a straightened posture.

"Slipping Rib Syndrome"

This is a rare disorder caused by trauma to the costal cartilages of the 8th, 9th and 10th ribs. Pain is sudden in onset, and is located under the ribs or in the upper abdominal quadrants. A clicking or popping sound is felt when lifting objects, flexing the trunk or even while walking. The pain is caused by one of the ribs hooking under the rib above and irritating the intercostals nerves. It may last for hours and may be followed by residual tenderness. The syndrome is confirmed by performing the "hooking maneuver", whereby the affected rib margin is grasped and then pulled anteriorly. Surgery is the only definitive management.

Gastroesophageal Reflux

This is very common in children and accounts for at least 7% of pediatric chest pain. The pain is usually worse in the recumbent position. History may reveal that the pain is "burning" in quality and may have developed after eating spicy food. A trial of antacids is often diagnostic and therapeutic.

Psychogenic Pain

Emotional stress or anxiety is the cause in about 10% of children with chest pain who present to a pediatric emergency department. Possible stressors includes school failure, recent death or illness in the family, recent loss of friends from moving to a new city or school, and school phobia.

The family history may be positive for angina, and the child may imitate the pain as an attention-getting mechanism. The symptoms usually do not fit into any specific pattern. The pain maybe recurrent or paroxysmal: it may relieved by distraction. Sleep is not disbursed. Play periods are not interrupted.

Hyperventilation may be associated with psychogenic chest pain. Stomach distention due to concomitant aerophobia can occur with hyperventilation and produce chest pain. Light headedness, headache, and paresthesias may also be found. Psychogenic chest pain should not be a diagnosis of exclusion. If significant stress is temporally related to the pain it is a reasonable diagnosis.

Those with chronic pain (and none of the worrisome features) do not necessarily need laboratory studies.

Respiratory Causes

Children with sudden onset of pain (within 48 hours of presentation) are more likely to have an organic etiology for the pain. It is not necessarily a serious etiology but pneumonia, asthma, trauma, and pneumothrax are more likely.

Pneumothorax: A pneumothorax should be suspected if the pain is sharp, of acute onset (less than 48 hours duration) and is associated with some respiratory distress. The pain is usually worsened by inspiration and may radiate to the shoulder, neck or even the abdomen. The patient will usually have dyspnea, tachycardia and decreased breath sounds on the affected side and sometimes even cyanosis. These signs and symptoms are dependent on the size of the pneumothorax and whether it is under tension. A small pneumothorax may produce minimal findings on examination.

A history of trauma may be there but many cases occur spontaneously or with exercise or cough. Underlying conditions that increase the risk of "spontaneous" pneumothrorax include asthma, cystic fibrosis and Marfan's syndrome.

Isolated pneumonia is not a common cause of chest pain in children.

Fever is much more likely to be associated with pneumonia, myocarditis, or pericarditis. Lobar pneumonia due to an encapsulated organism is a particular concern (H influenzae, pneumococcus). The pain is exacerbated by deep breathing or cough. There may be asymmetric excursions. Pain referred to right lower quadrant is frequent with lower lobe pneumonia.

Pleurisy may occur alone or with pneumonia . The pain is sharp, well localized over involved area and accentuated by deep breathing and coughing. Localized tenderness may be noted.

Pulmonary embolism: Pulmonary embolism is rare in children. It is usually seen in children with hypercoagulable state, deep vein thrombosis, teenage boys with minor trauma to lower extremity and very rarely in teenage girls who on oral contraceptives. Usually the patient has accompanying shortness of breath, pleuritic chest pain, fever, cough and hemoptysis. A swollen tender lower extremity on physical examination increases concern about venous thrombosis and a pulmonary embolism.

Pneumomediastinum. Free mediastinal air and subcutaneous emphysema are complications of asthma exacerbation and cystic fibrosis. It may also occur spontaneously or as a result of trauma. Pain characteristically is of sharp and stabbing nature. Some children have associated dyspnea and cough. Crepitation is often noted in the suprasternal notch and may extend to the neck, axilla and face. A chest radiograph confirms the diagnosis. The condition is usually benign and resolves within a few days.

Pleurodynia: It is an unusual cause characterized by paroxysms of sharp pain in the abdomen or thorax. It is caused by coxsackie virus and may occur in mini-epidemics. There is fever, and cephalgia. Pain may last for 2-3 days and then recur. Respiratory movements exacerbate the pain. Other family members may be affected.

Cardiac Chest Pain

Pediatric chest pain is rarely due to cardiac pathology. Only a small fraction of children who present to a pediatric ED have a cardiac etiology. Some of them have known heart disease at the time of presentation. A possibility of **supraventricular tachycardia (SVT) or premature ventricular beats** should be considered in older children complaining of palpitation and chest pain.

Pericarditis: The location, intensity , and character of pain in pericarditis is extremely variable. In general, it is dull and poorly located. It may be referred to the neck or shoulders. The pain may be increased by respiratory excursion or swallowing. Pulse paradoxus (lowering of the pulse pressure during inspiration) may be present. There may be a finding of Ewart sign, consisting of dullness and bronchial breath sounds over the left lower lobe, secondary to obstruction of the left mainstem bronchus by pericardial fluid, resulting in collapse of the left lung.

Some children with pericarditis have a sharp stabbing midsternal pain that is somewhat relieved when the patient sits up and leans forward. Distant heart sounds, neck vein distention and a friction rub may be found.

Rheumatic and Viral myocarditis: usually present with low grade fever, tachycardia out of proportion to the degree of fever and muffled heart sounds or a gallop rhythm. Tachycardia and hypotension may be worse with standing. A chest radiograph often reveals cardiomegaly.

Aortic valve stenosis, hypertrophic, cardiomyophathy and coronary artery disease can cause pain, especially with exercise because of ischemia.

Mitral valve prolapse is an unusual cause of thest pain in children. It causes dull or sharp, intermittent left-sided chest pain and is often accompanied by syncope/near syncope, and premature ventricular beats. Children with Marfan's syndrome may complain of chest pain due to rupture of an aortic aneurysm, which can be fatal.

Hypertrophic cardiomyopathy is generally inherited as an autosomal dominant disorder. A murmur may be heard best when the child is standing. These positions and exercise may exaggerate the chest pain.

Squatting or lying supine minimizes the obstruction and reduces the murmur.

Young children with sudden death frequently had preceding chest pain with exercise. Patients with chest pain that is worsened by exertion should be referred to a cardiologist for further testing including ehocardiogram, monitoring or exercise stress tests.

Tietz's Syndrome

This is a rare condition of unknown etiology that causes sternal chest pain. Physical examination may reveal tender, spindle-shaped swelling at the sternochondral junctions. The condition can last for months.

Esophagus

Chest pain secondary to esophageal inflammation is usually substantial and exacerbated by swallowing. They may be associated with vomiting or hematemesis. Dysphagia may be present.

Foreign Body in the Esophagus: Many young children ingest coins and other foreign bodies. If the foreign body lodges in the esophagus (especially in the upper esophagus), the child may complain of sudden pain and dysphagia. A chest radiograph or a metal detector usually confirms the diagnosis.

Herpes Zoster Infection

It is often associated with distressing chest pain when the lesions involve a chest wall dermatome. The pain sometimes precedes the vesicular rash by several days.

In a teenage girl with systemic lupus erythematouus, chest pain may be caused by pericarditis, myocarditis, endocarditis, pneumonia, pleural effision, and myocardial ischemia if they have renal disease and hypertension.

Vaso-occlusive crises may be the cause of acute chest syndrome.

FURTHER READING

1. Rowland TW. Richards MM: The natural history of idiopathic chest pain in children. A follow-up study Clin Pediatr 1986:25:612-614.
2. Selbst SM: Chest pain in children-consultation with the specialist. Pediatr Review 1997: 18:169-173.
3. Selbst SM. Ruddy R. Clark BJ. *et al.* Pediatric chest pain- prospective study. Pediatr 1988: 82:319-323.
4. Wiens L. Sabath R. Ewing L. *et al.* Chest pain in otherwise healthy children and adolescents is frequently caused by exercise-induced asthma. Pediatr 1992:90:350-353.
5. Rowe BH et al. Characteristics of children presenting with chest pain to a pediatric emergency department. CMAJ 1990; 143: 388-94.
6. Kocis KC.Chest pain in Pediatrics, Pediatr Clin North Am 1999; 46: 189-203.
7. Evangelista JA, Parsoon M, Renneburq AK. Chest pain in children: diagnosis through history and physical examination . J Pediatr Health Care 2000; 14 :3-8.
8. Massin MM. *et al.* Chest pain in pediatric patients presenting to an emergency department or to a cardiac clinic. Clin Pediatr 2001; 43: 231-8.

Sunit Singhi

14 Shock

Shock is a systemic disorder producing a state of circulatory dysfunction that results in a failure to provide adequate supplies of oxygen and nutrients to meet the demands of the tissue beds. It is commonly perceived that shock is a state of low cardiac output heralded by the development of hypotension. It is becoming increasingly clear that such a view of shock is too simplistic. .Shock occurs as a consequence of a complex intermixture of cellular, biochemical" and neuroendocrine responses interacting with local and circulating vasoactive mediators, products of cellular breakdown and exogenous agents such as endotoxin, to produce the resulting physiological state. The clinical manifestations of shock in any particular individual are the result of a complex combination of these factors, the precipitating etiologic agent, the preexisting state of health, and the effects and timing of therapeutic actions.

PATHOPHYSIOLOGY

Oxygen Derived Variables

To understand shock, it is helpful to define several factors associated with oxygen transport and utilization (Table 1). Oxygen availability is a direct function of cardiac index (CI) and arterial oxygen content (CaOl), the sum of hemoglobinbound oxygen and dissolved oxygen in arterial blood. The volume of hemoglobinbound oxygen is the product of the hemoglobin concentration, oxygen saturation, and the binding coefficient of oxygen to hemoglobin (1.34). Dissolved oxygen is the product of arterial oxygen tension (PaOl) and the solubility coefficient of oxygen in plasma (0.003).

Oxygen uptake (VOl) is a direct function of CI and the difference in oxygen content between arterial and mixed-venous blood. Oxygen extraction (ER) is the ratio of VOl to oxygen availability. Normally VOl by the tissues is determined by metabolic demand and is not determined or limited by the oxygen availability. Should oxygen availability fall, in the face of constant metabolic demand, ER increases as needed to maintain constant VOl. At some point, termed *critical oxygen availability*, ER will become limited by and dependent on oxygen availability. At levels of oxygen availability below this point, an oxygen deficit exists, anaerobic metabolism and lactate production rise and metabolic acidosis occurs. Severe or extended periods of tissue oxygen deficit will

Table 1: Hemodynamic and Oxygenation values

Variable	*Formula*	*Normal Range*
Hemodynamic		
Cardiac output	$CO = HR \times SV$	
Cardiac index	$CI = CO/BSA$	3.5-5.5 $L/min/m^2$
Systemic vascular resistance index	$SVRI = \frac{79.9\ (MAP - CVP)}{CI}$	800-1600 DYNE $SEC/CM^5/M^2$
Pulmonary vascular resistance index	$PVRI = \frac{79.9\ (MPAP - PCWP)}{CI}$	80-240 DYNE $SEC/CM^5/M^2$
Oxygen transport		
Arterial oxygen content	$Cao_2 = (Hb)(1.34)(\%sta) + (PaO_2)(0.003)$	17 - 20 ml/dl
Mixed venous oxygen content	$Cvo_2 = (Hb)(1.34)(\%sta) + (PvO_2)(0.003)$	12 - 15 ml/dl
Oxygen content difference	$A\text{-}vDO_2 = CaO_2 - CvO_2$	3 -5 ml/dl
Oxygen availability	O_2 avail $= CaO_2 \times CI \times 10$	550 - 650 ml/min/m2
Oxygen uptake	$VO_2 = CI \times A\text{-}VDO_2 \times 10$	120 - 200 ml/min/m2
Oxygen extraction ration	$\frac{A\text{-}VDO_2}{CaO_2}$	0.15 - 0.29

HR=heart rate; BSA= body surface area; MAP= mean arterial blood pressure; MPAP= mean pulmonary arterial blood pressure; BCWP= pulmonary capillary wedge pressure, SV= Stroke volume

Reprinted with permission of the publisher from Katz RW, Pollack MM, Weibley RE pulmonary artery catheterization in pediatric intensive care. Adv Pediatr 1983;30:169-190

result in damage to cellular function and structure with eventual cell death.

In many forms of shock, such as massive hemorrhage or pericardial tamponade, impaired oxygen availability is caused by impaired cardiovascular performance with low cardiac output. Cardiac output is a function of heart rate and the volume ejected per beat (stroke volume). Abnormalities of heart rate or rhythm such as bradycardia, extreme tachycardia, or dysrhythmias can produce shock. Stroke volume can be reduced by insufficient ventricular filling (inadequate preload), reduced cardiac contractility, or impeded ventricular emptying (increased afterload). Figure 1 depicts the interrelationship of factors determining cardiac output and blood pressure.

In some circumstances, such as sepsis or trauma, shock may occur with normal or increased cardiac output. Under these circumstances, oxygen and nutrient delivery may be inadequate for several reasons including increased demands for oxygen or nutrients, maldistribution of circulation at the organ or tissue level and failure of uptake or utilization of oxygen or nutrients at the cellular level.

Stages of Shock

Shock is not a single entity but rather a syndrome' with progressive stages of

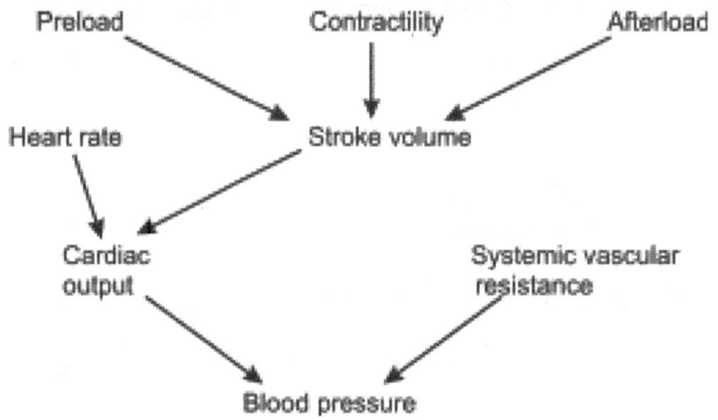

Fig. 1: Interrelationship of the factors determining cardiac output and blood pressure. (Reprinted with permission of the publisher from Perkin RM, Levin DL. Shock. In Levin DL, Norriss, eds. Essentials of pediatric intensive care. St. Louis. Quality Medical Publishers, 1990.)

severity: compensated, uncompensated, and irreversible. In compensated shock, intrinsic mechanisms restore and maintain vital organ function. This is achieved through a variety of neural, humoral, and cellular mechanisms. Compensatory mechanisms act to (1) preserve myocardial and cerebral blood flow at the expense of less vital organs such as skin, muscle, and splanchnic beds; (2) augment cardiac output through increased heart rate and contractility; and (3) restore circulating blood volume through vasocon-striction of capacitance vessels. Gross measures of cardiovascular homeostasis such as systemic arterial blood pressure, CI, heart rate, and peripheral perfusion may be normal or increased. Microcirculatory flow, how-ever, is reduced and maldistributed. The recognition of shock during the compensated phase with institution of effective treatment allows for the best prognosis for recovery. When shock is primarily caused by cardiac dysfunction, intrinsic responses intended to augment perfusion often further depress function (Figure 2). As such in shock of primary cardiac etiology, a compensated phase is rarely seen.

In uncompensated shock, compensatory mechanisms become exhausted and may contribute to further propagation of the shock state. The function of vital organs such as the heart, lungs, kidneys, and brain begins to fail. The hallmark of uncompensated shock is the vasodilation of various vascular beds allowing pooling of blood with ensuing coagulation, platelet aggregation, release of mediators of vascular tone, vascular and cellular permeability, and chemotaxis. Cellular function deteriorates in both local and remote tissue beds. Measures of cardiovascular homeostasis such as systemic arterial blood pressure, heart rate, cardiac output, peripheral perfusion, and urine output are clearly abnormal during uncompensated shock. Survival remains possible during uncompensated shock; but the course is usually prolonged and commonly complicated by single or multiple organ dysfunction. Invariably hospital costs, duration of hospitalization, morbidity, and mortality are increased in patients who progress to uncompensated shock.

Irreversible shock signifies damage to vital organ systems of such magnitude that, despite therapeutic interventions, death

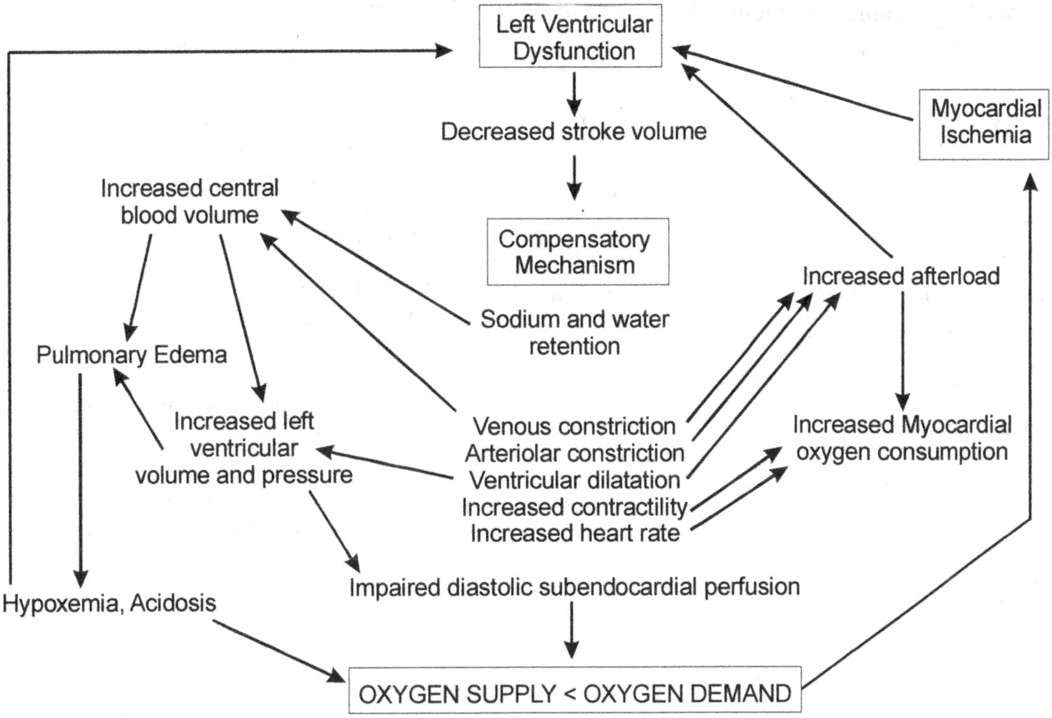

Fig. 2: Self-perpetuating pathways in cardiogenic shock. (Reprinted with permission of the publisher from perkin RM, Levin DL. Shock in the pediatric patient. K pediatrics 1982;101(6):16.6)

eventually occurs. Measures of cardiovascular homeostasis may be ameliorated by therapy but this improvement is transitory.

DIAGNOSIS AND DIFFERENTIAL DIAGNOSIS

Classifications of Shock

The prototypical classification system for shock was proposed by Hinshaw and Cox in 1972. Their system uses four subclasses of shock: (1) hypovolemic (due to insufficient circulating volume), (2) cardiogenic (due to pump failure), (3) distributive (due to a defect in distribution of blood flow), and (4) obstructive (due to extracardiac obstruction to blood flow). Although useful, this classification system overly simplifies the issues concerning some forms of shock. For example, septic shock is classified under distributive shock. As the mechanisms underlying septic shock are coming to be understood, however, septic shock would be better categorized as a mixed class with components of hypovolemic, cardiogenic, and distributive shock contributing to the overall pathology. In addition, since obstructive shock causes decreased cardiac performance, many authors consider it a subset of cardiogenic shock. Table 2 shows many of the etiologies producing each classification of shock.

Hypovolemic Shock

Hypovolemic shock is the most common cause of circulatory failure in pediatric patients. Major categories include losses of water and electrolytes such as with gastroenteritis or diabetes mellitus, hemorrhage as after trauma or surgery, and plasma losses as with burns or so-called *third spacing* as occurs after intraabdominal surgery (Table 3). Losses may be external as with hemorrhage from a laceration or thoracostomy tube or may be more occult as with hemorrhage into the soft tissues after a long bone or pelvic fracture.

Table 2: Classification of shock

I. Hypovolemic
   A. Hemorrhagic
      1. Gastrointestinal causes
         a. Meckel's diverticulum
         b. Esophageal varicies
      2. Trauma
      3. Internal bleeding
         a. Blunt trauma
         b. Long bone or pelvic fractures
         c. Retroperitoneal bleeding (any cause)
   B. Nonhemorrhagic
      1. Gastrointestinal losses
         a. Vomiting
         b. Diarrhea
      2. Renal losses
         a. Excessive diuretic effect
         b. Osmotic diuresis (diabetes mellitus)
         c. Diabetes insipidus
II. Cardiogenic
   A. Failure of contractile mechanism
      1. Myocardial contusion
      2. Cardiomyopathy
      3. Myocardial "stunning"
   B. Impedance to ventricular outflow
      1. Intrinsic
         a. Aortic stenosis
         b. Interrupted aortic arch
         c. Coarctation of the aorta
   C. Impedance to ventricular filling
      1. Intrinsic
         a. Mitral stenosis
         b. Atrial myxoma
         c. Atrial thrombus
      2. Extrinsic
         a. Pericardial tamponade b. Restrictive pericarditis
         c. Tension pneumothorax

Contd.

   D. Valve failure
      1. Acute mitral regurgitation 2. Acute aortic regurgitation
   E. Dysrhythmia
      1. Tachydysrythmias
      2. Bradydysrhythmias
   F. Myocardial rupture (trauma)
III. Distributive
   A. Sepsis
   B. Toxic shock
   C. Neurogenic
   D. Anaphylaxis
   E. Drug overdose
   F. Trauma without hypovolemia
   G. Hemorrhage shock and encephalopathy

Reprinted with permission of the publisher from Schuster DP, Lefrak 55. Shock in critical care. In Civetta JM, Taylor RW, and Kirby RR, eds. Critical care. Philadelphia: Lippincott, 1988;891.

Table 3: Causes of hypovolemic shock

Water and electrolyte loss	*Hemorrhage*
Diarrhea	Trauma
Vomiting	Surgery
Diabetes mellitus	Gastrointestinal bleeding
Diabetes insipidus	*Plasma losses*
Renal losses	Burns
Intestinal obstruction	Sepsis
Burns	
	Intestinal obstruction
	Peritonitis

The unifying mechanism of hypovolemic shock is a loss of circulating blood volume *(preload)* that results in reduced ventricular filling with a consequent fall in cardiac output. Compensatory mechanisms, mediated predominantly through the sympathetic nervous system, act to restore perfusion to vital organs by vasoconstriction of less vital tissue beds.

During the compensated phase of hypovolemic shock, patients characteristically demonstrate tachycardia, cutaneous vasoconstriction with pale or mottled skin and a prolonged capillary refill time, and diminished pulse pressure demonstrable as thready pulses. Systemic arterial blood pressure is maintained during the compensated phase by elevation of systemic vascular resistance. If appropriate and sufficient restitution of circulating volume is provided during the compensated phase of hypovolemic shock, recovery is usually complete.

If adequate volume replacement is not provided, progression to uncompensated shock will occur. Uncompensated hypovolemic shock is characterized by profound vasoconstriction with ischemia to key organ systems, intravascular stagnation and pooling, and eventual damage to key organs such as the heart and the brain, leading to irreversible shock. Patients in the uncompensated phase of hypovolemic shock may be obtunded or comatose, oliguric or an uric, and hypotensive.

Cardiogenic Shock

Cardiogenic shock is defined as hypoperfusion state in which the perfusion abnormality is due to primary cardiac dysfunction. Unlike adults, in whom coronary artery disease is common, primary cardiogenic shock is rare in children. All forms of shock as they progress into the uncompensated and irreversible stages, manifest cardiac dysfunction. Cardiogenic shock can be viewed as the final common pathway for all etiologies of shock.

Among the most common causes of primary cardiogenic shock in children is congenital heart disease. In several types of this disease, systemic blood flow depends on patency of the ductus arteriosus. These infants will present with cardiogenic shock on spontaneous ductal closure. Etiologies include hypoplastic left heart syndrome, critical aortic stenosis, interrupted aortic arch, and severe coarctation of the aorta. It may be difficult to distinguish these processes from the findings in shock due to neonatal sepsis. Another common cause of myocardial dysfunction associated with congenital heart disease is from myocardial injury during the postoperative period after repair of congenital heart lesions. Fortunately, the myocardium of the infant and child is surprisingly resistant to these insults and usually recovers except in especially severe or complex lesions.

Cardiogenic shock may occur as the consequence of a generalized hypoxicischemic insult. Etiologies include near-drowning, near-miss sudden infant death syndrome, and following cardiopulmonary arrest from other causes. Usually these patients also suffer severe brain injury because of hypoxia and ischemia. The myocardial effects can ordinarily be ameliorated, but death or severe disability in these patients is common because of their accompanying central nervous system (CNS) injury.

Other important etiologies of cardiogenic shock in children include dysryhythmias, drug intoxication, extrinsic inflow or outflow obstruction (tension pneumothorax or pneumopericardium, pericardial tamponade), metabolic disorders (hypoglycemia, cardiomyopathy), infectious disorders (constrictive pericarditis, myocarditis), and valvular disorders (regurgitant or obstructive).

Patients in cardiogenic shock rarely manifest a compensated phase in that compensatory mechanisms intended to support perfusion further impair cardiac output. These patients are as a rule tachycardic and hypotensive and have thready peripheral pulses and cold clammy skin. Further they may be mottled or cyanotic, have altered mentation, and are oliguric or anuric. Physical findings of hepatomegaly, jugular venous distension, and a gallop rhythm or findings such as cardiomegaly on chest radiograph, an increased central venous pressure or pulmonary artery wedge pressure may be helpful in differentiating cardiogenic shock from other varieties of shock.

Distributive Shock

Distributive shock results because of abnormal vascular tone producing a variable combination of venous pooling, physiologic shunting of vascular beds and increased vascular capacitance. Distributive shock, unlike other forms of shock, can occur in the face of normal or increased cardiac output. The various etiologies of distributive shock include anaphylaxis, neurogenic shock caused by cervical spinal trauma, drug overdose with an agent that causes vasodilation or vasomotor paralysis (barbiturates, antihypertensive agents, tricyclic antidepressants), and septic shock (Table 4). Septic shock, although historically included in the category of distributive shock, is more appropriately considered a mixed type of shock with components of hypovolemic, cardiogenic, and distributive shock. Patients with distributive shock are tachycardic and may have hypotension. They differ from patients with hypovolemic or cardiogenic shock in that during the early compensated phase they commonly have bounding pulses, wide pulse pressure, normal capillary refill time, warm distal extremities, and normal urine output. Findings also may include tachypnea, decreased systemic vascular resistance, low central venous pressure and pulmonary artery wedge pressure, and increased cardiac output. If not interrupted, later stages of septic shock are clinically similar to those in advanced hypovolemic or cardiogenic shock.

Patients with septic shock may be febrile or, especially in infants, hypothermic. They may have a leukocytosis with a preponderance of immature neutrophils or in severe cases may present with neutropenia. Hyperglycemia is common, and may occur, especially in young infants. In adults, septic shock is most commonly caused by gram-negative enteric bacteria. The offending organisms in children are more diverse and include both gram-positive and gram-negative bacteria, viruses, rickettsia, and protozoa (Table 5).

Table 4: Causes of distributive shock

Anaphylaxis	*Septic shock*
Antibiotics	Early phase
Vaccines	*Drugs*
Blood	Barbiturates
Local anesthetics	Phenothiazines
Iodine contrast media	Tranquilizers
Insects	Antihypertensives
Foods	
Neurologic Injury	
Head injury	
Spinal shock	

Table 5: Common pathogens causing septic shock

Neonates	*Children*
Group B β-hemolytic streptococci	S. pneumoniae
Enterobacteriaceae	Neisseria meningitidis
Listeria monocytogenes	S. aureus
Staphylococcus aureus	
	Immunocompromised
Infants	Enterbacteriaceae
H. influenzae	S. aureus
Peisseria meningitides	
Streptococcus pneumoniae	Psuedomonadaceae
S. aureus	Candida albicans

CLINICAL PRESENTATION

Effects of Shock on Organ Systems

Independent of etiology, shock is a process that affects all organ systems. The degree to which any particular organ system is affected will be a function of etiology, severity, and stage of shock.

Heart

Disturbed cardiac function may be the primary etiologic agent in shock as in children with congenital heart disease or cardiomyopathy. Under other circumstances, heart function may become disordered as a secondary manifestation of shock provoked by other mechanisms such as with trauma or sepsis. Secondary cardiac dysfunction can be broken down by the determinants of cardiac output noted earlier, specifically heart rate and rhythm, preload, contractility, and afterload.

Heart rate and stroke volume determine cardiac output. Young infants, especially neonates, have reduced amounts of myocardial contractile tissue and have very limited ability to increase cardiac output by increasing contractility. Therefore they are highly dependent on increased heart rate to improve cardiac output. As such, tachycardia is virtually always a manifestation of shock and represents a compensatory response. Excessive tachycardia, as may occur with extreme hypovolemia, hyperpyrexia, and high levels of either endogenous or administered catecholamines, is detrimental by reducing both diastolic ventricular filling time and coronary perfusion.

On occasion, especially in young infants subjected to hypoxic-ischemic injury to the myocardium or profound acidosis, *bradycardia* develops that dramatically embarrasses cardiac output. Atrial tachydysrhythmias can occur following myocardial injury or as a complication of pharmacological therapy (catecholamines, atropine). Ventricular tachydysrhythmias are rare but may occur in the face of severe disturbances of potassium or calcium concentrations, marked acid-base disturbance, hypoxicischemic injury, or direct myocardial traumatic injury, or drug overdose or from irritation caused by indwelling vascular catheters.

Preload is defined by the ventricular end-diastolic volume but can be estimated by the ventricular end-diastolic pressure. For the right ventricle, preload is estimated by the right ventricular diastolic pressure, right atrial pressure, or central venous pressure in decreasing order of accuracy. For the left ventricle, preload may be estimated by the left ventricular diastolic pressure or the left atrial pressure. In the absence of pathological intracardiac shunts or significant valvular pathology, the left ventricular preload may be estimated by the pulmonary artery wedge pressure, the pulmonary artery diastolic pressure, the right ventricular diastolic pressure, the right atrial pressure, or the central venous pressure in decreasing order of accuracy.

Preload is disturbed in all forms of shock. In hypovolemic shock, the primary disorder is a loss of intravascular volume with reduction in preload. In septic shock, anaphylaxis, or intoxication with a substance with vasodilatory properties, preload is reduced because vasodilation produces an expanded vascular space causing a relative hypovolemia. In primary cardiogenic shock, preload is commonly excessive due to the detrimental effects of renal compensatory efforts to augment cardiac output through reduced fluid excretion.

Diminished *myocardial contractility* causes shock with or without the presence of abnormalities of preload, afterload, or heart rate and rhythm. Decreased contractility may occur as a result of direct injury to the myocardium as in cardiomyopathy or myocarditis. Intracardiac surgery, such as for repair of congenital heart disease, especially procedures in which the ventricular muscle is incised, can result in decreased contractility. It may be diminished because of systemic consequences of shock that adversely affect myocardial performance including hypoxemia, lactic acidosis, myocardial ischemia, electrolyte abnormalities, and hypoglycemia and by the effects of endogenous circulating myocardial depressant agents (that is, myocardial depressant factor).

Afterload is the resistance against which the ventricle must eject its contents during systole. Systemic vascular resistance approximates afterload for the left ventricle as does pulmonary vascular resistance for the right ventricle (see Table 1). A few disease processes produce shock predominantly as a result of increased afterload. These include severe aortic stenosis and interrupted aortic arch anomalies that increase afterload of the left ventricle and pulmonary embolism, a rare cause of increased afterload of the right ventricle in children. Afterload is increased in all forms of shock except early phases of distributive and septic shock. This is especially true in primary cardiogenic shock as occurs with myocarditis and dilated cardiomyopathy.

Brain

Circulation to the CNS is protected during the compensated phase of shock.

Despite this, significant clinical abnormalities are common, ranging from agitation to stupor or coma. The mechanisms involved may include disturbed micro-circulatory flow, electrolyte and glucose abnormalities, and the release of both local and circulating factors with neurotransmitter properties. During uncompensated shock, cerebral blood flow may fall resulting in ischemic CNS damage. Ischemic brain injury may play a role in the development of irreversible shock.

Pulmonary

Early pulmonary manifestations of shock are tachypnea with hypocarbia and primary respiratory alkalosis. Later in the course of shock, tachypnea and hypocarbia persist as a compensatory response to metabolic acidosis from lactic acid accumulation. Eventually respiratory failure may occur primarily due to respiratory muscle fatigue consequent to inadequate supplies of oxygen and substrate to meet demands. Ventilatory demands may be increased due to altered pulmonary compliance secondary to interstitial and alveolar fluid accumulation. Fluid accumulation occurs because of capillary leak that commonly accompanies septic shock or from increased capillary hydrostatic pressure in left ventricular cardiogenic shock. Capillary leak and pulmonary hypertension are characteristics of the adult respiratory distress syndrome (ARDS), a potential complication of shock from any etiology but especially common following septic shock. Abnormalities of oxygen uptake within the lung are usually a consequence of intrapulmonary shunting caused by the development of pulmonary edema.

Kidneys

Through the renin-angiotensin system, the kidneys play a major role in the compensatory mechanisms of shock. The kidneys are also commonly damaged during shock. One of the most frequent causes of acute renal failure is hypoperfusion caused by shock states. Total renal blood flow is reduced during later stages of shock as the renal arteries are constricted, diverting blood flow to more vital organs such as the heart and brain. Oliguria is therefore caused by a combination of net decreased renal blood flow and increased tubular reabsorption.

Gastrointestinal Tract

Reduction of blood flow to the gastrointestinal (GI) tract is a major compensatory mechanism supporting systemic arterial blood pressure in shock. Several neural and humoral mechanisms are employed that result in vasoconstriction of the splanchnic vasculature. As a result, adverse conse-quences may result, including erosive gastritis, ischemic pancreatitis, and, perhaps most significantly, loss of the normal bacterial barrier function of the GI wall.

As a result of ischemia, GI bacterial flora and their products may translocate across the GI epithelium and into the portal circulation. These bacteria and bacterial products, particularly endotoxin, may be instrumental in the perpetuation of the shock state.

Liver

The liver is subject to ischemic injury during periods of reduced blood flow characteristic of shock. Ischemic hepatitis is typically marked by transient elevations in liver enzymes, particularly the serum transaminases, and moderate elevations in bilirubin.

Hematologic

Hemorrhagic shock with whole blood loss and subsequent mobilization of interstitial water results in decreases in hemoglobin and hematocrit proportional to losses. Shock from losses of body water or plasma, may result in variable degrees of hemoconcentration.

Coagulation

All forms of shock may include coagulation abnormalities. These abnormali-ties may take the form of mild elevations in prothrombin time (PT) and partial thromboplastin time (PTT) caused by hemodilution in hemorrhagic shock. Severe disseminated intravascular coagulation (DIC) with marked elevation in PT and PTT, thrombocytopenia, hypofibrinogenemia, and elevated circulating fibrin degradation products frequently accompany septic shock.

MANAGEMENT OF SHOCK

General Principles

It is important to emphasize that, since shock is progressive, management of the patient must be an ongoing process of evaluation, appropriate therapy, and reassessment of response to therapy. Repeated physical examinations concentrating on assessment of heart rate, blood pressure, peripheral perfusion (color and capillary refill time), respiratory pattern and effort, level of consciousness, and physical activity, as well as urine output, are the cornerstones in monitoring patients with shock. Many patients, especially those with hypovolemic shock from fluid and electrolyte losses, respond to initial therapy, obviating the need for more extensive monitoring techniques. Other patients, with later stages of shock or shock of other etiologies, will require more extensive monitoring techniques such as strict measurement of intake and output, arterial blood-gas measurement, monitoring of electrolytes and glucose, assessment of blood counts and coagulation profiles, continuous electrocardiographic monitoring, intraarterial pressure monitoring, and central venous pressure monitoring.

For all forms of shock, simultaneous with or soon after initial stabilization, treatment of the underlying cause of shock must be initiated. Hemorrhage, internal or external, must be stopped with surgery performed if necessary. Septic shock will require broad spectrum antimicrobial therapy guided by the clinical presentation and the age of the patient (see Table 5) and may require drainage of a septic focus. Cardiogenic shock from congenital heart disease may require treatment with prostaglandin E_1 to open the ductus arteriosus pending surgical correction.

Therapeutic goals (clinical endpoints) in management of septic shock are shown in Table 6. All these goals should be approached simultaneously in a timely manner.

Table 6: Therapeutic end points in the management of shock

- Normal pulses.
- Capillary refill time < 2sec
- Warm extremities.
- Normal mental status.
- Normal blood pressure.
- Urine output > 1ml/kg/hr
- Decreased serum lactate
- Reduced base deficit
- SvO2 > 70%

Cardiovascular Support

Support of the circulation is paramount in the treatment of shock. Central to shock therapy is the assurance of adequate flow of blood and delivery of oxygen to vital vascular beds such as the coronary, cerebral, and renal circulations. The cardiac output is dependent on heart rate, rhythm, and stroke volume; the latter is dependent on preload, contractility, and afterload. Therefore specific monitoring and therapy is presented for each of these factors.

Heart Rate and Rhythm

Patients with shock should have an initial assessment of heart rate and rhythm.

All patients require repeated assessment of heart rate and most should have continuous electrocardiographic monitoring.

The most common finding will be sinus tachycardia. Marked tachycardia will embarrass cardiac output by restricting ventricular filling but usually will respond to fluid administration. Preload therapy is discussed in the next section. Occasionally patients will present with dysrrhythmias that limit cardiac output. Therapy of dysrhythmias should include evaluation and treatment for hypoxemia; acid base abnormalities; electrolyte disturbances, especially hypocalcemia, hyperkalemia, or hypokalemia; and hypoglycemia. Patients with an indwelling central venous catheter should have a chest radiograph done to check the position of the catheter tip. Occasionally, catheters become malpositioned with the tip lying in the right ventricle producing rhythm disturbances. Treatment may require drugs that modulate cardiac rhythm such as atropine or isoproterenol for bradycardia; adenosine for supraventricular tachycardia, and lidocaine or amiodarone for ventricular tachydysrhythmias. On occasion, cardioversion or temporary pacemaker placement may be needed to achieve and maintain a stable perfusing rhythm.

Preload

Most forms of shock, with the exception of some types of cardiogenic shock, involve either an absolute or a relative hypovolemia that requires rapid therapy with intravascular volume expansion. Fluid administration should take the form of a rapid bolus of 10 to 20 ml/kg of fluid over 5-20 minutes, followed by an evaluation of response. Further therapy should be guided by response and ongoing losses. In patients requiring fluid therapy in excess of 60 to 80 ml/kg, CVP monitoring may be useful in evaluating the need for further fluid therapy. CVP should be interpreted in light of serial clinical assessment, as it is likely to be influenced by heart rate and intrathoracic pressure. A low CVP <10 cm H2O suggests need for further fluids.

The best choice of fluid for replacement in shock has been an area of ongoing debate in both the pediatric and critical care literature. A reasonable approach to fluid therapy is to use crystalloid in the form of 0.9 normal saline or lactated Ringer's solution for the first 40 to 80 ml/kg of replacement. If additional fluid resuscitation is required, consideration should be given to the type of fluid lost. If the cause of shock is hemorrhage, a transfusion of packed red blood cells may be necessary. With external losses of fluid and electrolytes, continued administration of crystalloid would be proper. If losses are of plasma, as in third spacing associated with septic shock, the use of colloid solutions such as five percent albumin, plasma protein fraction or hydroxyethyl starch (Hetastarch) may be suitable. There is no justification for the use of whole blood, plasma, cryo-precipitate or other transfusion subfrac-tions such as platelets for the purpose of fluid resuscitation. The use of these blood components should be reserved for patients requiring correction of specific coagulation abnormalities.

End points for fluid resuscitation should be based on clinical response. The criteria for satisfactory volume resuscitation include a reduction in heart rate toward normal for age; improved cutaneous perfusion as measured by skin color, skin turgor, and capillary refill time of two seconds or less; improved renal perfusion as gauged by a urine output in excess of one ml!kg per hour, stable blood pressure appropriate for age, and normal mentation. In patients with ongoing internal or external losses or in whom cardiac function is not stable, repeated assessments will remain mandatory to assure that appropriate preload is sustained.

In patients with septic shock, cardiogenic shock, adult respiratory distress syndrome, or multiple organ system dysfunction, preload augmentation must be administered cautiously and should be guided by invasive monitoring. If cardiac filling pressures rise without either direct or indirect evidence of improved cardiac output, further volume administration will probably be detrimental, resulting in worse cardiac function and increased peripheral and pulmonary edema formation. Under these circumstances, augmentation of cardiac contractility using pharmacologic means is required.

Caution should be exercised in fluid resuscitation of patients with shock and concurrent CNS injury who are at risk for cerebral edema formation. Vigorous fluid therapy may correct shock only to have the patient succumb to cerebral herniation from increased intracranial pressure. In these patients, early inotropic support may be warranted to reduce total fluid requirements.

Contractility

The use of agents to augment contractility is necessary when volume resuscitation has been optimized and cardiovascular function remains inadequate. The choices for agents to improve contractility are shown in Table 7. The proper choice of agent depends on the clinical circumstance.

Patients with hypovolemic shock rarely require inotropic support. Patients with cardiogenic shock benefit from agents that improve contractility but do not increase systemic vascular resistance *(vasopressor effect)*. Agents such as *dobutamine,* an analog of isoproterenol with potent inotropic effects, may be ideal for such patients. *Milrinone,* a noncatecholamine agent whose mechanism of action involves inhibition of phospho-diesterase type III, is a moderately potent inotropic agent with some vasodilatory effects. Milrinone may be helpful in patients with cardiogenic shock who have increased systemic vascular resistance. Patients with cardiogenic shock who fail to respond to these agents may require the use of more potent agents such as epinephrine or norepinephrine. Although these drugs may be effective, they exact a heavy toll on the heart in the form of increased myocardial work and oxygen consumption. They also act

Table 7: Inotropic agents and vasodilators

Drug	*Dose (μg/kg/min)*	*Predominant site of action*	*Comment*
Dopamine	0.5-5	Dopaminergic	Vasodilator to renal and cerebral beds
	5-10	β1	Inotropic dose
	>10	α1	Pressor dose
Dobutamine	5-20	β1, β2, dopaminergic	Inotrope, weak chronotrope, mild Vasodilator
Norepinephrine	0.05-1	α1, β1	Strong vasoconstrictor and inotrope; May cause splanchnic ischemia.
Epinephrine	0.03-0.1	β	Inotrope
	0.1-0.2	α1, β1, β2	Inotrope and pressor effect
	> 0.2	α	Vasoconstictor, arrhythmogenic
Dopexamine	0.5-6	β2, dopaminergic	Inotrope, vasodilator, improves splanchnic blood flow.
Phenylephrine	0.2-1	α1	Vasoconstrictor
Milrinone	0.75-1		Loading dose 50-75 mcg/kg iv; shorter t ½ and less effect on platelets as compared to amrinone.
Calcium chloride	10-20 mg/kg		Inotropy
Nitroglycerine	0.75-1		Venodilator
Nitroprusside	10-20 mg/kg		Vasodilator (A>V).

to increase afterload through vasoconstriction. This effect further increases myocardial oxygen demand and may offset any improvement in contractility. Patients in cardiogenic shock with markedly increased afterload and those with atrioventricular valve regurgitation often benefit from the use of a combination of an inotropic agent with a systemic vasodilator *(afterload reducing agent).*

The choice of vasoactive drug used in patients with septic shock would depend on patient's condition after adequate volume resuscitation. Some of pediatric patients have high cardiac output, vasodilation and hypotension manifesting as tachycardia, flush CFT, low to low normal blood pressure and wide pulse pressure. *Dopamine* is generally accepted as firest line vasopressor in this setting. It increases MAP through an increase in cardiac output and peripheral resistance.

Children with septic shock more often have myocardial dysfunction with compensatory vasoconstriction. This leads to a state of low cardiac output with high cardiac filling pressures and high systemic vascular resistance manifesting as tachycardia, prolonged CFT, cold extremities and low to low normal blood pressure and narrow pulse pressure. *Dobutamine* is the agent of choice in this setting. However, dobutamine alone may be inadequate in a hypotensive patient. Therefore, it is usually combined with dopamine or norepinephrine.

When a child in septic shock doesn't improve and the goals of treatment are not achieved even after dopamine and/or dobutamine infusion, the shock is labeled as *fluid refractory, dopamine/dobutamine resistant shock.* At this stage, children with shock can further be classified into 2 broad categories : warm shock and cold shock.

Children in cold shock may have low blood pressure. In these children, *epinephrine* should be titrated to achieve normal MAP for age. Once this is achieved but the child continues to have elevated systemic vascular resistance and low cardiac output, *nitrosovasodilators* are warranted. *Milrinone* should be strongly considered if low cardiac output and high vascular resistance state persists inspite of epinephrine and nitrosovasodilators.

Children with cold shock may also have normal blood pressure. In these children, *milrinone* would be the drug of choice if pulse pressure is low. However, if the pulse pressure is normal or high, *norepinephrine and dobutamine* should be titrated up.

Norepinephrine is the vasoactive agent of choice for the child with warm shock with poor perfusion or hypotension. It has potent á adrenergic vasoconstricting effects with little effect on heart rate or cardiac output. An infusion of *vasopressin* (0.3 to 2 milliunits/kg/min) may be useful in the setting of norepinephrine refractory shock. Vasopressin antagonizes the mechanisms of sepsis mediated vasodilation and acts synergistically with endogenous/exogenous catecholamines in stabilizing blood pressure.

Afterload

Patients with cardiogenic shock who manifest increased systemic vascular resistance or atrioventricular valve regurgitation, may benefit from the use of a systemic vasodilator. Caution must be taken when using vasodilators, especially in patients with low or normal blood pressure. Invasive cardiovascular monitoring, preferably using a Swan-Ganz catheter, is strongly advisable when the use of a vasodilator is contemplated.

The most commonly used drug is sodium nitroprusside. It has the benefit of a rapid onset of action and a short half-life, which facilitates titration. Sodium nitroprusside is a balanced vasodilator affecting arteriolar and venous capacitance vessels roughly equally. It should usually be used in combination with an inotropic agent such as dobutamine, dopamine, epinephrine, or norepinephrine. Nitroglycerine is a vasodilator whose effects are mostly on the venous capacitance vessels with less significant arteriolar effect. Nitroglycerine has the benefit of transcutaneous administration in more stable patients with congestive failure. As was noted earlier, amrinone afterloadreducing effects and may be helpful in the management of this patient subset.

Pulmonary

Virtually all patients with shock should receive oxygen supplementation. The adequacy of oxygen administration should be assessed using continuous pulse oximetry, arterial blood gases or both. Most patients with shock require endotracheal intubation and mechanical ventilation. Assisted ventilation is indicated in patients requiring an inspired oxygen concentration over 60 percent to achieve a Pa02 of 60 mmHg or an oxygen saturation of 90 percent and in those demonstrating evidence of respiratory failure. Indications of respiratory failure include marked tachypnea, dyspnea, apnea, or a Pac02 of 50 mmHg or greater. Patients with high oxygen requirements, rales on auscultation of the chest, and evidence of pulmonary edema on chest radiograph should receive increased positive end expiratory pressure (PEEP). Patients on mechanical ventilatory support usually will benefit from sedation using an infusion of a narcotic such as fentanyl (1 to 4 fLg/kg/hr) or a benzodiazepine such as midazolam (3 to 5 fLg/kg/min). Care must be exercised in giving sedatives and analgesics to hypotensive patients in that these drugs have vasodilatory effects. Some patients, especially those with ARDS, will require the use of neuromuscular paralysis with agents such as vecuronium or pancuronium.

Renal Support

Patients with shock should have a bladder drainage catheter (Foley catheter) placed for continuous monitoring of urine output. Blood urea nitrogen (BUN) and creatinine should be measured initially. Measurement should be repeated regularly for as long as shock or renal failure exist. Aggressive fluid replacement is necessary to support urine output. Patients with oliguria or anuria, especially those with evidence of low cardiac output, may benefit from administration of a loop diuretic such as furosemide (1 to 2 mg/kg/dose). Patients who develop acute renal failure may require dialysis (hemodialysis or peritoneal) or continuous arteriovenous hemofiltration (CA VH) to avoid fluid overload and to permit parenteral nutritional support.

Gastrointestinal Support

Patients with shock should have a nasogastric tube placed and applied at low intermittent suction. Measures should be taken to reduce the risk for gastrointestinal bleeding. Choices include the use of histamine blocking agents such as cimetidine or ranitidine or antacids administered through the nasogastric tube that act to prevent the production of gastric acid or to neutralize gastric acid respectively. There is evidence that the best method for reducing the risk of bleeding may be the use of sucralfate, a sulfated disaccharide-aluminum complex, that acts to protect the gastric mucosa from the effects of gastric acidity rather than by eliminating acid. This may be superior to the other methods because an acid milieu helps prevent growth of bacteria in the proximal bowel, the presence of which may promote bacterial translocation.

Hematologic Support

Shock patients should have a complete blood count (CBC) measured initially followed by repeated measurements until they are physiologically stable. Patients with hemorrhage and those receiving large amounts of asanguinous fluids should have CBCs measured more frequently. Ideally, to optimize oxygen availability, hemoglobin concentrations should be maintained at levels of 10 to 13 gm/dl. Concern about transmission of hepatitis or other viral agents may justify accepting lower hemoglobin concentrations in stable patients.

Recombinant human Activated Protein C (rhAPC) is recommended in adult patients at high risk of death such as those in setic shock, sepsis with MODS and sepsis induced ARDS. However, current data does not support its use in pediatric septic shock.

Coagulation Support

A coagulation profile, including a PT, a PTT, and a platelet count should be obtained initially on all patients with shock. If these are abnormal, the fibrinogen and fibrin degradation product concentrations should be measured, and the coagulation profile should be repeated at regular intervals until it is normal. Patients with isolated elevations of PT and PTT but with no evidence of bleeding may require no specific treatment. Patients who have active bleeding should receive fresh frozen plasma to replace clotting factors and vitamin K (1 mg/kg IV [intravenous]) to promote hepatic production of vitamin K-dependent clotting factors. Patients who have isolated thrombocytopenia should receive platelet transfusions if they are actively bleeding or if the platelet count falls below 10,000 per mm3. Disseminated intravascular coagulation, as may occur particularly in septic shock, may require repeated administration of fresh frozen plasma, platelets and cryoprecipitate until the underlying cause is eliminated.

Metabolic

A significant secondary complication of shock is development of metabolic acidosis. This impairs metabolic processes, impedes normal neurovascular interactions and interferes with action of vasoactive drugs administered to the patient. Correction is indicated when marked metabolic acidosis exists (arterial blood pH <7.15). Bicarbonate should be used only to partially correct the pH to levels which do not pose a serious immediate threat to life.

Pediatric sepsis patients frequently have hypoglycemia and hypocalcemia as their unique response to sepsis/septic shock. Hypoglycemia should be identified rapidly and corrected immediately as it is associated with negative inotropic effect and neurologic damage. A regular monitoring protocol should be followed and hyperglycemia should be avoided. Ionized hypocalcemia is common in children with sepsis admitted to PICU and may contribute to cardiac dysfunction. It should be corrected before cardiac output and perfusion pressure are restored with vasoactive drugs.

Serum sodium levels should be monitored and maintained within the normal range.

Nutritional Support

Excessive catabolism is the most common nutritional abnormality in shock states. Nutritional support should be started as soon as possible. Enteral nutrition is more physiologic and preferred.

Corticosteroid Therapy

Fluid refractory and dopamine or norepinephrine dependent septic shock defines the patient at risk for adrenal insufficiency. A random cortisol level of < 18 mcg/dL and rise in cortisol of < 9 mcg/dL following ACTH stimulation test indicates adrenal insufficiency. Children who have clear risk factors for adrenal insufficiency (patients on prolonged steroid therapy, with pituitary/adrenal abnormalities, with septic shock with purpura) should be treated with stress dose steroids (50mg/m2/d).

Intravenous Immunoglobulins

IVIg may be considered in children with severe sepsis, It acts by neutralizing endotoxins and attenuating the inflammatory cascade. However, large clinical trials do not recommend routine use of IVIg in patients with severe sepsis or septic shock.

Anti-inflammatory/Immunotherapy

Convincing evidence that septic shock and its morbid consequences are a direct result of endogenous protein and phospholipid mediators secreted by the host, has prompted the use of many anti-inflammatory and experimental immunomodulatory therapies (eg. Ibuprofen, pentoxyphylline, endotoxin antibodies, TNF antibodies, etc.). However, these efforts have not met with clinical success so far.

Extracorporeal Membrane Oxygenation

It may be used if other therapies have not worked. Limited success has been reported with this technique in patients with refractory shock or cardiac arrest.

FURTHER READING

1. Dellinger RP, Mitchell ML, Carlet JM, et.al. Surviving sepsis campaign : International guidelines for management of severe sepsis and septic shock. Crit Care Med 2008;36.
2. Zaritsky AL, Schexnayder SM, Berg RA, et.al. Pediatric Advanced Life support Provider Manual.Dallas : American Heart Association, 2006.

3. Rivers E, Nguyen B, Havstad S, et.al. Early goal directed therapy in the treatment of severe sepsis and septic shock. N Engl J Med 2001;345:1368-77.
4. Goldstein B, Giroir B, Randolph A, et.al. International consensus Conference on Pediatric sepsis : Definitions for sepsis and organ dysfunction in pediatrics. Pediatr Crit Care Med 2005;6:2-8.
5. Vallet B, Tavernier B, Lund N, et.al. Asssessment of tissue oxygenation in the critically ill. Eur J Anaesthesiol 2000;17:221-9.
6. Hatherill M, Waggie Z, Purves L, et.al. Mortality and the nature of metabolic acidosis in children with shock. Intensive Care Med 2003;29:286-91.
7. Carcillo JA, Davis AL, Zaritsky A, et.al. Role of early fluid resuscitation in pediatric septic shock. JAMA 1991;117:515-522.
8. De Bruin WJ, Greenwald BM, Notterman DA, et al. Fluid resuscitation in pediatrics. Crit Care Clin 1992;8:341-353.
9. Griffel MI, Kaufman BS. Pharmacology of colloids and crystalloids. Crit Care Clin 1992;8:235-253.
10. Finfer S, Bellomo R, Boyce N, et.al. A comparison of albumin and saline for fluid resuscitation in the intensive care unit. N Engl J Med 2004; 350:2247-56.
11. Ceneviva JA, Paschall JA, Maffei F, et.al. Hemodynamic support in fluid refractory pediatric septic shock. Pediatrics 1998;102:e19.
12. Pizarro CF, Troster EJ, Damiani D, et.al. Absolute and relative adrenal insufficiency in children with septic shock. Crit Care Med 2005;33:855-859.
13. Holmes CL, Wailey KR, Chittock DR, et.al. The effects of vasopressin on hemodynamics and renal function in severe septic shock: a case series. Intensive Care Med 2001;27:1416-1421.
14. Matok I, Vard A, Efrati O, et.al. Terlipressin as rescue therapy for intractable hypotension due to septic shock in children. Shock 2005;23:305-310.
15. Beale RJ, Hollenberg SM, Vincent JL, et.al. Vasopressor and inotropic support in septic shock : An evidence based review. Crit Care Med 2004;32:S445-S465.
16. Carcillo JA. Pediatric septic shock and multiple organ failure. Crit Care Clin 2003;19:413-440.
17. Carlotti AP, Troster EJ, Fernandes JC, et.al. A critical appraisal of the guidelines for the management of pediatric and neonatal patients with septic shock. Crit Care Med 2005;33:1182.
18. Sparrow A, Hedderley T, Nadel S, et.al. Choice of fluid for resuscitation of septic shock. Emerg Med J 2002;19:114-116.
19. Yunge M, Petros A. Angiotensin for septic shock unresponsive to noradrenaline. Arch Dis Child 2000;82:388-389.
20. Singhi S, Khilnami P, Lodha R et. al. Guidelines for treatment of septic shock in resource limited enviornment. J Pediatr Infect Diz 2009; 4:172-92.
21. Singhi S, Argent AC, Barannral AK et al. Septic shock: management in emergency department with available resournces. J Pediatr Infect Diz 2009; 4:85-98.

In the previous edition this chapter was written by Morris Gessouroun, MD Associate Professor, Pediatrics, Director—Pediatric Intensive Care Unit University of Oklahoma Health Sciences Center Oklahoma City, Oklahoma

Jagannath S. Surpure

15 Dysrhythmias

Cardiac dysrrhythmias are uncommon in children because of low incidence of ischemic heart disease. Almost every type of dysrrhythmia recognized in adults, however, has been reported in the pediatric age group. There have been major advances in diagnosis and management. Rhythm disturbance constitutes an acute emergency if it compromises heart rate, and it has the potential for degenerating into a lethal rhythm. The most important component is the adverse influence on the cardiac output. Cardiac output is the product of stroke volume and heart rate. The fast rates compromise adequate diastolic filling/stroke volume and thus reduce cardiac output. The abnormally slow rates also cause inadequate cardiac output. The other conditions, such as asystole, ventricular fibrillation, and electromechanical (EMD) dissociation have no cardiac output. There is no measurable heart rate, therefore no stroke volume and cardiac output. Pediatric cardiac arrest or asystole is usually the end result of longstanding hypoxemia and acidosis secondary to respiratory compromise. Primary cardiac arrest is infrequent and is more often a result than it is a cause (Figure 1).

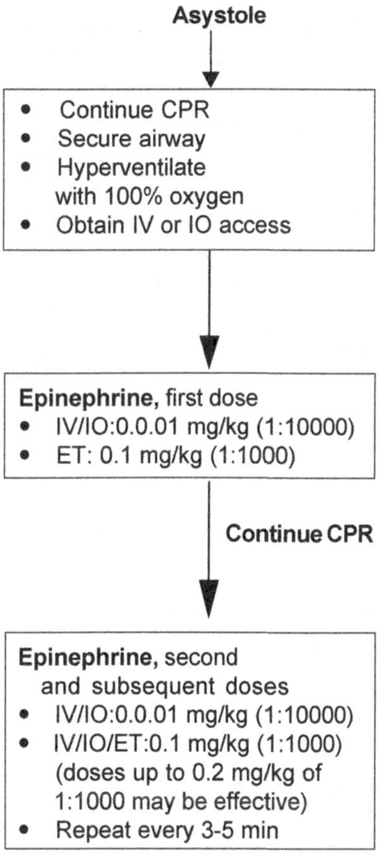

Fig. 1: Algorithm for asystole

The common abnormal rhythms can be conveniently classified for therapeutic purposes based on heart rate (Table 1).

PATHOPHYSIOLOGY

The normal heart rate in children is related to age and is influenced by several physiologic and pathologic conditions. Therefore clinicians should be aware of wide variations in normal rates. The cardiac heart monitoring system can cause potential artifacts emphasizing the importance of clinical assessment and correlation before therapeutic interventions.

The electrocardiogram (EKG) graphically represents the sequence of myocardial depolarization. This depolarization activity begins at the sinoatrial (SA) node and advances to the atrioventricular (A V) node, ultimately progressing to the endocardium of both ventricles via the bundle of HIS. The ventricular depolarization is represented on EKG as QRS complex while repolarizaton as S-T segment and T wave. The mechanisms that produce fast rates include reentry and ectopic pacemakers. The reentry pathway is more common and may be present anywhere along the conduction system. Slow rates are due either to a slowing of the intrinsic pacemaker (sinus) or to a block in conduction system that may be complete or incomplete. Most slow rates inchildren are the result of hypoxia and acidosis and therefore are present during either cardiac pre arrest or cardiac arrest situations.

Electromechanical dissociation (EMD) (Figure 2) is similar to asystole as there is no cardiac contraction and therefore no cardiac output. Even though the heart has electrical activity, it is ineffective in causing adequate muscle contractions. Ventricular fibrillation is rare in children. The myocardium has no effective contractions due to chaotic depolarization and repolari-zation.

CLINICAL ASSESSMENT

The patient may present with a variety of symptoms depending on age at presentation, including poor feeding, irritability, lethargy, pallor, dyspnea, sweating (evidence of congestive heart failure), syncope, dizziness, altered mental status (decreased cerebral blood flow), anginal pain (decreased coronary blood flow), palpitation, or missed beats (perception of cardiac rhythm disturbance). A clinical assessment must include a careful history, thorough physical examination, prompt analysis of the EKG, and determination and monitoring of hemo-dynamic status.

Table 1: Cardiac rhythm disturbances

Fast rates (tachyarrhythmias) Slow rates (bradyarrhythmias) Absent *or* disorganized	Sinus tachycardia (ST) Ventricular tachycardia (VT) Supraventricular tachycardia (SVT)
Slow rates (bradyarrhythmias)	Sinus bradycardia Atrioventricular blocks
Absent or disorganized	Asystole Ventricular fibrillation Electromechanical dissociation

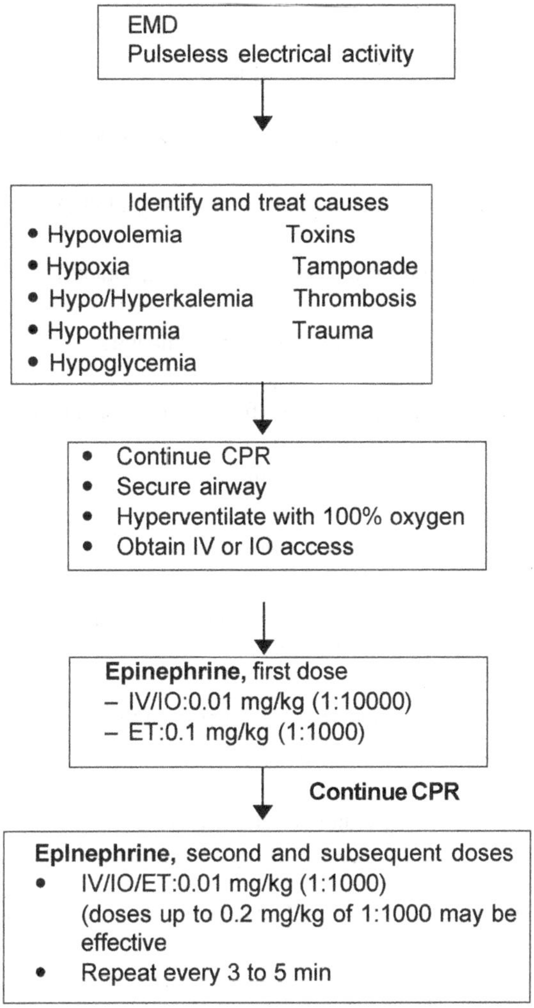

Fig. 2: Algorithm for EMD. (Adapted from American Heart Association, Guidelines for cardiopulmonary resuscitation and emergency care: Pediatric advanced life support).

The most common clinically significant cardiac rhythm disturbance in children is paroxysmal atrial tachycardia (PAT), also called SVT (Figure 3). Acute management is indicated when abnormal rhythm either compromises cardiac output or is unstable (Table 2), or when there is a potential for degeneration into a lethal, life-threatening rhythm disturbance such as ventricular fibrillation. The treatment may not be needed if the dysrhythmia is stable and does not compromise cardiac output.

Unstable

|

Synchronous cardioversion (0.2 joule/kg)

|

Synchronous cardioversion (0.6 joule/kg)

|

Synochronous cardioversion (1.2 joul/kg)

|

Correct underlying abnormalities

|

Pharmacology therapy adenosine (50-100) microgram/kg) IV, push

|

Stable

|

Vagal maneuvers

|

Adenosine (50-100 micrograms/kg)
(rapid push)

|

Adenosine (50-100 microgram/kg)
(rapid push)

|

Cardioversion, digoxin
beta blockers, pacing as indicated[b]

Figure 3: Algorithm 40 kg or less SVT. ([a]Note lesser second dose, [b]See text.)

Table 2: Unstable rhythms

Adolescent	Shock/collapse Chest pain-ischemia secondary to decreased perfusion of coronary arteries Congestive heart failure-resulting from decreased diastolic filling due to rapid heart rate
Child	Shock/collapse Congestive heart failure rare
Infant	Systolic blood pressure less than 60-70 mm/Hg Decreased peripheral perfusion
Newborn	Heart rate less than 80 per minute Blood pressure measurement difficult in newborn

All unstable slow rates are treated the same way regardless of the specific diagnosis. Initial therapy consists of proper ventilation and oxygenation. Medications (atropine and sympathomimetic) may be required. All unstable fast rates require cardioversion regardless of the specific diagnosis. Sometimes it is difficult to distinguish the origin of the fast rate, whether it is ventricular or supraventricular. The wide fast rates are usually ventricular in origin and may require lidocaine. Ventricular fibrillation requires defibrillation and lidocaine.

SUPRAVENTRICULAR TACHYCARDIA

SVT or PAT is the most common type of rhythm disturbance in children with or without cardiac disease. Its prevalence in children is estimated as 1 :25,000. Recently intracardiac electrophysiologic studies have resulted in better understanding of the mechanisms responsible for SVT. These mechanisms include reentry, enhanced automaticity, and triggered activity. Reentry is the most common form both in children and adults. The accessory pathways are the basis for reentrant fast rhythms seen in the preexcitation syndromes of which Wolff-Parkinson-White (WPW) is the most common. The mechanisms for atrial flutter and fibrillation are either reentry, automaticity, or both.

Clinical Presentation

This varies with age, rate and duration of tachycardia, and associated structural heart disease. In infants the symptoms include irritability/lethargy, pallor, poor feeding, vomiting, cold and moist skin, duskiness, upper respiratory infection, and tachypnea. An infant who has had tachycardia lasting more than 24 hours usually presents with symptoms of congestive heart failure. Rarely an infant may present in cardiovascular collapse or as a near-miss sudden death. In older children, symptoms may be palpitation, dizziness, or syncope. About 20 percent of SVT in children has congenital heart disease and 20 to 50 percent has a concealed accessory bypass tract. Other causes include myocarditis, trauma, postcardiac surgery or catheterization, electrolyte imbalance, and digitalis toxicity.

The Electrocardiogram

The EKG shows rapid heart rate varying with age. In infants, it is approximately 240 beats/min, but it can be as high as 300 beats/min. The rhythm is usually regular; P waves may not be identifiable at higher rates. QRS duration is normal most (more than 90 percent) of the time. A rare QRS from aberrant conduction may be difficult to distinguish from ventricular tachycardia. If tachycardia is of longer duration, STand T-wave changes may be consistent with myocardial ischemia. In severely ill infants (sepsis, hypovolemia), it may be difficult to distinguish ST from SVT. In ST, the heart rate is usually less than 200 beats/min, and the rate may vary from beat to beat. Clinicians may be able to identify P waves on an EKG. The chest X-ray is usually normal; in SVT, however, the heart size may be enlarged. The EKG changes in WPW syndrome include short PR interval, a delta wave, and a wide QRS complex. In Lown-Ganong-Levine (LGL) syndrome, the EKG shows short PR interval and a normal or narrow QRS complex (Table 3).

Therapy

In most cases, immediate intervention is not required (Table 4) as the rhythm dis-turbance is usually well tolerated and the patient is hemodynamically stable. If this is so, a cardiac consult is obtained for pharma-cologic intervention. SVT associated with hypotension or cardiovascular collapse, however, is a medical emergency and needs immediate

Table 3: SVT - Differential diagnosis

Type	*QRS Duration*	*Ventricular Rate/Rhythm*	*P Wave (II, III, AVF)*
ST	Narrow	120-230/min variable	Upright
SVT (A V nodal entry type)	Narrow	140-300/min regular	Inverted
Atrial fluter	Narrow	I5O-300/min variable	Saw-tooth pattern
Atrial fibrillation	Variable	I5O-300/min variable	Irregular

intervention. In infants, it is also an emergency because exact duration of the problem is unknown. An EKG (12-lead) and a long rhythm strip should be obtained immediately. This may help in accurate diagnosis and with the etiology.

The use of a diving reflex (immersion of the infant's face in a basin of water at 5°C or ice bag application to the face for 10 to 20 seconds) can be effective. Vagal maneuvers, that is, carotid artery massage, are not usually effective in young children.

Adenosine is considered the drug of choice. It has negative chronotropic, dromotropic and inotropic actions. It is effective for almost all reciprocating SVT and for both narrow and wide complex regular tachycardia. Its advantages include lack of adverse hemodynamic effects, lack of interaction with other drugs and a very short half life.

It is administered by rapid flush technique, starting at 0.1 mg/kg iv (maximum first dose 6mg). A second dose of 0.2 mg/kg (maximum 12 mg) may be given in absence of response. In the presence of cardiovascular collapse, emergency treatment is directed at immediate cadioversion. The initial dose is 0.5 J/kg with subsequent doses of 2 J/kg.

Propranolol, esmolol, other β adrenergic blockers, verapamil and digoxin have also been used with some success.

Table 4: Acute therapy of SVT in infants and children

Vagal maneuvers
- Diving reflex
- Unilateral carotid massage, Valsalva, vomiting/gagging

Pharmacological *
- Adenosine
- Propranolol
- Verapamil
- Digoxin

Cardioversion
- (0.5-2.0 joules/kg)

*See text for dosages.

CONCLUSIONS

The stable patient does not require immediate therapy. The hemodynamically compromised or collapse patient, however, needs immediate intervention with attention to underlying etiology. The most common rhythm disturbance, SVT, is described in depth. The other rhythm disturbances, that is, asystole and EMD commonly secondary to respiratory arrest (hypoxia and acidosis) are described in depth in Chapter 1 (Cardiopulmonary Resuscitation).

BRADYARRHYTHMIAS

Cardiac rhythm disturbances in children result, more often from noncardiac problem rather than steming form a primary cardiac disorder. Typically they arise as a result of hypoxemia and acidosis. Cardiac output is the product of stroke volume and heart rate. In children heart rates vary our a wide range and are age dependant. A heart rate of 100/min which may be considered slow for a neonate may be labelled a fast rate for an adolescent. In infants and children the cardiac output is rate dependant. In response to stress infants and children augment their cardiac output by increasing the heart rate rather than the stroke volume. Stroke volume increases with age as the heart rate decreases.

Arrhythmias in children can arise out of disturbance in impulse formation, impulse conduction or both in many children however no obvious cause can be found. Arrhythmias can result from congenital structural heart disease, post surgical problems, acquired heart diseases, dyselectrotylemias, endocrinopathies, neuromuscular disorders, renal and central nervous system diseases.

Drugs and toxic substance like digitalis, theophylline may also lead to rhythm disturbance. Cardiac rhythm disturbance frequently go unrecognized unless they develop acute decompensation. Hence the diagnosis has to be suspected from secondary manifestations like feature of CCF, features of decreased cerebral flow (syncope, dizziness), symptoms related to decreased coronary flow (anginal chest pain).

Sinus Bradycardia

Sinus Bradycardia arises from a slow generator potential of S.A. node or from diminished conduction of the generator impulse. Bradycardia can occur with or without escape rhythmus. The escape rhythm can arise from A-V node or the ventricles.

Sick Sinus Syndrome

This occurs either due to failure of the SA nodes to generate an impulse (sinus block) or from a decrease in impulse formation the S.A. node. This can occur in situations where there is injury to the SA node for eg post cardiac surgery patients. It may result secondary to ischemia, myocarditis and cardiomyopathies. The sick sinus syndrome can be associated with escape rhythms which can degenerate into fast rhythus (tachycardia). Patients present with Stokes Adam attack, hypotension and hypoperfusion. Those who become symptomatic require pacing. ECG may show evidence of sinus pause, escape rhythms and sometimes presence of bradycardia and tachycardia in the same patient.

Conduction Abnormalities

Bradycardia that arise out of conduction disturbances are the one in which normal impulse generated from the sinoatrial node is not conducted to the ventricles. Impulse generation at SA node and interatrial conduction is normal. The hazard associated with the conduction block is their propensity to progress on to conduction arrest. Depending on the level of the block, they are classified as 1st degree, 2nd degree and 3rd degree blocks.

In 1st degree heart blocks, all impulse formed in the SA nodes are conducted but slowly to the ventricles. This is manifested in the form of prolonged PR interval on the ECG. The rhythm is regular and the P and QRS morphology are normal. A PR interval greater than 0.14 sec. in infants, 0.16 sec. in children and more than 0.18 sec. in adolescent is considered prolonged.

In 2nd degree heart block some of the impulse fail to reach the ventricles owing to the conduction block. This is further subdivided as Mobitz type I and Mobitz type II blocks. In Mobitz Type 1 there is progressive prongation of the PR interval of successive beats and ultimately one beat is dropped. This can occur after every 3rd or 4th beat. The A.V. node is responsible for this conduction aberration. In Mobitz Type II there is intermittent and sudden dropping of QRS complexes not following any particular pattern like type I block. This rhythm has the dangerous potential to degenerate into complete AV block.

Third degree heart blocks, also known as complete heart block can be congenital or acquired. There is total lack of conduction of impulses from the atria to the ventricles. The atria and ventricle function independent of each other known as AV dissociation. The ECG will show bradycardia, abnormally slow QRS and irregular PR interval.

Bradycardia is quite commonly encountered in the ICU setting. This is usually secondary to increase in vagal tone as seen during pharyngeal and endotracheal suctioning, elevated intracranial tension, hypertension and abdominal distention hypoxia, metabolic acidosis, hypoglycemia, hypothermia can also frequently give rise to bradycardia.

Treatment of Bradyarrhythmia

Principles of therapy: Rhythm disturbances in children are trea-ted only if they are unstable. Unstable rhythms are defined as the ones which give rise to hemodynamic compromise or which have the potential to degenerate into a lethal rhythm. Since arrhythmia in children are often secondary to systemic illnesses, therapy should be directed towards the precipitating cause. Metabolic derangements like hypoxia, acidosis and dyselectrolytemia should be corrected. Ventilation, good oxygenation and adequate repletion of the intravascular volume are cornerstones of the therapy in any form of rhythm disturbances especially the bradyarrhythmia. Symptomatic bradycardias associated with features of hypoperfusion should be treated. Bradycardia unresponsive to oxygenation and ventilation should be treated with drugs. Epinephrine and atopine are the two drugs commonly used in the treatment of slow rhythm. No treatment is required for children with asymptomatic complete heart block with acceptable rate, narrow QRS complex and normal ventricular fuction.

Epinephrine

A sympathomimetic agent with both alfa and beta activity is useful in bradycardia associated with poor perfusion and hypotension. It can be given through intravenous, intraosseous and endotracheal route. The ET dose is 0.1mg/kg of 1:1000 solution diluted to a volume of 3-5 ml before installation. The IV route dose is .01 mg/kg (0.1ml/kg) of 1:10, 000.

Atropine Sulfate

It is a parasympatholytic agent which is useful in vagally mediated bradycardia, and in symptomatic conduction blocks (AV blocks.) The dose recommended for sue is 0.02mg/kg with a minimum dose of 0.1 mg. Smaller doses can produce paradoxical bradycardia. The dose can be repeated every 5 min to a maximum dose of 1.0 mg for a child. Same dose can be given endotracheally.

Isoproterenol has been found to be efficacious in patients not responding to atropine.

Pacing

Pacing as a form of therapy for symptomatic bradycardia is indicated in situations wherein the bradycardia is refractory to the above described forms of therapy. Non-invasive transcutaneous pacing has been used in adults, but experience in children is limited.

For AV blocks a cardiac pacing has to be at the ventricular level. The duration of temporary pacing may be as long as 1-2 weeks. If after 2 weeks AV conduction has not retrived back to normal, then permanent pacemaker has to be installed. Other route of pacing are transthoracic and transoesophageal.

FURTHER READING

1. O'Connor M, McDaniel N, Brady WJ. The pediatric electrocardiogram part II: Dysrhythmias. Am J Emerg Med 2008;26:348-58.
2. Tipple MA. Usefulness of the electrocardiogram in diagnosing mechanisms of tachycardia. Pediatr Cardiol 2000;21:516-21.
3. Berul CI. Defibrillator indications and implantation in young children. Heart Rhythm 2008;5:1755-7.
4. Bar-Cohen Y, Silka MJ. Sudden cardiac death in pediatrics. Curr Opin Pediatr 2008;20:517-21.
5. Samson RA, Atkins DL. Tachyarrhythmias and defibrillation. Pediatr Clin North Am 2008;55:887-907.
6. Denjoy I, Lupoglazoff JM, Guicheney P, Leenhardt A. Arrhythmic sudden death in children. Arch Cardiovasc Dis 2008;101:121-5.
7. Bouhouch R, El Houari T, Fellat I, Arharbi M. Pharmacological therapy in children with nodal reentry tachycardia: when, how and how long to treat the affected patients. Curr Pharm Des 2008;14:766-9.
8. Novo S, Barbaro G. Current trends in the treatment of supraventricular tachycardia in pediatric age. Curr Pharm Des 2008;14:722-22.

Charles Cooper

16 Congestive Heart Failure and Other Cardiac Emergencies

True cardiac emergencies in children are less common compared with the adult population. Cardiac diseases in infancy and childhood may be acquired or congenital. Acquired cardiac emergencies, such as cardiac tamponade, usually evolve acutely, and result in sudden alterations in cardiac physiology that may lead to rapid deterioration. Although 0.8% to 1% of infants have congenital heart disease, most are stable and do not present with acute decompensation in the perinatal period. Infants with obstructive cardiac lesions are exceptions, usually requiring emergency medical or surgical intervention. In infants, congestive heart failure usually is related to congenital heart disease, whereas in older children, it tends to be secondary to an acquired cause. Arrhythmias also may cause hemodynamic instability in infants and children. Supraventricular tachycardia is by far the most common emergently presenting arrhythmia in the pediatric population. Complete heart block is rare, but it can lead to congestive heart failure and occasionally to cardiovascular collapse and sudden death. Cyanotic spells, typically occurring in Fallot's tetrology, completes the list of the most frequent cardiac emergencies in pediatrics.

Successful management of pediatric cardiac emergencies requires an accurate diagnosis to institute an appropriate plan of therapy. The diagnosis, however, is not always straightforward, as evidenced by the nonspecific clinical picture that can be presented by congenital heart defects. Table 1 shows signs and symptoms which should raise suspicion of cardiovascular emergencies.

Table 1: When to suspect a cardiovascular emergency?

CCF :	Feeding difficulties, poor weight gain, poor exercise intolerance, chronic cough, increased sweating ; Tachycardia, tachypnea, hepatomegaly, cardiomegaly, gallop rhythm, crepts in lungs.
Cyanotic spell :	Restlessness, acute cyanosis, tachypnea, no crepts.
Tamponade :	Tachycardia, tachypnea, hypotension, cool extremities, mottled skin, oliguria, cardiomegaly, soft-distant heart sounds, hepatomegaly, raised JVP.

CONGESTIVE HEART FAILURE

Congestive heart failure in infants and children is a complex of symptoms originating from abnormal cardiac function. The symptoms may begin as barely perceptible to the parent; hence the children often present to the physician for medical care only after symptoms are far advanced.

In the young infant, congestive heart failure is most likely related to a structural defect of the heart. In the older child on the other hand, most often the congestive heart failure is secondary to an acquired illness or an acquired insult to the heart muscle itself.

A rapid determination that symptoms originate from abnormal cardiac function allows the prompt initiation of appropriate therapy (Table 2, Rapid cardiopulmonary assessment).

Pathophysiology

As part of a broad classification of structural defects of the heart, a delineation can be made between obstruction to flow from the ventricular chamber (for example aortic stenosis) and defects associated with too much pulmonary blood flow as a result of a large left to right shunt (for example, large ventricular septal defect).

Congestive heart failure symptoms may further be divided into those originating in the right side of the heart (the pulmonary circuit) and those that are left-sided in origin (the systemic circuit). The failure represents dilatation and loss of ventricular function and thus the abnormalities of either pulmonary or systemic circulation.

Presenting symptoms of heart failure reflect a combination of changes in both preload and afterload. *Preload* refers to the volume of blood returning to the heart for circulation. *Afterload* refers to the maintained pressure against which the heart must empty the normal circulating volume of blood. Either part of this system can fail.

Generally obstructive lesions, an abnormal afterload to the heart, lead to deterioration of the musculature itself. Hypertrophied muscle initially is very efficient in its performance of work, but begins to contract poorly as it fails and becomes unable to overcome the increased afterload. Likewise the increase in dimension of the muscle itself may preclude adequate nutrition from the myocardial circulation and foster myocardial failure. As a result, residual volumes following emptying of the ventricle begin to increase, reflecting a stretching of the muscle fibers to a length that no longer behaves according to the Starling principle and fails to contract either sufficiently or vigotously. The cycle is set, resulting in increasing diastolic volumes and end diastolic pressures. Thus the muscle starts failing.

The left-sided failure results in the inability of the ventricle to pump an adequate volume for perfusion of vital organs against elevated pressure. This results in multiple organ failure with deterioration in respiratory, kidney, and neurologic functions. The poor tissue perfusion results in altered metabolism. Anaerobic metabolism causes the accumulation of acid products further aggravating the failing cardiac muscle and other vital organ functions. The resultant elevation of ventricular end-diastolic pressures leads to the inability of the left atrium to empty so that its pressure becomes elevated. This leads to the development of pulmonary venous hypertension, increasing abnormal respiratory symptoms, and eventual respiratory failure. The initial ability of the respiratory system to compensate for metabolic acidosis fails with the worsening of the pulmonary edema.

Right-sided obstruction behaves in a similar manner. The elevation of the right-sided end-diastolic pressure as a result of obstruction is reflected in decreased pulmonary blood flow. Increasing right atrial pressure results in systemic venous

Table 2: Rapid cardiopulmonary assessment

Respiratory Assessment	*Cardiovascular Assessment*
Airway Patency	*Circulation*
Breathing	Heart rate
Rate	Blood pressure
Air entry	Peripheral pulses present/absent volume
Chest rise	Skin perfusion
Breath sounds	Capillary refill time
Stridor	Temperature
Wheezing	Color
	Mottling
Mechanics	
Retractions	*CNS (central nervous system) perfusion*
Grunting	Recognition of parents
Color	Reaction to pain
	Muscle tone
	Pupil size

Source: American Heart Assocciation. Textbook of pediatric advanced life support. Dallas: AA, American Academy of Pediatrics, 1990

congestion causing edema of body organs and spaces.

Large volumes of blood delivered to the pulmonary circuit through a congenital defect causes a left-to-right shunt and an initial plethora to the pulmonary circulation. Mean pulmonary artery pressure is elevated, and pulmonary edema is present. Increasing retention of carbon dioxide with decreasing exchange for oxygen result in respiratory acidosis. The combination of hypoxia and acidosis will further insult the failing myocardium. The stretched myocardial fiber no longer contracts adequately according to the Starling mechanism, and low cardiac output ensues. Poor tissue perfusion leads to multiple organ failure and the institution of metabolic acidosis. Ultimately early symptoms of respiratory distress become frank symptoms of respiratory failure.

A unique group of patients, ranging in age from infancy to teenage, present with congestive heart failure secondary to rhythm disturbances. The rapid rhythm tachycardia results in inadequate cardiac output as well as inadequate myocardial perfusion. Symptoms reflect the failure of both ventricles. Rapid conversion by cardioversion or defibrillation to a normal rhythm is essential for returning heart function to normal.

Drugs and viral and bacterial illnesses, affecting other organs of the body, may also attack the heart muscle, the conduction system, or the even heart valves. As a result, there may be a combination of symptoms suggesting both right and left heart failure.

Differential Diagnosis

Infants and children may present in heart failure without a known history of congenital heart disease. Presentation to the physician and parent may also be confused with acute respiratory illness because the signs of respiratory distress mask the symptoms associated with congestive heart failure. Any afebrile illness associated with respiratory distress certainly should alert the physician to consider heart failure as the etiology for the respiratory symptoms.

Table 3: Recognition of congestive cardiac failure

Symptoms	*Signs*
Rapid breathing	Tachycardia, gallop rhythm
Chronic cough	Tachypnea
Feeding difficulties	Hypotension
Failure to thrive	Enlarged heart
Sweating on forehead	Hepatomegaly, increased JVP
	Crepts in lungs
	Edema of dependent regions.

Clinical features that are helpful in recognition of congestive cardiac failure and criteria for diagnosis of neonatal cardiac failure are given in Tables 3 and 4 respectively.

Table 4: Criteria for diagnosis of Neonatal cardiac failure

A. Borderline : Any 3 of the following :
   - Cardiomegaly : CTR > 0.60
   - Tachycardia : HR >150bpm.
   - Tachypnea : RR > 60/min.
   - Wet lungs.

B. Moderate : A + any of the following :
   - Gallop rhythm.
   - Hepatomegaly > 3 cm
   - Frank pulmonary edema.

C. Severe cardiac failure : signs of vascular collapse :
   - Absent pulse.
   - Muffled extremities.
   - Gasping respiration.
   - Hypothermia.

D. Signs of antenatal CCF on USG :
   - Scalp edema.
   - Asites.
   - Pericardial effusion.
   - Decreased fetal movements.

Rarely an infant and child with nephritis and generalized edema may present mimicking congestive heart failure. Appropriate laboratory studies can help delineate the etiology quickly.

Rapid heart rates can be associated with many conditions and may not necessarily be abnormal rhythms. Treatment of the illness will cure the rapid heart rate. When in doubt, an electrocardiogram (EKG) can help clarify the presence or absence of an abnormal cardiac rhythm. Table 5 outlines abnormal assessments and physical findings and gives appropriate interventions.

Laboratory Evaluation

The laboratory evaluation for the patient with congestive heart failure is designed to help delineate the etiology and the initial steps of management.

A chest X-ray will reveal heart size, abnormal configuration, and pulmonary vascular pattern. Pulmonary pathology can also be ruled out as the etiology for the acute symptoms.

An EKG will rule out rhythm disturbances and chamber enlargement as etiology for the symptoms. In addition, the EKG serves as a baseline to further therapy.

A complete blood count (CBC) will reveal the absence of anemia and may help delineate infection as the etiology.

An electrolyte profile, including glucose and calcium, is to be determined.

Electrolyte maintenance and replacement may be important in both the etiology as well as the treatment of the patient.

When possible blood-gas determination should be obtained.

Table 5: Differential diagnosis.

Examination	*Assessment*	*Intervention*
Respiration		
Tachypnea	Rapid rate Clear lung fields	Oxygen
Dyspnea	Rales and wheezes on auscultation	Lasix
Cyanosis	Rales, decreased breath Sounds	Evaluate further; may need intubation and artificial ventilation
Continuing deterioration in any of these indicates need for intubation and artificial ventilation.		
Respiratory arrest	No respiratory effort	CPR (cardiopulmonary resuscitation) Intubation and artificial ventilation.
Circulation Heart rate	Auscultation of heart sounds Timing of rhythm Counting of rate	Medications Cardioversion Defibrillation (rare)
Central pulses	Palpation of quality to estimate Cardiac output	Inotropes
Peripheral pulses	Comparison of quality and strength to central pulses	Inotropes
Capillary refill (more than 3 seconds)	Determined in extremity as a measure of cardiac output and perfusion	Inotropes
Edema	Accumulation of tissue fluid as a result of decreased cardiac output	Inotropes

This is a particular problem with smaller infants and children. Warmed capillary beds may be the source for the blood sample when arterial sticks are neither feasible nor successful. A $PaCO_2$ of greater than 50 mmHg may indicate need for urgent intubation and ventilation.

Pulse oximetry is useful in determining the success of peripheral oxygenation as well as a deterioration in the cardiac output. Poor cardiac perfusion will result in decreased readings.

Diagnostic studies, not part of the lifesaving management of the patient, are to be pursued when doing so is feasible. The patient who is not improving may require more sophisticated evaluation earlier in the course in order to determine the precise etiology and if possible the reason for limited improvement.

An echocardiogram is helpful in delineating structural abnormalities. It will be helpful in looking at and following myocardial function and is most diagnostic in the presence of a pericardial effusion.

Invasive cardiac catheterization with placement of the Swan Ganz cardiac output catheter may be necessary in order to monitor pulmonary artery pressures as well as cardiac output and vascular resistance during fluid management.

Management

Management of the patient with congestive heart failure requires frequent reevaluation and assessment of the patient to determine the need for further interventions. Rapid cardiopulmonary assessment as outlined previously in Table 1 is used to reassess the patient condition and progress of therapy frequently.

Cyanosis and respiratory distress not responsive to delivery of oxygen may warrant further intervention with intubation and ventilation. Deteriorating vital signs, decreased saturations on oximetry, and increasing work of ventilation are also indicators for further intervention.

Temperature control is an often neglected but important vital sign to follow. Body temperature in sick infants and children is frequently abnormally low and warrants frequent assessment to determine the need for warming procedures.

Heart rate may be rapid and is the body's response to maintaining an adequate cardiac output in the light of a failing myocardium. Digoxin in children remains the most used drug in the management of acute congestive heart failure. Apart from slowing heart rate, improved myocardial contractility increases cardiac output. In the patient with acute congestive heart failure, digoxin is given intravenously according to the following regimen:

Digitalizing Dose: Administration:

40 micrograms/kg iv using the following schedule:
1/2 dose initially
1/4 dose six to eight hours later depending on condition 1/4 dose six to eight hours after the second dose

Approximately 12 hours after the last dose, 10 micrograms/kg, (maintenance dose) is given as 1/2 dose every 12 hours. This results in a pharmacokinetic steady state in 3-5 days.

When a child is in mild heart failure, the maintenance dose may be administered orally without loading doses; this results in a steady state in 5 to 8 days.

Diuretic therapy to remove fluid accumulation in the tissues, including the lung interstitial spaces, improves the patient significantly. The initial drug can be Lasix given as a dosage of 2 mg/kg intravenously. The drug may be repeated every four to six hours. The close monitoring of electrolytes is essential. Bumex, a newer diuretic, is used frequently when the response to Lasix is less than expected. Sometimes alternating these two drugs produces the desired effect.

Maintenance fluids are usually given at approximately 60 percent of normal. In order to maintain an adequate output, an adequate stroke volume must be maintained. The patient in congestive heart failure may have a diuresis that decreases the preload. Therefore a delicate balance between fluid input and output must be maintained carefully, specifically during the frequent, large doses of diuretics use period.

Depending on the severity of the congestive heart failure, the use of inotropic agents and afterload-reducing agents (such as Dobutamine, Dopamine, milrinone, hydralazine, nitroglycerine, ACE inhibitors) might be indicated. These drugs require intensive management of the patient's vital signs, including urinary output and neurologic status. Combined use of an inotropic agent, a vasodilator and a diuretic produces most improvement in both inotropic state and congestive symptoms. Experience with the use of newer agents like Levosimendan and Ibopamine in children is limited.

The patient with rhythm disturbances precipitating congestive heart failure, that is, atrial or ventricular tachyarrythmias, require quick intervention with either cardioversion or defibrillation. An appropriate defibrillator with small enough joules should be available for the small infant and child. Recommended joules for cardioversion start at ½ joule/kg. Recommended joules for defibrillation start at 2 joules/kg. Rarely the child or infant will require electrical pacing of the heart in order to maintain an adequate rhythm.

PERICARDIAL TAMPONADE

Pericardial tamponade is one of the principal syndromes of cardiac compression characterized by increased intrapericardial pressure, impaired diastolic pressures, decreased ventricular volume and consequently decreased cardiac output. The spectrum of cardiac tamponade is wide ranging from asymptomatic elevations of intrapericardial pressures to symptomatic circulatory collapse.

Pathophysiology

The pericardial cavity normally contains about 15-50 ml of fluid, the normal intrapericardial pressure is zero or slightly sub atmospheric. The intrapericardial pressure shows variations with cycles of respiration, becoming more negative during inspiration and less negative during expiration. The magnitude of hemodynamic embarrassment caused by a pericardial fluid collection depends on the interplay of the following factors.

a) The rapidity with which the fluid accumulate in the pericardial cavity: It is an important determinant of symptomatic cardiac tamponade. Small volumes (150-200 ml) which have accumulated rapidly can impair cardiac filling markedly eg. traumatic effusions. Gradual accumulation of fluid on the contrary gives enough time for the pericardium to stretch and accommodate large quantities of fluid up to 1000-1500 ml.
b) The thickness of the overlying parietal pericardium: A greatly thickened pericardium due to any cause will require less quantity of fluid to produce signs of compression.
c) Ventricular muscle mass thickness: Thicker muscle mass require more fluid to produce cardiac tamponade.
d) The total intravascular blood volume: the greater the intracardiac volume, the less the tamponade.

Once the intrapericardial pressure reaches the right heart pressures, the transmural filling pressures decrease, resulting in impaired right atrial and right ventricular filling and a drop in right ventricular output. There is a secondary fall in left ventricular output. The initial compensatory mechanisms include increased ejection fraction, tachycardia, increased peripheral vascular resistance; all resulting from symapathoadrenal stimulation. Hypotension is a late feature, which reflects the failure of the compensatory mechanisms.

The *common causes* of cardiac tamponade in children are tuberculosis, neoplasms, trauma, uremia and idiopathic pericardial effusion is an exclusion diagnostic state.

Clinical Features

Children with tamponade may present with tachypnea, syncope, chest pain, hypotension and shock. The Beck's triad of low arterial pressure, elevated CVP and silent heart on examination is very rarely encountered in a given patient. In children sometimes, the only, clinical clue might be tachypnea and hepatomegaly. The physical findings which can be appreciated in older children are a increased central venous pressure and pulsus paradoxus.

Normally the systolic pressure drops by 10-12 mmHg with inspiration. A fall greater than this indicates pulsus paradoxus. This can be estimated with a sphygnomanoimeter or by direct intraarterial pressure monitoring, which is more aceurate. It may be difficult to assess in patients with hypotension sever tachypnoea or irregular rhythm. Localized fluid collection may not give rise to pulsus paradoxus. Pulsus paradoxus may also be seen in absence of in patients with obstructive airway disease, constrictive pericarditis, pulmonary embolism and hypovolemia. The degree of paradoxical pulse does not correlate well with severity of cardiac tamponade.

Central Venous Pressure is invariably elevated, although it may be difficult to detect in children. In some patients with tamponade, in early stages or with associated volume depletion, the CVP may be normal (low pressure tamponade). Kussmaul's sign, an increase in jugular venous pressure with inspiration, may be seen in some patient.

Diagnosis

Besides the clinical signs a raised central venous pressure, pulsus paradoxus, tachypnoea and hepatomegaly, presence of circulatory insufficiency in the context of a disease involving the pericardium may aid in the diagnosis. X-ray chest shows an enlargement of the cardiac silhoutle with moderate- to large effusions. The heart shadow is globular with smooth continuous boarders and a narrow pedicle. Another sign on the plain x-ray chest that is specific for pericardial effusion is the fat line, usually seen in the lateral projection. It is based on the principle that a layer of fat on the epicardial surface of the heart has a lower radiodensity than does the myocardium or the pericardial fluid on either side.

The EKG may show diffuse low voltage complex. Serial EKG with diminishing voltages are more useful than isolated EKG tracings. Non specific ST-T changes can also be seen in pericarditis, and do not necessarily indicate the presence of tamponade.

Echocardiography is a very useful tool in the diagnosis of pericardial effusion tamponade. It helps in determining the location, and amount of fluid in the pericardial sac. The findings that are considered specific for tamponade are right ventricular and right atrial collapse in diastole.

Treatment

The principal option available to the physician in the management of tamponade is the urgent removal of the fluid and to prevent reacumulation. The various modalities which can serve the above purpose are pericardiocentesis, pericardiostomy (periparдial window), partial pericardiectomy and complete pericardioctomy. In the emergency pericardiocentesis can serve both the therapeutic and diagnostic purposes. It should be done under local anesthesia with cardiac monitoring. Surgical modalities as stated above are indicated in situations where there is rapid accumulation requiring repeated pericardiocentesis, adhesions in fluid, evidence of loculations, early features of constriction and where pericardial biopsy is needed for specific diagnosis. Improving preload with crystalloid or colloid infusions may have hemodynamic benefit. Use of preload reducers like diuretics should, however, be avoided.

CYANOTIC SPELLS

Children with cyanotic congenital heart disease with decreased pulmonary blood flow, especially tetralogy of Fallot, develop episodes of increased cyanosis and tachypnea. These episodes have been described by various names including cyanotic spells, hypoxic spells, anoxic spells, blue spells and syncopal episodes. Apart from the fact that these are frightening for the parents, they may result in serious CNS complications and rarely, death.

Definition

The literature throws little light on what actually constitutes a spell. However, episodes characterized by intense cyanosis and paroxysmal hyperpnea in children with congenital heart disease are recognized as cyanotic spells. No correlation exists between the resting arterial PO_2 and hence the presence or absence of cyanosis and the occurrence of cyanotic spells.

Pathophysiology

The central event that results in a spell is a decrease in pulmonary blood flow relative to systemic blood flow. Several hypothesis have been postulated fro the causation of these spells. These include (1) right ventricular infundibular spasm (2) Sudden changes in systemic vascular resistance and venous return, which increase right-to-left shunting (3) Alterations in sensitivity of the respiratory centre (4) marked changes in heart rate.

Most spells are precipitated by crying, defacation or feeding, especially soon after awakening from sleep. During sleep, oxygen consumption is reduced considerably and there is reduction in respiratory rate. Relative hypercarbea results and the respiratory centre becomes oversensitive to any further increases in carbon-dioxide$_2$. Soon after waking up, any increase in activity or crying/ defaecation (Valsalva – like manouvre) results in an increase in oxygen demand and a fall in systemic vascular resistance. Right to left shunting increases causing a fall in PaO_2 and a further increase in $PaCO_2$. The respiratory centre gets excessively stimulated by this rise in CO_2 and increased oxygen demand and hyperpnea occurs. Hyperpnea, in turn, results in sympathetic stimulation leading to a rise in heart rate and an increase in cardiac output. Any increase in heart rate increases the functional obstruction to the right ventricular outflow and thus increased the right-to-left shunting of blood, decreasing the pulmonary blood flow. Thus, a vicious cycle is set. Atrial tachycardias due to increased sympathetic tone, also increases right – left shunting.

Clinical Features

Cyanotic spells occur in upto 40% of infants and young children with decreased pulmonary blood flow. Age at onset varies between 1 month to 2 years with a peak incidence between 2-3 months age. Spells continue to occur in children as old as 12 year, though spontaneous remission has been described between 2-6 years age. Although, these episodes can occur at any time of the day, the majority occur in the morning soon after awakening. They are often precipitated by crying defacation or feeding. Other significant stresses such as anemia, polycythemia, dehydration, invasive medical procedures and infections may also precipitate cyanotic spells. An episode may last from minutes to several hours; most of them last between 15 to 60 minutes.

Clinically, a cyanotic spell is recognized by obvious cyanosis, hyperpnea and the history of heart disease. However, a preceding history of overt cyanosis may not be forthcoming as spells can occur in children with little or no cyanosis otherwise. During a spell, the child is initially irritable and crying followed by limpness, generalized stiffness and even unconsciousness. Seizures may occur occasionally. Hyperpnea is a constant features of spells. The cardiac murmur is notably shortened or may even be absent during the episode.

Investigations

Generally, investigations should be avoided during the spell as attempts to obtain blood may cause agitation and further aggravate the spell.

The hematocrit should be checked as both anemia and polycythaemia are not desirable. Iron deficiency anemia should be ruled out on a peripheral blood smear. Arterial blood gas determination is required to assess the acid-base balance and ventilatory status, especially if the attack is prolonged.

Once the patient is stabilized, the underlying heart disease and its severity must be ascertained.

Management

A child with a cyanotic spell requires immediate attention. The aim of management is to improve the arterial PO_2 and acidosis by improving the pulmonary blood flow.

1. The baby is calmed and placed in a knee-chest position (physiologically similar to squatting.) This position redistributes the systemic blood flow to the upper body and increases the systemic vacular resistance and hence improves pulmonary blood flow.
2. Supplemental oxygen should be administered as PaO_2 may be quite low and some benefit may be obtained from even small increased in dissolved oxygen.
3. Subcutaneous morphine (0.1 – 0.2 mg/kg) is usually effective in relieving a spell. Its mechanism of action is not clear. Morphine probably aborts the cycle of hyperpnea and vasomotor changes by depressing the respiratory centre. It may also have inhibitory action on catecholamines at the cardiac level.
4. Correction of acidosis by the administration of sodium bicarbonate is indicated. Initially 2 mEq/kg of $NaHCO_3$ solution is given over 5 min. Subsequent doses may be needed depending on the arterial PH.
   The majority of children with cyanotic spells respond to these initial therapeutic measures. In prolonged attacks, further measures are required.
5. Beta-adrenergic blockade with intravenous propnolol (.1 mg/kg over 4-5 min) yields prompt improvement. Its action is hypothesized to be reduction in the sympathetic tone (and hence decrease in heart rate) and relaxation of the RV infundibular spasm, thus decreasing R-L shunting.
6. Administration of IV fluids in maintenance doses is required in severe spell as the pulmonary blood flow and RV output are volume dependant.
7. Vasopressors increase the systemic vascular resistance and thus reduce the R – L shunting and improve oxygenation. Phenylephrine, which relatively specifically increase SVR as compared to pulmonary vascular resistance can be given intravenously. Heart rate should be monitored during the infusion. Digitalis, epinephnine and morepinephrine are contraindicated in this setting.
8. Correction of precipitating factors such as polycythaemia, anemia, dehydration or infection should be undertaken.

Once a spell has been successfully managed, it is important to prevent the recurrence of these episodes, chronic oral propranolol therapy (1-2 m/kg 4 times daily) has been shown to prevent recurrences.

However, the occurrence of spells is an indication for surgical correction of the underlying heart disease. Where total correction is not possible, a shunt surgery should be undertaken to improve pulmonary blood flow.

Complications

The complications of cyanotic spells are related to the hypoxic injury to the central nervous system. Convulsions, cerebrovascular accidents leading to hemiparesis and coma have been described following cyanotic spells. Rarely, they may even be fatal. Recurrent spells may lead to hypoxic brain damage and hence, mental retardation.

Conclusion

Cardiac emergencies can cause mortality if an acute problem is not recognized and treated promptly. Since the symptom is merely part of a complex disease process, the patient will need to be admitted or transported to a facility that can delicately manage and diagnostically evaluate the care of these very sick infants and children.

FURTHER READING

Congestive Cardiac Failure

1. Margossian R. Contemporary management of pediatric heart failure. Expert Rev Cardiovasc Ther 2008;6:187-97.
2. Frobel AK, Hulpke-Wette M, Schmidt KG, Läer S. Beta-blockers for congestive heart failure in children. Cochrane Database Syst Rev 2009;(1):CD007037.
3. Kaufman BD, Shaddy RE, Shirali GS, Tanel R, Towbin JA. Assessment and management of the failing heart in children. Cardiol Young 2008;18 Suppl:63-71.
4. Working Group on Management of Congenital Heart Diseases in India, Saxena A, Juneja R, Ramakrishnan S. Drug therapy of cardiac diseases in children. Indian Pediatr 2009;46:310-38.
5. Hunt EA, Brunetti M, Nelson KL, Shilkofski NA, Peddy SB. Recognition and initial management of cardiac emergencies in children. Minerva Pediatr 2009;61:141-62.
6. Schweigmann U, Meierhofer C. Strategies for the treatment of acute heart failure in children. Minerva Cardioangiol 2008;56:321-33.
7. Foerster SR, Canter CE. Pediatric heart failure therapy with beta-adrenoceptor antagonists. Paediatr Drugs 2008;10:125-34.

Pericardial Temponade

1. Lee C, Mason LJ. Pediatric cardiac emergencies. Anesthesiol Clin North America 2001;19:287-308.
2. Bowers P, Harris P, Truesdell S, Stewart S. Delayed hemopericardium and cardiac tamponade after unrecognized chest trauma. Pediatr Emerg Care 1994;10:222-4.
3. Askegard-Giesmann JR, Caniano DA, Kenney BD. Rare but serious complications of central line insertion. Semin Pediatr Surg 2009;18:73-83.
4. Scarfone RJ, Donoghue AJ, Alessandrini EA. Cardiac tamponade complicating postpericardiotomy syndrome. Pediatr Emerg Care 2003;19:268-71.

Cyanotic Spell

1. Grech V, Goldman A. Acute respiratory distress syndrome due to cyanotic spell in an infant with tetralogy of Fallot. Pediatr Pulmonol 2001;32:406-7.
2. DiMario FJ Jr. Prospective study of children with cyanotic and pallid breath-holding spells. Pediatrics 2001;107:265-9.
3. Kothari SS. Mechanism of cyanotic spells in tetralogy of Fallot—the missing link? Int J Cardiol 1992;37:1-5.
4. Rao PS. Diagnosis and management of cyanotic congenital heart disease: part I. Indian J Pediatr 2009;76:57-70.
5. Yee L. Cardiac emergencies in the first year of life. Emerg Med Clin North Am 2007;25:981-1008.

17

Sunit Singhi

Hypertensive Emergencies

Hypertension is defined as a blood pressure (BP) above 95 percentile for the age (1). Blood pressure readings between 90th and 95th percentile values for the age on at least 3 occassions is labels as high normal BP, while a systolic or diastolic BP> 99th percentile is termed severe hypertension (Table 1).

Prompt recognition of the clinical manifestations and early implementation of individualized treatment is of critical importance. To emphasize proper approach to clinical evaluation and treatment of high blood pressure in the emergency setting it is differentiated into Hypertensive Urgency and Emergency (2).

Hypertensive Emergency

Hypertensive emergency (HTE) is a BP high enough to cause acute end organ damage requiring reduction of arterial pressure within one hour. The end –organ damage may manifest as encephalopathy, intracranial bleed, acute left ventricular failure and pulmonary edema, acute renal failure, and retinopathy. It may occur at lower levels of BP in patients with recent onset hypertension than in those with long standing hypertension. Thus, there is no specific BP level that constitutes a HTE.

Hypertensive encephalopathy is the most common manifestation of HTE in children

Table 1: 95th percentile limits for pressure at different ages, adopted from task force recommendations(1)

	95th – 99th Centile		*>99th Centile*	
Age	*Systolic*	*Diastolic*	*Systolic*	*Diastolic*
< 7 days	> 96	-	106	- >110
7-30 days	104	-	110	- >120
1 mon – 2 yrs	112	74	118	82-134/96
3 yrs – 5 yrs	116	77	124	84-134/96
6 yrs – 9 yrs	112	78	130	86
10 yrs – 12 yrs	126	82	134	90-144/96
			13-184	160-104

and is defined as transient cerebral dysfunction that occurs when blood pressure rapidly increases.

Hypertensive Urgency

Hypertensive Urgency (HTU) is defined as high blood pressure which does not pose any immediate risk to cardiovascular or other end organs; the blood pressures may be reduced slowly in 24 hours. These patients, in contrast to those of HTE, may be managed on ambulatory basis.

Table 2 gives the common causes of hypertensive emergencies and urgencies in children. In our population it affects 1%-4% of all children, secondary causes are more frequent than primary in children < 6 years. Severe hypertension is most likely to be secondary hypertension of renal etiology or vascular cause; essential hypertension is uncommon.

MANAGEMENT

Initial Assessment

A symptomatic hypertensive patient constitutes hypertensive emergency which needs immediate attention. The initial assessment should be directed towards identification of affected end-organs and possible cause (Table 3). The history taking and examination should be brief and relevant. The symptoms are typically nonspecific. BP should be measured in both the limbs. It is best measured with help of a mercury manometer. The cuff should cover at least two-third of child 's upper arm circumference. The diagnostic work up must be individualized according to the history and physical examination findings (Table 4). Complicated diagnostic tests and transport of the patient to other departments for evaluation should not be done until BP is adequately controlled.

Table 2: Etiology of hypertensive crises in Pediatrics

Renal	*Renovascular diseases*
1. Glonerulonephritis: Acute poststreptococcal, Henoch –Schonlien or chronic Pylonephritis : Acute and chronic.	1. Coarctation ofAorta 2. Aorto- arteritis 3. Renal artery anomalies 4. Vasculitis
ENDOCRINE	
Hemolytic Uremic Syndrome Congenital malformations (polycystic disease, dysplasia, hypoplasia)	1. Pheochromocytoma 2. Neuroblastoma 3. Adrrnogenital disease 4. Cushing's syndrome
Obstructive Uropathy.	
MISCELLANEOUS	
1. Corticosteriod administration 2. Gullain- Barre Syndrome 3. Raised intracranial pressure 4. Essential Hypertension	

Table 3: Clinical findings in presence of which hypertensive emergency must be looked for.

Symptoms	*Signs*
Headache	Short stature,peripheral edema,pallor
Dizziness	Trachcardia,increased sweating,flushing
Excessive crying	Moon faces, obesity
Epistaxis	Absent or delayed femoral pulses, leg pressure Significantly lower than arm pressure.
Failure to thrive	Abdominal bruit
Joint pain	Hypertensive funduscopic changes
Convulsions	Neurologic deficit, eg, absent papillary refles, Hemiparesis
Hemiplegia	Encephalopathy, occipital blindness, (HSEB)
Irritability, confusion Visual disturbances Personality changes	

Table 4: Diagnostic workup in hypertensive emergency

General	*Specific*
Hemogram :	Ultrasound abdomen
Renal disease – low hemoglobin.	Intravenous pyelography
Urine microscopic and routine for	Echocardiography
Albumin, RBCs, pus cells and castes	CT Scan
Renal parameters- urea, creatinine	Plasma Renin
Electrolytes-renal disease	Urinary 17 ketosteroids Vanil-Mandelic
Mineralocorticoid excess.	acid and Catecholamines
Chest X-ray	
ECG	

Phase I: Urine-complete, CBC
Urea & eletrocytes, Lipid profile, ECG, X-ray. Echocardiography,

Phase II: Plasma Renin activity (PRA)
Isotope Scan with ACE inhibitors, Flow study, Endocrine screen, cortisol

Phase III: Voiding CUR, Renal Biopsy, renal vein sampling if severe elevation or response to antihypertensive drugs.

General Principles

The patients with HTE should be hospitalized, have an intravenous access established and placed on a BP monitor. The drug therapy should be initiated without delay.

Each patient need a precise and individualized management and choice of medications. The two most important considerations in the treatment are etiology and duration of hypertension. Etiology determines the selection of the most effective antihypertensive agent, while acuteness of BP elevation defines the rapidity and degree by which it should be reduced.

Therapeutic Goal

The decision to rapidly lower BP is dependent on benefit to be derived from treating HT and risk of medication. The goal of emergency management of THE with an acute rise in BP is to lower the mean arterial pressure by 20% over a period of minutes to one hour(4). It is preferable to use on e drug when the patients condition is acute. The BP in HTU (severely hypertensive but asymptomatic patients) should be decreased by one third of planned reduction in first 6 hours, by another third during the next 12-36 hours and the last third during next 48-96 hours. Precipitous reduction of BP to normotensive levels provokes an end organ ischemia or infarction due to loss of auto-regulation. More gradual reduction using oral drugs obviates this problem. Complications of hypertension should be managed appropriately.

Monitoring

Vigilant Neurologic monitoring: After medication for the effectiveness of therapy should be monitored by serial measurement of BP, ideally by direct intra-arterial monitoring. Serial neurologic examinations are also important in the child with hypertensive encephalopathy -early symptoms of vertebral hypoperfusion, blindness, paralysis, coma and death have been reported because of inappropriately aggressive therapy.

Drugs Used

The drugs used in management of hypertensive emergency fall in two groups : direct vasodilators (such as sodium nitroprusside, diazoxide, hydralazine, nifedepine etc.) and sympathetic inhibitors (labetolol). The important advantages and disadvantages, and the dosage of the drugs are listed in Table 5. Diazoxide, parenteral hydralazine and prazosin which have been used in HTE are not included in the discussion. Of the drugs available for hypertensive urgency nifedepine, clonidine, captopril and labetalol are safest and most useful.

The Choice of Drugs

This depends on patient's condition, present medication, suspected etiology and the end-organ involved. Hypertension due to pain is best treated with analgesics.

In HTE it is preferable to use the drugs that allow close monitoring of reduction of BP, such as those given by incremental infusions. If intracranial bleed is suspected one would avoid drugs that increase cerebral blood – blocker should be avoided. Nitroprusside is generally recommended as the drug of first choice.

Sodium Nitroprusside

Nitroprusside causes direct vasodilatation of capacitance and resistance vessels, it is the most potent and predictable antihypertensive drug. It does not evoke tachycardia, any be reducing the preload, it improves borderline myocardial dysfunction and cerebral blood flow. It is preferred drug for severe long standing hypertension, hypertensive encephalopathy, hypertensive emergency associated with acute LV failure, head injury and pheochromocytoma.

It requires an infusion pump for administration, and careful and constant bedside monitoring. Since the light causes rapid degradation of the drug, the bottle and the tubings need to be covered with a black sheet. Although thiocyanate, a by-product of nitropruside metabolism, gradually accumulates in oliguric patients, it does not preclude the use of the drug for up to 2 days even in anephric patients. Thiocyanate toxicity (toxic levels > 100 mg/L) results in nausea, weakness, disorientation, tinnitus, muscle spasm, acidosis and psychosis.

Nifedipine: Nifedipine, a calcium channel blocker has a powerful vasodilator action

Table 5: Drugs used in Hypertensive emergencies.

Drug	*onset of action; duration*	*dose & route*	*advantages/ disadvantage*
Sodium Nitorpruside	< 30 seconds ; 1-5 min.	0.5-8 ug/kg/min. by continous drip	Requires continous monitoring Thiocyanate poisoning If > 72 hrs. use. Solution photosensitive
Nifedipine	10 min; 4-6 hours	0.25-05 mg/kg/dose (aspirate in syringe) Sublingual	- Occasional hypotension.
Labetolol	<5 min;	Bolus : 0.5 mg/kg Over 2 min. I/V	- Contraindicated in Asthma,CCF, heart-block
	upto 24 hours	Double dose q 10 min. Max: 5 mg/kg and Total 300 mg.	Hypotension, rash. –Easy to titrate
Captopril	15 min; 8-12 hours	Age > 6 months 0.3-2.0 mg/kg, oral	Very useful for renal hypertension.
Diazoxide	< 30 min ; Peak at 30 min.	0.1 –0.5 mg/kg IV push at 10-15 min. Interval	Potent and convenient
Hydralazine	< 30 min ; 4-12 hours	0.1-0.5 mg/kg IV Maximum –25 mg.	Trachycardia, flushing, Acute hypotension.

with little effect on cardiac conduction. In clinical practise the potential negative chronotropic, inotropic and dromotropic effects are seldom a problem. Its dilating effect on the coronary vessels and the decrease in afterload results in a lesser myocardial oxygen demand. The impaired renin and aldosterone secretion may also contribute to its antihypertensive action.

Hypotension is the most serious side effect. It is likely after high dose or when it is used in patient who is on beta-blocker or ACE inhibitors. Minor side effects are related to vasodilatation; these include peripheral edema, headache, flushing and parasthesias which usually diminish with the use.

The drug has been considered to be a safe and effective antihypertensive agent for infants and children. In a study involving 21 children sublingual nifedipine in the dosage 0.25-0.5 mg/kg decreased arterial pressure from 183/136 to 132/98 mmHg in 30 minutes. The antihypertensive effect started within 10 minutes, peaked at 30 minutes and continued for 6 hours. An increase in heart rate was reported in most of the patients in this study. In our experience, with use of sublingual nifedipine it was possible to achieve a 25% reduction in BP within 30 minutes with a sublingual dose of 0.5 mg/kg in most of the children.

Labetolol : Labetolol is a combined nonselective antagonist of beta and alpha adrenergic receptors. It decreases heart rate, total systemic vascular resistance and rennin activity while renal perfusion is maintained. It must be used with caution in heart failure, heart block and bronchial asthma due to its beta-antagonism. Its experience in pediatric age group is limited though its considered to be safe for use.

Captopril : Captopril is a angiotensin converting enzyme inhibitor and therefore particularly useful in rennin dependent hypertension. It is started in a dose of 0.3 mg/kg orally, and doubled every two hourly till the desired effect or a dose of 2 mg/kg is reached. It does not affect CNS.

OUTCOME

The exact mortality of hypertensive emergency in children is not known, but the risk of death has diminished with early recognition of the condition and use of more efficacious drugs. The patients may require further management after initial control of BP such as correction of renal artery stenosis, removal of tumour, correction of coarctation of aorta, or it may be incurable as in chronic glomerulonephritis.

FURTHER READING

1. The Seventh report on the Joint National Committee on prevention, delection, evaluation, and treatment of high blood pressure JAMA. 2003; 289.
2. Brady TM, Feld LG. Pediatric approach to hypertension. Semin Nephrol. 2009; 29 (4): 379-88.
3. Update on the 1987 Task force on blood pressure in children and adolescents: a working group report from the national high blood pressure education program. National high blood pressure education program working group on hypertension control in children and adolescents. Pediatrics 1996; 98 (4 pt 1); 649-58.

Deepti Suri and Sunit Singhi

18 Limp

Limp is one of the common presentation to emergency department. It may be difficult to localize source of pain (e.g., hip pain may be referred to knee). Young children often are not able to localize pain.

EVALUATION

Useful diagnostic clues in the history could be obtained from the age, onset of pain (sudden vs insidious), duration of pain: (intermittent vs constant), quality of pain: (severe vs mild), location of pain: (reproducible/localizable for referred pain), history of trauma (accidental vs nonaccidental) and presence of constitutional symptoms such as fever, weight loss, night sweats, malaise (neoplasms and infections) (Table 1).

Physical examination should include general and local assessment. On general examination presence of lymphadenopathy, skin changes, hepatomegaly and splenomegaly should be noted. On local examination stance (pelvic tilt, scoliosis, knee flexion, leg asymmetry, rotation of foot), gait: (shortened stance phase, gait associated with pain, antalgic gait, Trendelenburg gait), muscle strength: (Trendelenburg test: children>3 yrs, school age: heel-toe walk), passive/active range of motion, pain during motion,and signs of limb shortening and muscle wasting (calf and thigh diameter) should be looked for. *Trendelenburg* gait is side lurching gait, with shifts of trunk toward weak/painful extremity and pelvis tilts away from the affected side. It occurs in conditions where there is a decreased force transmitted through extremity, such as in congenital hip dislocation, Legg-Calve-Perthes disease, slipped capital femoral epiphysis.

Table 1 : Differential diagnoses of limp: Systems approach

Infectious
Common: osteomyelitis, septic arthritis, cellulitis
Uncommon: discitis, CNS infections, appendicitis,
Musculoskeletal
Slipped capital femoral epiphysis (SCFE), Legg-Calve-Perthes disease, Congenital Dislocation of Hip (CDH), Osteochondroses (Osgood-Schlatter Disease, Sinding-Larsen-Johansson Syndrome), Fractures, Child Abuse, Neoplasm
Inflammatory
Transient synovitis, juvenile rheumatoid arthritis (JRA), myositis,
Hematological
Sickle cell crisis, hemophilia, leukemia
Neuromuscular
Guillain-Barre syndrome.

DIFFERENTIAL DIAGNOSIS

1. Transient Synovitis

Transient synovitis is acute self-limiting aseptic inflammation of synovial lining.

It is the most common non-traumatic cause of sudden limp and inability to walk in children and is believed to be a post-infectious reactive arthritis. It most commonly affects the hip, but occasionally affects the knee or ankle. Peak incidence is seen between 3-8 years of age, predominently in boys. Typically the child has 1-to 2-days history of limp, complains of severe unilateral pain in the hip, thigh, or knee, often with a history of viral symptoms within the past 1-2 weeks. There is little or no fever, and the child appears well on general physical examination. On local examination, the joint (usually hip) is painful on passive range of motion. The hip is abducted and externally rotated. Thigh and knee is flexed. Rotation and extension of hip are restricted.

Transient synovitis is a diagnosis of exclusion. Another diagnosis is likely if the patient is below 2 years or older than 10 years, has high grade fever, or if the symptoms have lasted for more than 2 weeks.

Laboratory tests or imaging studies are not very helpful in distinguishing transient synovitis from septic arthritis of the hip. White blood cell counts are normal in the majority of patients with both conditions. Erythrocyte sedimentation rate (ESR) is elevated (>20) in most patients with septic arthritis and about half of patients with transient synovitis. Fluid in the joint space is common in both conditions. The definitive test is joint aspiration, and may be necessary to exclude bacterial infection.

Management includes rest and position of the extremity in the position preferred by the patient, non-steroidal anti-inflammatory agents, and re-evaluation in 24-48 hours. Some patients may have recurrence within 6 months (4-17%).

2. Osteomyelitis

For details see chapter—.Osteomyelitis usually presents with slow, insidious progression of symptoms. Neonates present with fever (in 50%), and pseudoparalysis of limb. On examination, there is restriction of movement, local edema, erythema and point tenderness.

3. Developmental Dysplasia of the Hip (DDH) or Congenital Dislocation of Hip (CDH).

It includes a spectrum of acetabular dysplasia, hip subluxation, and hip dislocation. When missed, the limp associated with CDH manifests as the infant starts walking. It is usually painless and is associated with a Trendelenburg gait, often with toe walking on the affected side to accommodate the limb shortening. Bilateral involvement, which occurs in about 20% patients, produces a waddling gait with out-toeing.

4. Legg-Calve-Perthes Disease

Legg-Calve-Perthes disease (LCPD) is an avascular necrosis of the femoral head that presents as hip or knee pain, most often in boys. Onset of limping is insidious, with limitation of internal hip rotation and flexion. The peak incidence is between 4-9 years of age (range 3-12 years).

Pain is usually mild, intermittent and referred to thigh/knee. The limp could be related to pain, limb-length discrepancy, or limited internal rotation and abduction of hip. Muscle atrophy may be present.

Hip X-ray: In initial phase shows small radiodense femoral head and widened medial joint space due to cartilage hypertrophy. Changes are best seen in frog-leg lateral view. After a few months, crescent-shaped subchondral radiolucent line makes its appearance. In the later phases areas of radiodensity and radiolucency (fragmentation phase), and abnormally shaped femoral head are seen.

Management requires orthopedic clinic follow-up and conservative treatment.

5. Juvenile Rheumatoid Arthritis (JRA)

The diagnosis is made clinically based on unexplained persistent arthritis in one or more joints for more than 6 weeks in a child under the age of 16 years. The disease is subclassified into systemic, pauciarticular (4 or fewer joints), or polyarticular (>4 joints). Rheumatoid factor is virtually never positive in patients with pauciarticular JRA, and will be positive in fewer than half of patients with polyarticular JRA. On the other hand, ANA is positive in about 50% of patients with pauciarticular disease.

6. Slipped Capital Femoral Epiphysis (SCFE)

SCFE refer to displacement of proximal femoral metaphysis anterolaterally and superiorly. It presents in early adolescence, most commonly in obese boys. Often there is a history of minor trauma. The usual presentation is with non-radiating, dull aching pain in thigh, groin, hip or occasionally knee. The pain worsens with activity. Symptoms are progressive, not severe, and lead to a mild antalgic gait with external rotation of the affected leg. Sometimes, acute slips with sudden, severe pain also occur.

On examination, hip is tender to palpation, with limitation of internal rotation and flexion. Mild atrophy of thigh may occur in longstanding pathology. SCFE is bilateral in 25-40%. It has been associated most with hypothyroidism, and rarely with acromegaly, excess growth hormone, hypopituitarism, and hypogonadism. Hypothyroidism is especially important to consider if the SCFE occurs in a patient under the age of 10 years.

On investigations, blood counts and ESR are normal. Hip X-ray shows slip; more obvious on frog-leg lateral view, and Klein's line. If a line is drawn along superior border of proximal femoral metaphysis, it normally transects femoral epiphysis by 20%. A line touching lateral margin of epiphysis indicates slippage of femoral epiphysis inferiorly and medially.

Management includes orthopedic consult, bed rest, traction and surgical fixation. Risk of avascular necrosis increases with delay in diagnosis.

7. Osgood-Schlatter Disease

It occurs from chronic microtrauma to tibial tuberosity secondary to overuse of quadriceps and is usually seen in adolescent boys, 11-18 years old. Heterotopic bone formation occurs at tendon insertion site. The pain is precipitated by trauma in 50%. Clinical presentation is generally with pain for months, continuous or intermittently, exacerbated by running, jumping, kneeling, and relieved by rest, and restriction of exercise. The pain is reproducible by extending knee against resistance, stressing quadriceps, or squatting with knee in full flexion.

On examination: tenderness and soft-tissue edema is seen over proximal tibial tuberosity at patellar tendon insertion. A visible lump is present and a firm mass may be palpable.

Lab evaluation is not indicated unless other etiologies are being considered. Plain film lateral view of knee in slight internal rotation shows irregular ossification of proximal tibial tuberosity, and calcification and thickening within patellar tendon.

The condition is benign and self-limited. Corticosteroid injections are not recomm-ended. Treatment includes analgesic-anti inflammatory drugs, avoidance of pain-producing activities, and vigorous exercise, and muscle strengthening.

8. Toddler's Fracture

Typically child presents with refusal to walk after jumping off of a toy box. He is tender over the distal portion of his tibia. It refers to nondisplaced spiral fracture of the tibia.

This type of fracture may be seen in children from the age they start walking up to 6 years. The fracture is usually seen on the anteroposterior (AP) view, rarely on the lateral. Even with normal radiographs if clinical suspicion is high, presumptive treatment with follow-up films in 10-14 days is indicated. In the absence of trauma, occult osteomyelitis is included in the differential diagnosis.

9. Salter Harris Fracture

Salter Harris Fracture refers to type 1 fracture of the distal fibula. Child typically presents with limping and pain over the lateral malleolus after twisting the ankle while playing. Typically the child is able to bear weight. Plain radiographs of the ankle are negative.

Closely mimicking Salter-Harris fracture in clinical presentation is **Jones fracture**, which refers to avulsion fracture of fifth metatarsal bone. Typically, the child–a teenage boy, presents with pain and limp after twisting his ankle. On examination, palpation of lateral aspect of foot reveals the fracture.

10. Osteochondroses

Osteochondroses are a group of lesions that occur in the lower extremity in growing bones, with a clinical picture of localized pain and limp. Radiographic changes include irregularity, increase in density, or decrease in size of the affected bone.

Sever's disease typically presents in a young child (8-12 years) at the insertion of the Achilles tendon on the calcaneus.

Sinding-Larsen-Johansson Syndrome (SLJS)

SLJS occurs in preadolescent children at the attachment of the patellar tendon to the inferior pattelar pole. Osgood-Schlatter disease is found at the insertion of patellar tendon on the proximal tibial tuberosity of adolescents.

Kohler's disease affects the tarsal navicular, and is typically seen in children 2-9 years old.

Freiburg's disease most commonly involves the 2nd metatarsal head, but can also be seen in the 3rd and 4th with decreasing frequency. It is most common in adolescent girls.

Sometimes limp may be caused by pathology outside the lower extremities. There include discitis in lumber region. The child, typically under 5 years, presents with progressive limp, and eventually refuses to sit or walk over a few weeks.

CONCLUSION

Causes of limp vary with age (Table 2). Clinical evaluation of limp should include onset, history of trauma and constitutional symptoms, quality of pain, type of gait, and muscle bulk. Transient Synovitis is by far the commonest cause in young children, but it requires exclusion of septic arthritis and sometimes osteomyelitis. Systemic symptoms and signs may point to a systemic cause or JRA. Initial laboratory investigations in emergency room should include a complete blood count and X-rays. Further tests may be planned later. Management includes relief of pain with analgesic-anti-inflammatory agents and rest and use of antibiotics wherever indicated.

Table 2: Differential diagnosis of limp with respect to age:

Birth-2 Years	*2-10 Years*	*10-18 Years*
Septic arthritis	Septic arthritis	Fractures
Toddler's fracture (SCFE)	Transient synovitis	Slipped capital femoral epiphysis
Osteomyelitis	Osteomyelitis	Osteomyelitis
Congenital hip dislocation	Legg-Calve-Perthes	Patello-femoral problems
Nonaccidental trauma	Juvenile idiopathic arthritis	Tumors
	Leukemia	Sickle cell crisis
	Fractures	
	Sickle cell crisis	

FURTHER READING

1. Eich GF, Superti-Furga AS, Unbricht FS, Willi UV. The painful hip: evaluation of criteria for clinical decision-making. Eur J Pediatr.1999;158:923-928.
2. Lawrence LL. The limping child. Emerg Med Clin North Am. 1998;16(4):911-929.
3. Sawyer JR, Kapoor M. The limping child: A systematic approach to diagnosis. Am Fam physician 2009; 79: 215-224.

William A. Herndon

19 Acute Osteomyelitis and Septic Arthritis

Acute hematogenous septic arthritis and osteomyelitis can cause significant morbidity if they are not promptly diagnosed and properly managed. The character of these infections is changing. In the past, bone and joint infections in children have been responsible for significant mortality. The advent of antibiotics, the availability of newer diagnostic techniques, a better understanding of the pathophysiology of these infections, and advances in anesthetic and surgical management, however, have changed the course of these diseases. Despite these advances, diagnosis is often delayed. Outcome is directly related to time from onset of symptoms to institution of treatment. It is imperative that a high index of suspicion be present when a neonate, infant, or child presents with a limp, inability to bear weight, or refusal to use a limb.

Although they are sometimes present at the same time, this chapter will cover acute hematogenous osteomyelitis and acute hematogenous septic arthritis separately.

ACUTE HEMATOGENOUS OSTEOMYELITIS

Acute osteomyelitis is an infection of bone most often caused by the hematogenous spread of bacteria. It may occur in adults but is primarily seen in children. Osteomyelitis may also be caused by trauma or by penetrating wounds with subsequent direct inoculation of the bone by bacteria.

Acute osteomyelitis most commonly is caused by hematogenous spread. Staphylococcus aureus is the most common causative agent, followed by β-hemolytic streptococcus, Streptococcus pneumoniae, Escherichia coli, and Pseudomonas aeruginosa.[1, 2, 3] The incidence of infection by haemophilus influenzae has declined dramatically because of widespread HIB vaccination.[3, 4, 5]

Pathophysiology

The most common site is the metaphyseal region of a long bone. An understanding of the pathophysiology of this condition requires knowledge of the vascular supply of this region. The nutrient vessel enters the diaphysis and branches to send small arterioles to the metaphysis. These vessels empty into venous lakes that in turn drain into the medullary cavity. In neonates, some of the arterioles cross the growth plate to supply the cartilaginous epiphysis. With time, the epiphysis develops its own blood supply and communication between the metaphysis and epiphysis is no longer present. This distinct separation of metaphyseal and epiphyseal circulation continues until closure of the physis.

Hobo demonstrated that bacteria injected into the osseous circulation caused infection in the metaphysis of a long bone.[6] Some physicians hypothesize that two factors are responsible for this occurrence: (1) bacteria lodge in the sluggish venous lakes of the metaphysis and (2) reticuloendothelial cells are sparse in that area. After bacteria have become lodged in the region, an inflammatory response develops. Pus forms and may spread in several directions. Spread toward the medullary canal may occur but is readily walled off by the diaphysis. The direction of remaining spread depends to some extent on the age of the child. In neonates, pus may spread to the epiphysis via the blood vessels that cross the physis. In infants and children, pus spreads through the cortex and becomes subperiosteal. The periosteum in the child is thick and easily elevated by pus allowing spread along the shaft of the bone. Pus in the bone destroys the endosteal circulation, while the periosteal circulation to the bone is destroyed when the periosteum is elevated. The cortex becomes devascularized and forms a sequestrum. The well vascularized peri-oseum lays down reactive new bone in an attempt to wall off the spreading infection and forms an involucrum.

Clinical Presentation

The most common complaint is pain. Neonates and infants usually will not use the involved extremity due to pain. The older child often will not use the extremity or, if the lower extremity is involved, will limp severely or refuse to bear weight. There may or may not be a history of trauma or of recent infection elsewhere in the body. It must be remembered that children fall every day, usually with very little sequelae. Often parents or the child may attribute symptoms to an injury. Trauma may causally be related to the production of osteomyelitis. Besides pain and refusal to use the limb, initial complaints may include fever, malaise, and decreased or absent appetite.

Pain, tenderness, erythema, and warmth over the metaphyseal region of a long bone indicates acute hematogenous osteomyelitis until proven otherwise. Swelling, erythema, and warmth are usually demonstrable in joints other than the hip. Fever is usually, but not always, present. Examination of the child must be careful, systematic, and above all gentle. In infants and young children, the first examiner often has the best chance at a reliable exam. Considerable patience is required. Very gentle joint range of motion should be performed and the metaphysis should be evaluated for tenderness. Careful, slow movement of the joint is usually tolerated with osteomyelitis, but not with septic arthritis.

Laboratory Evaluation

The diagnosis of early hematogenous osteomyelitis cannot be made with any single noninvasive test. The white blood cell count (WBC) is often, but not always, elevated. The erythrocyte sedimentation rate (ESR) is more consistently elevated but is not specific.

Radiographic bone changes (rarefaction, lysis, periosteal elevation) are not seen for 7 to 14 days after the onset of symptoms (Figure 1). Deep soft tissue swelling may be seen early and is good evidence of the presence of osteomyelitis. Comparison radiographs are helpful[7].

The technetium 99m bone scan is a sensitive test for the presence of osteomyelitis. The intensity of uptake becomes more focal and intense at the area of interest, and when positive on all three phases is highly sensitive for osteomyelitis (73% to 100% sensitivity). [8, 9, 19]. It is not specific, hower, and carrier a significant incidence of false positives and

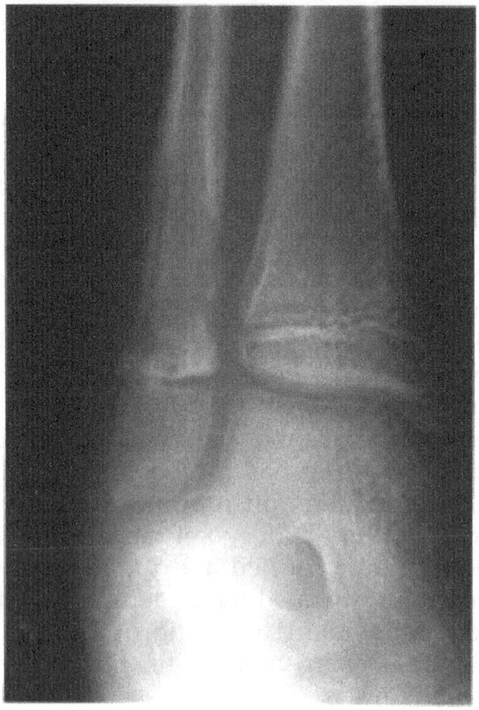

Fig. 11.1: Advanced radiographic changes of acute hematogenous osteomyelitis of the distal fibula.

negativesIn a recent metaanalysis the pooled sensitivity reached 61% but the specificity was the lowest (25%) compared with leukocyte scintigraphy and MRI.[11]

Since the radioisotope localizes in areas of increased vascularity or new bone formation, a positive scan may be seen in fractures, tumors, and inflammatory processes. Unfortunately the bone scan has developed a reputation as the single best test for the diagnosis of osteomyelitis. In the right situations, it can be useful. It can be, and often is overused. There is no reason to get a bone scan when radiographic changes are present. The scan is often unreliable in neonates and in the distal extremities. Nuclear imaging is most helpful in the diagnosis of axial skeletal infections and when multiple foci of infection are suspected.

Gallium scan has improved specificity compared with the three-phase bone scan alone.[12, 13] The reported sensitivity for gallium scan has ranged from 25% to 80%, with a specificity of 67%.[14, 15] A gallium scan can be obtained in conjunction with technetium (Tc) scan in the same patient, and the information that is obtained may be more useful than that of either examination alone[16]

The use of radiolabelled antibiotics is fast emerging as a promising diagnostic test for the detection of infective lesions because of their specific binding to the bacterial component.[17] The main advantage of these agents may be the differentiation between infection and sterile inflammatory lesions.[18,,19] The normal Infecton (ciprofloxacin labelled with Tc-99m) image shows high uptake by the kidneys with excretion to the urinary bladder, moderate uptake by the liver and spleen, and no uptake by bone or bone marrow.[20] In a population of 102 patients who had various infections undergoing an Infecton scan, the authors reported an overall sensitivity and specificity of the method of 83% and 91%, respectively.[20]

Serial blood cultures are positive in 30% to 60% of cases.[21-24] Cultures of blood and material aspirated by needle of the involved bone yield positive findings in up to 87% of cases[25, 26] and the yield from sub-periosteal aspiration approaches 90%.[27]

Aspiration should be done before nuclear imaging. It does not interfere with later bone scanning and may make it unnecessary. Figure 2 demonstrates a logical workup for patients with suspected bone or joint infections.

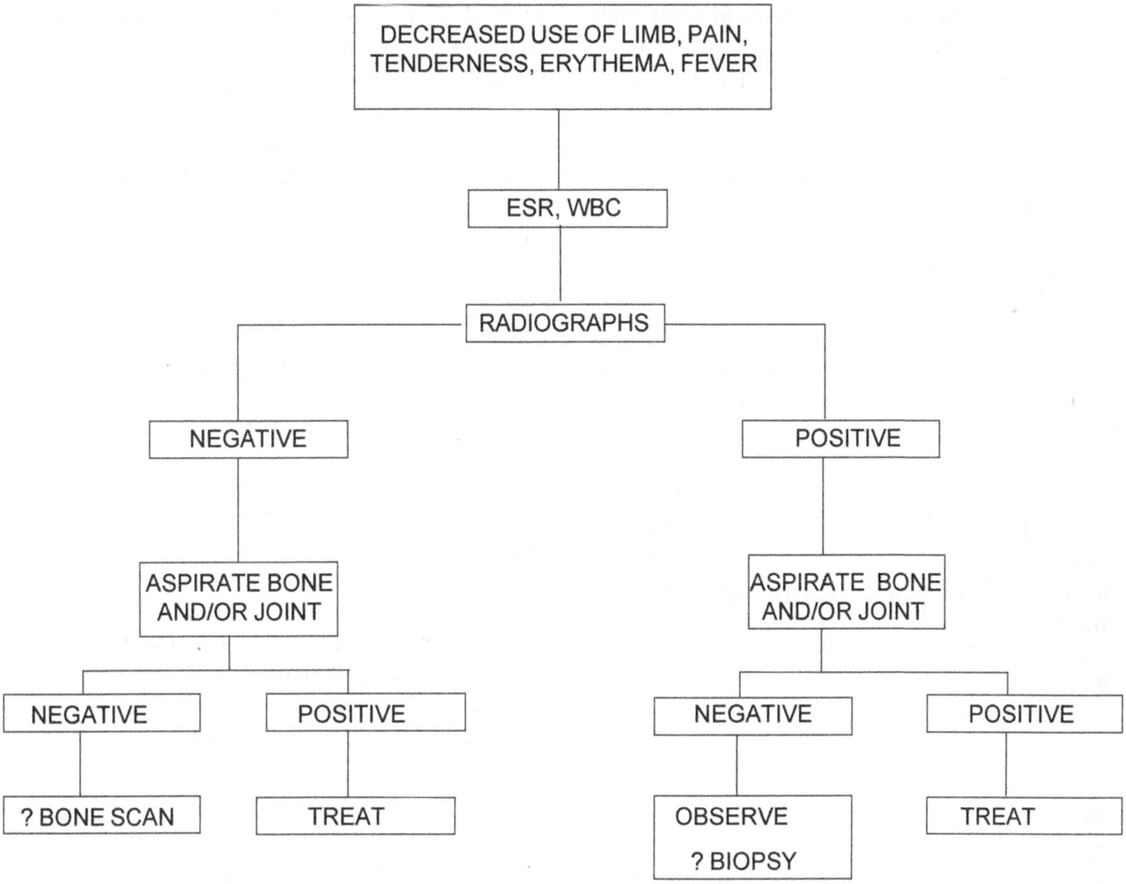

Fig. 2: Suggested workup of suspected bone and joint infections in children

Differential Diagnosis

The diagnosis of osteomyelitis is usually not difficult when a high index of suspicion is maintained. The presence of trauma may lead one away from the correct diagnosis. Clinically erythema and swelling may be attributed to cellulitis, which is usually caused by a penetrating wound or bite and which tends to be well localized and not associated with deep bone tenderness. As was stated previously, tenderness, swelling and erythema near the metaphyseal region of a long bone must be considered to be osteomyelitis until it is proven to be otherwise. Septic arthritis may be confused with osteomyelitis or may be present in addition to osteomyelitis.

Radiographically osteomyelitis is most often confused with a bone tumor or fracture. The clinical history and laboratory findings will usually be helpful, but in some instances, only a biopsy will establish the diagnosis when tumor is suspected.

Management

The proper management of bone and joint infections in children continues to be controversial. There is little disagreement, however, that outcome is improved with early diagnosis and rapid institution of treatment. Antibiotics are the mainstay of treatment for acute osteomyelitis. The place of surgery is more controversial.

Antibiotics alone are often sufficient for the treatment of acute osteomyelitis. This requires early institution of treatment with the right antibiotic. It is often necessary to begin antibiotic therapy before an organism has been identified. The choice of antibiotic depends on the age of the patient. Neonates require coverage against penicillin resistant *Staphylococcus aureus, Group B Streptococcus,* and enteric organisms. Initial therapy therefore usually consists of a penicillinase-resistant penicillin in combination with an aminoglycoside. More recently, cefotaxime alone has been used in this age group. In infants and older children, *Staplococcus aureus* is responsible for at least eighty percent of all cases of osteomyelitis, and initial use of a penicillinase-resistant penicillin is recommended.

In a French nationwide survey, 80% of centres used an association of 3rd generation cephalosporin plus fosfomycin or an association of penicillin M and aminoglycoside, followed by oral penicillin M or pristinamycin. Intravenous therapy lasted 7 to 14 days in 72% of the centres.[28] Similarly, Belgian authors recommend oxacillin (>5 years) or a combination of oxacillin with cefotaxime (< 5years) in the empirical treatment of osteoarticular infection.[29] For treatment of MRSA infections, clindamycin, vancomycin and linezolid are commonly prescribed antibiotics.[30]

At present, there seems to be a general consensus that a short period of intravenous (IV) therapy can be followed by oral therapy.

In general, oral therapy requires good initial response to intravenous therapy, identification of a specific organism, and patient compliance. The time of treatment required for adequate treatment has not been well documented. In the absence of good prospective studies, most authors use a course of six weeks of therapy.[31-33]

Most authors agree that at least some form of surgical therapy is useful in certain cases of osteomyelitis.[1,31,32] Indications for surgery include the demonstration of an abscess (from subperiosteal or bone aspiration) and unresponsiveness to medical therapy after two to three days. Figure 3 summarizes a recommended treatment protocol for acute osteomyelitis.

ACUTE SEPTIC ARTHRITIS

Early diagnosis and early institution of treatment is even more important in cases of septic arthritis than in osteomyelitis since pus rapidly destroys joints. Infection may be established in one of three ways: (1) by hematogenous spread to the synovium, (2) by direct extension from an adjacent osteomyelitis, and (3) by direct traumatic introduction of bacteria into the joint. It most commonly involves the joints of the lower extremity, especially the knee and the hip. Spread from a focus of osteomyelitis occurs by two possible mechanisms depending on the age of the patient. In neonates, the infection spreads across the physis into the epiphysis. This explains the association of osteomyelitis with almost every case of neonatal septic arthritis. In infants and children, spread occurs directly from the bone into the joint space when the metaphysis is intra-articular (hip, shoulder, elbow).

Pathophysiology

After introduction of bacteria into the joint by either direct inoculation or hematogenous spread, bacteria are phagocytized by the synovium, and an intense inflammatory response occurs. The synovium produces an exudate of synovial fluid and white blood cells. Pus forms in the joint, and destructive enzymes released by the synovium, white

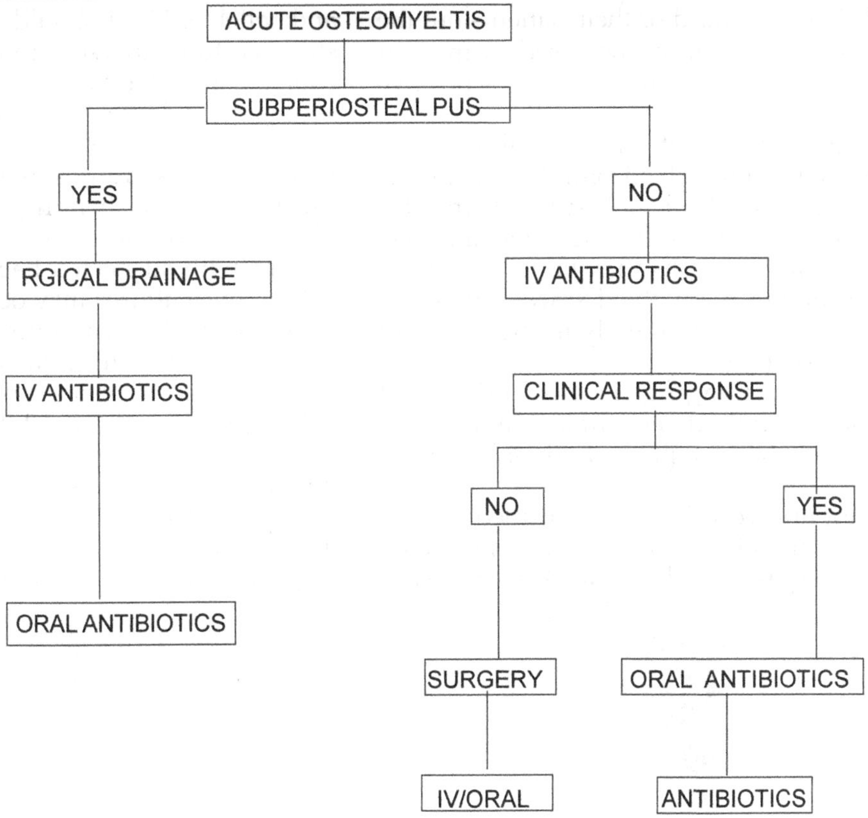

Figure 3

cells, and some bacteria begin to destroy the cartilage matrix. The loss of ground substance changes the mechanical properties of the cartilage and the collagen becomes susceptible to mechanical destruction. As intra-articular pressure increases, further damage occurs. This is most pronounced in the hip where avascular necrosis can occur following tamponade of the retinacular vessels. It is important to remember that septic arthritis is initiated by bacterial invasion but that joint destruction is in most part caused by the body's response to the infection.

Clinical Presentation

Patients with acute septic arthritis present in a similar fashion to those with acute hematogenous osteomyelitis. Diagnosis in the neonate may be extremely difficult, and bone/joint infection may be identified as part ot a sepsis workup. The neonate usually will not move the involved extremity *(pseudo-paralysis)*. The infant or child usually has extreme pain and tenderness and will not allow active or passive movement of the joint. Children will not bear weight if the lower extremity is affected. The hip joint, if it is involved, is held in flexion, abduction, and external rotation. Rotation of the joint will elicit crying from the child due to pain. More superficial joints are usually swollen, erythematous, and warm. Any joint motion causes pain and guarding. The patient appears ill and is irritable. Fever is usually; but not always, present.

Laboratory Evaluation

Morrey and associates found an elevated

WBC in only a third of their patients but the ESR was significantly increased in most of the patients.[35] Blood cultures may be positive in a third of cases.

Radiographs of the involved and contralateral uninvolved joint should be done but are not often helpful.[36] Capsular distention or deep soft tissue swelling may by seen. Radiographs may be more helpful when the hip is involved since joint space widening can be seen early in the course of the disease (Figure 4).

Nuclear imaging is not useful. It characteristically demonstrates mild diffuse uptake of the isotope on both sides of the joint.

Suppurative arthritis is confirmed by joint aspiration. Failure to aspirate a suspected septic joint is inexcusable as it is easy, safe, and reliable. Fluid should be sent for gram stain, culture, and sensitivity and for a cell count. Using blood culture bottles to culture synovial fluid specimens may increase the yield of the offending microorganism.[37] Blood cultures are positive in about half of the patients with nongonococcal septic arthritis and should be obtained in any patient with suspected bacterial arthritis.[38, 39] Negative cultures may occur in those who have received recent antimicrobial therapy or are infected with a fastidious organism, such as some streptococci or mycoplasma. A WBC greater than 50,000 is strongly suggestive of septic arthritis although inflammatory arthritis may also present with very high WBCs. Both septic arthritis and inflammatory arthritis have a predominance of polymorphonuclear leukocytes (greater

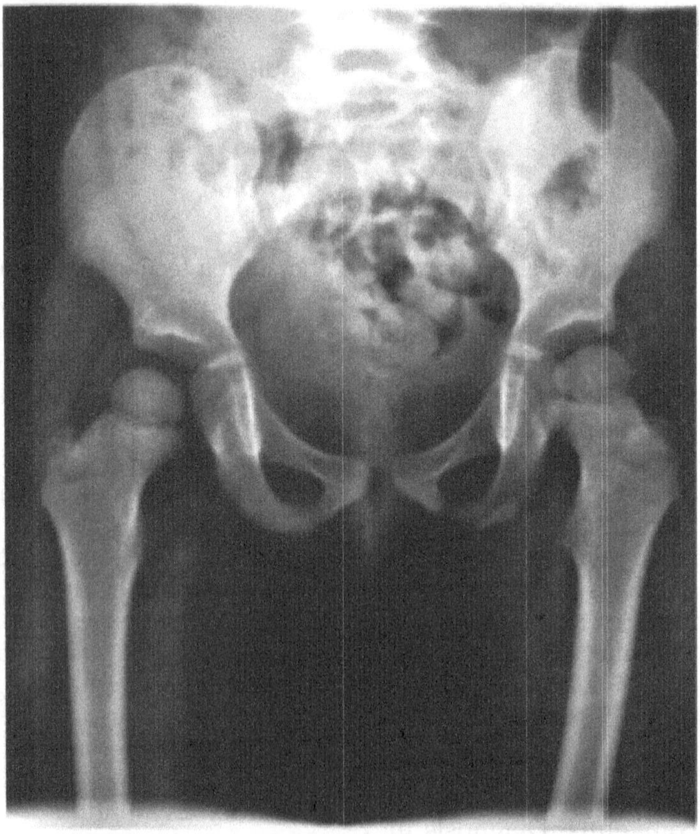

Fig. 4: Widened joint space in a child with septic arthritis of the right hip

than 75 percent). Any remaining fluid may be sent for protein and glucose determinations. In septic arthritis, the former should be elevated (greater than 2.5 percent gm) while the glucose level will be 40 to 50 mg/ 100 ml less than the serum value (drawn simultaneously).

If synovial fluid cannot be obtained with closed-needle aspiration, the joint should be aspirated under CT or fluoroscopic or ultrasound guidance. Certain joints, such as the hip or sacroiliac joints, may require surgical arthrotomy for diagnostic aspiration.

The usefulness of polymerase chain reaction in the diagnosis and management of many infectious diseases, including septic arthritis, is still being defined.[40]

Scintigraphy, CT scanning, or MRI is far more sensitive than plain films in early septic arthritis. CT is more useful to detect effusions and inflammation in joints that are difficult to examine, especially in the hip, sternoclavicular, and sacroiliac joints. MRI demonstrates adjacent soft tissue edema and abscesses and may be especially helpful in detecting septic sacroiliitis. [41-43]

Differential Diagnosis

The clinical presentation of the child with septic arthritis may be mimicked by several other conditions. Cellulitis and osteomyelitis may present in a similar fashion. Juvenile rheumatoid arthritis, acute rheumatic fever, transient synovitis, and even Legg-Perthes disease may present with a sensitive joint. Joint aspiration usually will readily differentiate septic arthritis from the other conditions.

Management

Treatment has two aims: (1) that the joint must be sterilized and (2) that products of the inflammatory response must be removed. Antibiotics easily cross the synovial barrier and reach sufficient concentration in the joint. Intra-articular antibiotics are not necessary. The method of removal of pus and debris from the joint is controversial.

As with osteomyelitis, adequate antibiotic management requires a short course of IV antibiotics followed by oral therapy . Optimal treatment times have not been well established. In addition, helpful clinical guidelines include the initial response to antibiotics as well as the status of the ESR.

Treatment must often be initiated before an organism has been identified. Initial management depends therefore on patient age. Neonates are usually infected with enteric organisms, *S. aureus*, or *Group B Streptococcus* so that a course of either a penicillinase-resistant *penicillin* combined with an *aminoglycoside* or the use of *cefotaxime* alone is appropriate. In the age range from 6 to 24 months, both *S. aureus* and *H. influenzae* are common, and initial treatment needs to cover both organisms. Cefotaxime or cefuroxime cross the blood-joint barrier, and therefore both are effective against resistant strains of S. *aureus* and *H. influenzae.* Children older than five years are treated with a penicillinase-resistant penicillin. Of course after precise organism identification the antibiotic regimen should be changed when necessary.

The method of joint drainage possibly remains the most controversial issue in the treatment of bone and joint infections in children. Choices include multiple needle aspirations, open arthrotomy, and arthroscopy. Virtually all authors concur with immediate arthrotomy for the hip joint.[43-45] Disagreement exists when treating joints other than the hip. The most important factor determining the outcome of septic arthritis is time from onset of symptoms to initiation of treatment.[46] If treatment is begun less than five days after the onset of symptoms, a single aspiration accompanie by appropriate antibiotics will frequently lead to a good result. If the patient does not show a rapid clinical response or if fluid reaccumulates rapidly, drainage by arthrotomy or arthroscopy should be performed, and will ultimately produce a satisfactory result. Multiple needle aspirations are not recommended. They are painful and can further damage the joint. Early institution of treatment is more important than the method of drainage. The protocol (Figure 5) summarizes a recommended treatment regimen for acute septic arthritis of joints other than the hip.

CONCLUSIONS

The advent of antibiotics, newer diagnostic techniques, and perhaps the changing character of the infections has improved the outcome of the treatment of acute hematogenous osteomyelitis and acute septic arthritis. Mortality in the otherwise normal patient is virtually nonexistent today. Sequelae from the delayed diagnosis and improper treatment of these conditions, however, are still present. These include joint destruction, chronic osteomyelitis, and length and angular deformities of bone — each of which can be permanently disabling. A high index of suspicion combined with treatment based on the pathophysiology of the disease will lead to a satisfactory result in the majority of cases. This approach recognizes that not all cases can be treated medically and that not all cases require surgery and emphasizes early diagnosis and rapid institution of treatment.

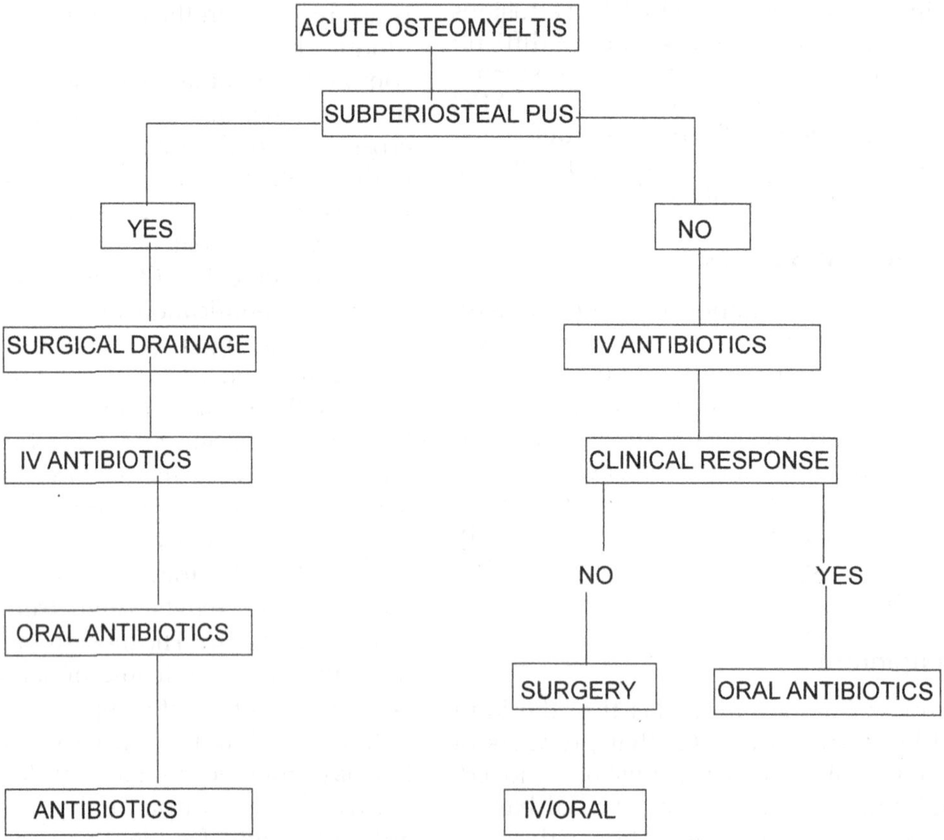

Fig. 5: Suggested treatment protocol for acute hematogenous septic arthritis

REFERENCES

1. Kaplan S. Osteomyelitis in children. Infect Dis Clin N Am 2005; 19:787–97.
2. Nelson JD. Acute osteomyelitis in children. Infect Dis Clin N Am 1990; 4:513.
3. Karwowska A, Davies H, Jadavji T. Epidemiology and outcome of osteomyelitis in the era of sequential intravenous-oral therapy. Pediatr Infect Dis J 1998; 17:1021.
4. Bowerman S, Green N, Menco G. Decline of bone and joint infections attributable to Haemophilus influenzae type B. Clin Orthop 1997; 341:128.
5. Christiansen P, Frederiksen B, Glazowski J, *et al.* Epidemiologic, bacteriologic and long term follow up data of children with acute hematogenous osteomyelitis and septic arthritis. J Pediatr Orthop 1999; 8:302.
6. Hobo T. Zur pathogenese der akuten haemotogenen osteomyelitis. Medicinalis Universitatis Imperialis in Kioto. Acta Scholae 1921;4:1-30.
7. Pineda C, Vargas Al, Rodri guez AV. Imaging of Osteomyelitis: Current Concepts. Infect Dis Clin N Am 2006: 20; 789–825.
8. Maurer AH, Chen DCP, Camargo EE, *et al.* Utility of three-phase skeletal scintigraphy in suspected osteomyelitis: Concise communication. J Nucl Med 1981; 22:941–9.
9. Alazraki N, Dries DJ, Datz F, *et al.* Value of a 24 hour image four phase scan in assessing osteomyelitis in patients with peripheral vascular disease. J Nucl Med 1985; 26:711–7.
10. Schauwecker DS. The scintigraphic diagnosis of osteomyelitis. AJR Am J Roentgenol 1992; 158:9–18.
11. Termaat MF, Raijmakers PG, Scholtein HJ, *et al.* The accuracy of diagnostic imaging for the assessment of chronic osteomyelitis: A systematic review and Meta-analysis. J Bone Joint Surg 2005; 87:2464–71.
12. Concia E, Prandini N, Massari L, *et al.* Osteomyelitis: Clinical update for practical guidelines. Nucl Med Commun. 2006;27:645-60.
13. Peters AM. The use of nuclear medicine in infections. Br J Radiol 1998;71:252–61.
14. Al-Sheikh W, Sfakianakis GN, Mnaymneh W, *et al.* Subacute and chronic bone infections: Diagnosis using In-111, Ga-67 and Tc-99m MDP bone scintigraphy and radiography. Radiology 1985;155:501–6.
15. Schauwecker DS, Burt RW, Park HW, *et al.* Evaluation of complicating osteomyelitis with Tc-99m MDP, In-111 granulocytes, and Ga-67 citrate. J Nucl Med 1984; 25: 848–53.
16. Lewin JS, Rosenfield NS, Hoffer PB, *et al.* Acute osteomyelitis in children: Combined Tc-9m and Ga-67 imaging. Radiology 1986; 158:795.
17. Singh B, Mittal BR, Bhattacharya A, *et al.* Technetium-99m ciprofloxacin imaging in the diagnosis of postsurgical bony infection and evaluation and the response to antibiotic therapy: A case report. J Orthop Surg (Hong Kong) 2005; 13:190–4.
18. Singh AK. 99mTc-4 flouroquinolone: Evaluation as a specific infection imaging agent. Indian J Nucl Med 1997; 12:148.
19. Britton KE, Wareham DW, Das SS, *et al.* Imaging bacterial infection with 99mTc-ciprofloxacin (Infecton). J Clin Pathol 2002; 55:817–23.
20. Britton KE, Vinjamuri S, Hall AV, *et al.* Clinical evaluation of technetium—99m Infecton for the localization of bacterial infection. Eur J Nucl Med 1997; 24:553–6.
21. Riise OR, Kirkhus E, Handeland KS, *et al.* Childhood osteomyelitis-incidence and differentiation from other acute onset musculoskeletal features in a population-based study. BMC Pediatr 2008; 8:45.
22. Rasmont Q, Yombi JC, Van der Linden D, Docquier PL. Osteoarticular infections in Belgian children: A survey of clinical, biological, radiological and microbiological data. Acta Orthop Belg 2008; 74:374-85.
23. Saavedra-Lozano J, Mejías A, Ahmad N, *et al.* Changing trends in acute osteomyelitis in children: Impact of methicillin-resistant Staphylococcus aureus infections. J Pediatr Orthop 200; 28:569-75.
24. Dieckmann R, Hardes J, Ahrens H, *et al.* Treatment of acute and chronic osteomyelitis in children. Z Orthop Unfall 2008; 146:375-80.
25. Howard CB, Einhorn M, Dagan R, *et al.* Fine-needle bone biopsy to diagnose osteomyelitis. J Bone Joint Surg Br 1994; 76:311.
26. Willis RB, Rozencwaig R. Pediatric osteomyelitis masquerading as skeletal neoplasia. Orthop Clin N Am 1996; 27:625.

27. Karwowska A, Davies H, Jadavji T. Epidemiology and outcome of osteomyelitis in the era of sequential intravenous oral therapy. Pediatr Infect Dis J 1998; 17:1021.
28. Milcent K, Guitton C, Koné-Paut I. French nationwide survey about management of acute osteomyelitis in children. Arch Pediatr 2009; 16:7-13.
29. Rasmont Q, Yombi JC, Van der Linden D, Docquier PL. Osteoarticular infections in Belgian children: A survey of clinical, biological, radiological and microbiological data. Acta Orthop Belg. 2008; 74:374-85.
30. Saphyakhajon P, Joshi AY, Huskins WC, Henry NK, Boyce TG. Empiric antibiotic therapy for acute osteoarticular infections with suspected methicillin-resistant Staphylococcus aureus or Kingella. Pediatr Infect Dis J 2008; 27:765-7.
31. Zaoutis T, Localio AR, Leckerman K, Saddlemire S, Bertoch D, Keren R. Prolonged intravenous therapy versus early transition to oral antimicrobial therapy for acute osteomyelitis in children. Pediatrics 2009; 123:636-42.
32. Weichert S, Sharland M, Clarke NM, Faust SN. Acute haematogenous osteomyelitis in children: Is there any evidence for how long we should treat? Curr Opin Infect Dis 2008; 21:258-62.
33. Cohen R. Shorten treatment of severe osteomyelitis in children Arch Pediatr 2007; 14:S128-30. 37.
34. Ogden JA, Lister G. The pathology of neonatal osteomyelitis. Pediatrics 1975 ;4:474-479.
35. Morrey BF, Bianco AJ, Rhodes KH. Septic arthritis in children. Orthop Clin North Am 1975;6:923-934.
36. Welkon CJ, Long SS, Fisher MC, *et al.* Pyogenic arthritis in infants and children: A review of 95 cases. Pediatr Infect Dis 1986;5 :669-676.
37. Von Essen R. Culture of joint specimens in bacterial arthritis: Impact of blood culture bottle utilization. Scand J Rheumatol 1997; 26:293–300.
38. Kortekangas P, Aro HT, Lehtonen OP. Synovial fluid culture and blood culture in acute arthritis: A multi-case report in 90 patients. Scand J Rheumatol 1995; 24:44–7.
39. Esterhai JL Jr, Gelb I. Adult septic arthritis. Orthop Clin North Am 1991; 22:503–14.
40. Post JC, Ehrlich GD. The impact of the polymerase chain reaction in clinical medicine. JAMA 2000; 283:1544–6.
41. Garcia-De La Torre I. Advances in the Management of Septic Arthritis. Infect Dis Clin N Am 2006; 20: 773–788.
42. Forrester DM, Feske WI. Imaging of infectious arthritis. Semin Roentgenol 1996; 31:239–49.
43. Zimmerman B III, Mikolich DJ, Lally EV. Septic sacroiliities. Semin Arthritis Rheum 1996; 26:592–604.
44. Bynum DR, Nunley JA, Goldner JL, *et al.* Pyogenic arthritis: Emphasis on the need for surgical drainage of the infected joint. South Med J 1982;75:1232-1235.
45. Goldenberg DL, Brandt KD, Cohen AS, *et al.* Treatment of septic arthritis. Comparison of needle aspiration and surgery as initial modes of joint drainage. Arth Rheun 1975;18:83-90.
46. Howard JB, Highgenboten CL, Nelson JD. Residual effects of septic arthritis in infancy and childhood. JAMA 1976;236:932-935.
47. Herndon WA, Knauer S, Sullivan JA, *et al.* Management of septic arthritis in children. J Pediatr Orthop 1986;6:576-578.

Dipak Sheth

20 Major Multiple Trauma

Major trauma is defined as a severe, potentially life-threatening injury to one body system or serious multisystem injuries. Almost every child who sustains injuries of these types will require hospitalization for operative intervention, intensive care, or close observation. The physician in the emergency department should anticipate specific patterns of injuries associated with common mechanisms of trauma (for example, high-speed motor vehicle occupant, fall from significant height) and should be prepared to manage the child during the first hour in the hospital. This management includes assessing the extent of injuries, resuscitating the child in the trauma bay, intervening for abnormal vital signs or laboratory values, and developing a general plan for the patient's care after leaving the trauma room.

Children die from injuries more than from any other cause after the first year of life. More than 45% of all death in children from 1 to 14 years is the result of trauma. Over 5000 traumatic deaths per year occur within this age group; 805 of this mortality were unintentional and 47% directly related motor vehicle collisions (MVC). Injury accounts for approximately 5% of infant death as well.[1,2] In US, The most fatalities occur in the field before arrival at a health care facility.

The most common single organ system injury associated with death in injured children is head trauma.[3,4] Because multiple trauma is common in children, the emergency physician must evaluate all organ systems in any injured child, regardless of the actual mechanism of injury.

Because of the high annual incidence of childhood trauma, the emergency physician should be prepared to manage the severely injured child. Preparation also implies institutional readiness—a fully equipped location in the Emergency Department and a coordinated response team. No health care provider alone can adequately deliver care to the child with severe injuries. A team of individuals are necessary to perform various functions in the trauma room: manage the airway, establish vascular access, obtain blood specimens, monitor and record frequent vital signs, and intervene to stabilize the child. The other half of the support team outside the trauma room should include an individual to talk with family members in a quiet room, a radiology technologist, transport personnel, a security officer, and a nursing supervisor who controls traffic and functions as coordinator of communication with consultants, the operating room, and the central laboratory. At the Children's

National Medical Center in Washington, D.C., 16 people respond to "trauma stats" with subsequent assessment and stabilization of most trauma patients within 15 minutes. In the general hospital setting where adult trauma assumes the larger role, the trauma team should practice occasional drills in response to different pediatric trauma scenarios.

PATTERNS OF INJURY

While each child is an individual, injury patterns repeat themselves. Some common injury mechanisms and their outcomes are:

1. Unrestrained occupant in a motor vehicle travelling over 25 mph
   a. Closed head injury.
   b. Maxillofacial trauma.
   c. Cervical spine injury.
   d. Blunt trauma to chest and abdomen.
2. Restrained occupant of a motor vehicle travelling over 40 mph
   a. Whiplash.
   b. Abdominal lap-belt injuries (abdominal contents compressed against lumbosacral spine).
   c. Lumbar spine fractures or dislocations.
3. Pedestrian or cyclist struck by motor vehicle travelling over 25 mph
   a. Lower extremity fractures (femur, tibia, and fibula fractures).
   b. Deep lacerations with significant blood loss.
   c. If the child is thrown into the air: skull fracture, open or closed head injury, cervical spine injuries, blunt abdominal trauma.
   d. If the child is run over: blunt chest and abdominal trauma, rib fractures, pneumothorax and pelvic fractures.
4. Fall from height greater than 10 feet
   a. Central nervous system (CNS) trauma (skull fracture, spinal cord injuries).
   b. Long bone and foot fractures.
   c. Blunt abdominal trauma including injuries to the liver, spleen or kidney.
5. Penetrating trauma from stabbing or firearm injury.
   a. Disrupted arterial or venous blood supply.
   b. Perforated viscus.
   c. Pneumothorax.
6. Child abuse
   a. Fractures of the ribs, skull, long bones (spiral fractures and metaphyseal chip fractures).
   b. Ecchymoses, lacerations, sphincter tears.
   c. Shaken baby syndrome (unresponsive child, seizures, full fontanelle, retinal hemorrhages, intracerebral bleed).

THE INJURY EVENT AND ACTIVATION OF RESPONSE

There are major anatomic, physiologic, and psychological differences in the pediatric and adult patients. These play a major role in the evaluation and management of the pediatric trauma patient. Compared to adult, the child's body size allows for a greater distribution of traumatic injuries, causing multiple trauma. The child has a greater relative body surface area causing greater heat loss as a result of evaporation. Therefore there is greater requirement of free water, trace minerals and metals in a child with injury. The internal organs like liver and spleen of the child are placed anteriorly subjecting them to more susceptible to injury. This is compounded by the lack of musculature and subcutaneous tissue to protect these organs. The kidney is highly susceptible to deceleration injury because it is not well protected and more mobile. The Salter Harris type fracture is common in children because the growth plates are not closed. These fractures if not treated properly can cause limb-length discrepancy with healing. The head-to-body ration is greater in child, the cranial bones are thinner and brain is less myelinated resulting in more serious injury to head. Physiologically, children respond to pain differently than adults depending on the age and maturation of the child and the severity of the injury. Unlike adults, children have a greater capacity to maintain blood pressure despite significant acute blood losses (25%). Therefore any subtle change in heart rate, blood pressure and extremity perfusion may indicate impending cardiorespiratory failure and should not be overlooked. Psychologically, they are often dispropor-tionately irritable relative to their degree of injury, making assessment more difficult. Schafer has shown that about 25% of children will show signs of posttraumatic stress disorder after discharge from the hospital.[9]

A serious injury event occurs involving a child. Witnesses activate the emergency medical service (EMS) system; paramedics arrive and begin a field assessment and stabilization (Table 1). Depending on the geographic locale, the child is transported to the medical center as a "scoop and run" or a well-packaged, immobilized patient with an intravenous (IV) line established. Ideally the hospital is alerted and given an estimated time of arrival prior to the patient's appearance. The hospital physician in charge assesses the potential severity of the child's injuries and determines the level of institutional response. For example, in the child with relatively minor injuries and stable vital signs, no loss of consciousness, or an isolated injury such as a supracondylar fracture with good distal pulse, the trauma team is not required. The endotracheal tube intubation may not be the most effective means of ventilation in the prehospital setting. BVM is as effective and may be safer than endotracheal intubation in prehospital setting[10]. In the more severely injured child, the trauma team is alerted. Institutional criteria vary on when to activate the trauma team. Some of the guidelines used at the Children's National Medical Center in Washington, D.C., are included in Table 2.

FIRST FIVE MINUTES IN THE HOSPITAL PRIMARY SURVEY AND RESUSCITATION

When a child arrives in the trauma bay, multiple functions take place simultaneously. A paramedic provides a concise thirty-second report. The child is immobilized on a back-board with protection of the cervical spine by an appropriately-sized collar. The patient is disrobed and personnel apply cardio-respiratory monitor leads, a blood pressure cuff and pulse oximeter. Universal precautions are taken by everyone dealing with a bleeding child, handling blood specimens, or performing phlebotomy.

Table 1: Pediatric trauma score

Component	*+2*	*+1*	*– 1*
Size	> 20 kg	10-20 kg	< 10 kg
Airway	Normal	Maintainable	Unmaintainable
Central nervous system	Awake	Obtunded	Comatose
Systolic blood pressure	> 90 mmHg	90-50 mmHg	<50 mmHg
Open wounds	None	Minor	Major or penetrating
Skeletal	None	Closed fracture	Open/multiple fracture
Palpable pulse*	At wrist	At groin	Not palpable

* "Used only if a proper sized blood pressure cuff is not available.

Adapted from McCarty DL, Surpure JS. Pediatric trauma: Initial evaluation and stabilization. Pediatric Annals 1990;19:584.

Table 2: Criteria for trauma stat

1. Mechanism of injury
   a. Unrestrained occupant at speeds of 25 mph or greater
   b. Restrained occupant at speeds of 40 mph or greater
   c. Hit by vehicle at speed of at least 20 mph
   d. Occupant ejected from vehicle
   e. Fall from height of 10 feet or greater
   f. Prolonged vehicle extrication of 20 minutes of more
   g. Dragged underneath vehicle or run over by vehicle wheels
   h. Any injury requiring helicopter evacuation from the scene
2. General location of injuries
   a. Shock following injuries
   b. Respiratory distress following injuries
   c. High suspicion of C-spine injury
   d. Uncontrolled traumatic hemorrhage
   e. Open fractures
   f. Severe maxillofacial injuries
   g. Unstable chest injuries
   h. Major pelvic injuries
   i. Blunt abdominal trauma with hypotension, rigidity, or significant tenderness
   j. Penetrating wound or crush injury to the head, neck, chest, abdomen, pelvis, or groin
   k. Neurological injuries producing prolonged loss of consciousness, altered mental status, posturing, seizures, lateralizing signs, or paralysis
   l. Major amputations
   m. Fracture of long bone in association with other injuries
   n. Two or more proximal long bone fractures
   o. Tracheal and laryngeal injuries
   p. Burns
      1) 20% or greater BSA for children under 2 years
      2) 25% or greater BSA for children from 2 to 4 years
      3) 40% or greater BSA for children 5 years and older
      4) Any burn where smoke inhalation is suspected
3. Physiological distress
   a. Patients with a trauma score of 12 or less
   b. Patients with a Glasgow coma scale (GCS) score of 12 or less
   c. Patients with an injury severity score of 15 or greater
   d. Patients with a history of respiratory or cardiopulmonary arrest following injury

First, the examining physician looks at the entire child for 5 to 10 seconds to determine the overall extent of injuries, level of consciousness, and viability of the patient. The highest priority in the approach of injured child is ruling out the presence of life- or limb-threatening injury. The next the physician begins a systematic approach as described by the American College of Surgeons following the mnemonic "ABCDEFGH": Airway maintenance with C-spine control, breathing, circulation with control of hemorrhage, disability (neurologic status), exposure/ extremities, Foley catheter, gastric tube, history (Figure 1).

The primary survey (ABCDE) rapidly identifies and intervenes for lifethreatening conditions. The resuscitation phase begins almost immediately: providing supplemental oxygen, obtaining vascular access, administering volume-expanding fluids, and eventually completing the mnemonic "FGH" (Foley catheter, gastric tube, and history). Any child or infant with a potentially serious or unstable injury requires continual reassessment. Vital signs should be repeated every 5 minutes during the primary survey and every 15 minutes thereafter until the patient is considered stable. Following the primary survey and resuscitation phase, the secondary survey includes a more thorough physical examination.

Airway with Cervical Spine Control

Compared to adult, children have major differences in the anatomy of airway which has significant implications in a child with multiple trauma. Children have relatively larger tongue which can cause airway obstruction. Therefore they need better head positioning or use of airway adjunct (oropharangeal airway or nasopharangeal airway). Children have large mass of adenoid

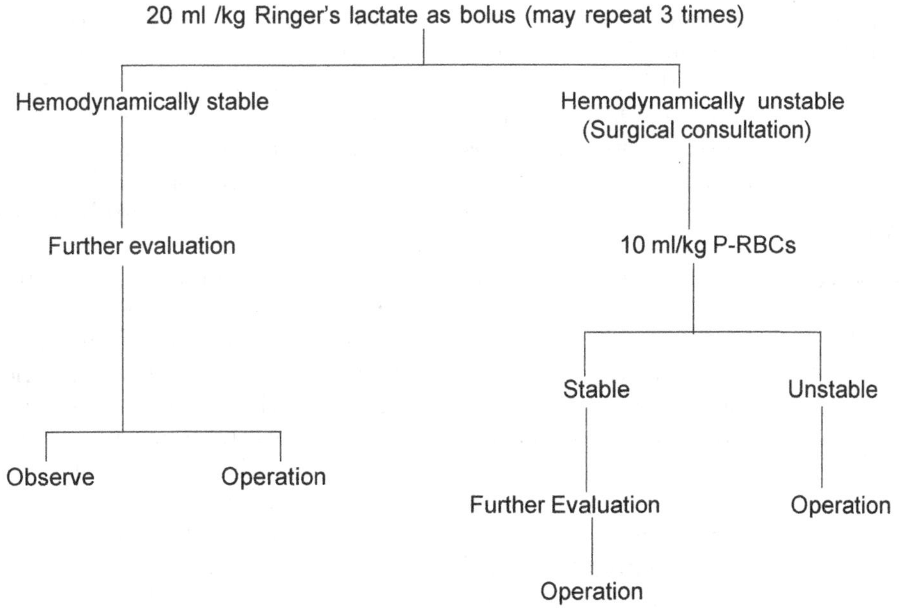

Fig. 1: Resuscitation flow diagram for the stable and unstable pediatric patient (Adapted from American College of Surgeons, Advanced trauma life support manual, 1989)

tissue making nasotracheal intubation more difficult. In children epiglottis is floopy and more omega shaped therefore straight blade is more useful than curved blade for intubation. Larynx is more cephalad and anterior making it more difficult to visualize the vocal cords. The physician may need to get lower than the patient and look at 45-degree angle while intubating. In children the length of trachea is short leading to intubation of right main stem or dislodgement of endotracheal tube.

Assess the patency of the oropharynx. A lusty cry is a welcome sound as it implies an unobstructed airway. Suction blood, saliva, or vomitus from the mouth and throat. The tongue often falls backwards obstructing the pharynx and glottis. A jaw thrust under the angles of the mandible pushes the tongue anterior, reduces noisy respirations, and unblocks the airway.

If the child is already intubated, determine that a proper size endotracheal tube has been used, that it is inserted to a proper depth, and that it has minimal air leak. The endotracheal tube should be securely attached to the patient's face. Other children will require intubation based on indications discussed in the next section.

Breathing

Place 100 percent oxygen on the patient by either mask or nasal cannula.

Inspect the chest for rate and regularity of breathing. Are there periods of apnea-bradypnea, periodic breathing, or Cheynes-Stokes respirations? Are chest excursions symmetric and sufficient to ventilate? Remember that infants are abdominal breathers. Auscultate air movement bilaterally noting asymmetry, decreased breath sounds, or lack of air movement. Suspect a pneumothorax when little or no air exchange is heard and there is poor chest wall movement, cyanosis, or hyperresonant percussion of the thorax. Agitation may be a sign of hypoxia. Hemothorax presents with decreased breath sounds and dullness to percussion. In the child with a suspected pneumothorax who is physiologically stable, obtain a stat chest radiograph. In the unstable patient, an emergent needle thoracocentesis is performed in the fourth intercostal space at the anterior axillary line. Tube thoracostomy with continuous negative pressure is then required. If a hemothorax is suspected, make certain to establish IV access first then give adequate fluid volume prior to evacuating the chest. Any open chest wound must be covered with vaseline gauze to reestablish the integrity of the chest wall.

Patient respirations can be supported with a bag-valve mask and 100 percent oxygen. Be careful to provide only the volume necessary to cause the chest to rise, because excessive volume or rate of ventilation can increase the likelihood of gastric distension and further impair ventilation. Intubation should be performed when a combination of airway, breathing, and neurologic factors are present. Some of the indication to intubate are[1] any inability to ventilate by bag-valve-mask (BVM) methods or the need for prolonged control of airway;[2] Glasgow coma scale (GCS) score of 8 or less to secure the airway and provide controlled hyperventilation if needed;[3] Any patient in uncompensated shock resistant to initial fluid administration.[4] Another common reason to intubate is respiratory failure resulting from either mechanical (flail chest) or neurological factors. Injuries or burns to the face, mouth, or neck often lead to edema and a compromised upper airway.[5] Loss of protective laryngeal reflexes can result into pulmonary aspiration from gastric contents in the vomiting child is another indication for intubation. Intubate whenever optimum control of the airway is paramount such as in the paralyzed child (traumatically or pharmacologically) or in the child with increased intracranial pressure that requires hyperventilation. Rarely cricothyroidotomy is necessary in pediatric patients. In general orotracheal approach is recommended. Problems associated with nasotracheal intubation include inherent difficulties in children, impairment of tube passage by the acute angle of the posterior pharynx, and the probability of causing bleeding within oral cavity and causing increase intracranial pressure with insertion.

Circulation With Control of Bleeding

Apply pressure to any spurting or oozing wounds and maintain pressure on those areas. Assess circulation by looking at skin color and capillary refill, which should be two seconds or less. Listen to the heart to determine pulse rate, quality of heart sounds, or friction rubs. To assess the effectiveness of cardiac contractions, feel central and distal pulses on extremities. In a child, maintenance of a systolic blood pressure does not ensure that the patient is not in shock. This is an effect of the ability of the pediatric vasculature to constrict and increase systemic vascular resistance in an attempt to maintain perfusion. In general palpable peripheral pulse correlates with a systolic blood pressure greater than 80 mm Hg and a palpable central pulse with a pressure greater than 50 mm Hg[12].

Intravenous access is often not obtained in the field, especially in the infant or younger child. Vascular access should be obtained with the largest feasible catheter; success with a 24-gauge catheter, however, is far superior than no access at all. In infants, favored sites are antecubital fossa, saphenous, and dorsum of the hand. Upper extremity is the preferred site of intravenous line, in the absence of available upper extremity peripheral site, lower extremity site could be used. Femoral vein is a preferred site for insertion of a central line, by use of guide wire technique. The external jugular vein is an alternative but is often inaccessible when the cervical spine has not been cleared radio-logically. In the critically injured child, if percutaneous access cannot be obtained in a few minutes, consider an intraosseous route or vascular cut down. Intraosseous access is secured in the proximal tibia on the flat, medial portion two cm below the knee, aimed perpendicularly and away from the tibial growth plate. Use a bone marrow needle with stylet but remember that marrow is often not able to be aspirated, but the needle accepts manual pushes of fluid and medication. Later after volume resuscitation, the usual veins become more readily accessible by percuta-neous attempts. A fractured leg precludes that extremity for intraosseous access. Cut-downs are best performed on saphenous or femoral veins. Cut-down is a skilled technique and takes longer to achieve the line compared to intraosseos route, hence it may not be a preferred procedure during initial resuscitation.

Begin fluid resuscitation in the hypo-volemic patient with Ringer's lactate solution at 20 cc/kg body weight. Remember that hypotension is a late sign of shock, and earlier signs (tachycardia, tachypnea, confusion, delayed capillary refill) require prompt management. If necessary, fluid boluses may be repeated three times and then whole blood (20 cc/kg) or packed cells (10 cc/kg) are administered (Figure 1). In a patient who present in a decompensated shock or cardiopulmonary failure, occult bleeding is a potential cause for the shock, administer crystalloid and blood product simultaneou-sly.[13]

In contrast to the adult, cardiogenic shock is a rare event in the face of childhood injury. However, any degree of chest trauma associated with the presence of shock must alert the clinician to the possibility of concomitant myocardial contusion or rupture. The classic presentation of neurogenic shock, involving hypotension without an increase in heart rate, should be considered in patient with head or neck injury.

Disability

Neurologic disability is briefly assessed. The level of consciousness can be categorized as *alert*, responsive to *voice*, responsive to *pain*, or *unresponsive* (AVPU). The Glasgow Coma Scale (GCS) (ranging from 3 to 15) scores the patient in three areas best motor response, best verbal response, and eye opening (Table 3), A GCS score below 8 is predictive of serious head injury and poor outcome. It is important to rule out hypoglycemia in any patient with altered mental status. This is particularly important in younger children since their glycogen stores are easily depleted, predisposing them to hypoglycemia. In any unconscious child, the examiner should look for signs of increased intracranial pressure and of impending herniation. A more detailed neurologic evaluation can be conducted in the secondary survey.

Exposure/Extremities

The child should be completely disrobed to evaluate all regions of the body. Use trauma scissors to cut away clothing without disturbing the cervical spine or IV lines. This function should begin immediately on admission to the Trauma Room. Remember that children lose heat rapidly and need to be kept normothermic with heating lamps or warmed blankets. Extremities are examined for gross deformities, discoloration, swelling, amputations and lacerations.

At this point the primary survey is complete. The resuscitation phase has begun. Vascular access has been established; monitoring equipment is in place; vital signs have been assessed more than once; blood specimens have been drawn; the airway has

Table 3: Glasgow Coma Scale

Activity	*Score*	*Infants (Best response)*	*Children/Adults*
Eye opening	4	Spontaneous	Spontaneous
	3	To speech or sound	To speech
	2	To painful stimuli	To pain
	1	None	None
Verbal	5	Appropriate words or sounds; social smile; fixes and follows	Oriented
	4	Cries but consolable	Confused
	3	Persistently irritable	Inappropriate words
	2	Restless/agitated	Incomprehensible words
	1	None	None
Motor	6	Spontaneous movement	Obeys commands
	5	Localizes to pain	Localizes pain
	4	Withdraws to pain	Withdraws to pain
	3	Abnormal flexion (decorticate)	Abnormal flexion (decorticate)
	2	Abnormal extension (decerebrate)	Abnormal extension (decorticate)
	1	None	None (flaccid)

been stabilized; and the patient has been intubated if necessary. The FGH of the mnemonic is completed with Foley catheter, gastric tube and history.

Catheter

Urine output is a good measure of adequate perfusion. In young children and unconscious victims, place a Foley catheter to monitor urine production (minimum 2 cc/kghr) accurately. Gross hematuria or severe perineal ecchymoses preclude insertion of a catheter until urethral integrity can be established with an excretory urogram (IVP). Cooperative older children and adolescents may not require an indwelling bladder catheter.

Gastric Tube

A nasogastric tube should be inserted to decompress the stomach and reduce the volume of acidic fluid that could be aspirated. Bloody gastric contents are an early clue to serious abdominal injury. Use an orogastric tube if a cribriform plate fracture potentially exists.

History

Obtain additional history regarding allergies, medication, past illnesses and hospitalization, last meal, and events (mnemonic AMPLE) preceding the injury. Also obtain the history of tetanus immunization, use antibiotics as indicated. Patient should be monitored continuously as needed and ensure urine output of 1 ml /kg/hr.

THE SECOND FIVE MINUTES SECONDARY SURVEY

The secondary survey is a head-to-toe evaluation of the child. Special attention should be paid to the presence or absence of traumatic findings.

Head

Inspect the head for scalp lacerations that can bleed profusely. Is there any visible deformity or open defect? Palpate for asymmetry, depressions, defects, crepitus, and fontanelle size and tension. Large hematomas have raised edges and depressed centers, mimicking depressed skull fractures.

Eyes

Note the position of the eyelids and globes at rest along with any spontaneous movements. Determine if the globe has sustained a penetrating injury or subconjunctival hemorrhage and whether there is bleeding in the anterior chamber. A hyphema in a supine patient distributes around the limbus of the iris. Feel around the orbital rims for signs that indicate fracture such as tenderness, crepitus, or irregularity. Lid ptosis may be a preexisting condition or represent a cerebral hemispheric lesion. Spontaneous blinking indicates an intact pontine reticular formation. Provoked blinking from sound or light implies relevant sensory pathways are intact.

In the unconscious child, the eyes are a helpful gauge of CNS injury and its approximate location. Pupils should be symmetrical and reactive to bright light. Small pupils require close observation or magnification to detect reactivity. Some children have congenital anisocoria, which can explain unequal pupils in the patient without any obvious head trauma. A nonreactive, dilated pupil unilaterally raises the immediate concern of ipsilateral epidural (or subdural) bleeding requiring immediate intervention. If ipsilateral pupil dilation is associated with contralateral hemiplegia, lateral (uncal) herniation is occurring. Bilateral pupillary dilation is associated with central (tentorial) herniation, prolonged hypoxia, and brain death. Remember that some illicit drugs such as cocaine and amphetamine cause large nonreactive pupils as do pharmacologic agents such as atropine. Opiates, barbiturates, and psychotropics cause bilaterally small but reactive pupils.

An intact corneal reflex (lid closure, upward deviation of gaze) implies a normal brain stem from midbrain to lower pons. Oculocephalic (doll's eye) reflexes should never be tested until the cervical spine is deemed uninjured. Similarly oculovestibular reflexes (calorics) should not be performed if tympanic membranes are perforated. Finally the fundi should be examined for retinal hemorrhages, especially in an infant where a shaking injury is a possibility.

Ears

Look for bruising overlying the mastoid (Battle's sign), pathognomonic for basilar skull fracture (along with raccoon eyes or hemotympanum). Blood or gelatinous matter from the ear canals can be an ominous sign of CNS injury. Clear liquid in the ear canals can be spinal fluid or tears, most commonly the latter. Using an otoscope, examine the canal and tympanic membranes, noting perforations or hemotympanum. Hemotympanum has a subtle blue-purple hue rather than bright red. A red, injected tympanic membrane implies infection, a coincidental finding that may explain the presence of fever in many traumatized infants and preschool-aged children.

Nose and Mouth

Are cartilage and nasion aligned or misshapen? Is blood or cerebrospinal fluid (CSF) leaking from nostrils? Are nares patent? A septal hematoma will require evacuation.

The gums, lips, and tongue bleed readily and clot slowly. Attempt to determine the source of any blood loss from the oropharynx. Examine teeth for excess mobility, pain, crown fractures, and intrusions. Completely avulsed teeth can become foreign bodies in the mouth or airway. Disrupted orthodontic hardware in an adolescent may cause bleeding inside the lips as well as great anxiety to the patient and parents. A sublingual hematoma is associated with a midline mandibular fracture. Palpate the temporomandibular joint for tenderness and subluxation on movement.

Neck

If lateral cervical spine films do not rule out fracture, dislocation, compression, or subluxation, leave the collar in place. The radiograph should be reviewed by the treating physician and should expose the complete cervical spine and first thoracic vertebrae. If spinal cord injury without radiologic abnormality (SCIWORA) is suspected, leave the collar in place. Pseudo-subluxation of C2 on C3 is a common finding in children. When the collar is removed, palpate the cervical spine for irregularities or pain. Often the sterno-cleidomastoid muscles are sore after a whiplash event. If discomfort cannot be isolated to the strap muscles only, replace the collar until more definitive studies can be performed, including open mouth views, swimmer's view, and/or computed tomography (CT).

Chest

An anteroposterior (AP) chest radiograph should be performed in all patients to detect bony injuries and pulmonary or cardiac problems. Palpate the length of both clavicles for deformity or crepitus often found in falls and sports injuries. Rib fractures may present with point tenderness but are unusual because the chest wall is so compliant in children. When rib fractures are present, large forces have impacted the thorax. In one study of blunt chest trauma, the presence of four or more rib fractures had a high correlation with mortality.

Heart

Reassess heart sounds. If the heart sounds muffle, neck veins distend, and pulsus paradoxus occurs (exaggerated drop in systolic blood pressure during inspiration), consider the possibility of cardiac tam-ponade. Tamponade is rare in children but should be considered when there has been a direct blow to the chest or any penetrating thoracic injury. Pericardiocentesis is per-formed with a plastic-sheathed needle entering subxy-phoid and aiming toward the heart. A positive pericardiocentesis necessitates open thoracotomy.

Abdomen

Inspect the abdominal wall for distention and ecchymoses. A horizontal band of bruising can occur in the vehicle occupant wearing a lap belt and provides a clue to underlying injury. Similarly ecchymoses on the left or right upper quadrant can indicate spleen or liver lacerations respectively. Listen for the presence of bowel sounds. Palpate for tenderness in each quadrant and flanks. Push downward simultaneously on the anterior iliac spines to check the stability of the pelvic rim in addition to palpating the pubic ramus. Bladder injuries are commonly associated with pelvic fractures. Obtain a urine sample to determine whether hematuria is present; hematuria is defined as greater than ten red blood cells per high power field on microscopy.

Penetrating trauma to the abdomen with violation of the peritoneum will require exploration in the operating room.

Genitalia/Rectum

Look at the integrity of external genitalia. If bruising, swelling or burns have affected the area, insert an indwelling Foley catheter before a urethral obstruction occurs. Perform a digital rectal examination for anal sphincter tone and detection of blood (obvious or occult) in the stool.

Extremities

Obtain AP radiographs of suspected limb fractures. Immobilize arms and legs with suspected fractures and determine the integrity of distal pulses. Absence of distal pulses should prompt a gentle attempt to realign the limb and an urgent arteriogram. A displaced femoral fracture presents with a painful swollen thigh that can hold a significant volume of blood. When a lower leg is broken, tibia and fibula are both commonly affected. If the patient was transported in traction or antishock trousers, use these devices for splinting and immobilization until definitive orthopedic care is rendered.

FURTHER DIAGNOSTIC STUDIES

In the trauma bay, the treating physician must determine which additional studies and consultations are necessary. All children, deserve radiographs of lateral cervical spine, AP chest, and AP pelvis. Any limb deformity should also be radiographed. Additional plain films are indicated to evaluate the lumbosacral spine in children with lap belt injuries. Maxillofacial injuries can be delineated with plain radiographs.

In any child in whom vascular integrity has been compromised, consider contrast angiography. This modality is particularly helpful in penetrating injuries.

CT scans are important diagnostic studies that are invaluable in assessing head injuries and blunt abdominal trauma. Any child with a suspected skull fracture, loss of consciousness, or ongoing coma requires a CT scan of the head. With questionable findings on plain films, a CT can clarify issues surrounding the cervical spine.

Serious abdominal trauma occurs in one quarter of all multiply traumatized children. Peritoneal lavage, used more frequently in adult victims, has been supplanted by CT scans in children. While deep peritoneal lavage can be performed quickly in the trauma room, it is a nonspecific test, unable to pinpoint the origin of bleeding (Any deep penetrating injury will require operative intervention no matter what) The CT identifies specific organs injured and the extent of their damage. Many organ injuries such as liver lacerations and splenic hematomas are treated expectantly, and the CT provides a baseline assessment to which further studies can be compared. Indications for CT scans of the abdomen include:[1] localizing signs to the abdominal examination—abdominal pain, distention, absence of bowel sounds;[2] a hematuria of greater than 10 red blood cells per high power field (RBC/HPF) or blood in the stool;[3] an unconscious child with mechanism of injury consistent with abdominal trauma;[4] pelvic fracture; or[5] abused child with suspected abdominal injury.

The final role of the physician in the trauma bay is to coordinate consultations with subspecialists and help in reaching a decision regarding the hospital disposition of the patient. Invaluable consultants include all of the surgical subspecialities: orthopedics, neurosurgery, cardiothoracic surgery, urology, plastic surgery, ophthalmology, and oral surgery. Orthopedists are frequently needed in approximately one third of cases to provide definitive care of injured bones and joints following resuscitation and stabilization phases. Urgent orthopedic consultation is necessary with open fractures and loss of distal pulses resulting from fractures. The trauma physician should remember to administer tetanus toxoid and antibiotics to any child with an open fracture. When a neurosurgeon is required, it is often on a *stat* basis for such injuries as penetrating skull wound, depressed skull fracture, severe closed-head injury or spinal cord trauma. If the child demonstrates signs of increased intracranial pressure and impending herniation, the trauma physician must intervene immediately by elevating the head of the bed to 30°, intubating the patient, hyperventilating, and giving an osmotic diuretic to reduce brain swelling. If these temporizing measures do not work, the neurosurgeon may be required to reduce pressure with a burr hole prior to intervention in the operating room.

There are four general dispositions for the child who survives in the trauma room: operative intervention, intensive care unit (ICU), admission to a general ward or discharge home. The latter occurs infrequently and is generally not recommended. For the stable child with an isolated injury, a minimum of 24 hours of in-hospital observation is recommended. For the child with unstable vital signs following volume resuscitation, especially following a blood transfusion exceeding half the estimated blood volume, the child should be explored in the operating room to locate sites of hemorrhage and to control them. Open limb fractures, most depressed skull fractures, extensive lacerations and tendon injuries, orthopedic pinnings, and definitive thoracic and abdominal injury repair—all require transfer to the operating suite. The child who is stable following initial resuscitation in the trauma bay but who has sustained serious injuries with the potential for deterioration requires admission to an ICU with close nursing observation.

The "golden hour" begins at the time of injury, so it is important to transfer the seriously injured child to a regional trauma center promptly. A rapid response from a coordinated team of individuals assesses the extent of injuries, resuscitates the child, stabilizes vital signs, calls appropriate consultants, and arranges for the best hospital disposition of the child.

REFERENCES

1. Jaffe, D. emergency management of blunt trauma in children. N. Engl. J Med 1991;324:1477-82.

2. Minirio A, Heron M, Smith B, et al. Death: final data for 2004. National vital statistics reports, Hyattsville (MD). National Center for Health Statistics.
3. Cooper A, Floyd T, Barlow B, et al. Major blunt abdominal trauma due to child abuse. J Trauma 1988;28:1483.
4. Eichelberger MR, Pratsch GL, eds. Pediatric trauma care. Rockville, Md.: Aspen, 1988.
5. Eichelberger MR, Randolph JG. Progress in pediatric trauma world. J of Surg 1985; 9:222.
6. Garcia VF, Gotschall CS, Eichelberger MR, *et al.* Rib fractures in children: A marker of severe trauma. J Trauma 1990;30:695.
7. Jaffe D. Wesson D. Emergency management of blunt trauma in children. N Engl J Med 1991;324:1477.
8. McCarty DL, Surpure JS. Pediatric trauma: Initial evaluation and stabilization. Pediatric Annals 1990;19:584.
9. Schafer I, Barkman C, Riedeser P. et al. Postraumatic sundromes in children and adolescents after road traffic accidents-a prospective cohert study, Psychpathology 2006: 39(4): 159-64.
10. Gaushe M, Lewis RJ, Stratton SJ et al. Effect of out-of-hospital pediatric endotracheal intubation on survival and neurological outcome: a controlled clinical trial. JAMA 2000;283:783-789.
11. Taylor GA, Eggli KD. Lap-belt injuries of the lumbar spine in children: A pitfall in CT diagnosis. Am J Radiology 1988;150:1355.
12. Young GM, Klein BL, Ochsenschlager DW, et al. The child with multiple injuries: Resuscitation priorities. Indian Journal of Pediatrics 1988; 55:705.
13. American College of surgeons. Advanced Trauma Life Support (ATLS) student course manual. American College of surgeon 2004.

In the previous edition this chapter was written by Douglas A. Boenning, MD Associate Medical Director Emergency Medicine Trauma Center Children's National Medical Center Washington, District of Columbia

21 Head Trauma

Sonia Singh and Yuri Gilhotra

Head injury is a major cause of morbidity and mortality in the pediatric population. Over 1.5 million pediatric head injuries are reported each year. Mild traumatic brain injury (TBI) appears to be the most common and generally has a good outcome. Head injury is more common amongst males in all age groups. The mechanism of head injury varies depending on the age of the child. In patients under the age of four, automobile passenger-related trauma, and falls account for a majority of head trauma. Between the age of five and nine, pedestrian accidents become the most prominent mechanism of trauma, accounting for 39.3 percent of injuries. In adolescents, 51.8 percent of head traumas are caused by motor vehicle accidents (1). MVA associated head trauma has the highest morbidity and mortality in all age groups.

SPECTRUM OF INJURIES

Scalp Lacerations

Lacerations of the scalp are among the most common types of tissue injuries following trauma to the head. The scalp is a very vascular structure made up of five layers that include: skin, subcutaneous tissue, aponeurosis, *loose* areolar tissue, and the pericranium (SCALP). The large vessels that supply the scalp run just above the galea aponeurosis, and injury to this layer may result in significant blood loss. Debris from the accident site, as well as hair or clothing, may become entangled in the wound and should be removed meticulously prior to wound closure. All scalp lacerations should be explored to rule out a skull fracture prior to closure.

In rare instances, an injury to the scalp may lead to bleeding into the subgaleal space. The degree of trauma may be very minor or completely unrecognized by the patient. The area of swelling associated with the subgaleal hematoma may be variable and is frequently associated with headache. Subgaleal hematomas cross the suture lines, and can lead to significant blood accumulation and hypovolemia. In general, these hematomas will resolve spontaneously. No attempt to tap the fluid should be made since they frequently re-accumulate and, if infected, may lead to very serious complications (2).

Skull Fracture

Children often present with skull fractures that are described as linear, depressed, or basilar. About 75% of skull fractures are linear, with the parietal bone being the most common site. The significance of a skull fracture is as a marker of the amount of energy that was applied to the patient's head. A large amount of concentrated force is necessary to crack both tables of the skull, and one must be concerned about the amount of this energy that was transmitted to underlying structures. Thus the fracture may be an indication of a more severe injury to the brain, and approximately 48% of patients have associated intracranial lesions. In almost all cases, a simple fracture of the skull (Figure 1) will heal with time. This is because the edges of the fracture are naturally fixed into rigid approximation by the very nature of the skull itself and very little is necessary to promote the proper union of the bony edges.

In all skull fractures, the dura, which is closely approximated to the inner table of the skull, may be lacerated. In children under the age of two a dural laceration may result in herniation of the leptomeninges into the bony cleft. At this age, as the brain is growing at a very rapid rate the bony edges may not have time to heal completely. The growth and pulsation of the brain may lead to a growing skull fracture or leptomeningeal cyst. Repair of these cysts can be very difficult if they are left to grow to a large size. Children who sustain a skull fracture under the age of two should be followed up in by neurosurgery to ensure that the fracture closes and does not progress to a growing cyst.

Depressed Skull Fracture

Depressed skull fractures (Figure 2) result from forces applied to a small cross sectional area and often requires surgical repair. The skin over the injury site may be open, closed, contused, or absent. Brain may be present in the wound, or on rare occasions, severe cortical bleeding from a lacerated artery or vein may also be present. All depressed skull fractures should be evaluated by a neurosurgical specialist to determine the appropriateness of surgical decompression and repair. Minor depressions of the skull, less than bone skull thickness, may be

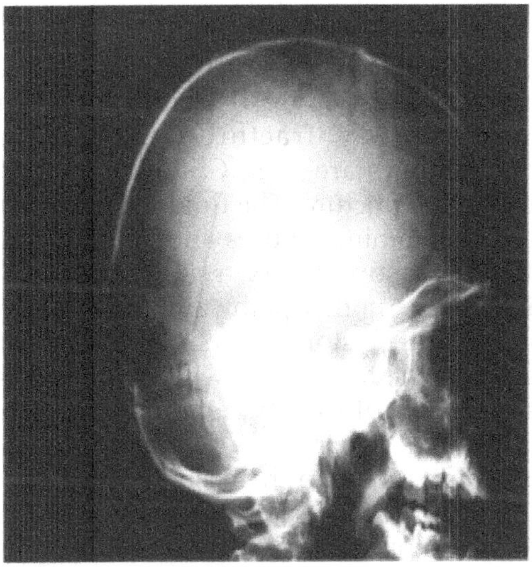

Fig. 1: Photograph of a simple linear skull fracture

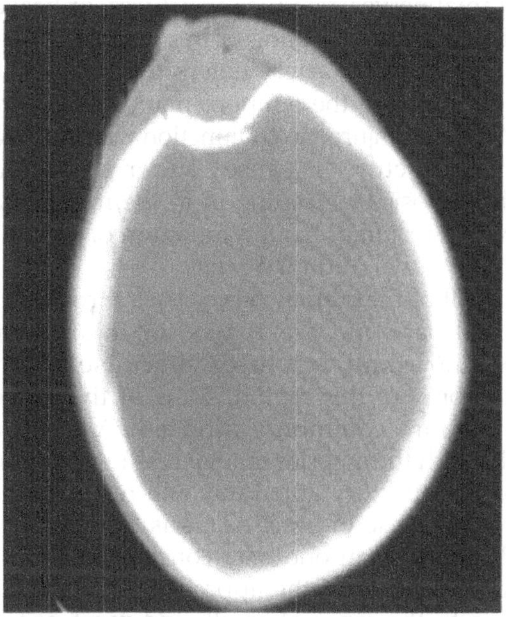

Fig. 2: Compound depressed skull fracture caused by a hammer blow.

observed since they will heal in a manner similar to a simple skull fracture. The more complicated injuries usually will require vigorous debridement and closure. In those injuries with exposed brain, the wound should be covered with saline-soaked gauze to prevent drying of the brain prior to surgical repair. Children with depressed skull fractures are at higher risk for developing seizures, and will often be put on prophylactic anticonvulsants.

Basilar Skull Fracture

Fractures of the skull through the base are not seen well on plain X-ray films but should always be considered in patients with head trauma. In these patients, the fracture almost always heals without surgical intervention except in the most severe cases. The factor that differentiates the basilar skull fracture from a fracture over the convexity of the brain is the associated structures that run through the base of the skull. Injury to the cranial nerves, vascular structures, or basilar dura may be disabling or in some cases fatal.

The carotid artery enters the base of the skull deep to the temporo-mandibular joint. When it is injured in conjunction with a basilar skull fracture, it causes either a vascular thrombosis or bleeding in to the middle ear with a resultant hemotympanum or blood in the external auditory canal.

All of the cranial nerves pass through the skull base and are at risk for injury from basilar skull fractures. Because of the anatomy of this region, some of the nerves are more commonly affected. A fracture through the anterior cranial fossa with injury to the olfactory apparatus will result in loss of the sense of smell. This is a far greater disability than one may consider at first. A large portion of the appreciation of taste is due to the sense of smell, and most people with total anosmia will complain of a loss of the taste of food.

Anterior fossa fractures may also lead to injury to the optic nerves or the nerves of ocular control passing through the superior orbital fissure. Probably the most commonly injured cranial nerves are the seventh, leading to a facial paralysis, and the eighth, leading to a sensorineural hearing loss. In the traumatized patient, the seventh nerve may also develop a delayed dysfunction, and therefore it is very important to document careful examination of facial movement. Injury to the lower cranial nerves, passing through the jugular or hypoglossal foramen, is relatively uncommon.

Basilar skull fractures are often associated with venous bleeding in the soft tissues behind the ear. This is called the *battle sign* and an accumulation of blood in the periorbital region is known as the *racoon sign.* Either of these signs should alert the clinician to the possibility of a basilar fracture and a computerized tomography (CT) scan should be performed with bone windows. Patients with basilar skull fractures are admitted in the hospital for close observation.

Cerebrospinal Fluid Leak

At the base of the skull, the dura is tightly adhered to the bony structure in a number of places. This leaves it at risk for a tear should a bony fracture occur. If the leptomeninges are torn, CSF may leak out through the fracture. The fluid may leak into the air-containing sinuses and subsequently into the nasopharynx, resulting in CSF rhinorrhea. Another pathway of CSF flow is through the mastoid or floor of the middle fossa into the middle ear where it may pass through a ruptured tympanic membrane, producing otorrhea, or through the eustachian tube into the nasopharynx.

In most cases, a CSF leak will stop within two weeks but should be watched carefully. The use of prophylactic antibiotics for this type of injury is controversial. Some suggest that bacterial flora is reduced by the use of antibiotics and therefore the risk of infection is reduced. Others suggest that antibiotic usage encourages resistance without protection, and if meningitis were to result from a CSF leak, the organism would be more difficult to treat. CSF leakage should be addressed and followed by a neurosurgeon, who may elect to either drain CSF with a lumbar catheter or opt for surgical repair of the site of leakage.

Intracranial Lesions

The cranium is a closed space in which only a limited amount of volume may accumulate. The layers of the skull above the brain are the arachnoid, which contains the CSF, the dura, and the skull. Blood may accumulate in each of these areas, producing distinctive radiological and clinical syndromes.

An epidural hematoma (Figure 3) results from blood accumulating between the dura and the skull. The classic clinical presentation of a lucent period following head trauma with a subsequent rapid deterioration of consciousness is rare in children. This is because most epidural hematomas result from bleeding of diploic veins.

The more characteristic source of blood causing the epidural hematoma is arterial. The middle meningeal artery runs within the structure of the temporal bone and in the first part of its course may be completely surrounded by bony investiture. Fracture of the bone across this bony canal will commonly lacerate the artery and cause a hematoma under pressure. This rapid accumulation of blood is the reason for the classical lucent period following head trauma prior to the onset of unconsciousness. In general, the relatively focal nature of the epidural hematoma and mechanism of injury leading to less diffuse brain trauma herald a better outcome than would be expected with other forms of hematoma accumulation.

If the small bridging vessels of the subdural space are torn, a subdural hematoma results Fig 4. The plane of dissection for this

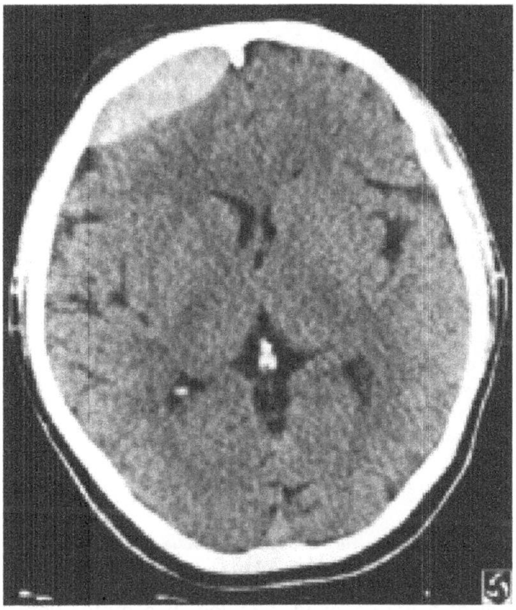

Fig. 3: Epidural hematoma.

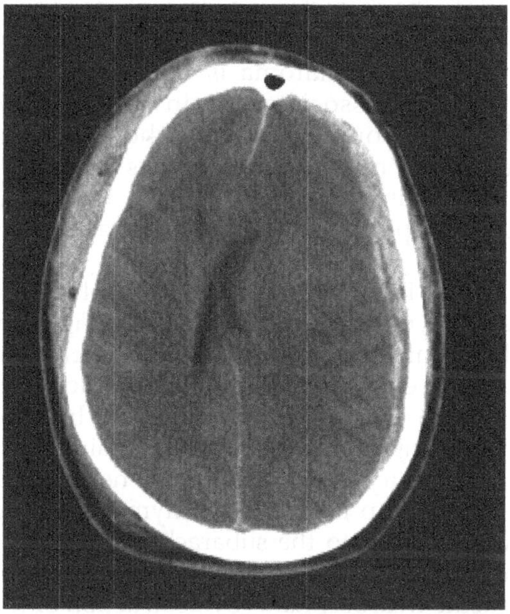

Fig. 4: Left subdural hematoma with a mass effect

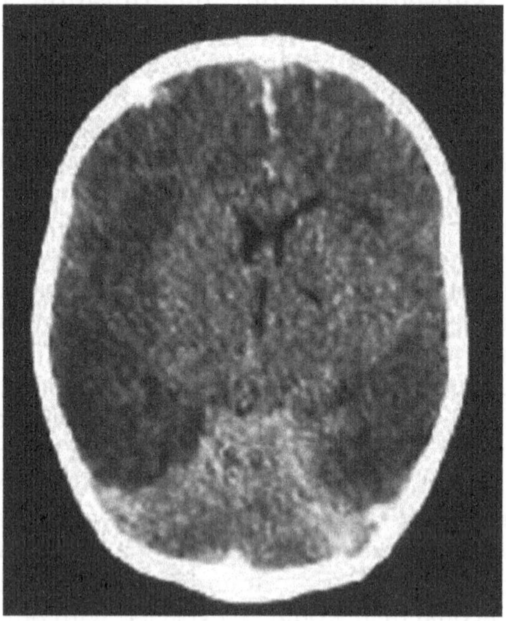

Fig. 5: Intraparenchymal bleed

blood is along a path of much less resistance than that for the epidural hematoma and leads to the characteristic crescent shape seen on the CT scan. In general, the outcome from a subdural hematoma is worse, perhaps because of associated brain trauma. The bleeding source, like in the epidural hematoma, may be either venous or arterial, and the clinical course will vary depending on the rapidity of accumulation and mass effect.

Bleeding may also occur within the parenchyma of the brain as seen in Figure 5. The common areas for intraparenchymal bleeds are the frontal and temporal lobes. It is not uncommon in the traumatized brain to observe injury in one area of the brain with a similar injury directly across the head called a contra coup injury. Parenchymal bleeding may extend into the subarachnoid space or into the ventricles and may occasionally lead to acute hydrocephalus by obstruction of the outflow pathways. This should be carefully monitored and followed.

Penetrating Trauma

Penetrating trauma is relatively rare in children. It can result from a gunshot with its transferred torque effect to surrounding brain tissue, or foreign body introduction along the path of injury. Skull x-rays often show these foreign bodies; see (Figures 6 and 7).

Penetrating trauma is managed as any other form of head trauma. A CT scan is essential to determine the extent of injury and associated intracranial bleeds. In addition, an arteriogram may be indicated in some patients where major vascular structures are at risk. Figure 8 shows a laceration of the anterior portion of the superior sagittal sinus.

The foreign body should not be "pulled out" until there has been adequate assessment of the injury. In most cases, the foreign body should be removed in the operating room with blood available for

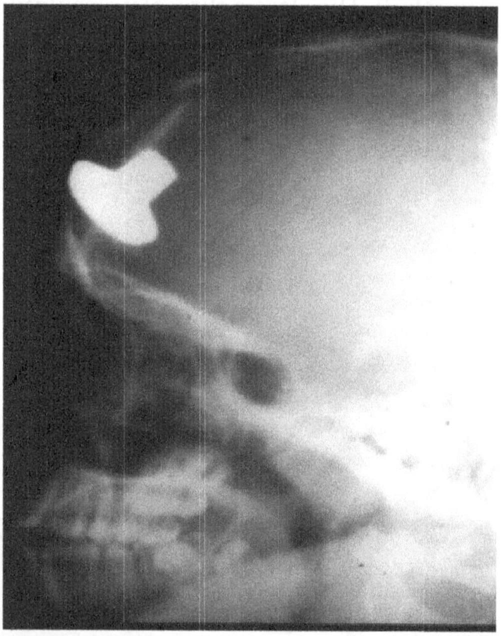

Fig. 6: Photograph of a radio knob foreign body in the skull of a young child involved in a motor vehicle accident.

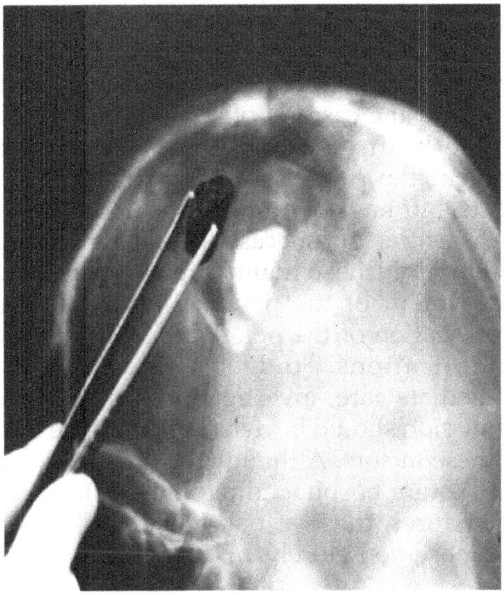

Fig. 7: Photomicrograph of gravel removed from the skull of this child involved in a motorcycle accident.

immediate transfusion. Laceration of a major dural sinus may bleed profusely or allow air entry into this area, causing a major air embolism that could be more easily controlled in the operating room.

Concussion

The syndrome of concussion following impact injury to the head is poorly appreciated. Many patients are seen on a single visit and sent home after being found to be neurologically intact. Many of the patients will develop headaches, concentration or memory problems, or dizziness that may persist for weeks or even several months. Confusion and amnesia are the hallmarks of concussion. Imaging studies of the brain may show minor changes on magnetic resonance imaging (MRI) or be normal. Some patients will experience problems with school performance or athletic participation. Reassurance and time are the only treatment, but alerting the patient to the possibility of a post-concussive syndrome and the need for follow-up is very important in avoiding problems that may develop.

Closed-Head Trauma

The term *closed head trauma* implies an injury that does not penetrate the covering of the brain. The main pathophysiology of the injury is a concussive force, with resultant

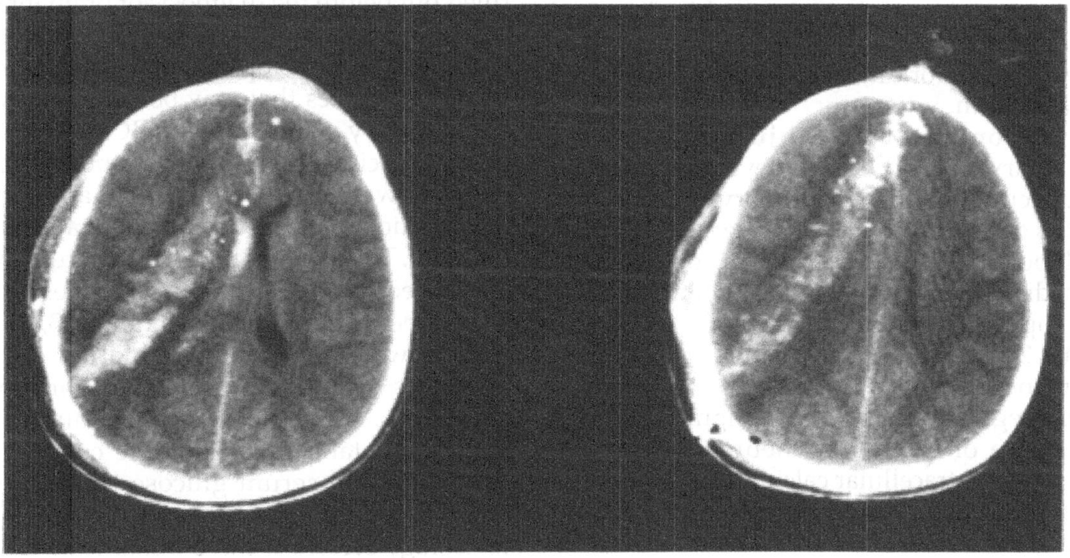

Fig. 8: Gunshot wound in the head of this teenager with associated in-driven bone.

dysautoregulation of blood flow. These areas will subsequently change their blood flow in response to the blood pressure and not in response to $PaCO_2$ and will subsequently produce mass by their enlarged vascular space.

Cerebral perfusion depends on an adequate arterial pressure to force blood through the brain vasculature. An increase in the intracranial pressure above the mean arterial pressure will effectively stop the flow of blood into the brain and result in death of the tissue. In all cases, the cerebral perfusion must be protected, which can be most easily accomplished by maintaining intracranial pressure (ICP) below 20 mmHg. Control of the patient's blood pressure and intracranial pressure is essential in bringing about a good outcome. Early control of ICP may help reduce the amount of injury that the patient experiences.

Pathophysiology

Brain injury can be primary and secondary:

Primary injury results from the direct force of impact. In children, this tends to be diffuse in contrast to adults. Higher head to torso ratio and unique biochemical properties, like high brain water are responsible for diffuseness of the injury seen in children.

Secondary brain injury follows the primary impact. It may develop acutely or subacutely following primary brain injury. This occurs as a result of decrease in cerebral blood flow as a result of neurochemically mediated vasospasm and astrocytic swelling compressing the microcirculation within the first 24 hours of injury. Disruptions of blood brain barrier, alteration in cerebral autoregulation also play a significant role. Release of excitotoxic neurotransmitters, elevated intracellular calcium and potassium concentrations, formation of free radicals and apoptosis also contribute to the secondary injury. Hypoxia, hypotension and intracranial hypertension act as secondary insults and exacerbate the primary injury.

Goals of emergency management are to prevent these secondary events and try to interrupt the cascade of secondary injury of viable brain. Experimental therapies to prevent the progression of primary injury exists, but has not found any clinical use.

Essential for successful management of children with head trauma are a proper clinical assessment of the primary injury and an appreciation of the potential for intracranial complications. Indeed, the need for immediate care, investigations and hospital admission should be determined on the basis of these factors. Although most patients will not require hospital admission or diagnostic procedures, those at risk must be identified and observed closely

CLINICAL PRESENTATION

The typical patient presents to the emergency department with a history of trauma and has an altered level of consciousness that alerts the clinician to the possibility of a head trauma. A variety of factors may contribute to the alteration of mentation and should be ruled out before the diagnosis of brain injury is made. In many traumatic situations, the patient may develop hypotension from a variety of causes that may be unrelated to a head injury. The basic ABCs (airway, breathing, circulation) of life support should be followed first to ensure adequate oxygenation of the blood and adequate blood pressure. The patient's body temperature may also affect the level of consciousness and should be taken into consideration (3,4).

Following the initial evaluation of the patient's status, the potential for toxic substances, most notably alcohol, causing an altered mental status should be considered as well as the serum glucose. These tests should be followed by a comprehensive toxicology screen. If these initial tests fail to demonstrate a reason for the patient's altered mental status, a diagnosis of head injury should be entertained.

HISTORY AND PHYSICAL

The history and physical are very important in the assessment of the patient with closed head trauma. Details regarding the mechanism of injury allow an assessment of the amount of energy that the patient received during the trauma and how that energy was directed to various areas of the body. The initial response of the patient to the injury and at-the-scene reports of the patient's mental status, seizures and vomiting are important in assessing the progression of the head trauma. If the patient was confused at the scene and is now normal, there is less reason for concern than there is with a patient in a reverse scenario. Detailed medical history is frequently unavailable during the initial assessment of the patient, and associated medical conditions such as insulin-dependant diabetes may not be known.

The physical examination should begin with a primary survey of airway, breathing circulation, disability and exposure including c-spine immobilization and mini neurological exam (A-alert, V-verbal, P-pain, U-unresponsive) (Table 1). This should be followed by the secondary survey to include a formal assessment of the level of consciousness and assessment using the Glasgow Coma Scale (GCS) (Table 2). Patients are described as having a severe head injury if the GCS score is 8 or less. A moderate head injury is considered when the GCS is 9-12 and minor head injury correlates with a GCS score of 13 to 15. These classifications guide therapy as well as prognosis. Severity of intracranial injury may also be classified as mild, moderate and severe based on clinical examination (Table 3).

Table 1: Features of physical and neurologic examination of children with head trauma

Physical examination
Determination of vital signs
Investigation for signs of skull fracture
Hematotympanum
Periorbital or postauricular eccymosis
Cerebrospinal fluid otorrhea or rhinorrhea
Depressed fracture or penetrating injury
Neurologic examination
Glasgow Coma Scale
Pupillary light reflexes
Cranial nerve examination
Movement of extremities
Plantar responses

Table 2: Glasgow Coma Scale

Score	*Response*	*Response*	*Response*
Eye opening	< 1year	0-1 year	
4	Opens spontaneously	Opens spontaneously	
3	Opens to a verbal command	Opens to a shout	
2	Opens in response to pain	Opens in response to pain	
1	No response	No response	
Best motor response	> 5 years	2-5 years	0-23 months
5	Oriented and able to converse	Uses appropriate words	Cries appropriately
4	Disoriented and able to converse	Uses inappropriate words	Cries
3	Uses inappropriate words	Cries and/or screams	Cries and/or screams inappropriately
2	Makes incoprehensible sounds	Grunts	Grunts
1	No response	No response	No response
Best verbal response	> 1 year	0-1 year	
6	Obeys command	Spontaneous	
5	Localizes pain	Localizes pain	
4	Flexion withdrawal	Flexion withdrawal	
3	Flexion abnormal (decorticate)	Flexion abnormal (decorticate)	
2	Extension (decerebrate)	Extension (decerebrate)	
1	No response	No response	

Best upper limb motor response	
Obeys commands	6
Vocalizes	5
Withdraws	4
Abnormal flexion	3
Extensor response	2
None	1

Eye-opening response	
Spontaneous	4
To speech	3
To pain	2
None	1

Verbal response*	
Oriented	5
Confused conversation	4
Inappropriate words	3
Incomprehensible sounds	2
None	1

Table 3: Classification of severity of intracranial injury

Mild
Asymptomatic
Mild headache
Three of fewer episodes of vomiting
Glasgow Coma Scale score of 15
Loss of consciousness for less than 5 minutes
Moderate
Loss of consciousness for 5 minutes or more
Progressive lethargy
Progressive headache
Vomiting protracted (more than three times) or associated with other symptoms
Post-traumatic amnesia
Post-traumatic seizure
Multiple trauma
Serious facial injury
Signs of basal skull fracture
Possible penetrating injury or depressed skull fracture
Suspected child abuse
Glasgow Coma Scale score of 11 to 14
Severe
Glasgow Coma Scale score of 10 or less or decrease of 2 points or more not clearly caused by seizures, drugs, decreased cerebral perfusion or metabolic factors
Focal neurologic signs
Penetrating skull injury
Palpable depressed skull fracture
Compound skull fracture

MANAGEMENT PRIORITIES

Primary Survey: Assesment of Airway, Breathing and Circulation

Airway, breathing and circulation should be assessed as soon as the child enters pediatric emergency unit. Primary and secondary survey should be performed as for any other child with multiple traumas.

Rapid sequence intubation should be performed if patient is comatose with due attention to cervical spine stabilization. Head lift and chin thrust maneuver should be avoided. Airway opening should be done with jaw thrust. Lignocaine (1-2 mg/kg) should be administered 2-5 minutes before laryngoscopy. Thiopentone, etomidate or propofol can be used as sedative agents as they have cerebroprotective effect. Midazolam is a useful alternative especially in hypotensive patients. For paralysis, non depolarizing agent like rocuronium (0.6 – 1.2 mg/kg) should be used. Prevention of hypoxia and hypercapnia are vital in improving outcome in such patients. Assisted ventilation to maintain normoxia and normocarbia are then required along with continued sedation in such patients.

Hypovolemia is a frequent problem noted in pediatric trauma victims. Signs of hypoperfusion include increased heart rate, loss of peripheral pulses, decreased urine output and prolonged capillary refill. Children often maintain systolic blood pressure despite significant blood loss until they develop acute hypotension. Ideal fluid for volume resuscitation is still debated. However, most use a crystalloid. Isotonic normal saline is preferred to lactated Ringer solution. Colloid, mainly hydroxyl ethyl starch could be advantageous because it does not increase cerebral edema and lesser volume is needed compared with normal saline. Persistent hypotension refractory to volume resuscitation should be treated with vasoactive agents like dopamine or epinephrine to ensure adequate cerebral perfusion.

Management of Intracranial hypertension (Table 4)

Head injury patients are prone to develop raised ICP which can potentiate secondary injury. Careful neurological monitoring helps in early detection of cerebral herniation. A set of treatment protocol which can be used in emergency department.

The goal of treatment is to lower the ICP to a level that is adequate to increase cerebral perfusion pressure (CPP) as this is key to improve cerebral oxygenation and prevent cerebral ischemia.

General Maneuvers

The general measures used for all patients with raised ICP is to keep head in midline and elevate it to 30^0, treatment of fever, avoidance of jugular venous outflow obstruction, maintenance of normovolemia, normoxia and normocarbia (p_aCO_2=35mm Hg). Adequate sedation and analgesia should be maintained with opioids and benzodiazepines to avoid anxiety and pain which may cause spikes in intracranial pressure. In children, propofol as a sedative is avoided owing to the risk of metabolic acidosis. Optimization of mean arterial pressure (MAP) with fluid therapy and vasoactive drugs is crucial for maintaining CPP.

Table 4: Management of raised intracranial pressure

1. Place head and neck in midline
2. Elevate head end of the bed not more than 30 degrees.
3. Minimise stimulation (suctioning and movement)
4. Maintain normoxia and normocarbia.
5. Give normal maintenance IV fluids.
6. Maintain normal blood sugar and serum electrolytes.
7. Osmotic diuretics like mannitol (0.5 g/Kg intravenously),
8. Use controlled hyperventilation (avoid PaCO2 fall less than 30mmHg) if clinical signs of impending herniation appears.

First line ICP-targeted Therapy

CSF drainage: CSF drainage provides immediate but transient effect and is especially indicated in situations where the raised ICP is secondary to hydrocephalus. However biffuse brain swelling as in TBI may cause chinked ventricles making CSF drainage difficult.

Osmotic therapy: Mannitol (bolus doses of 0.5-1 g/kg every 4-6 h) remains the cornerstone of therapy especially in acute rise of ICP. Adequate preload and MAP are an important prerequisite for Mannitol therapy. However there is little data on use of mannitol in children. There are very few studies on use of hypertonic saline (HS) in children. It has been shown that an increase in serum sodium concentration significantly decreases ICP and increases CPP in severe TBI. In addition, sustained hypernatremia and hyperosmolarity were safely tolerated in these patients. At the present time, there is limited experience with continuous infusion of 3% hypertonic saline 0.1-1.0 ml/kg/h but has a reasonably good performance in contemporary clinical trials.

Hyperventilation: Mechanical ventilation should provide adequate oxygenation

(Oxygen saturation >90%) and avoid hypercarbia ($PaCO_2$>38 mmHg). In children, hypocarbia ($paCO_2$<35mmHg) decreases cerebral blood flow and can induce cerebral ischemia hence hyperventilation should be avoided. Mild hyperventilation may be considered case of intracranial hypertension refractory to general maneuvers, cerebrospinal drainage and hyperosmolar therapy.

Continuous EEG (if possible) is helpful to detect sub-clinical/subtle seizures especially in sedated patients so that adequate anticonvulsants can be given.

Second line ICP-targeted Therapy

Profound hyperventilation ($PaCO_2$ <35mm Hg), barbiturates and moderate hypothermia are the modalities used for refractory intracranial hypertension. Profound hyperventilation however, requires cerebral blood velocities or oxygenation monitoring to detect cerebral ischemia.

Moderate hypothermia: Hyperthermia (body temperature >38^0 C) may worsen outcome by increasing metabolic demand, inflammatory changes, lipid peroxidation, neuronal excitoxicity cell death and acute seizure. Cooling on the other hand reduces the cerebral metabolic rate and oxygen consumption. There is limited evidence for its use though one pediatric study has demonstrated the safety of the method, but the effects on functional outcome and intracranial hypertension were not assessed. There is no recommendation as of now to use hypothermic strategy in children with severe TBI.

Surgery: Surgery is not a first-line treatment except to evacuate compressive subdural or epidural hematomas. Refractory intracranial hypertension can be treated with decompressive craniectomy. Children likely to benefit from surgery are those with diffuse cerebral swelling, within 48 h of injury, no episodes of sustained ICP>40 mmHg, secondary clinical deterioration, evolving cerebral herniation syndrome.

LABORATORY AND RADIOLOGY

Laboratory evaluation is essential to the evaluation of any patient who has undergone a major trauma. Blood counts and chemistries, arterial blood gasses and serum alcohol levels, routine clotting studies (PT [prothrombin time] and PTT [partial thromboplastin time]) should also be performed. Indications for X-ray skull are given in Table 5 and for neuroimaging are given in Table 6. When severe injury to the brain occurs, factors released into the blood can lead to a fulminant disseminated intravascular coagulopathy. This complication is a hallmark of a bad outcome and indicates the degree of brain injury that may be present.

Table 5: Indications for skull radiography

(a) Possible penetration,

(b) Possible depressed fracture,

(c) Compound fracture,

(d) Previous craniotomy with indwelling shunt,

(e) Child less than 2 years of age with "boggy" scalp hematoma

(f) Suspected child abuse

Computerised Tomography

Computed axial tomography (CAT or CT) of the brain is the most important radiological evaluation to be performed. This test will help determine the presence of a surgically removable mass lesion or identify a patient with an injury more severe than clinical examination indicated and will require expectant observation. There is no role for

Table 6: Indications for urgent cranial CT

Clinical suspicion TBI with

- Any neurological deficit or abnormality
- Seizure after head injury in a patient who has no history of epilepsy
- Observed LOC > 5 minutes or defined amnesia > 5 minutes
- Suspicion of penetrating cranial injury or depressed skull fracture
- Signs of base of skull fracture
- Depressed LOC = GCS < 14 (any drowsiness if age one year or less)
- Age one year or less with scalp bruise, swelling or laceration > 5 cm or tense fontanelle OR MAJOR IMPACT MECHANISM WITH ANY CLINICAL CONCERN
- Head trauma in the setting of a high speed (> 60 km/hr) MVA as either pedestrian, cyclist or occupant
- Head trauma in the setting of a fall > 3m in height
- Head trauma related to a high speed injury from a projectile or an object.
- Any intentional head trauma associated with possible child management

→ OBTAIN NEUROSURGICAL CONSULT ASAP → **URGENT CRANIAL CT**

CONSIDER CRANIAL CT

CLINICAL SUSPICION TBI

- Persisting headache
- Irritability or altered behaviour
- Impact seizure or possible amnesia
- LOC < 5 minutes
- Vomiting or dry retching in absence of fever or diarrhoea
- Unable to rouse to alert state. Young infants that present late evening or night may be difficult to assess because of normal sleep patterns and should be observed if not scanned

OR

MODERATE IMPACT MECHANISM

- Blow to head
- Head trauma in the setting of a fall > 1 m in height
- Injury to head from a projectile or an object

→ **OBSERVE FOR 6 HOURS**

DETERIORATION AT ANY TIME → **URGENT CRANIAL CT**

STABLE → **REVIEW AT 6 HOURS**

ANY OF THE FOLLOWING PRESENT ?

- Headache
- Persistent irritability
- Abnormal behaviour
- Persisting vomiting
- Unable to rouse to alert state after a sleep

Yes → **CRANIAL CT BEFORE DISCHAGE**

NO → **HOME WITH HI ADVICE IF NO SUSPICION OF CHILD MALTREATMENT**

(Consider cranial CT: NO → **HOME WITH HI ADVICE IF NO SUSPICION OF CHILD MALTREATMENT**)

Adapted from Dunning J. *et al.*. *Arch Dis Child* 2006;91:885-891 (CHALICE) Consider your local medical resources, access to cranial CT and transport capability when applying these guidelines.

contrast enhanced head CT in the acutely injured child, unless an angiogram is being performed to evaluate for concomitant vessel injury. CT scanning is a safe and accurate investigation for older children who are able to lie still for the procedure. In younger children, particularly those under 5 years, general anesthesia or procedural sedation may be required to achieve CT scanning. In addition, the risks of cranial irradiation need to be considered. Therefore, particularly in younger children, the risk of CT should be balanced against the risk of delayed diagnosis. Observation in the emergency department, for a period of at least 6 hours from the time of injury, may be used as an alternative approach in children whose indications are marginal. Vomiting, amnesia, and impact seizures require particular consideration. Vomiting is very common especially in young children and vomiting secondary to raised ICP is difficult to determine. It is also difficult to ascertain the true length of amnesia. Impact seizures must be differentiated from seizures after the head injury as they are not associated with intracranial pathology. In these children CT should be considered if symptoms persist despite a period of observation. Because of these practical considerations, below is a guideline based on modified CHALICE criteria to give a more realistic but safe approach to the management of suspected traumatic brain injury.

Skull X-rays

There is some controversy over the usefulness of plain skull films. For almost all types of head trauma, the CT scan provides more information than do plain skull films, but in limited instances (associated mandible or facial fractures) skull films may be indicated in addition to CT scanning. Many studies have illustrated that the presence of a skull fracture significantly increases the risk of intracranial injury. However, the absence of a skull fracture has a poor negative predictive value, as approximately 50% intracranial injuries will not have an associated skull fracture.

The patient with serious head trauma should also have routine cervical spine X-rays to rule out associated injury. In the child with a relatively disproportionate head mass, associated injury to the cervical spine should always be suspected.

CONCLUSIONS

The long term neuro-cognitive and behavioral consequences of head trauma can vary widely, based of extent of injury. Overall, children have a better prognosis and improvement in function may continue for years after injury. Those patients with a GCS score less than 3 have a high mortality and morbidity. Children with coma that lasts less than 2 weeks have considerable better neurocognitive outcome and fewer developmental and behavioral sequelae.

Head injury education and prevention ie. car seats, seat belts, and helmets help reduce the incidence and severity of head injury. Children who have suffered mil-moderate concussions should not return to contact sports until they are completely symptom free, both at rest and with exertion. Any child with symptoms persisting greater than a week after a head trauma, should be referred for neurocognitive evaluation.

The ideal imaging modality for assessing head injury is a non-contrast CT, which can reliably detect both intracranial and skull fractures. However, we need to be aware of the long-term risks associated with radiation exposure associated with CT. Great advances have been made in the initial evaluation and stabilization of the pediatric patient with head trauma associated with improvement in outcome.

FURTHER READING

1. Mazzola CA, Adelson PD. Critical care management of head trauma in children. Crit Care Med. 2002 Nov;30(11 Suppl):S393-401.
2. Meyer PG, Ducrocq S, Carli P. Pediatric neurologic emergencies. Curr Opin Crit Care. 2001 Apr;7(2):81-7.
3. Canadian Paediatric Society (CPS) Management of children with head trauma Canadian Medical Association Journal 1990; 142(9): 949-952.
4 National Collaborating Centre for Acute Care. Head injury: triage, assessment, investigation and early management of head injury in infants, children and adults. London (UK): National Institute for Clinical Excellence (NICE); 2003 Jun. 248 p. [373 references].
5. Orliaguet GA, Meyer PG, Baugnon T. Management of critically ill children with traumatic brain injury. Pediatric Anesthesia 2008;18:455-461.

In the previous edition this chapter was written by David J. Gower, MD Assistant Professor of Surgery, Section of Neurosurgery, University of Oklahoma Health Sciences Center, Oklahoma City, Oklahoma

Shiva Kalidindi

22 Abdominal Trauma

Trauma is the leading cause of death in children aged 1 through 14 years. Blunt abdominal trauma occurs frequently and is second to head trauma as a cause of death in childhood accidents, but it is responsible for the majority of preventable deaths. Abdominal trauma accounts for 8-10% of all trauma admissions to pediatric hospitals. At least 25 % of children with multisystem injury have significant abdominal injury. Motor vehicle crashes, auto-pedestrian injury, bicycle injury(e.g., handlebar injury) and falls are the major causes of blunt abdominal injury in children; More than 80% of traumatic abdominal injuries in children result from blunt mechanisms[1-5]. Child abuse should be suspected if the history is inconsistent with the injury. Penetrating injuries in children are less common and result in 8-12% of the abdominal trauma admissions in most trauma centers.

Appropriate triage, careful initial evaluation, rapid and appropriate diagnostic procedures, and vigorous management of immediate life-threatening conditions are essential to achieve the best results. The mortality of blunt abdominal trauma in children is directly related to the level of involvement: it is < 20 % in isolated liver, spleen, kidney, or pancreatic trauma; increases to 20 % if the gastrointestinal tract is involved; and increases to 50 % if major vessels are injured [7].

PATHOPHYSIOLOGY

Proper evaluation and management of abdominal trauma in children requires knowledge of certain unique anatomic and physiologic characteristics of children. Children are more vulnerable to abdominal injury caused by blunt forces than are adults.

Compared to adults, children have a relatively smaller anteroposterior abdominal diameter, which provide a smaller area over which the force of injury can be dissipated. The diaphragm inserts into the rib cage horizontally, providing a shallower, less spacious dome within which a comparatively large liver and spleen reside. The ribs, which are incompletely mineralized and more flexible than they are in adults. However, this increase in compliance makes them less effective at energy dissipation and, therefore, less effective at protecting the upper abdominal structures (e.g., spleen, liver). In addition, they have relatively larger viscera, less overlying fat, and weaker abdominal musculature that of an adult[1]. Thus providing less protection to underlying structure. Also the close proximity of many vital organs in the child's small abdomen results in more severe injuries per amount of force in children than in adults who experience blunt abdominal trauma.

Children have diaphragmatic breathing. When the diaphragm is injured or irritated, ventilatory compromise results. The bladder extends to the level of the umbilicus at birth and is, therefore, more exposed to a direct impact to the lower abdomen. With age, the bladder descends to its retropubic position. The rapid growth of the spine during adolescence influences its anatomy and biomechanical properties, particularly in the lumbar area. In a child with a thin abdominal wall and who is poorly restrained (lap belt only), the fulcrum of a flexion injury would be at the body of the spine, which exposes it to a flexion-distraction injury (Chance fracture).

Injury to the highly vascular organs such as the spleen, the liver, or blood vessels produces significant loss of blood. The hemorrhagic shock resulting from injury to intra-abdominal organs is the most serious and immediate threat to the child's life. Because of the unique compensatory mechanisms of the injured child, hypotension secondary to hypovolemic shock is a late and ominous event. Early aggressive fluid resuscitation is indicated in injured children. Potentially life-threatening peritonitis and sepsis follow peritoneal contamination by ruptured hollow viscera. Because young children have a disproportionately larger body surface area and less thermoregulation, preserving core temperature during the care of an injured child is important.

INITIAL ASSESSMENT

The basic principles of initial assessment and resuscitation for a traumatized child remain the same as for an adult. The first priority in the management of any trauma patient is A focused primary survey aimed at rapidly assessing the ABCs (airway, breathing, and circulation) remains the initial priority. In addition, at the time of the primary survey, performing an abbreviated neurologic assessment (D) and completely exposing (E) the child to thoroughly search for injuries is appropriate. After stabilization of cardiorespiratory status, the secondary survey, a fully exposed head-to-toe examination with emphasis on the abdomen, is performed. Rapid identification of life-threatening conditions is the goal of this initial assessment. When profuse bleeding reduces circulating volume, the remaining blood must be fully oxygenated by administration of 100 % oxygen and proper maintenance of ventilation. Fluid resuscitation is an important component of the management of abdominal injuries in children. The cervical spine must be protected by a semirigid cervical collar until a cervical spine injury is properly excluded.

Exsanguinating intra-abdominal bleeding occurs without significant external evidence of injury. Hypovolemic shock is readily diagnosed when children present with signs of overt shock such as cold clammy skin, prolonged capillary refill, tachycardia, and hypotension. However severe intraabdominal hemorrhage in children can be masked by their ability to maintain normal blood pressure with large volume blood loss [8]. These children may initially have tachycardia, irritability, or confusion but only when the compensatory mechanisms are overwhelmed by the continuous loss of blood, does profound shock occur. Overt or evolving shock is vigorously treated by replacement of lost intravascular volume with type-specific whole blood. Ringer's lactate or normal saline provide volume support until blood is available. As fluid may leak intra-abdominally, two large-caliber intravenous (IV) lines are established above the diaphragm and samples for laboratory analysis are obtained. If transcutaneous vascular access cannot be readily established, a venous cut-down is placed. A fluid bolus of 20 ml/kg should be administered over 5 to 10 minutes. Patient's hemodynamic status should be closely monitered and repeat boluses may be administered and type O Rh-negative blood may be transfused if type-specific blood is unavailable. Children with abdominal trauma and hemodynamic instability should undergo immediate emergent laparotomy[8]. Repeated, serial examinations are necessary in children with abdominal trauma because life-threatening abdominal injury may not be apparent upon the initial examination [9].

Once the ABCs have been addressed, monitors for heart rate, respiration, blood pressure, and oxygen saturation are placed. The physical examination should include inspection, auscultation, and palpation. A nasogastric or orogastric tube (in patients with maxillofacial trauma) should be placed before abdominal examination. Gastric decompression may facilitate abdominal examination and prevent aspiration of gastric contents if vomiting occurs [8]. Inspection of the abdomen may reveal distention associated with bleeding or intraperitoneal air. When a traumatic diaphragmatic hernia is present, a scaphoid abdomen might be observed. All abrasions and contusions should be documented and may indicate associated intra-abdominal injury. For example, skin ecchymosis from a lap belt injury may indicate a hollow organ injury and spinal fracture. Abdominal palpation reveals tenderness associated with injury in children who are neurologically healthy. Findings may include focal tenderness, which is often a result of abdominal wall contusion, or rebound tenderness, which suggests an intraperitoneal process, such as hemorrhage or perforation. The presence of blood on rectal examination may indicate bowel perforation. Decreased rectal sphincter tone may indicate spinal cord injury. Additional signs of spinal cord injury include priapism, hypotension with relative bradycardia, and decreased strength and sensation [10,11]. Boys with abdominal trauma should be examined for testicular injury. Perineal or vaginal laceration should be suspected in children with pelvic fractures [12].

Abdominal injury also can be obscured by concurrent extraabdominal injury (eg, head trauma, thoracic trauma, extremity fracture) [13]. In addition, the examination may be unreliable if the patient's neurologic status is impaired due to brain or spinal cord injury or substance use, and in children younger than one year of age [14].

Laboratory Evaluation

Laboratory testing is a routine component of the trauma evaluation. The baseline tests performed are typically determined according to the suspected severity of injury and individual institutional guidelines. A CBC count and urinalysis (UA) are routinely performed in most children with suspected intra-abdominal injuries. The CBC count provides a baseline blood count, and urinalysis is often performed as a screening test for genitourinary trauma [15]. A positive UA for blood should prompt further evaluation because even microscopic hematuria can be associated with significant renal trauma.Liver function tests (LFTs) and pancreatic enzyme tests have variable sensitivity and specificity for abdominal organ injuries. In all cases in which significant abdominal injury is suspected or present, a blood specimen for type and cross-match should be obtained.

Diagnostic Peritoneal Lavage

With the availability of CT scanning and FAST examination, the utility of diagnostic peritoneal lavage (DPL) for the assessment of the injured abdomen has significantly diminished. Although very sensitive for the detection of intra-abdominal blood and hollow visceral injuries, DPL is nonspecific and invasive and has associated morbidity. Diagnostic peritoneal lavage (DPL) may be useful in the evaluation of a hemodynamically unstable child, particularly if he or she requires emergent surgery (e.g., craniotomy), and time does not permit abdominal CT scan or when CT scan is unavailable. Some surgeons prefer performance of emergent laparotomy to DPL. Positive DPL includes greater than 100,000 RBC/mm3, greater than 500 WBC/mm3, bacteria, vegetable fiber, and bile or amylase in excess of serum levels(>175 IU/L). Any of these may indicate the need for celiotomy[8].

Ultrasonography

Although the focused assessment by sonography in trauma (FAST) examination has become a standard part of the initial evaluation of bluntly injured abdomens in adult trauma centers[16] its role in pediatric trauma is still unclear. Ultrasonography is useful for the rapid evaluation of stable children with blunt abdominal trauma. FAST is highly sensitive for the detection of free intra-peritoneal fluid, but it is operator-dependent and lacks specificity.

Computed Tomography

Abdominal CT is the preferred diagnostic imaging modality to detect intraabdominal injury in hemodynamically stable children who have sustained blunt abdominal trauma [17]. CT is sensitive and specific in diagnosing liver, spleen, and retroperitoneal injuries, which may be managed nonoperatively [15]. CT is less sensitive in detecting injuries of the pancreas, intestinal tract, bladder, and lumbar spine [18,19].The oral and IV contrast agents may be needed for optimal evaluation but have some hazards.

Intravenous Pyelography

IV pyelogram (IVP) identifies significant parenchymal disruption and potential renovascular injury. A single-shot IVP can be performed prior to abdominal exploration in unstable patients. CT, however, is more specific and as scan time decreases, the IVP will become less useful.

SPECIFIC INJURIES

Splenic Injuries

The spleen is the organ most commonly injured in blunt abdominal trauma[1]. Splenic trauma often occurs with little or no outward evidence of injury and may result from low energy impact. Rib fractures, pain from associated injuries, and the sensory loss from spinal cord trauma or altered mental status increase the difficulty of recognizing splenic rupture. Patients with splenic injuries may present with hemorrhagic shock, diffuse abdominal tenderness, left upper quadrant pain, or left shoulder pain(Kehr's Sign) due to diaphragmatic irritation from subphrenic blood[20]. Plain abdominal radiographs can show the gastric air bubble shifted to the right because of compression from the splenic hematoma. CT is preferred because of the frequent association of other injuries (Figure 1). CT delineates splenic injury with high accuracy, and the degree of disruption noted aids in decision making. Traumatic spleen injuries are graded according to severity . Most other children with splenic trauma can be managed nonoperatively. Nonoperative management consists of bed rest with intensive observation, IV fluids and judicious blood transfusion with frequent reevaluation. This is preferred because splenectomy or splenorrhaphy predispose the child to sepsis. Laparotomy is indicated in children with splenic injury and hemodynamic instability.

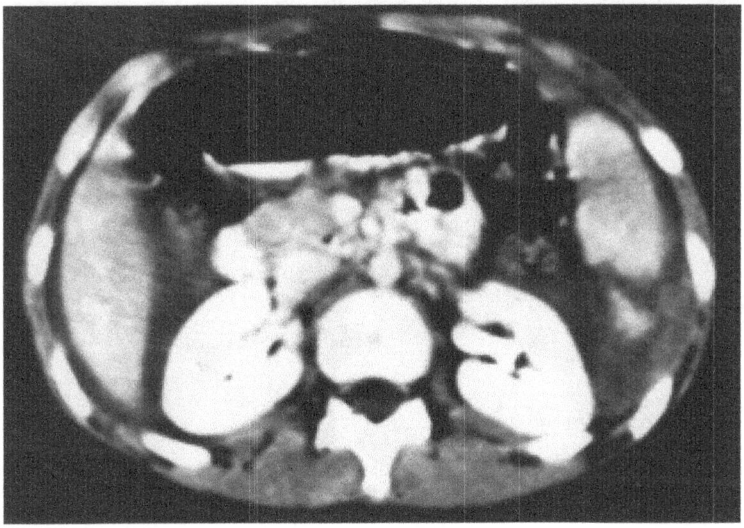

Fig. 1: Contrast enhanced abdominal CT scan of a 12-year-old female, victim of motor vehicle accident, showing extensive splenic laceration with hemoperitoneum around the liver.

Hepatic Injury

The liver, the largest organ of the abdomen, is frequently the site of significant hemorrhage. Liver injury is usually more severe than splenic injury, and is the most common fatal abdominal injury, with a mortality rate of 10 to 20 percent[23]. Right upper quadrant tenderness and abdominal distention may indicate hepatic injury but these signs are also commonly found in multiply injured and frightened children who cry and swallow large amounts of air. Occult liver injury may be identified by elevated serum concentrations of serum aspartate aminotransferase (AST) and serum alanine aminotransferase (ALT). CT of the abdomen should be performed if AST concentrations are greater than 450 IU/L and ALT levels are greater than 250 IU/L and the child does not require immediate laparotomy [1]. CT, however, is the best diagnostic tool for detecting and staging hepatic injury (Figure 2). Immediate operation is necessary to control major hemorrhage(transfusion requirement of greater than 40 cc/kg of packed red blood cells) or hemodynamic instability. Hemobilia, or bleeding from the hepatobiliary tractis rarely associated with blunt abdominal trauma, particularly of the liver . The classic triad of hemobilia includes biliary colic, obstructive jaundice, and occult or acute GI bleeding[25]. The diagnosis is confirmed with cholangio-graphy. Treatment usually consists of embolization although hepatic resection may be necessary.

For isolated liver or spleen injury, current recommendations for length of stay and observation are per Stylianos and the American Pediatric Surgical Association (APSA)[21]. These recommendations are based on CT grade of injury. For grade 1 injury, no ICU stay, 2 total hospital days, and 3 weeks activity restriction. For grade 2 injury, no ICU stay, 3 total hospital days, and 4 weeks activity restriction. For grade 3 injury, no ICU stay, 4 total hospital days, and 5 weeks

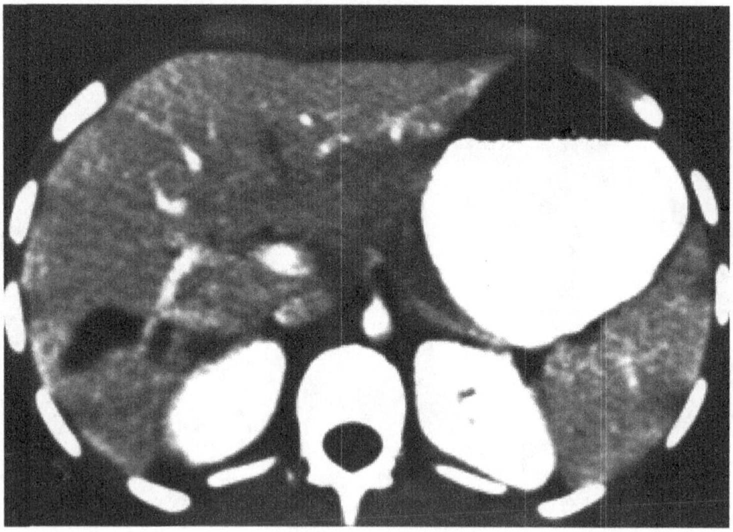

Fig. 2: Abdominal CT scan of a 10-year-old female victim of motor vehicle accident showing hepatic laceration.

activity restriction. For grade 4 injury, 1 day of ICU stay, 5 total hospital days, and 6 weeks of activity restriction. These guidelines have been prospectively evaluated and demonstrate significant reduction in length of stay without adverse sequelae.

Pancreatic Injury

Pancreatic injury usually occurs in less than 3 percent of children as a result of compression of the pancreas against the spinal column, which produces contusion or transection. Bicycle handlebar injuries, motor vehicle accidents, and child abuse account for most of the injuries to the pancreas. Pancreatic injury usually presents with signs of pancreatitis such as abdominal pain, vomiting, fever, and epigastric tenderness. Patients with delayed presentation of pancreatic trauma may have findings suggestive of pancreatic pseudocyst, including epigastric pain, palpable abdominal mass, and hyperamylasemia [8]. Amylase levels may or maynot be elevated, however serial amylase levels are more helpful than a single measurement. Abdominal ultrasound and a contrast-enhanced CT may help to establish the diagnosis although the accuracy of these imaging modalities is low.

The initial management consists of rest, nasogastric suction, and administration of fluids. Pancreatitis pseudocyst, abscess, and fistula are complications that may require surgical intervention.

Renal Injuries

Blunt abdominal trauma involves renal injury in 10-20% of cases and 90% of these injuries are from a blunt mechanism of injury. Auto-pedestrian accident victims, automobile accident victims, and cyclists struck by motor vehicles frequently sustain renal injuries. Children with renal injuries may complain of flank pain. A renal mass, a flank hematoma, and tenderness of the costovertebral angle may be present. Gross hematuria usually occurs with major renal trauma [26].

IVP is the quickest, most readily available, and most cost effective means of evaluating suspected renal injury [26]. Associated hepatic and splenic injuries make CT more useful as an investigating modality, and the extent of renal injury is better defined (Figure 3).

Conservative management with bed rest, monitoring, and antibiotics is standard for low-grade renal injury. Absolute indications for renal exploration are an expanding or pulsatile renal hematoma. Acute renal failure, shock, urinary extravasation with or without urinary ascites, and abscess formation may complicate the management of renal injury. Hypertension, hydronephrosis, cyst, renal stone, renal atrophy, and renal intestinal fistula may manifest as late complications.

Intestinal Injuries

Overall, hollow viscus injuries are present in 3% of abdominal injuries. The risk for hollow visceral injuries significantly increases with pancreatic injury or when multiple intra-abdominal organs (eg, liver, spleen) are affected. Most blunt intestinal injury results from motor vehicle or bicycle related trauma. In young children (particularly those less than four years who have duodenal injuries), child abuse must also be considered[27]. The vast majority of detected hollow organ injuries require operative intervention, with the exception of some intestinal wall hematomas (i.e, duodenal), which can be first treated nonoperatively[24].

Bruising of the abdominal wall after a motor vehicle collision is an important finding. This is usually the result of a lap seat belt or a restraint device. A seat belt syndrome has been described as the concurrent findings of abdominal wall bruising, intra-abdominal injury, and vertebral fracture[28].

A large duodenal hematoma usually produces signs of high intestinal obstruction and mesenteric tears may cause significant intraperitoneal hemorrhage. Severe peritonitis and sepsis follow perforation of the intestinal tract. Abdominal pain, vomiting, and tenderness herald the onset of peritonitis. Free air under the diaphragm on an upright plain radiograph of the abdomen is diagnostic of intestinal perforation and mandates immediate surgical repair.

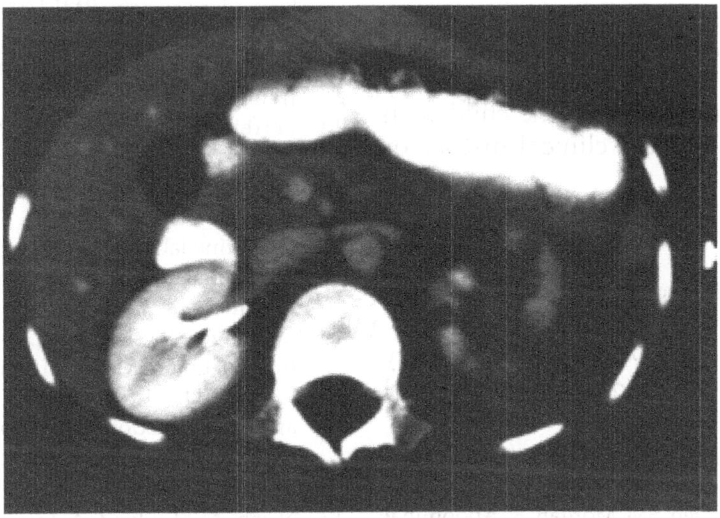

Fig. 3: Abdominal CT scan of a 9-year-old male, who fell from a tree, showing lacerations of left kidney.

Duodenal hematoma usually resolves with conservative management involving nasogastric suction, bowel rest, and parenteral nutrition. The risk of infection in cases of intestinal perforation is high, dictating early and liberal use of antibiotics. Management of intestinal perforation includes fluid resuscitation, antibiotic therapy, and surgical repair.

Urinary Bladder Injury

Blunt trauma, usually motor-vehicle-related accidents, causes most pediatric bladder injuries. Diagnosis is confirmed by IVP and cystogram. Before a retrograde cystogram is performed, however, urethral injury must be ruled out with a retrograde urethrogram.

Child abuse

Children with abdominal trauma secondary to assault or abuse have the highest mortality rate out of all causes of abdominal trauma. Abdominal trauma related to child abuse also carries a particularly high risk of hollow viscus injury. Anorectal injuries in children usually result from sexual abuse. In all children with suspected inflicted injury, the abdomen must be thoroughly evaluated. The possibility of inflicted abdominal injury should also be considered in the child with unexplained or unusual clinical history or physical findings.

REFERENCES

1. Schafermeyer, R. Pediatric trauma. Emerg Med Clin North Am 1993; 11:187.
2. Cooper, A, Barlow, B, DiScala, C, et al. Mortality and truncal injury: the pediatric perspective. J Pediatr Surg 1994; 29:33.
3. Wright, MS. Update on pediatric trauma care. Curr Opin Pediatr 1995; 7:292.
4. Rothrock, SG, Green, SM, Morgan, R. Abdominal trauma in infants and children: prompt identification and early management of serious and life-threatening injuries. Part I: injury patterns and initial assessment. Pediatr Emerg Care 2000; 16:106.
5. Cooper A, Thomas F, Barlow B, et al: Major blunt abdominal trauma due to child abuse.J Trauma 1988;28(10):1483-1487.
6. Zorlundemir U, Ergren Y, Yucesan S, et al. Mortality due to trauma in childhood. J Trauma 1988;28(s):669-671.
7. Cantor, RM, Leaming, JM. Evaluation and management of pediatric major trauma. Emerg Med Clin North Am 1998; 16:229.
8. Saladino, RA, Lund, DP. Abdominal Trauma. In: Textbook of Pediatric Emergency Medicine, 5th ed, Fleisher, GR, Ludwig, S, Henretig, FM (Eds), Lippincott Williams and Wilkins, Philadelphia, 2006. p.1453.
9. Saladino, R, Lund, D, Fleisher, G. The spectrum of liver and spleen injuries in children: failure of the pediatric trauma score and clinical signs to predict isolated injuries. Ann Emerg Med 1991; 20:636.
10. Jaffe, D, Wesson, D. Emergency management of blunt trauma in children. N Engl J Med 1991; 324:1477.
11. Driscoll, P, Skinner, D. ABC of major trauma. Initial assessment and management—II: Secondary survey. BMJ 1990; 300:1329.
12. McAnena, OJ, Moore, EE, Marx, JA. Initial evaluation of the patient with blunt abdominal trauma. Surg Clin North Am 1990; 70:495.
13. Ferrera, PC, Verdile, VP, Bartfield, JM, et al. Injuries distracting from intraabdominal injuries after blunt trauma. Am J Emerg Med 1998; 16:145.
14. Isaacman, DJ, Scarfone, RJ, Kost, SI, et al. Utility of routine laboratory testing for detecting intra-abdominal injury in the pediatric trauma patient. Pediatrics 1993; 92:691.
15. Boulanger, BR, McLellan, BA. Blunt abdominal trauma. Emerg Med Clin North Am 1996; 14:151.
16. Coley BD, Mutabagani KH, Martin LC, et al. Focused abdominal sonography for trauma (FAST) in children with blunt abdominal trauma. J Trauma. May 2000;48(5):902-6.
17. Neish, AS, Taylor, GA, Lund, DP, Atkinson, CC. Effect of CT information on the diagnosis and

management of acute abdominal injury in children. Radiology 1998; 206:327.
18. Udekwu, PO, Gurkin, B, Oller, DW. The use of computed tomography in blunt abdominal injuries. Am Surg 1996; 62:56.
19. Taylor, GA, Eggli, KD. Lap-belt injuries of the lumbar spine in children: a pitfall in CT diagnosis. AJR Am J Roentgenol 1988; 150:1355.
20. Choong, RK, Grattan-Smith, TM, Cohen, RC, Cass, DT. Splenic injury in children: a 10 year experience. J Paediatr Child Health 1993; 29:192.
21. Stylianos S. Compliance with evidence-based guidelines in children with isolated spleen or liver injury: a prospective study. J Pediatr Surg. Mar 2002; 37(3):453-6.
22. Hennes HM, Smith DS, Schneider K, et al. Elevated liver transaminase levels in children with blunt abdominal trauma: A predictor of liver injury. Pediatrics 1990;86(1):87-90.
23. Pryor, JP, Stafford, PW, Nance, ML. Severe blunt hepatic trauma in children. J Pediatr Surg 2001; 36:974.
24. Oldham KT, Guice KS, Ryckman F, et al. Blunt liver injury in childhood: Evolution of therapy and current perspective. Surgery 1986; 100(3):542-549.
25. Sax, SL, Athey, PA, Lamki, N, Cadavid, GA. Sonographic findings in traumatic hemobilia: report of two cases and review of the literature. J Clin Ultrasound 1988; 16:29.
26. Bass DH, Semple PL, Cywes S, et al. Investigations and management of blunt renal injuries in children: A review of 11 year's experience. J Pediatr Surg 1991;26(2):196-200.
27. Gaines, BA, Shultz, BS, Morrison, K, Ford, HR. Duodenal injuries in children: beware of child abuse. J Pediatr Surg 2004; 39:600
28. Achildi O, Betz RR, Grewal H. Lapbelt injuries and the seatbelt syndrome in pediatric spinal cord injury. J Spinal Cord Med. 2007;30 Suppl 1:S21-4.

In the previous edition this chapter was written by E. Stevers Golladay, MD Professor of Surgery, Head of the Section of Pediatric Surgery, Louisiana State University Medical Center, New Orleans, Louisiana
and
Dileep R. Vyas, MD, Assistant Professor of Pediatrics University of Arkansas for Medical Sciences Arkansas Children's Hospital Little Rock, Arkansas

Sonia Singh and Yuri Gilhotra

23 Thoracic Trauma

Thoracic injury is relatively less frequent in children than it is in adults; its incidence, however, appears to be rising. In children, these injuries are usually due to blunt trauma, but penetrating injury is becoming more common in preadolescents and teenagers. Mechanisms of injury follow a different pattern for various age groups. From birth to four years of age, child abuse and motor vehicle accidents predominate. In the 5- to 9-year-old age group, autopedestrian injuries are common and from 10 to 17 years of age, falls and bicycle injuries increase in frequency. Thoracic injuries are more common in boys.

The highly compliant chest wall of children allows for significant intrathoracic injuries to occur without ribs being fractured; therefore rib fractures which are a common indicator of injury severity in adults are not as useful in children. Associated injuries involving multiple organ systems increase the mortality of children with chest injuries. The mobility of the mediastinum in children dissipates force with a resultant lower incidence of injury to the airway and blood vessels, but conversely the faster mediastinal shift causes cardiovascular compromise more rapidly. The first few hours after injury yield the highest mortality, and therefore early diagnosis and therapy is essential.

INITIAL APPROACH

The initial priority to any child with a serious injury begins with the maintenance of a patent airway, adequate ventilation, and oxygenation. The cervical spine must be protected by a semirigid cervical collar until injury is excluded by clinical examination and adequate radiography. Patency of the airway can be maintained by displacing the mandible forward with a jaw thrust and by opening the mouth. Obstructing objects such as a foreign body or clot should be immediately removed. The airway must be suctioned free of blood and debris.

The adequacy of ventilation is assessed by the rate and the depth of respirations, activity of the accessory muscles, stridor, wheezing, grunting, cyanosis, and pallor. Administration of supplemental oxygen by face mask or nasal cannulae or in conjunction with a bag-valve mask device is used when these signs are noted. The adequacy of oxygenation is judged initially by the color of the skin and mucosa and confirmed by pulse oximetry and blood-gas studies. Inadequate ventilation or oxygenation, rising oxygen requirements, rising $PaCO_2$, and falling PaO_2 dictate the need for intubation.

Hypoxemia despite a patent airway and supplemental oxygen may herald severe pulmonary or cardiac injury such as pneumothorax, tension pneumothorax, hemothorax, or hemopneumothorax, cardiac contusion, pericardial tamponade, and vascular or septal rupture. Evacuation of the pleural or pericardial space with needle aspiration followed by the placement of a drainage tube is required for improvement in oxygenation and ventilation.

The adequacy of circulation must be assessed by mental status, heart rate, quality of the pulses, color and temperature of the skin, capillary refill, and blood pressure. Inadequate perfusion or shock causes further tissue hypoxia in children with chest injury. Loss of blood into the pleural space, abdomen, pelvis or thigh or an open wound can each exceed 40 percent of the blood volume and result in poor perfusion as can myocardial contusion and pericardial tamponade because of decreased cardiac output and hypotension.

Establishing two secured large-caliber intravenous *(IV)* lines is the next priority in any severely injured child. A type and crossmatch is obtained, and blood is sent to the laboratory for the investigations listed in Table 1 as soon as venous access becomes available. Intraosseous lines in infants and young children can be placed rapidly in the tibia or femur. Venous cut-down (saphenous, femoral, cephalic, or external jugular) provides reliable access early in the management of severe shock when percutaneous access is so difficult. Infusion of 20 ml/kg of Ringer's lactate or 0.9% saline over 5 to 10 minutes should be initiated after access is obtained to treat hypotension. A second bolus of 20 ml/kg over a similar period allows sufficient time for type-specific blood to be available for transfusion. Transfusion of O negative unmatched blood may be used prior to availability of type-specific blood. A detailed search for the extent of chest injury, other associated injuries, and the degree of physiologic derangement follows the management of ventilation and circulation. The child is exposed and examined completely. Catheters and monitors to record the heart rate, respiratory rate, electrocardiogram (EKG), blood pressure, urinary output, and pulse oximetry are then established. The stomach is decompressed with a nasogastric tube to prevent gaseous distention, subsequent vomiting, and possible gastropneumonic reflux in a patient with compromised ventilation. An orogastric tube is preferred if there is a nasal fracture or bleeding.

A child's surface area is larger in proportion to their body weight than is an adult's, and therefore children must be protected from hypothermia by warm blankets and overhead heaters.

A portable chest radiograph can be performed for unstable children although upright and lateral radiographs in the radiology department are preferred. Entrance and exit sites of penetrating wounds are marked. 12-lead EKG should be obtained. Need for further studies such as esophagograms or aortogram are dictated by

Table 1: Laboratory Studies for Thoracic Injury

CBC[a] blood type and crossmatch	Arterial blood gas
Electrolytes-BUN[b]-blood sugar	Coagulation studies, urinalysis

[a]CBC = complete blood count
[b]BUN = blood urea nitrogen

the signs attendant to abnormalities of these structures.

The following mnemonic may help memorize the initial approach.

Primary Survey/Resuscitation

A. Airway, "C" spine
B. Breathing
C. Circulation/hemorrhage control
D. Detailed examination (Data collection [vital signs, monitors, dextrostix])
E. E. Exposure, environmental control/ (hypothermia, fever)
F. Foley
G. Gastric tube, blood gases

SPECIFIC INJURIES

Rib Fractures

The reported incidence of pediatric rib fractures in extensive trauma varies between 30 and 50 percent and implies that a significant fall, traffic accident, severe injury, or child abuse has occurred. Occupants as passengers in motor vehicles involved in accidents in older children and motor vehicle pedestrian accidents in younger children account for most pediatric rib fractures. Fractures of the first three ribs are often associated with bronchial, cardiac, or large-vessel injuries. The fractures of the lower three ribs are associated with hepatic and splenic injury. As the number of fractured ribs increases, so does the severity of injury and the extent of associated organ injuries thus increasing morbidity and mortality. Patients with rib fractures have localized pain on deep breathing, cough, or positional changes. The respiratory excursions may be diminished. A chest radiograph helps define the extent of injury. If pain is not controlled by analgesics, intercostal nerve block with a small volume of bupivacaine (0.25 percent) with epinephrine(1:200,000) is useful. As much as 1 ml/kg may be injected at the lower margin of the fractured rib and the ribs above and below the fracture level posterior to the fracture site.

Pneumothorax

Traumatic pneumothorax can follow penetrating or blunt injury and is usually associated with hemothorax. A small pneumothorax may be asymptomatic. A significant pneumothorax produces respiratory distress, tracheal shift, hyperresonance to percussion, and decreased breath sounds. Mediastinal shift, asymmetrical chest wall movement, tracheal shift, distended neck veins, and hyperresonance to percussion are signs of tension pneumothorax. Rapid respiratory deterioration of a mechanically ventilated patient with a well-placed endotracheal tube should arouse suspicion. Plain chest radiograph and lateral decubitus radiographs (with the suspected side upward) are diagnostic. Anterior second intercostal needle thoracostomy must be performed immediately if the child is severely stressed. A thoracostomy tube is placed posteriorly to evacuate the frequently present hemothorax better and aid in reexpansion of the collapsed lung. The thoracostomy tube allows evacuation of pneumothorax, hemothorax, and facilitates the re-expansion of the collapsed lung. Traumatic pneumothorax can yield as much as 15 percent mortality.

Open Chest

Open chest is an unusual injury in children with impailment on a fixed object as the most common cause. Penetrating injury to the thorax usually seals itself. If the penetrating object is large enough to leave a defect, a "sucking chest wound" may result. The pressure gradient between the thoracic cavity and the atmospheric pressure necessary for air exchange and venous return is destroyed, resulting in hypoxia and hypotension. If the chest wall hole is two thirds the diameter of trachea, air passes preferentially through the opening with respiration. The management of open pneumothorax requires its prompt closure with an occlusive dressing (a sterile towel or a gloved finger). This should be followed by a dressing with multiple layers of vaseline gauze extending at least five cm beyond the wound's edges. Securing the dressing with tapes on three sides with one side left open creates a flutter valve effect to prevent the development of tension pneumothorax. Definitive care requires placement of a chest tube through a separate wound followed by the surgical closure of the defect.

Hemothorax

Both blunt and penetrating injuries may result in hemothorax. Lacerations of the intercostal, internal mammary, and pulmonary vessels and occasionally rupture of a cardiac chamber or aorta are the causes of hemothorax. Parenchymal lacerations, because of the elastic recoil of lung tissue, low pulmonary artery pressure and the release of vasoactive substances, do not usually cause large volume blood loss. Forty percent of the calculated blood volume may be lost into one hemithorax. A large hemothorax produces the compression of the ipsilateral lung, contralateral mediastinal shift, and shock. Tracheal shift to the contralateral side, dullness to percussion and decreased breath sounds are the usual signs. Upright chest or lateral decubitus chest radiographs show a collection of fluid in the costophrenic, cardiophrenic, or subpulmonic sites (Figure 1). Rapid infusion of fluid and blood is necessary to resuscitate the child. The vast majority of patients will require evacuation of blood by tube thoracostomy to provide effective air exchange, monitor ongoing loss and reduce the risk of fibrothorax. Traumatic hemothorax has a 2 percent incidence of empyema. Isolated traumatic hemothorax has low mortality, but for children with associated head and abdominal injury, the mortality rate approaches 70 percent.

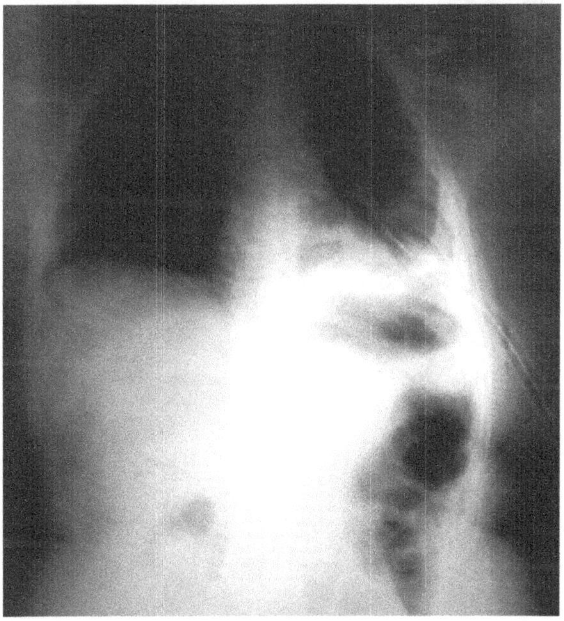

Fig. 1: Chest radiograph of a 12-year-old female, victim of motor vehicle accident showing left pleural effusion with a chest tube in place.

Pulmonary Contusion

The most common serious intrathoracic injury in children is pulmonary contusion.

Pulmonary contusion, although associated with rib fracture or flail chest, often occurs without rib fractures. The lesion can be fairly localized or widely disseminated. The response of the lung to injury varies from minimal interstitial edema to rapid intra-alveolar extravasation of blood and fluid. Early institution of measures to limit interstitial pulmonary edema is important. These include judicious use of intravenous infusions, control of pain, and careful pulmonary toilet. Use of diuretics, bronchodilators, and prophylactic antibiotics should also be considered. Dyspnea, hemoptysis, dullness to percussion, wheezing, and crepitance develop with progression to respiratory failure. This mandates constant surveillance for hypoxemia and hypercarbia.

Chest radiographs may demonstrate peribronchial and/or perivascular infiltrate that can progress to consolidation (Figure 2). Arterial blood gases will establish the degree of respiratory compromise. Patients needing an FiO_2 of 0.4 to 0.5 by mask to maintain oxygen saturation will usually require endotracheal intubation and administration of positive end-expiratory pressure. Rapid institution of ventilatory support is critical in children with multiple contusions and multiple rib fractures and with those who require large-volume fluid resuscitation and those with deteriorating arterial blood gases. The arterial oxygen saturation should be maintained at about 90 percent. Pneumonia, fat embolism, and pulmonary embolism are common complications. The mortality varies with the severity of injury but may be as high as 70 percent when associated with other extra thoracic injuries.

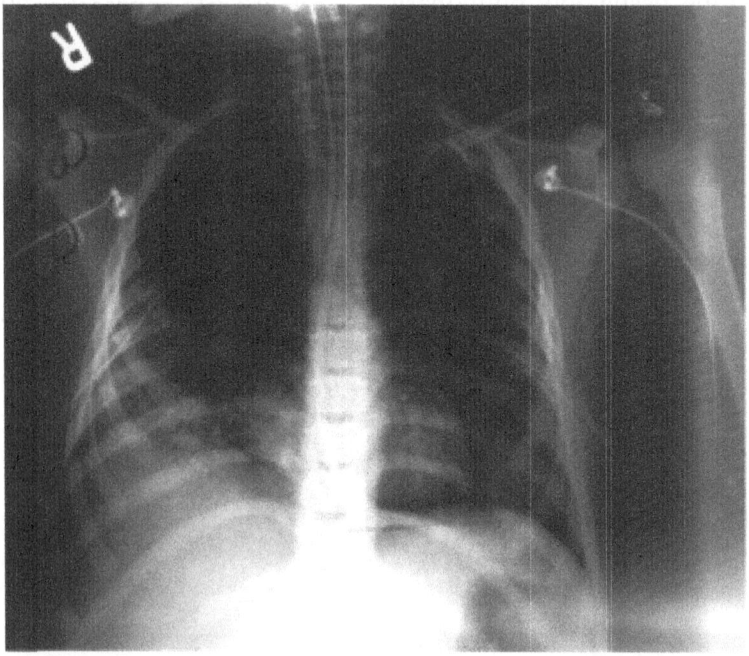

Fig. 2: Portable chest radiograph of a 6-year-old male, victim of motor vehicle accident, showing right lower lung infiltrate compatible with pulmonary contusion.

Flail Chest

Although rib fractures are not unusual in childhood, flail chest is rare. Lateral rib fractures and fractures of the sternum, pneumothorax, hemothorax, and pulmonary contusion are common associates of flail chest. Several contiguous ribs fractured at more than one point, may create a flail chest. Multiple rib fractures on chest radiograph do not constitute a flail chest. A section of chest wall must exhibit paradoxical motion during the respiratory cycle. Associated pneumothorax, hemothorax, or pulmonary contusion demand increased work of breathing, which increases paradoxical chest wall motion. Flail chest may not be apparent until the work of breathing is increased. In addition, chest wall muscle spasm may temporarily stabilize the flail segment, which becomes sympto-matic as the muscles tire.

Initial therapy demands attention to ventilation and oxygenation. Not all patients with flail chest require endotracheal intubation and mechanical ventilation. The decision for such intervention depends on clinical and laboratory factors such as shock, hypoxia, hypercarbia, respiratory rate, associated head injury, and the necessity for general anesthesia for other injuries. Careful attention should be paid to fluid resuscitation. The lungs of a child with flail chest are very sensitive to fluid overload. Careful monitoring of pulmonary and cardiac function is necessary to optimize fluid administration. Treatment is primarily directed at pain control and underlying pulmonary contusion. Pneumonia is a common complication. In children with two or more associated injuries, fractures of more than seven ribs, bilateral flail chest, and shock, the mortality can be as high as 95 percent. Late mortality is usually associated with pulmonary sepsis.

Tracheobronchial Disruption

Intrathoracic tracheobronchial injuries are rare. These injuries occur in a setting of high-energy impact and are usually associated with other injuries. Acute mortality is high. Timely diagnosis of these injuries is essential.

Three main mechanisms of injury are: (1) Sudden compression of the chest pulls the lungs apart, creating traction at the carina that results in a tear of the tracheobronchial tree. (2) A force applied while the glottis is closed causes high intrabronchial pressure that ruptures large bronchi. (3) Rapid deceleration generates shearing force at the areas of fixation such as the carina and causes rupture of the bronchus. Subcutaneous emphysema, dyspnea, hemoptysis, sternal tenderness, and positive *Hamman's sign* are common. Common radiographic findings include pneumothorax, pneumomediastinum, subcutaneous emphysema, accompanying fractures of clavicles and ribs, and pulmonary contusion. Bronchoscopy will confirm the diagnosis. The immediate treatment requires ventilatory support and a placement of a tube thoracostomy. The definitive treatment consists of primary suture of the lacerations. Overall mortality is appro-ximately 30 percent.

Diaphragmatic Injury

Traumatic diaphragmatic injury is uncommon. Falls from heights and automobile accidents are the usual causes of blunt injury to the diaphragm. Gunshot wounds and stab wounds to the chest below the fourth intercostal space account for most of the penetrating injuries to the diaphragm and produce small holes with delayed presentations. Blunt trauma produces large radial tears. The gradient of peritoneal-pleural pressure facilitates the herniation of abdominal viscera into the chest, usually on the left side. Scaphoid abdomen, dullness to percussion on the chest, and the presence of bowel sounds in the chest establish the diagnosis.

Chest radiographs may show mediastinal shift, herniated viscera and elevation of the diaphragm or the presence of a nasogastric tube in the intrathoracic stomach. Bowel contrast studies and positive contrast peritoneography may be helpful in difficult cases. If ventilatory support is necessary, bag-valve-mask ventilation should be avoided because insufflation produces further distention of the herniated gastrointestinal tract and causes further compromise of ventilation. Placement of a nasogastric tube helps to decompress a herniated stomach. Immediate surgical repair should be undertaken.

Chest pain or dyspnea in a child who has had blunt or penetrating trauma can signify a chronic diaphragmatic hernia and should warrant a chest radiograph. Chronic diaphragmatic hernias are better repaired by a thoracic approach. Acute diaphragmatic injury from blunt trauma has a 90 percent association with intra-abdominal injuries. Associated fractures of the lumbar spine are common.

Myocardial Concussion and Contusion

Cardiac concussion from blunt chest injury causes transient dysrhythmias and/or nonspecific ST-segment changes. There is no histopathologically identifiable lesion in this condition and the electrocardiographic abnormality is usually of no significance. Cardiac contusion results from forceful blunt injury that causes histopathologically identifiable lesions. The true incidence of myocardial injury after blunt injury is unknown. Signs and symptoms suggestive of myocardial contusion include precordial pain, diaphoresis, bruised precordium, tachycardia, low blood pressure, dyspnea, heart murmur, and precordial rub. Chest radiographs may demonstrate suggestive findings such as first rib or sternum fracture. Although many different tests suggest the diagnosis, there is no gold standard. Serial EKGs, serial creatinine phosphokinase isoenzyme (CK-MB) ratios, echocardiogram, pyrophosphate scan, multiple-gated acquisition (MUGA) cardiac scan and radionuclide angiograms are used to investigate cardiac function and perfusion. Common EKG abnormalities associated with myocardial contusion include ST-T wave changes and conduction abnormalities. Abnormalities of the other tests described here should enhance suspicion. Although most children will recover without serious problems, they should be admitted to a pediatric intensive care unit and closely monitored as signs of pump failure, hemodynamic instability, or cardiac arrhythmia may arise and must be treated appropriately. The morbidity from myocardial contusion in a hemodynamically stable patient without conduction abnormality is minimal.

Aortic Rupture

Aortic rupture is a common cause of death in automobile accidents in adults. Its occurrence in children is rare. It is usually caused by blunt injury such as a fall from a height of more than 20 feet or a pedestrian motor vehicle accident. The tear often occurs near the aortic isthmus, although some tears extend to involve the aortic arch or a cardiac chamber. Associated injuries are common, and immediate mortality is high. The survivors of aortic rupture have a contained hematoma or an intact adventitia. The child may complain of midscapular pain that radiates to the back and dyspnea and dysphagia are frequent. Hypertension in the upper extremity and hypotension in the lower extremities results from inadequate perfusion distal to the site of aortic rupture. Supraclavicular hematoma and deviation of trachea to the right can also be present. Obliteration of the aortic knob, widened mediastinum, fracture of the first or second rib, deviation of trachea, and/or esophagus (nasogastric tube) to the right on chest radiograph are suggestive of aortic rupture. A high index of suspicion, complimented by clinical and radiologic findings, will provoke aortography and lead to the correct diagnosis. Blood pressure should be continously monitored. Hemodynamic decompensation from blunt aortic injury is usually very rapid and massive, causing death from exsanguina-tion. In a child with suspected blunt aortic trauma, immediate left anterolateral thoracotomy and repair may reduce the mortality. The mortality for patients who arrive alive in the emergency department is about 30 percent.

Hemopericardium

Hemopericardium can result from penetrating or blunt injury to the pericardial, epicardial, myocardial, or coronary vessels, intrapericardial great vessels, or cardiac chambers. Even a small amount of blood in the pericardial sac restricts cardiac activity and interferes with cardiac filling, producing cardiac tamponade. The presence of distended neck veins, low blood pressure, narrow pulse pressure, and distant heart sounds suggest the diagnosis. A decrease in systolic blood pressure in excess of 10 mmHg during inspiration, called *pulsus paradoxus,* is associated with pericardial tamponade. Widened cardiac shadow on chest radiograph, low voltage complexes on EKG, and peaked T-waves in the precordial leads with flat Ts laterally may also be present.

The initial management of hemopericardium consists of IV fluids to raise the central venous pressure followed by inotropic support of the blood pressure. Pericardiocentesis may temporarily relieve the symptoms, but open pericardiotomy must then be performed. Pericardial aspiration may not be diagnostic or therapeutic if there is clotted blood in the pericardial sac.

Esophageal Injury

Esophageal trauma can be caused by penetrating or blunt trauma. Blunt epigastric injury causes forceful ejection of gastric contents into the esophagus, significantly raising the intraluminal pressure that causes linear tears in the lower esophagus. Transmural rupture produces the leakage of gastric and esophageal content into the mediastinum, causing mediastinitis. Rupture from the mediastinum into the pleural space quickly follows, producing multifloral empyema.

The history of a severe blow to the lower sternum or epigastrium, pain or shock disproportionate to the severity of injury, fever, subcutaneous emphysema, pleural effusion, and the appearance of particulate matter or saliva in the chest tube drainage are suggestive or predictive of esophageal injury. Salivary amylase may be found in the chest tube drainage. Methylene blue, when it is swallowed, will also appear in the thoracostomy tube. The diagnosis may be confirmed by a water soluble contrast esophagogram. The initial treatment is directed toward drainage and the administration of fluid and antibiotics. The definitive treatment consists of the repair of the esophagus via thoracotomy.

The mortality of esophageal rupture is high when the diagnosis is delayed or the perforation of the esophagus is intra-abdominal.

Traumatic Asphyxia

Traumatic asphyxia occurs when the chest is flattened between a compressant force and a hard surface during maintenance of a closed glottis. It is most typically seen after an automobile passes over a child's chest. The resilient chest wall of a child allows compression of the heart, the lungs, and the great vessels to occur without rib or sternal fractures. A sudden, sharp rise in the intrathoracic pressure causes the pressures in the supraclavicular vessels and the head and neck capillary pressures to rise. The classic feature of traumatic asphyxia is a supraclavicular cyanosis of the neck and the face and a V-shaped distribution of the cyanosis in the posterior interscapular area. Other frequently associated clinical features include petechiae of the head and neck, subconjunctival hemorrhage, epistaxis, hemoptysis, hematemesis, blurred vision, mental dullness, and hyperpyrexia. Cardiac injury and pulmonary contusion may also be associated. Post-obstructive pulmonary edema, peripheral or spinal paralysis occur rarely. The treatment is largely supportive and consists of elevation of the head of the bed, oxygen supplementation, and fluid limitation. Associated injuries may dictate more invasive procedures to maintain homeostasis and are largely responsible for the associated morbidity and mortality. More than 90 percent of the cases, however, recover completely without specific treatment.

SPECIAL PROCEDURES

Tube Thoracostomy

Emergency tube thoracostomy may be necessary to drain air, fluid, or both from the pleural cavity and help reexpand the lung. The usual site for the placement of a chest tube is the fifth intercostal space anterior to the midaxillary line on the affected side (Figure 3). The diameter of the selected tube should approximate the width of the intercostal space through which it is to be placed. A wide area of skin around the placement site is antiseptically prepared and draped. The proposed incision site, usually the skin overlying the seventh rib in the midaxillary line, is infiltrated with local anesthetic. A 1 to 3 cm skin incision is used to develop a craniad posterior tunnel. The pleural space is entered through the fifth intercostal space. The chest tube is directed by a hemostat through the tunnel so that the tip of the tube is located at the posterior third intercostal space. The tube is connected to an underwater seal or suction at negative 10 to 20 cm water pressure. The tube is secured to the skin with nonabsorbable sutures. A chest X-ray verifies the tube position, adequacy of pleural space drainage, and the re-expansion of the lung. It may also reveal previously unrecognized lung pathology.

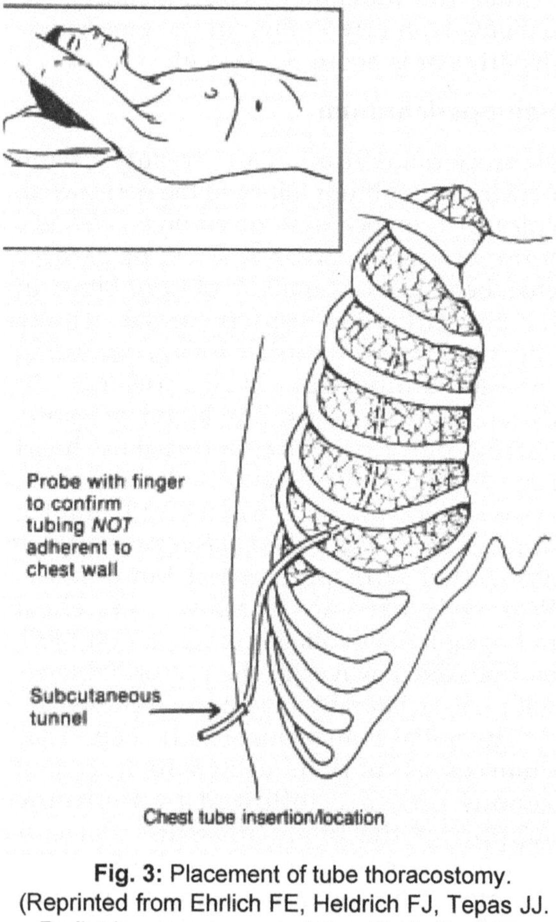

Fig. 3: Placement of tube thoracostomy. (Reprinted from Ehrlich FE, Heldrich FJ, Tepas JJ. Pediatric emergency medicine. Rockville, MD.: Aspen, 1987; 73, with permission from Aspen Publishers, Inc. © 1987.)

Pericardiocentesis

Pericardiocentesis is used for aspiration of cardiac tamponade. It is best done in the operating room with continuous EKG monitoring. The xiphisternal area is antiseptically prepared and draped. A long large-caliber over-the-needle cannula is inserted in the left xiphocostal angle and advanced toward the left shoulder at a 30 to 45 degree angle to the plane of the body (Figure 4). A 20 ml syringe maintains a small negative pressure as the needle is advanced. When the needle tip penetrates the pericardial sac, blood will appear in the syringe. If the needle is advanced into the myocardium, an injury pattern (ST-T changes or QRS widening) will appear on the EKG monitor. The needle should be withdrawn slightly if an injury pattern appears. Once the needle tip is in the pericardial space, the cannula is advanced into the pericardial sac, and the needle is withdrawn. The cannula is connected to a syringe and stopcock, and the pericardial space is drained.

CONCLUSIONS

Thoracic injuries are uncommon in children, yet remain a significant source of mortality and morbidity. A thorough physical exam

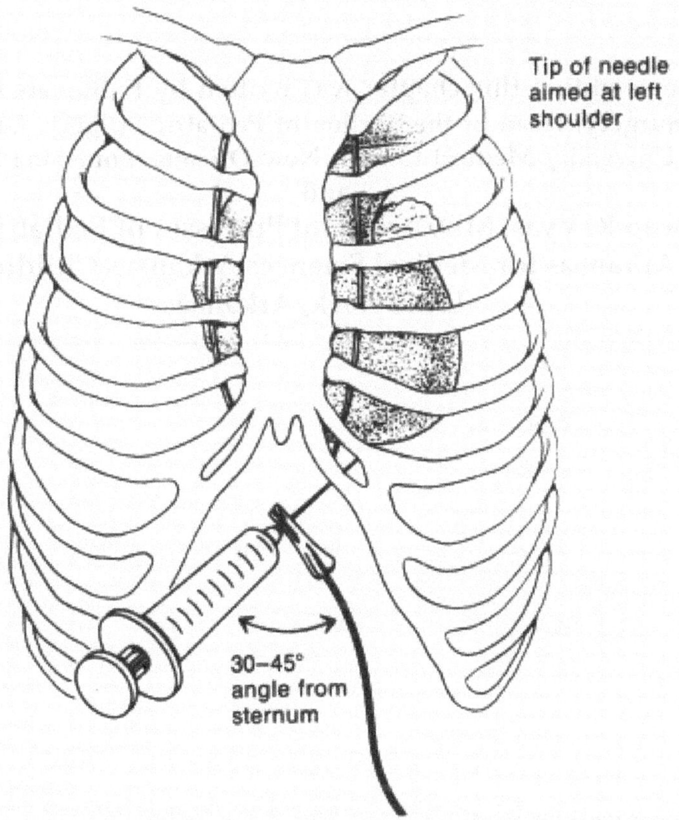

Fig. 4: Location and technique of pericardiocentesis. (Reprinted from Ehrlich FE, Heldrich FJ, Tepas JJ. Pediatric emergency medicine. Rockville, Md.: Aspen, 1987; 73, with permission of Aspen Publishers, Inc., © 1987.)

with attention to anatomic and physiologic differences in children, and expeditious care of life-threatening emergencies has improved outcome. The majority of injuries are safely managed with expectant observation alone or with tube thoracostomy for blood orxt decade air.

FURTHER READING

1. Tovar JA. The lung and pediatric trauma. Semin Pediatr Surg 2008;17:53-9.
2. Donnelly LF. Imaging issues in CT of blunt trauma to the chest and abdomen. Pediatr Radiol 2009;39 Suppl 3:406-13.
3. Sartorelli KH, Vane DW. The diagnosis and management of children with blunt injury of the chest. Semin Pediatr Surg 2004;13:98-105.
4. Moore MA, Wallace EC, Westra SJ. The imaging of paediatric thoracic trauma. Pediatr Radiol 2009;39:485-96.
5. Bliss D, Silen M. Pediatric thoracic trauma. Crit Care Med 2002;30:S409-15.
6. Avarello JT, Cantor RM. Pediatric major trauma: an approach to evaluation and management. Emerg Med Clin North Am 2007;25:803-36.
7. Mendelson KG, Fallat ME. Pediatric injuries: prevention to resolution. Surg Clin North Am 2007;87:207-28.
8. Westra SJ, Wallace EC. Imaging evaluation of pediatric chest trauma. Radiol Clin North Am 2005;43:267-81.
9. Neal MD, Sippey M, Gaines BA, Hackam DJ. Presence of pneumomediastinum after blunt trauma in children: what does it really mean? J Pediatr Surg 2009;44:1322-7.

In the previous edition this chapter was written by E. Stevers Golladay, MD Professor of Surgery, Head of the Section of Pediatric Surgery, Louisiana State University Medical Center, New Orleans, Louisiana

and

Dileep R. Vyas, MD, Assistant Professor of Pediatrics University of Arkansas for Medical Sciences Arkansas Children's Hospital Little Rock, Arkansas

Dipak Sheth

24 Spine Injuries

Fortunately, injuries to the spine and spinal cord are rare in children. They deserve serious attention, however, for several reasons. If they are not recognized and treated appropriately, they can have devastating consequences, including paralysis, deformity and pain. Also they are not easy to recognize, particularly because of the numerous normal radiographic appearances of the child's spine that may resemble fracture or instability. Finally these injuries may assume different patterns and require different treatment than do their adult counterparts.

The true incidence of pediatric spinal injury is not known. It has been estimated that 2.5 to 3.3 percent of all spinal injuries occur in children and it consist of less than 2-4% of all childhood injuries. Thoracolumbar spinal injury, accounts for up to 75% of all pediatric spine fractures. While the majority 80% of thoracolumbar vertebral fracture do not have concomitant neurologic deficits, it is a major source of functional disabilities in children who survive the initial injury the incidence is usually reported to be higher in males, and it increases with age, probably due to vehicular trauma, sports activities, and other risk-taking behaviors. Cervical spine birth trauma should be considered in a newborn with decreased tone, a nonprogressive neurologic deficit, and a negative history of a familial neurologic disorder. During ages 3 to 5 years, falls from heights, motor vehicle accidents, and child abuse are the most common causes. From 6 to 15 years, they are usually the result of motor vehicle accidents and sports injuries. The number of spine injuries in children that result in spinal cord injury (SCI) is also unknown. Paraplegia is three times more common than quadriplegia. The importance of SCI in producing paralysis is obvious.

Another sequela of SCI in children is spinal deformity. This is most common in younger children, with higher levels of injury, with spasticity, or when a laminectomy has been performed. Children with simple fractures and no SCI tend to remodel, and deformity is seldom progressive.

PATHOPHYSIOLOGY

Injuries to the spine and spinal cord in small children may assume different patterns and behave differently than they do in adults. This may be explained by some basic anatomical and physiological differences between children and adults. First the cartilaginous plates in the child's spine are still growing. This explains certain injury patterns peculiar to children since the growth plates constitute an area of mechanical weakness in a motion segment; also injury to the plate or further growth in the presence of paralysis or spasticity can lead to progressive deformity. On the other hand, the child's spine has some ability to remodel after simple fractures. Second the child's spine has more inherent ligamentous laxity than does the adult spine, accounting for the fact that SCI can occur without fracture or dislocation. Third the child's head is proportionately larger than is the adult's thus imparting more energy to the spine. This also requires different positioning in the child to achieve reduction of cervical spine injuries. Fourth, the facet joints are oriented more horizontally in the child, allowing more motion normally, especially in the cervical spine. Most cervical spine injuries in children occur at the upper end, as opposed to adult injuries, which often occur in the lower cervical spine. By around ages 8 to 10, the child's spine has achieved nearly adult proportions, and the injury patterns more closely resemble those seen in adults. The last difference between children and adults is fortunate in that children have a greater potential to recover from SCI.

It is possible for children to sustain SCI without a visible fracture on plain radiographs, linear tomograms, or computed tomography (CT). This is known as spinal cord injury without radiographic abnormality (SCIWORA). The SCI may be complete or incomplete. The incidence of SCIWORA among all SCIs in children is reported to be between 5 and 67 percent. Proposed mechanisms of SCIWORA include physeal separation,ligamentous disruption, and ligamentum flavum compression of the spinal cord secondary to in folding in hyperextension. Spinal cord infarction from compression of collateral blood supply or disruption of the artery of Adamkiewicz supplying the spinal cord, hematoma formation from soft-tissue bleeding, and direct contusion of the thoracic spinal cord also contribute to nonosseous injury. The proportionately larger head-to-body size ratio and the relatively poorly developed neck musculature explain why the injury is more common in the younger age groups and in the upper cervical spine. The onset of paralysis may be delayed, or the paralysis may be precipitated or exacerbated by a second episode of trauma. The injury may be recognized by myelography or magnetic resonance imaging (MRI). Somatosensory evoked potentials (SSEP) may be useful in the presence of concomitant head injury or as a baseline.

CLINICAL PRESENTATION

Injury to the spine and spinal cord should be immediately suspected in any child who has sustained multiple trauma, especially from a motor vehicle accident (Figure 1). This is especially true if a head injury has occurred. Lacerations, abrasions, or contusions around the head and neck should alert one to the possibility of cervical spine injury and may serve as valuable clues as to the mechanism of injury. In the unconscious patient, a diligent search must be made to rule out injury to the spinal column and to assess the status of the spinal cord. Radiographs of the entire spine should be obtained. The motor and sensory levels and the presence or absence of reflexes should be determined (to serve as a baseline). The spine should be protected by log rolling and positioning with such devices as sandbags or soft collars. Anyone complaining of neck or back pain following injury should be evaluated. Similarly any complaint of numbness or weakness, even if it is transient, should be taken seriously. Some patients with an injury to the upper cervical spine (such as an odontoid fracture) will complain of

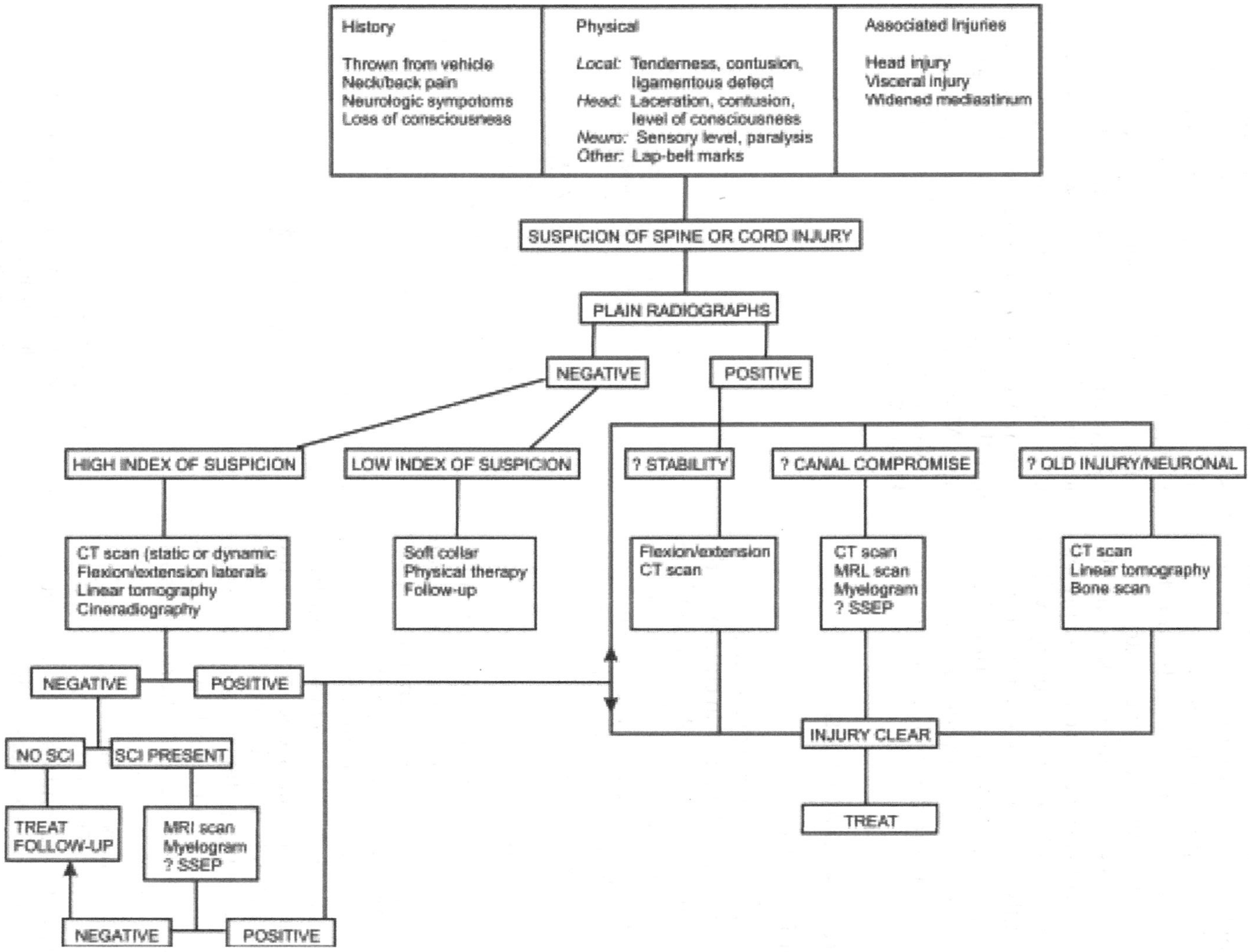

Fig. 1: Clinical presentation of spine and spinal cord injuries in children

numbness or paresthesias in the occipital nerve distribution. Any patient with significant visceral injury from blunt trauma should be suspected of spinal injury. A widened mediastinum may be the first indication of a thoracic spine injury and is thought to result from bleeding at the fracture site. Occasionally a child will present with torticollis following a minor injury. This is especially common following an upper respiratory infection and is often due to atlantoaxial rotatory fixation (AARF). The laboratory evaluation will be considered further later.

DIFFERENTIAL DIAGNOSIS

Normal Findings

The most frequent source of confusion in the evaluation of spinal injuries in children is the rather common occurrence of normal findings or variations that may resemble fractures or instability. It is necessary to have some familiarity with these to avoid confusion that can result in overtreatment.

Growth Centers

There are numerous secondary ossification centers in the immature spine. These can resemble fractures, but can usually be recognized by their positions, by their smooth sclerotic margins, and by the absence of soft tissue swelling. Most vertebrae form from three ossification centers, one in the centrum and one in each neural arch. The arches usually fuse in the midline posteriorly by age two to four years and are seldom a source of confusion (Figure 2(a)). There is also a cartilaginous line between the neural arch and its junction with the central ossification center on each side. These are known as the neurocentral synchondroses and are usually closed by three to six years of age. They can be mistaken for fractures of the neural arch. The ring apophyses form during adolescence, disappearing by skeletal maturity, and appear as small points of ossification at the superior and inferior ends of the vertebral bodies (Figure 2(b)). They are seldom mistaken for fractures but may themselves be subject to injury during adolescence. There is a horizontally oriented growth plate at the base of the dens, which is contiguous laterally with the neurocentral synchondroses. This usually disappears by five to seven years of age. Most fractures of the odontoid in children occur through this growth plate (Figure 2(c)).

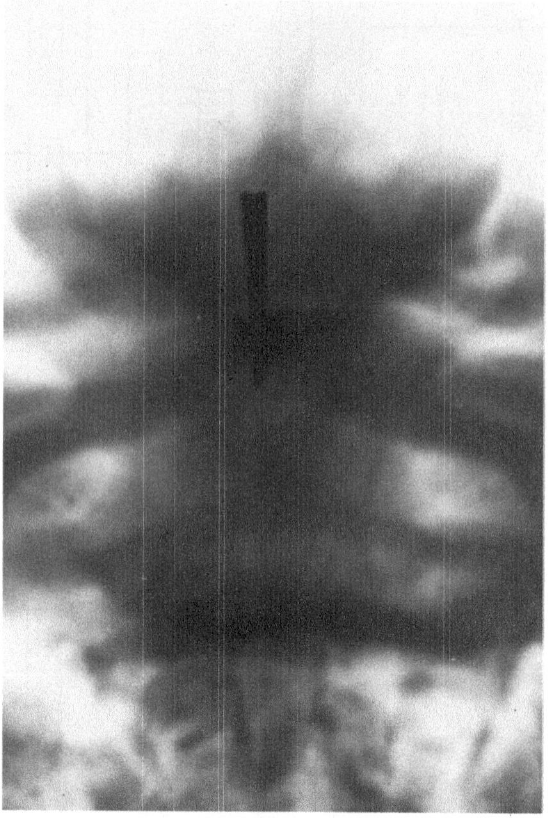

Fig. 2: Normal appearances in the child's spine. (a) Open-mouth odontoid view in a six-month-old. The arrow indicates the synchondrosis between the two neural arches

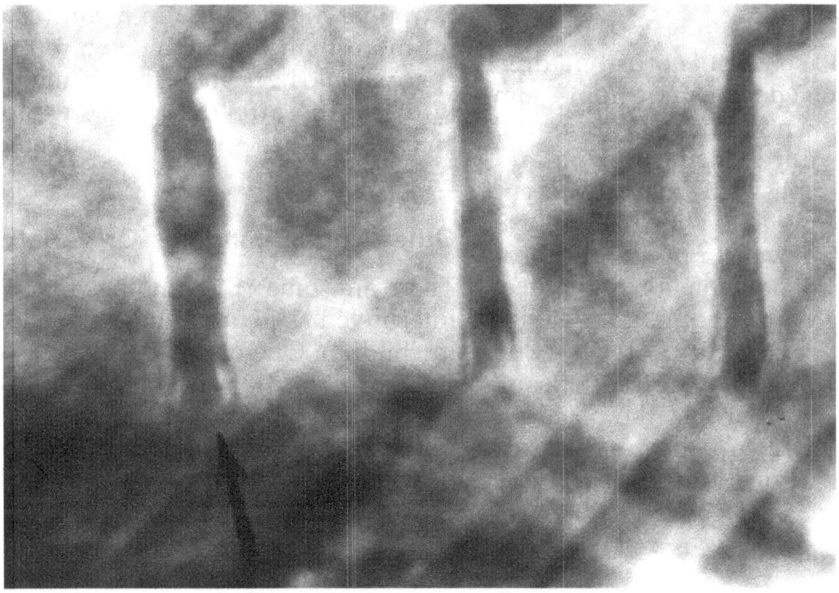

Fig. 2: (continued) (b) Ring apophysis. The arrow indicates the normal appearance. This is the site of the endplate fracture seen in adolescents although the injury involves the posterior portion of the ring

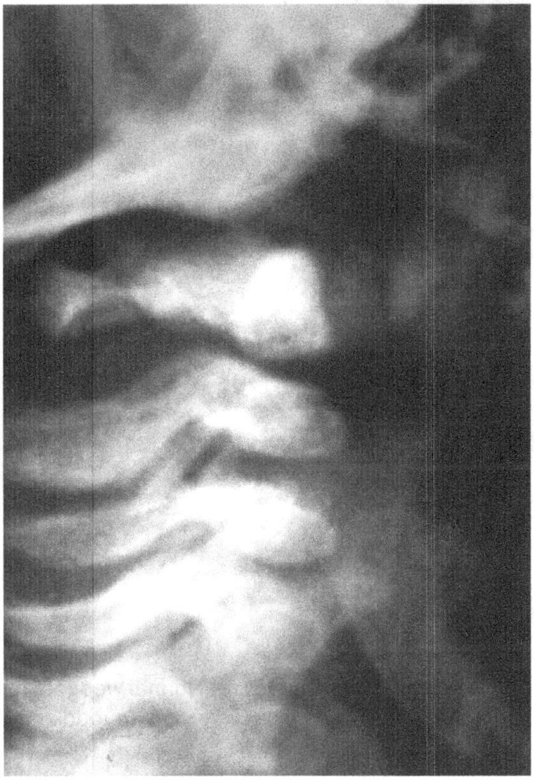

Fig. 2: (continued) (c) Odontoid growth plate can be mistaken for a fracture. In fact, most odontoid fractures in children occur through this area of weakness

Pseudosubluxation

Between 19 and 40 percent of normal children under age eight will demonstrate upto 4 mm of anterior movement of the second cervical vertebra on the third during flexion and extension radiographs. This may also occur at the segment between the third and fourth vertebrae. It is believed to be the result of the normal horizontal orientation of the facet joints and the greater ligamentous laxity present in this age group. It may be recognized by the absence of soft tissue swelling and by the fact that the posterior elements align, even in the position of apparent subluxation (Figure 2(d)). The retropharyngeal space in a child should be no more than 7 mm, and the retrotracheal space should be no more than 14 mm although both can be affected by crying, position changes, and the amount of adenoid tissue present.

Other Normal Findings Or Variations

There are some other findings that might be interpreted as injury but are actually normal in children. One of these is that the cervical vertebral bodies are normally wedged anteriorly until about age eight (Figure 2(e)). There are also indentations in the vertebrae, both anteriorly and posteriorly that are

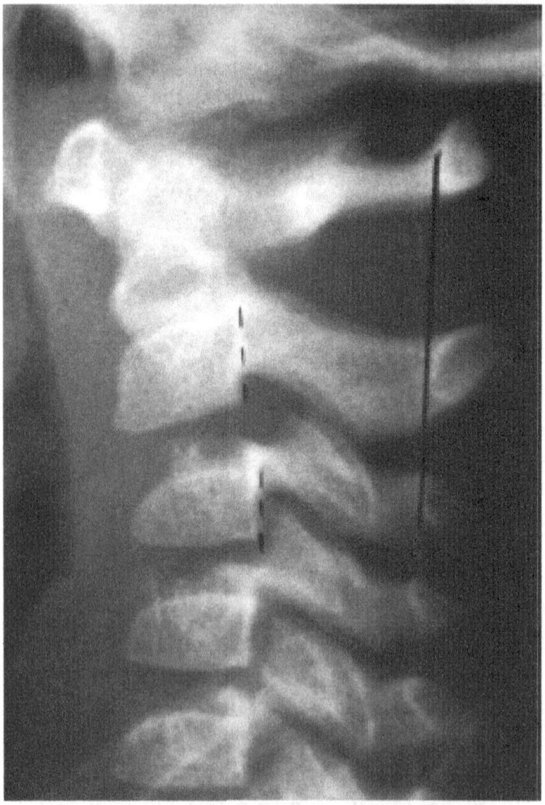

Fig. 2: (continued) (d) Pseudosubluxation in a 2½-year-old. Note the absence of soft tissue swelling anteriorly and that the posterior elements maintain their normal alignment

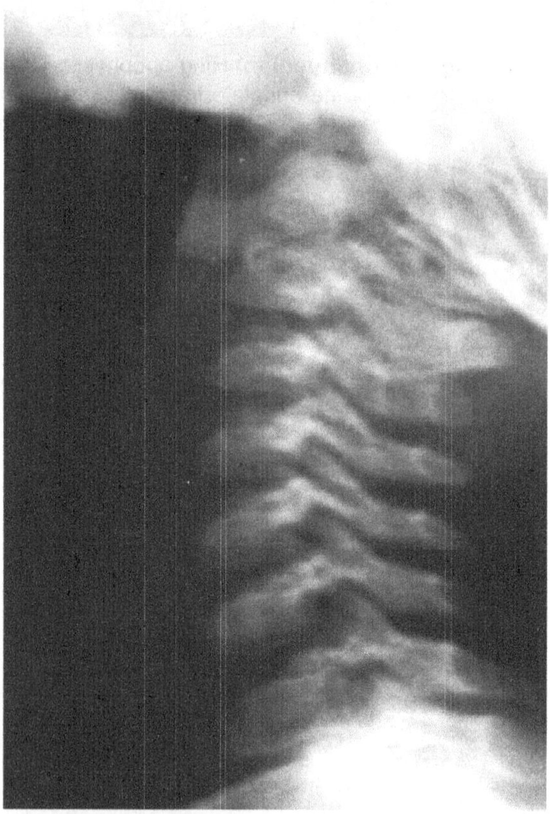

Fig. 2: (continued) (e) Normal wedged appearance of cervical vertebrae in toddler

normal in children. There is normally no lordotic curve in the cervical spine in 15 percent of children (This would suggest muscle spasm and significant injury in an adult).

Other Nontraumatic Findings

There are some other findings that are not normal but that are not traumatic in origin and need be of no concern in an emergency setting. Atlantoaxial instability often develops in Down's syndrome and in certain types of dwarfism (Figure 3(a)). There are also abnormalities associated with the formation of the odontoid process. Aplasia is the total absence of the odontoid, and hypoplasia is the incomplete formation of the odontoid. Either of these may be associated with atlantoaxial instability. Os odontoideum has the appearance of the tip of the odontoid being separated from its base. This is thought to be due to a non-united fracture sustained earlier in childhood and is often associated with atlantoaxial instability (Figure 3b). The tip of the odontoid moves with the anterior arch of C1. Vertebra plana can be seen in eosinophilic granuloma and can be mistaken for a traumatic compression fracture (Figure 3(c)).

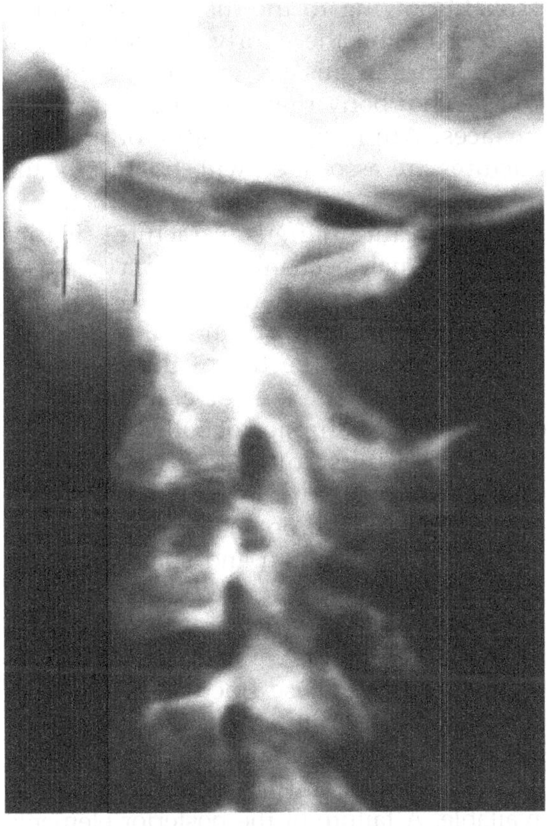

Fig. 3: Nontraumatic abnormalities. (a) Atlantoaxial instability in a five-year old with Down's syndrome. Note the interval between the anterior cortex of the dens and the posterior cortex of the anterior ring of the atlas, which in this case measured 7 mm

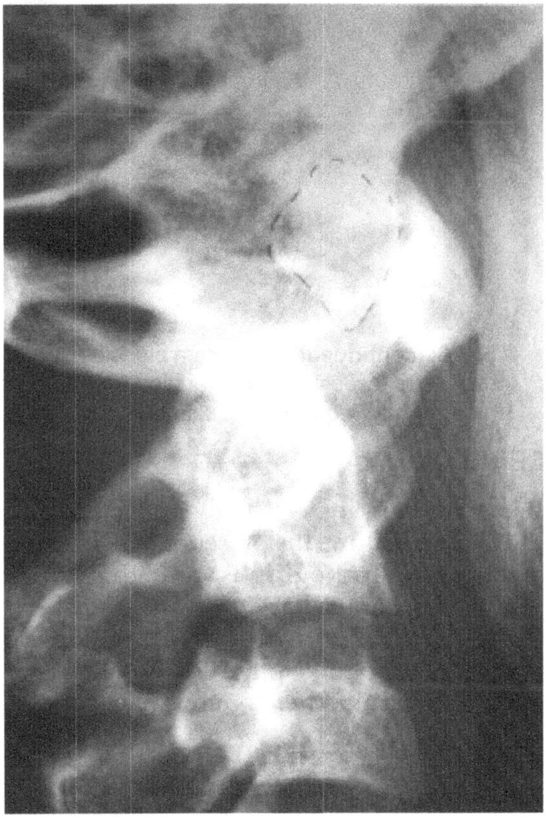

Fig. 3: (continued) (b) Os odontoideum (outlined) with C1-C2 instability. Note that the dens moves with the atlas

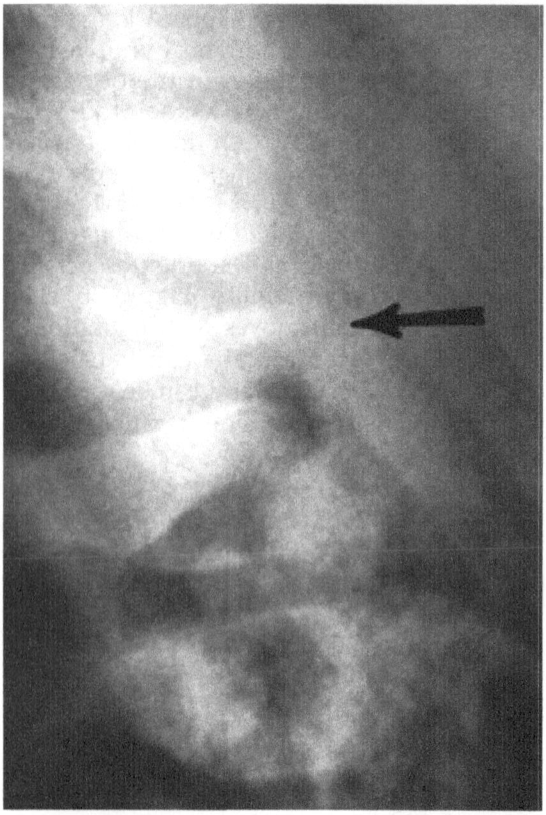

Fig. 3: (continued) (c) Vertebra plana of T12 (arrow) due to eosinophilic granuloma. This usually requires no treatment

SPINE TRAUMA

Injury to the spine is usually apparent from the clinical picture, the presence of soft tissue swelling on radiographs, and the radiographic appearance of a fracture or dislocation. Neurologic findings may also be present. The following are some patterns of spine trauma that are commonly encountered.

Spinal Cord Injury

Injury to the spinal cord or nerve roots is commonly associated with a fracture or dislocation. A neurologic injury may be present, however, without any apparent injury to the spine. There are varying degrees of neurologic injury. Most authors group SCIs into those that are complete and those that are incomplete. The incomplete injuries are then often subclassified by degree of neurologic involvement or by anatomic pattern of involvement. The prognosis for recovery is fairly good in an incomplete injury and dismal in a complete one, but this is not as certain in children as it is in adults.

Osseoligamentous Injuries/Fractures/ Cervical Spine

Most injuries to the cervical spine in children are seen in the upper three segments, probably owing to the disproportionately large head and the poorly developed neck musculature in this age group. The atlas or C1 is a thin bony ring with broad articular surfaces. Approximatlely 40% of all atlas fractures are associated with fracture of the C2 fracture. The most common C1 fracture is a burst fracture (Jefferson fracture) (Figure 4a). The usual mechanism of injury is axial loading, such as when a large load falls vertically on the head, or in a fall where the patient lands on the top of the head in a neutral position. The Jefferson fracture consists of the disruption of both anterior and posterior rings of C1 with latreral displacement of the lateral masses. The fracture is best seen on an open-mouth view of the C1 to C2 region and axial CT scans. These are unstable fractures.

The *Hangman's fracture,* involves the posterior elements of C2, i.e. the pars interarticularis. These fractures are due to extension type of injury. Patients with this fracture should be maintained in external immobilization until specialized care is available. A failure of the posterior elements of the C2 vertebra is sometimes associated with anterior subluxation of C2 on C3 (Figure 4(b)).

Odontoid fractures are seen in children, but they usually fail through the growth plate, and their healing potential is better than it is

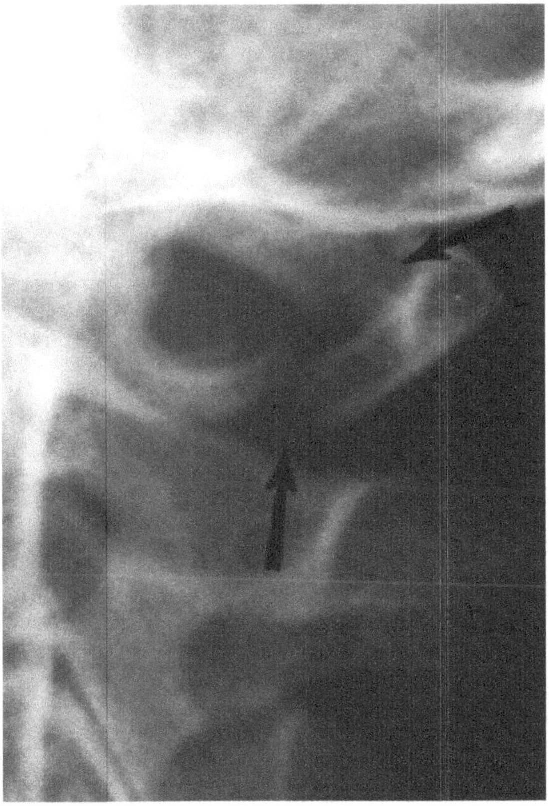

Fig. 4: Traumatic appearances.
(a) Jefferson fracture, two fractures with jagged eduges are seen in the arch of C1

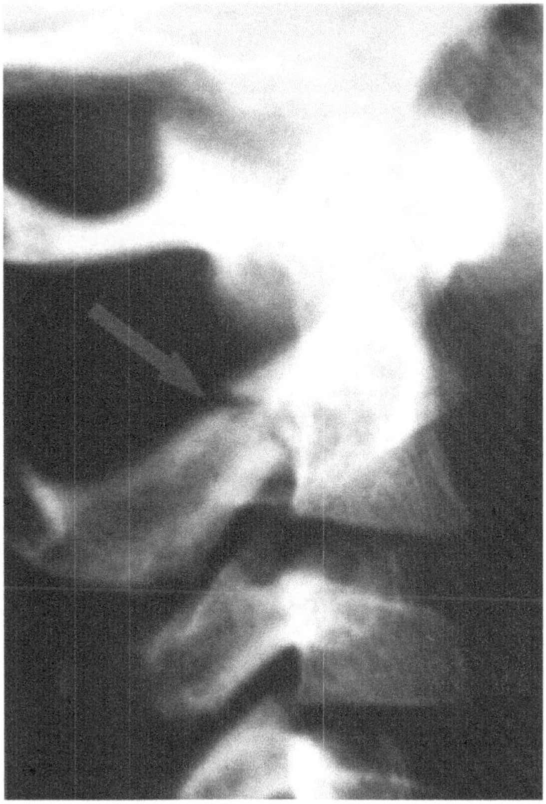

Fig. : (continued) (b) Hangman's fracture

in adults. They are identified on open-mouth view or lateral cervical spine view. There are some fractures that are peculiar to children. One example is an avulsion fracture that occurs through the ring apophysis as one might see in the cervical spine from a hyperextension injury. In children past the age of ten, the patterns more closely resemble those seen in adults; for example, more lower cervical spine injuries are seen. Anterior compression fractures are rarely seen in the cervical spine, and when they do occur, they are usually in the lower segments (Figure 4(c)).

They are usually stable injuries. More often the appearance of wedging in a child's cervical spine is the normal pattern of ossification. Fracture dislocations in the older age groups are seen in the lower segments and are virtually the same as adult injuries. Burst fractures are the result of axial compression and are often associated with encroachment on the spinal canal by retropulsed fragments of the vertebral body. They are prone to late collapse and deformity and require prolonged traction or spinal fusion. They are usually seen only in patients who are past puberty.

Thoracolumbar Spine

Compression fractures and burst fractures are also seen in the thoracolumbar spine, although rarely in small children (Figure 4(d)). A flexion-distraction injury (Chance fracture)

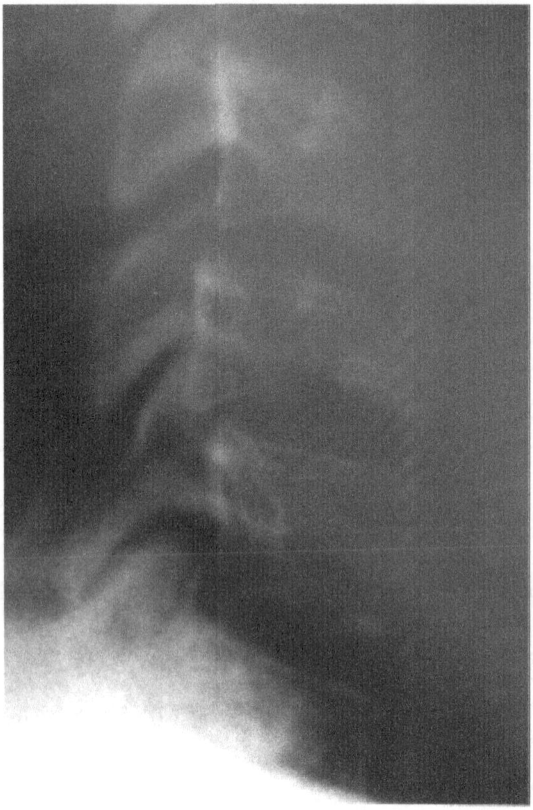

Fig. 4: (continued) (c) Compression fracture of C6 in a 20-year-old. This is basically an adult injury

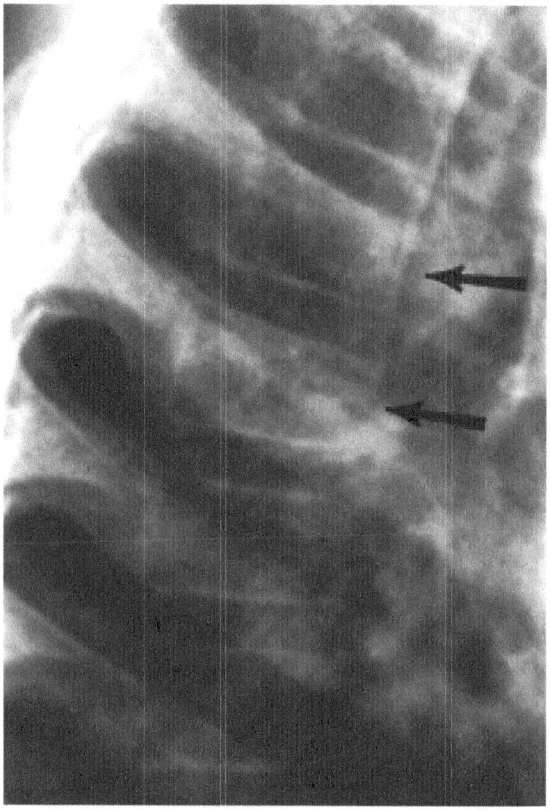

Fig. 4: (continued) (d) Compression fractures of T5 and T6 (arrows). Note the loss of anterior height compared to adjacent vertebrae

results when a passenger is thrown forward while restrained only by a lap seatbelt. The torso is flexed forcibly around the lapbelt with the axis of rotation anterior to the spine. The spine then fails in a tension mode. The fracture classically occurs through the interspinous ligaments posteriorly and through the disc space anteriorly, but the failure can occur through the spine at any level of the motion segment. Another injury peculiar to childhood is a fracture of the endplate, seen particularly in the lumbar spine in adolescents. These often mimic disc protrusions, and a CT scan, MRI scan, or myelogram is necessary to make the diagnosis.

Dislocations

Dislocations commonly occur in conjunction with fractures and, when they do, are termed *fracture-dislocations*. It is very rare for them to occur by themselves in children. One instability pattern that is seen in childhood, however, is atlantoaxial instability. The transverse ligament is the first line of defense, and its rupture is denoted by an atlantodens interval (the distance between the anterior cortex of the dens and the posterior cortex of the anterior ring of the atlas on a flexion lateral radiograph) of greater than five mm. Only three mm is acceptable in an adult, but more of the dens and the atlas are cartilaginous in the child. Greater than 10 to 12 mm indicates that the alar, apical, and cruciate ligaments have also failed. Overriding of the atlas on the dens of as much as two-thirds on the extension radiograph is normal and is seen about 20 percent of the time. The *rule of thirds* states that the odontoid process occupies about one-third of the spinal canal as does the spinal cord, leaving one-third empty. Knowing this and the amount of displacement, one can estimate the space available for the cord (SAC), thus determining if the position or the existing instability is acceptable.

OTHERS

Atlantoaxial Rotatory Fixation

AARF is a condition in which one of the facets of Cl subluxes forward on C2, resulting in some amount of fixed rotation between Cl and C2. It often follows an upper-respiratory infection. It is usually apparent on plain radiographs, showing asymmetry of the lateral masses of Cl, both in their size and in the distance between them and the odontoid process (Figure 5(a)). The lateral view shows a true lateral of the head and Cl, but an oblique of the remainder of the cervical spine, or vice versa. The anterior ring of Cl on the lateral view 'appears larger than normal' because one is really viewing the lateral mass (Figures 5(b) and 5(c)). It is often impossible to obtain routine radio-graphic views because of the torticollis posture, but the diagnosis can be confirmed by CT or by cineradiography, either of which demonstrates that Cl is locked on C2 with

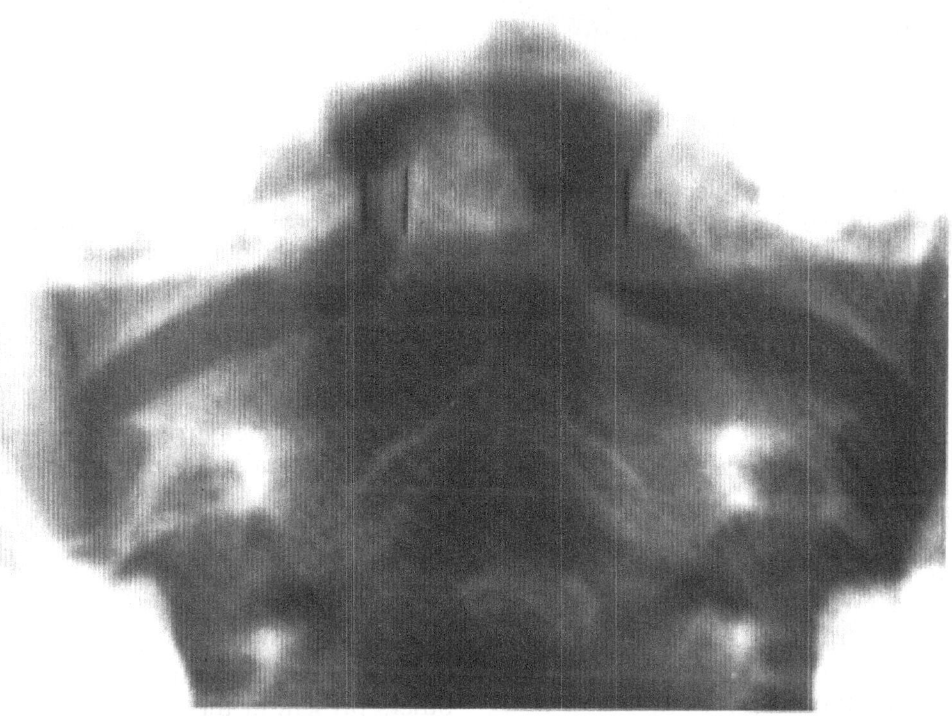

Fig. 5: AARF. (a) Open-mouth odontoid view. Note the difference in the interval between the dens and the lateral masses

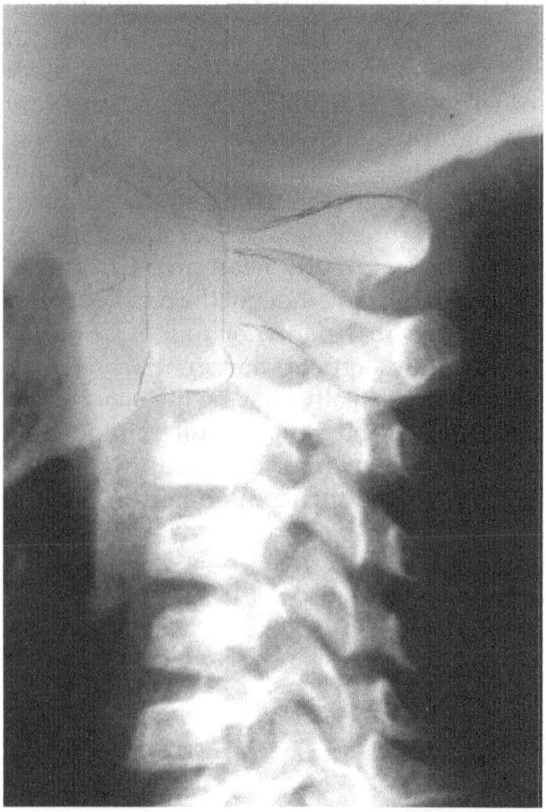

Fig. 5: (continued) (b) Lateral view. Note how large the anterior ring of C1 appears (because one is really viewing the lateral mass)

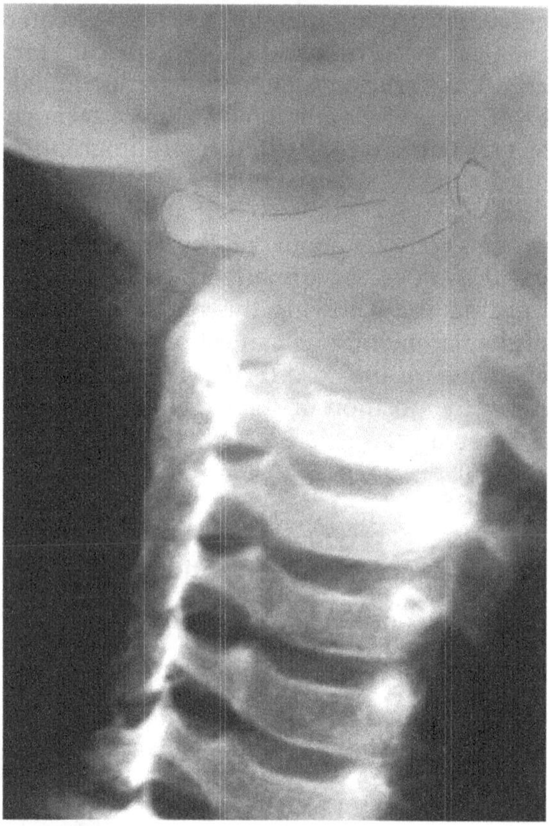

Fig. 5: (continued) (c) Oblique view. Note that a true lateral of the C1 vertebra is obtained with an oblique projection of the remainder of the cervical spine

respect to rotation in one direction or the other. Dynamic CT scanning is the most reliable modality.

Soft Tissue Injury

Soft tissue injury without instability, commonly known as *whiplash injury*, can occur in children as well as in adults. The etiology is unknown but probably results from tearing of soft tissue structures such as muscles and ligaments insufficient to cause demonstrable instability. Others may be due to occult fractures not seen with the modalities commonly employed. Just as in adults, the symptoms can become longstanding in children but usually respond to simple conservative measures and reassurance. Children generally do better than adults.

HISTORY AND PHYSICAL EXAMINATION

History

It is invaluable to obtain an accurate history of what caused the injury from the patient or others present at the scene for determining the mechanism of an injury.

Direct injury can occur from a direct blow or from a penetrating wound. Indirect injury can result from flexion, extension, axial loading, distraction, or flexion-distraction or from a combination of some or all these.

If there is no recognized trauma, one would want to know whether the patient has had any recent infections, particularly of the upper respiratory tract. Next physicians should inquire about symptoms, particularly pain in the neck or back, and numbness or weakness, even if transient. Has the patient been able to void since the time of the injury? Those with upper cervical spine injuries sometimes complain of pain or numbness in the distribution of the occipital nerves.

Physical Examination

A thorough examination for other injuries must be done, especially in a patient with sensory loss or decreased level of consciousness. This helps to assess the general condition of the patient and may provide important clues regarding the likelihood and/or nature of spinal injury.

Signs of injury to other areas may give some information regarding the mechanism of injury. For example, a laceration, an abrasion, or a contusion on the forehead may indicate that the patient sustained a blow to the head that resulted in an extension stress to the neck. Similarly lap-belt marks should lead to suspect a flexion-distraction force.

There may be some local indicators in the area of the injury. Tenderness or ecchymosis should raise a high index of suspicion. Palpable ligamentous defects or step-offs can provide useful information regarding stability at the fracture site.

A thorough neurologic evaluation is mandatory. Motor and sensory levels should be determined and carefully recorded to serve as a baseline. Perianal sensation in patients with apparently complete injuries should be specifically tested because even a small amount of sparing indicates that the lesion is partial, vastly changing the prognosis. Also if an injury is apparently complete at first presentation, the clinician should look for reflexes, including abdominal, cremasteric, anal wink, and bulbocavernosus. As long as they are absent, the patient is in spinal shock, and the prognosis is indeterminate.

ADJUNCT STUDIES

Refer once again to Figure 16.1. Plain radiographs are usually sufficient to determine the presence or absence of significant spinal injury. The standard views generally obtained for the cervical spine are the AP, lateral, odontoid and oblique views. It may not be necessary to obtain all of these views on every patient, depending on the level of suspicion. Every victim of blunt trauma from a motor vehicle accident with midline neck pain, tenderness on palpation, neurologic deficits referable to the cervical spine, an altered level of consciousness, or who is suspected of being intoxicated should have a lateral cervical spine X-ray, unless the victim is conscious and gives a reliable history of no neck injury.

The lateral should include the C7 vertebra, which may be difficult to see in obese or heavily muscled patients. A swimmer's view, lateral linear tomography, or sagittal reconstruction from CT can be helpful in this instance. Lateral views in flexion and extension can demonstrate instability, but should only be performed in an awake patient, ideally with a physician in attendance, and should be curtailed if any neurologic symptoms occur.

The open-mouth odontoid view should include the entire odontoid process and the right and left C1, C2 articulations. The AP view of the c-spine assists in the identification of a unilateral facet dislocation in instances where there is little or no dislocation identified on the lateral film. Axial CT scans at 3-mm intervals should be obtained through suspicious areas identified on the plain films or through the lower cervical spine if it is not visualized on the plain film. The complete series of cervical radiographs must be reviewed by a doctor experienced in the proper interpretation of theses films before they are considered normal and the cervical collar is removed.

If the plain radiographs are positive and clearly demonstrate the injury, proceed directly to treatment. If there is a question regarding stability, flexion-extension laterals or CT will be useful. If canal compromise is suspected, it can be evaluated by CT, myelography, CT-myelography, or MRI scanning or in certain select cases by SSEP monitoring. To know whether the appearance is possibly that of a normal variant, computed or linear tomography may show a growth plate or the ragged edges of a fracture more clearly. If there is still uncertainty about whether the fracture is old or new, a bone scan may help but may not be positive for two or three days.

If the plain radiographs are normal and there is a low index of suspicion of significant injury, symptomatic treatment as with a soft collar and analgesics and follow-up are appropriate. If there is high suspicion of significant injury, CT is very useful in the cervical spine. Static images are good for delineating fractures; dynamic images may be necessary to show an AARF or to demonstrate an instability resulting in cord impingement. Linear tomography is better at showing fractures in the horizontal plane (for example, odontoid fractures). If these studies are negative and there is no spinal cord injury, proceed to treatment and follow-up. If a spinal cord injury is present, however, obtain an MRI scan and/or myelography. This may demonstrate a source of continuing cord impingement (such as a disc herniation or an endplate fracture) that would be amenable to surgery with a positive effect on the long-term prognosis. These studies also will help to delineate the level of injury by the demonstration of bleeding Or edema in the cord Or by a block to flow Or extravasation of contrast medium. Extravasation of contrast at the level of a SCIWORA injury carries an extremely poor prognosis. If a partial cord injury is recognized, a second episode of injury with catastrophic consequences can be prevented.

MANAGEMENT

The goals of management should be to prevent further injury, to relieve cord compression, to ensure stability, and to avoid deformity and pain in the future. Some differences in treating children are worth mentioning. First, they heal better and more quickly. Second, their potential for recovering useful function following a neurologic injury is greater. Even in an apparently complete injury, the prognosis is not necessarily nil at the time of initial presentation. Third, some deformities from fractures are able to remodel with growth. Finally, children tolerate prolonged immobilization and bedrest better than adults do. Therefore surgical treatment is less often necessary in children. On the other hand, children have a much greater tendency to develop spinal deformity following SCI. Therefore they are more likely to require long-term bracing or spine fusion for late deformity.

Initial Management

The initial management should include optimal positioning to prevent further injury. The neck should be immobilized with a soft or hard collar and/or sandbags. The patient should be moved by log rolling and transported on a board. Extension of the neck for intubation should be avoided. In small children, the head is proportionately larger than it is in adults. Placing a child on a flat surface will tend to place the cervical spine in a flexed position or result in anterior translation at the site of injury. Therefore small children should be positioned with the head somewhat posterior to the trunk by placing bolsters under the trunk or the head in a depression.

For SCI patients, there is some evidence for the use of *methylprednisolone* in the acute management. All patients with SCIs should receive antacids to protect them from stress ulceration. A Foley catheter should be placed immediately, followed by an intermittent catheterization program if recovery of bladder function does not occur. Decubitus precautions should begin immediately.

Surgical Management

Figure 6 presents an algorithm describing a reasonable approach to the management of spinal injuries. Usually the first consideration is whether the injury is displaced; if so, a reduction should be achieved. This can often be done by merely positioning the patient in such a way that the spine becomes better aligned. Sometimes traction is necessary to achieve a reduction, and rarely it may be necessary to perform an open reduction.

After the injury is reduced, one must maintain the reduction and provide stability if it is lacking. Some injuries are intrinsically stable and require only symptomatic treatment or a collar. Those that are less stable may require external support in the form of either a cast or orthosis or either prolonged bedrest or traction to maintain alignment while healing occurs. The halo brace can be considered a form of ambulatory traction. Surgical fusion is sometimes the best way to provide stability, particularly when an open reduction or decompression is necessary, when deformity is present, or when rapid mobilization of the patient is desirable (as in a poly trauma patient or an SCI patient in need of rehabilitation).

The third consideration is compromise of the spinal canal and neural elements. The indications for decompression are a progressive neurologic deficit, possibly persisting compression of the cauda equina or conus medullaris (because of their increased potential for recovery), and possibly incomplete cord lesions with persistent compression, particularly if a plateau in neurologic recovery can be demonstrated. A final consideration might be canal compromise with intractable pain. Usually all that is necessary to decompress the spinal canal is realignment of the spine, especially when the injury is new. If decompression is necessary, a vertebrectomy through an anterior approach is more often appropriate. If an SCI is complete, the prognosis for recovery is very poor and probably is not improved by canal decompression. In this case, decompression is probably unwarranted, and consideration can be given to restoring alignment and providing stability.

The treatment of SCIWORA is no different from the treatment of SCI with fracture or dislocation, but it is very important to recognize partial injuries after the first episode, so that measures necessary to prevent further injury are taken.

MANAGEMENT OF SPECIFIC INJURIES

Atlantoaxial Rotatory Fixation

Most of these injuries are seen early and respond to bedrest, a soft cervical collar, and a mild relaxant such as diazepam or a nonsteroidal anti-inflammatory medication. If this is unsuccessful, a few days in head halter traction is usually successful. Some of these injuries are associated with temporary C1-C2 instability as is demonstrated on flexion-extension radiographs. They should be protected with a soft cervical collar for six weeks. When the condition has been

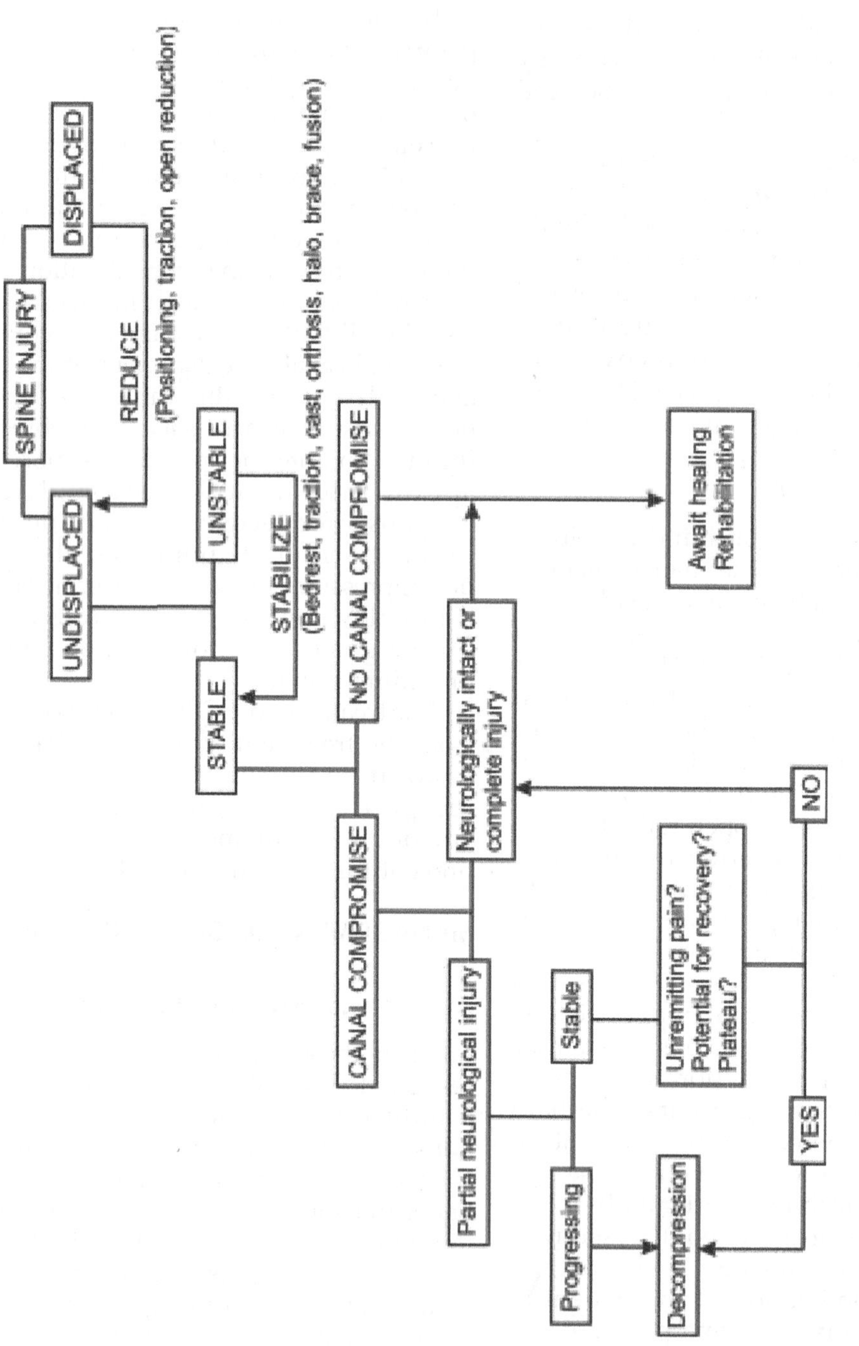

Fig. 6: Management of spine and SCI in children

present for longer than a month, it may not reduce, or it may recur after a reduction in traction. In this case or when instability persists for longer than six weeks, a C1-C2 posterior in situ fusion is occasionally indicated.

Atlas Fracture

Fracture of the atlas Oefferson fracture} usually results from axial compression and is a stable injury. Most of these fractures will heal in a Minerva cast or a halo brace. Three months is usually sufficient for healing although six months may be necessary.

Axis Fractures

A fracture of the posterior elements of the C2 vertebra (Hangman's fracture) will usually heal with a cast or brace but, if it is significantly displaced, may require a fusion.

Odontoid fractures can usually be treated with a halo brace or a Minerva cast for six to eight weeks, and surgery is seldom necessary. The results in older children are similar to those seen in adults. Fractures through the odontoid near the tip (type I) and those through the body of C2 (type III) generally heal well. Those at the base of the odontoid (type II), however, frequently proceed to a nonunion and may require a fusion to restore stability.

Lower Cervical Spine

Fracture-dislocations in the lower cervical spine (C3-C7) are seen mainly in older children and are treated in a similar manner to treatment of the same injuries in adults. One should consider the mechanism of the injury since they can occur from flexion or extension. Most are adequately managed in a cast, an orthosis, or a halo. Surgery is usually done for flexion injuries, which can lead to late kyphosis, and generally consists of posterior wiring and fusion. Anterior fusion is not indicated because disruption of the anterior longitudinal ligament renders them more unstable. Primary anterior vertebrectomy and fusion is sometimes indicated for burst fractures from axial compression, because they commonly involve canal compromise, and because they have a tendency toward late collapse. Laminectomy is not indicated for any of these injuries because it produces further instability and may lead to a swan-neck deformity.

Ligamentous Disruption

Ligamentous disruption is less common in children than it is in adults. A loss of the normal lordosis and a stiff neck are constant features, but children commonly have no lordosis as a normal finding. Lateral radiographs in flexion may show a widened interspace posteriorly, a loss of parallelism of the facet joints, kyphosis of the disc space, posterior opening, or calcification of the disc space as a delayed feature. A delay in diagnosis is common, and it may be worthwhile to repeat the flexion film three to six weeks after the injury because increased mobility may be masked initially by splinting. Surgery is done for persistent or worsening deformity.

Thoracolumbar Injuries

Compression fractures occur at multiple levels more commonly in children than they do in adults. Pathologic fractures are seen in children and should be considered. They can result from an aneurysmal bone cyst, leukemia, or other myeloproliferative disorder. They are usually stable and can be treated with a cast or orthosis. Sometimes only symptomatic treatment is necessary. Most should be admitted to the hospital for observation because they are prone to developing ileus or urinary retention. They also often require pain management and should be observed for the development of a progressive neurologic deficit.

Flexion-distraction injuries (Chance fractures) are usually stable and can be managed by bracing although fusion may occasionally be required. One should also suspect injuries to visci from the lap belt.

Fracture of the vertebral limbus in adolescents occurs between the ring apophysis and the vertebral endplate. It most commonly involves the superior endplate in the midlumbar spine and often produces compression of the neural elements. Treatment is excision of the loose body through a laminotomy.

CONCLUSIONS

1. The recognition and understanding of spinal injuries in children is important if catastrophes are to be avoided.
2. Spinal injuries in children share some similarities with adult injuries but also have some important differences.
3. Significant neurologic sequelae are possible without radiographic abnormalities.
4. Treatment must be appropriate from the beginning to prevent compli cations.
5. Laminectomy should be avoided except in very special circumstances.

The author would like to thank Doctors Theresa Stacy and Timothy Tytle for their help in locating figures for this manuscript.

FURTHER READING

1. Akbarnia BA. Disorderes of the pediatric and adolescent spine: Pediatric spine fractures. Ortho clin north America 1999; 30:521-535.
2. Ferguson RL. Thoracic and spinal trauma of the immature spine. Rothman –Simeone. The spine: 5th edition 2006.
3. Trumble J, Myslinski J. Lower thoracic SCIWORA in a 3-year old child: Case report Ped Emergency Care 2000; 16:91-93.
4. Yazici M, Alanay A, Aksoy MC, et al. Traumatic L1-L2 dislocation without fracture in a 6-year old girl: Spine 1999: 24:1483-1486.

25 Coma and Altered Mental Status

Consciousness is a complex neurophysiologic process, involving the integrity of the reticular activating system in modulating interactions between the cerebral cortex and the brainstem. Suppression of the reticular activating system (RAS) produces alterations in mental status leading to coma. The RAS is an ill-defined group of neurons extending from the rostral medulla to the midbrain which has a primary role in arousal of the cerebral cortex. Whereas large bilateral lesions are required to produce coma in the cerebral hemispheres, small lesions in critical areas of the brainstem may produce pronounced changes of consciousness. The ultimate neurologic outcome and quality of survival depends on whether cellular integrity of the central nervous system (CNS) and supporting mylenation have been damaged during coma. In general, transient metabolic derangements of the CNS are well tolerated in children, provided that the flow of oxygen and glucose is uninterrupted.

PATHOPHYSIOLOGY

Loss of consciousness occurs after only six seconds of complete global ischemia and signifies the neurons' intolerance of anaerobic metabolism. The point at which irreversible damage from hypoxic-ischemic injury occurs is still controversial. Traditional clinical observations have noted irreversible damage occurring after approximately six minutes of complete global ischemia. Some children, after prolonged cardiac arrest, however, have a transient period of eye opening, recognition of parents, and response to verbal command followed by deterioration to brain death. Such clinical observations lend support to experimental evidence that irreversible neuronal injury occurs primarily during the period of reperfusion after complete global ischemia, due to the damage done to cellular membranes by superoxide radicals and by the influx of calcium ions.

Although the exact mechanism continues to be debated, there is universal agreement about the importance of preventing hypoxic-ischemic injury when possible by continuously delivering oxygen and glucose to the CNS. In addition to correcting hypoxemia, anemia, and hypotension, management of increased intracranial pressure is important in maintaining neuronal perfusion and integrity. Intracranial pressure (ICP) reflects a balance between the four intracranial fluids: blood, cerebrospinal fluid (CSF), interstitial fluid, and intracellular fluid.

After the sutures and fontanels close, the Kelly-Monroe hypothesis states that one of these fluids can increase only at the expense of the other three. During the early phases of cerebral edema, ICP remains normal or mildly elevated because of displacement of blood and CSF out of the intracranial compartment. The lateral ventricles collapse, and CSF is reabsorbed or displaced downward into the spinal canal where the dura has a limited capability of expansion. Cerebral blood volume, on the other hand, can be lowered by arterial constriction from hyperventilation or by increasing venous drainage with head elevation.

After compensatory mechanisms are exhausted, ICP elevates abruptly since liquids are not compressible substances. If the difference between the mean arterial pressure and the ICP falls to 30 torr, the electroencephalogram (EEG) becomes isoelectric, signifying global ischemia due to the collapse of small arterioles. Although it is invasive, monitoring of this type is used in children to determine the cerebral perfusion pressure as an indirect assessment of cerebral blood flow. Blood pressure and ICP are modulated to maintain the cerebral perfusion pressure in a safe range, usually above 50 torr.

Coma can also lead to either cardiopulmonary arrest or brain death. Respiratory failure progressing to arrest occurs secondary to suppression of the respiratory center in the medulla. Alterations in respiratory drive results in hypoventilation or central apnea, both of which present insidiously as a decreased work of breathing. Less commonly, coma can also be associated with a distributive form of shock. Thalamic dysfunction can produce decreased sympathetic tone and increased venous capacitance. The hemodynamic consequences are a relative hypovolemia, decreased venous return and decreased cardiac output.

CLINICAL PRESENTATION

The onset of altered mental status leading to coma is often insidious, producing vague symptoms from the parents, such as, "My child is acting funny or different," "She is not herself", "Something is wrong", or "He is not acting right". The first clinical task is to determine the child's level of responsiveness or consciousness. There is a continuum of altered consciousness and this can be subdivided depending on the degree of severity. Plum and Posner subdivide this continuum into clouding of consciousness, delirium, obtundation, stupor and coma. While specific definitions have been suggested for each of these states, they are not uniformly applied and easily confused. Thus, for clinical management and communication: Clinicians should not rely on single world descriptions of a patient with altered mental status, instead, the patients' state should be carefully described including: orientation, verbal output, eye opening and response to environmental stimuli. Useful in quantitating these observations is the Glasgow Coma Scale which measures and provides a numerical score for three parameters: motor responses, eye opening and verbal response. In the earliest phases of an abnormal physical examination, the child is awake and ambulatory, appears normal on first inspection, and answers questions appropriately. But on a closer look, the patient has an expressionless facies and appears dazed, perhaps glassy eyed. The ability to answer questions, though appropriate, is a bit sluggish. The term *cloudy sensorium* describes this condition. When it is associated with high fever, the neurotoxin produced by Shigella is one of the classic causes of this altered status, which can precede the diarrhea phase of the disease.

During the next lower phase, the patient is inappropriately sleepy, but can be aroused and is oriented. Failure to recognize parents is a cardinal symptom and sign which always points to a serious underlying disease process, whether it is due to coma, seizure, respiratory failure, or shock. At the beginning of this phase, the symptomatology is likely to be vague and perhaps even misleading, but if they are asked the specific question, "Does your child recognize you?" parents will respond "no" after a thoughtful pause. Failure to recognize parents is also a sign as judged by the nature of the child's eye contact and ability to follow their parents to whom they look for security. Ability to recognize and interact with parents can be judged and assessed as early as one month of age. Failure to recognize parents is often accompanied by being confused and combative, as well as by failure to respond to verbal commands. New onset of enuresis in a child who has been previously toilet trained can occur during this phase as well.

As the level of consciousness further deteriorates, the response to noxious stimuli becomes the critical factor. The degree of noxious stimuli can vary from light touch to moderate or severe pain. Failure of an infant to respond to a lumbar puncture or venipuncture rapidly alerts the clinician to a low level of consciousness.

The common causes of coma in children are illustrated in Table 1. *Appropriate responses to pain* vary in level of defensiveness. When *combative,* the patient is able to find and to fend off the noxious stimuli. *Localization* refers to the ability to reach and to touch the noxious stimuli, but the patient is too comatose to struggle against it. *Withdrawal* refers to a single extremity response to move away from the pain. If pain is applied to an extensor surface, the patient will flex away from it, and vice versa.

Table 1: Common causes of non-traumatic coma in children

Infections
- Meningitis (Bacterial, Tubercular)
- Encephalitis
- Brain abscess
- Subdural/epidural empyema
- Cerebral malaria
- Enteric encephalopathy
- Severe systemic infection, sepsis

Metabolic
- Hypoglycemia—Insulin excess
- Hyperglycemia—Diabetes mellitus
- Reye's syndrome
- Acidosis, alkalosis
- Hepatic failure
- Uremia
- Hypercapnia
- Dyselctrolytemia-Hyponatremia, hypomagnesemia
- Hypermagnesemia, hypocalcemia, hypercalcemia
- Hyperosmolar states
- Hyperammonemia

Drugs and Poisons
- Opioides
- Barbiturates
- Salicylates
- Sedatives
- Snake bite

Miscellaneous
- Postictal-status epilepticus
- Hypoxic-ischemic injury, shock, postcardiac arrest
- Pulmonary edema, severe anemia
- Hypertensive encephalopathy

Withdrawal becomes an *inappropriate response to pain* when the patient flexes into pain applied on the flexor surface of the extremity. Inappropriate responses, however, are most obvious when the patient has a spastic, four-extremity reaction, which is non-purposeful in nature. *Decorticate posturing* consists of extension of the lower extremities with simultaneous flexion of the upper extremities at the elbows. *Decerebrate posturing* involves extension of all four extremities. True posturing needs to be distinguished from appropriate withdrawal or combativeness with increased muscle tone. The distinction is usually obvious by the purposeful nature of the latter.

Decorticate and decerebrate posturing can be produced in laboratory animals by creating a surgical lesion at the level of cerebral hemispheres and brain stem respectively. In children, posturing rarely signifies a structural lesion such as a brainstem hemorrhage but is more commonly associated with a physiologic disturbance caused by a metabolic problem, inflammation, or increased ICP. In the deepest stages of coma, the child has no response to painful stimuli. The child's extremities are usually flaccid and are flexic at this point.

Children in shock, on the other hand, have a fluctuating level of consciousness. Their mental status can vary from being unresponsive during painful procedures to being alert and recognizing their parents. These fluctuations are indicative of the varying levels of cerebral blood flow and cortical perfusion. Obvious signs of posturing are usually absent during this process, so the severity of the child's condition can be underestimated if the clinician becomes falsely reassured by the child's best neurologic response instead of determining the reason for the child's worst neurologic response.

The clinical presentation of increased ICP varies. Signs of impending herniation must be picked up as early as possible (Table 2). Subacute or chronic elevation of ICP presents as headaches, vomiting and papilledema. Since papilledema takes 48 to 72 hours to develop fully, it is often absent in coma with acute increased pressure. In this situation, increased ICP is suspected when there is a rapid onset of coma with a working diagnosis compatible with this problem. It is especially suspected when the level of consciousness has deteriorated to the point of posturing or there are pupillary changes compatible with cerebral herniation.

Table 2: Signs suggestive of impending herniation

1. Decorticate or decerebrate posturing
2. Abnormalities of vital signs: Tachycardia or bradycardia, hyperventilation, Cheyne Stokes breathing or irregular respiration, hypertension or hypotension
3. Pupillary abnormalities: Unilateral or bilateral fixed dilated pupils, unequal pupil

Central herniation begins when bilateral pressure on the midbrain causes loss of sympathetic tone, and the pupils constrict in a pinpoint fashion. Uncal herniation occurs when pressure in one cerebral hemisphere causes a unilateral impingement on the third cranial nerve by the uncal gyrus at the level of the tentorium. Loss of parasympathetic tone causes dilation of the ipsilateral pupil. If the increase in ICP continues and is irreversible, both central and uncal herniation end in the pupils being irregular, fixed, and dilated in a midposition after both uncal gyri herniate downward through the tentorium.

The focus from which the pressure originates is also important in determining the clinical presentation. Increased ICP from hydrocephalus produces the *sunset sign.* Dilation of the lateral ventricles compresses nearby nerve tracts, causing a downward deviation of the eyes. This upper motor neuron sign presents as a gaze deficit, the earliest form of which consists of loss of upward gaze. Acute shunt obstruction in hydrocephalus can present as loss of upward gaze and altered mental status before progressing to coma.

Other forms of supratentorium increased ICP, such as that produced by the intracellular edema of Reye's syndrome, presents as *rostrocaudal deterioration.* In this situation, the level of consciousness deteriorates sequentially as has already been described, followed by progressive cranial nerve dysfunction, culminating in cerebral herniation. Compression of the respiratory center in the medulla finally leads to a permanent cessation of respiration. This process is exactly opposite of the return of function that can occur after a resuscitation from cardiac arrest. Return of respiration, followed by pupillary function and possibly by cortical function reflects the pattern of reperfusion.

Increased pressure, originating in the posterior fossa, is relatively uncommon but has a distinct clinical presentation. Etiologies include cerebellar infarction and tumors that cause secondary hemorrhage or edema. In the early phases, cortical perfusion remains intact. The patient is usually semialert but is confused or has an altered sensorium. The child is no longer ambulatory and can manifest unusual motor movements of the extremities that are neither posturing nor seizure activity. Occasionally pressure in the posterior fossa can slowly build to a critical point at which all circulation suddenly becomes compromised and global ischemia occurs. The patient has a sudden loss of consciousness with apnea. If it is witnessed, the respiratory arrest is rapidly reversible with assisted ventilation, but the neurologic examination reveals findings consistent with brain death. The various respiratory patterns in coma with relation to the site of lesion are shown in Table 3.

Table 4 summarizes the rapid examination of the cranial nerves. Presence of the pupillary, oculocephalic, corneal, and gag reflexes confirms the basic function of all but the cranial nerves I and XI. Rapid lateral turning of the head stimulates a vestibular reaction and subsequent eye movement. This doll's eye maneuver is normal when eye movement occurs and is referred to as the *oculocephalic reflex.* The oculovestibular reflex has a similar motor component but is elicited by ice water irrigation of the tympanic membranes. For clarity of charting, these reflexes are best described as "present" when eye movement occurs or as "absent" when it does not. "Normal doll's eyes", on the other hand, means different things to different observers.

The presence of focal neurologic signs can be helpful in localizing discrete lesions when they are present or in signifying asymmetrical intracranial events. Examples of the latter include generalized seizures with prominent clonus on one side only and generalized cerebral edema with early uncal herniation. Focal cranial nerve signs include anisocoria, ophthalmoplegias and facial asymmetry.

Table 3: Respiratory pattern in coma, relation with site of lesion

Pattern		*Site of Lesion*
Cheyne Stokes	:	Bilateral cerebral hemispheres with intact brain stem, Midbrain, Pons (Impending transtentorial herniation), Metabolic viz uremia, hypoxia, hypertensive encephalopathy
Neurogenic hyperventilation	:	Mid brain, pons (Diffuse raised ICP), acidosis, hypoxia
Apneustic breathing	:	Mild or caudal pons, pontine infarction (Meningitis, hypoglycemia, anoxia)
Cluster breathing	:	Low pons or high medulla
Ataxic breathing	:	Medulla (dorsomedial), cerebellar tonsillar herniation, Pontine or cerebellar hemorrhage

Table 4: Rapid neurologic assessment

Level of consciousness	
Appropriate to verbal command	*Inappropriate response to pain*
Alert, oriented	Decorticate
Confused	Decerebrate
	No response
Inappropriate to verbal command	*Focal neurologic signs*
Fails to recognize parents	Anisocoria
No response to verbal command	Hemiplegia
	Facial
	Extremity
Appropriate response to pain	Paraplegia
Combative	Quadriplegia
Localizes	
Withdraws	

Cranial nerve reflexes	*Sensory*	*Motor*
Pupillary reflex	II	III
Oculocephalic reflex	VIII	III, IV, VI
Corneal reflex	V	VI
Gag reflex	IX, X	IX, X, XII

The rapid neurologic assessment can be performed in less than two minutes and is helpful in determining the neurologic stability of the patient as well as in creating a differential diagnosis.

Monoparesis, hemiplegia, paraplegia or quadriplegia can be detected by examination of the extremities for movement, tone, and reflexes.

DIFFERENTIAL DIAGNOSIS

The first diagnostic task is to separate the altered mental status leading to coma from those produced by seizures and postictal phenomenon. In the case of witnessed grand mal epilepsy, the distinction is clear. The physician only needs to check for return of purposeful responses to painful stimuli during postictal drowsiness to confirm that the seizure has stopped. If the patient fails to respond to painful stimuli appropriately, an EEG can be helpful in the diagnosis of ongoing electrical status without corresponding abnormal motor movements. Other forms of seizure activity, such as frequent petit mal and partial complex seizures, can present with altered mental status without the obvious abnormal motor movements and the loss of consciousness characteristic of grand mal. Once the possibility of seizures has been excluded, the differential diagnosis of coma can be divided into four categories, based on focal neurologic signs and increased ICP.

1. No Focal Signs and Normal Intracranial Pressure

This category contains the most common cause of childhood coma and is the least likely to be associated with any mortality or permanent sequella. It includes concussions from mild head trauma, toxins, metabolic abnormalities, mild CNS infections, and postictal states. Metabolic conditions include uremia, hyponatremia, hypernatremia, hypercapnia, hypocalcemia and global ischemia. The latter is usually associated with cardiac or respiratory arrest and can vary from transient to permanent. The severest forms, leading to brain death or survival in a persistent vegetative state, can be accompanied by a delayed onset of increased ICP after 12 hours or more. Managing this form of pressure with intracranial monitoring, however, has not been shown to improve outcome.

Children with small pupils and coma usually have a toxic ingestion that belongs in this category. Opiates produce these findings, but exposure to ethanol, phenothiazines, and organophosphates also presents in this fashion. The prognosis is usually favorable for all of these conditions. The possibility of pontine hemorrhage and early central herniation from cerebral edema also needs to be considered in these patients.

2. No Focal Signs and Increased Intracranial Pressure

This category has the highest mortality. It includes severe head trauma, Reye's syndrome, fulminant bacterial meningitis, and diabetic ketoacidosis. All of these conditions are reasonable candidates for monitoring intracranial pressure in order to prevent or minimize ischemic damage. Hydrocephalus with shunt obstruction also belongs in this category.

3. Focal Signs and Normal Intracranial Pressure

The most common cause in this category is benign. A Todd's paresis is a transient, postictal hemiparesis that resolves completely within 24 to 72 hours after the seizure. Cerebral vascular accidents, on the other hand, are relatively uncommon in the pediatric age group. The more frequent etiologies are sickle cell anemia and bacterial meningitis. Rare conditions include homocysteinuria and embolic phenomena from acute bacterial endocarditis or left atrial myxoma.

4. Focal Signs and Increased Intracranial Pressure

This category includes the mass lesions: intracranial hemorrhage, tumors, brain abscess, and arteriovenous malformations. Prognosis depends on location and surgical accessibility. Herpes encephalitis, which can produce cystic degenerations in the temporal region and generalized cerebral edema, also needs to be considered in this category.

PHYSICAL EXAMINATION

A rapid cardiopulmonary assessment is first performed in order to determine the adequacy of airway, breathing, and circulation (ABCs). If trauma is suspected, cervical immobilization should be performed simultaneously with this initial inspection. Next a rapid neurologic assessment should be performed to determine the child's level of consciousness, cranial nerve status, and the presence of any focal neurologic signs (Table 4). Determination of the exact heart rate, respiration, blood pressure, temperature, transcutaneous saturation, and glucose by bedside testing follows next.

With this information, the physician is able to build a working differential diagnosis based on one of the four categories already outlined. If the patient is neurologically and hemodynamically stable, the diagnosis can usually be made by taking a quick problem-oriented history from the parents. According to the index of suspicion that evolves from the working differential, questions can be directed toward recent onset of infectious symptoms, ingestion-related behaviors and risk factors, abnormal motor movement suggestive of seizures, complaints of headache and vomiting, changes in behavior, underlying medical illnesses, and occult forms of trauma. If the history is totally benign and does not help define the etiology of the coma, unwitnessed seizure, drug ingestion, and child abuse need to be given thorough consideration.

LABORATORY EVALUATION

Laboratory evaluation of altered mental status and coma can be thought of in terms of both general screening tests to be performed on all patients and specific tests directed at further defining the categories in the differential diagnosis already outlined. Basic screening tests include electrolytes, glucose, blood urea nitrogen, arterial blood gases, and at least one liver enzyme. In regards to the latter, the gamma Guatemala transferase (GGT) and serum glutamate pyruvate transaminase (SGPT) are more liver-specific than serum glutamic-oxaloacetic transaminase (SGOT), which can be found in skeletal and cardiac muscle as well. If hepatic coma is likely, determination of serum ammonia and prothrombin time (PT) is also important. Hyponatremia and hypernatremia can present as coma or seizures. Disturbances of potassium, calcium, and magnesium, however, are more likely to present as alterations in muscle tone and possibly as dysrhythmias.

For toxicology screenings, samples from the urine, blood, and gastric contents are important for analysis. When indicated, carbon monoxide, serum lead level and tests for inborn errors of metabolism can be considered. Although many of the tests for inborm errors will not be helpful in the acute management, some of these disorders are intermittent and evaluation is more informative when performed during a symptomatic period. Occasionally, a plain film of the abdomen can be helpful in quantifying the severity of the ingestion if a radiopaque substance such as iron tablets or substances containing lead are in question.

Lumbar puncture for diagnosis of meningitis and encephalitis is important but is deferred in situations in which the patient has focal neurologic signs or is suspected of having significant increased intracranial pressure. In severe meningitis with increased intracranial pressure, cerebral herniation and brain death can occur in the field or in the emergency department even before a lumbar puncture has been performed. If a child presents with a high fever, coma, and posturing, antibiotics can be started and the lumbar puncture postponed until it is clearly safe to perform it.

When increased intracranial pressure is suspected, an emergency computerized tomography (CT) or magnetic resonance imaging (MRI) scan is the procedure of choice, both to rule out mass effect and to document signs of cerebral edema. Obliteration of the quadrigeminal plate cistern correlates highly with pupillary changes of uncal herniation. Small lateral ventricles and obliterations of fissures can also indicate increased pressure.

MANAGEMENT

The management of coma should be approached as a medical emergency. First, medical stability should be ensured. Supportive care of the comatose child is ultimately directed at continuous delivery of oxygen and glucose to the neurons while maintaining oxygenation, ventilation, and perfusion to the other organ systems (Table 5). Unless the possibility fo trauma can be excluded, the cervical spine should remain stabilized until appropriate radiolological evaluation excludes injury Further evaluation ensures as a combination of history, physical examination and treatment which must occur concurrently and requireds a team of caregivers. When the cause of coma is known

Table 5: General management of children in coma

Rapid cardiopulmonary assessment	*Rapid neurological assessment*
Airway	Level of consciousness
Normal	Focal neurologic signs
Spinal immobilization if trauma suspected	Cranial nerve reflexes
Clear secretions	Increased intracranial pressure
Maintainable by simple maneuvers	*Quick history*
Chin lift or jaw thrust	*Initial blood work*
Nasopharyngeal airway	Dextrostix at bedside
Unmaintainable	Complete blood count (CBC)
Rapid oral intubation	Electrolytes and blood urea nitrogen (BUN)
Breathing	Glucose
Normal Spontaneous	Liver enzymes
Increase FiO_2	
Maintainable by bag-valve-mask device	
Intubation necessary to protect airway	
Maintain (hyper-) ventilation	
Circulation	
Normal	
Obtain vascular access	
Monitor heart rate	
Transcutaneous 02 saturation	
Neurogenic Hypotension	
Trendelberg position	
Volume expansion	
Alpha agonists	

(e.g. medication ingestion, near drowing, etc.) work-up is more limited and treatment can be immediately focused. Management decisions and interventions are made concurrently with performance of the physical examination. Once the initial assessment and stabilization have been performed, confirmation of the working diagnosis is performed by taking the history and performing selective laboratory procedures (Table 6).

The degree of supportive care necessary in each case needs to be individualized according to the child's level of consciousness and the pathophysiology involved. The decision to perform endotracheal intubation to protect the airway, for instance, is based on the state of the child's protective reflexes more than on the level of consciousness and is modified by factors such as the presence of respiratory compromise or increased ICP.

CONCLUSION

The etiology of childhood coma can be either obvious (such as from witnessed trauma) or obscure and difficult to determine. In either event, initial stabilization in the emergency department is critical to prevent secondary cerebral ischemia whether it is from

Table 6: Management based on four working diagnostic categories

1. No *focal signs and normal ICP*	
Toxins	Blood and urine screen
CNS infections	CT scan for ICP signs
Lumbar puncture	
Concussion	CT scan to rule out hemorrhage
Metabolic	Correct specific defect
Anoxic about	Anticipatory counseling of family
outcome	
Small pupils	Narcan for opiates
	Also consider:
	Ethanol
	Phenothiazines
	Organophosphates
	Pontine hemorrhage
	Early central herniation
	Rule out mass effect
	Rule out acute hydrocephalus
	Evaluate basal cisterns
2. No *focal signs and increased ICP*	
CT scan	Rule out mass effect
	Rule out acute hydrocephalus
	Evaluate basal cisterns
Medical therapy	Head elevation
	Hyperventilation
	Mannitol
	Thiopental
	Muscle relaxation
3. *Focal signs and normal ICP*	
Todd's paresis	Reassure parents
Cerebrovascular accident	MRI scan
	Possible angiogram
4. No *focal signs and increased ICP (CT scan)*	
Hemorrhage	Emergent surgery
Tumor	Urgent surgery
	Possible emergent ventriculostomy
Abscess	Antibiotics
	Possible emergent surgery
A VM/subarachnoid hemorrhage	Observation
	Delayed surgery
Herpes encephalitis	EEG
	Lumbar puncture
	Acyclovir
	Monitor ICP

After stabilization of the patient, a working differential diagnosis of coma is based on categorization determined by ICP and focal neurologic signs. Specific diagnostic and therapeutic procedures follow and are summarized in this table.

AVM = arterial venous malformation.

respiratory failure, shock, or increased ICP. (These mnemonics are helpful both for quick initial assessment and for management.) Once the patient is stabilized, the diagnostic work-up proceeds on lines determined by the presence or absence of increased ICP and focal neurologic signs. Except for anoxic encephalopathy incurred during an episode of asystole and for severe head trauma, the prognosis is usually favorable.

FURTHER READING

1. Ashwal S. Brain death in the newborn. Clin Perinatol 1989;169(2):501-518.
2. Coulter DL. Neurologic uncertainty in newborn intensive care. N Engl J Med 1987;316(14):840-844.
3. Drake B, Ashwal S, Schneider S, *et al.* Determination of cerebral death in the pediatric intensive care unit. Pediatrics 1986;78(1):107-112.
4. Goodwin SR, Friedman WA, Bellefleur M, *et al.* Is it time to use evoked potentials to predict outcome in comatose children and adults? Critical Care Medicine 1991;19(4):518-524.
5. Rowland TW, Donnelly JH, Jackson AH, *et al.* Brain death in the pediairic intensive care unit. A clinical definition. American Journal of Diseases of Children 1983;137(6):547-550.
6. Strickbine-Van Reet P, Glaze DG, Hrachovy RA, *et al.* A preliminary prospective neuro physiological study of coma in children. American Journal of Diseases of Children 1984; 138(5):492-495.
7. Tasker RC, Boyd S, Harden A, *et al.* Monitoring in non-traumatic coma. Part II: Electro encephalography. Archives of Disease in Childhood 1988; 63 (8) : 895-899.
8. Tasker RC, Matthew DJ, Helms P, *et al.* Monitoring in non-traumatic coma. Part I: Invasive intracranial measurements. Archives of Disease in Childhood 1988;63(8):888-894.
9. Bansal A, Singhi SC, Singhi PD, *et al.* Non-traumatic coma. Indian J Pediatr 2005;72 (6): 467-73.
10. Plum and Posner's Diagnosis of Stupor and Coma (Contemporary Neurology 71) by Posner JB, Saper CB, Schiff N, Plum F. New York, Oxford University Press, 2007.
11. Sacco RL, VanGool R, Mohr JP, Hauser WA. Nontraumatic coma. Glasgow coma score and coma etiology as predictors of 2-week outcome. Arch Neurol 1990; 47(11):1181-4.
12. Seshia SS, Johnston B, Kasian G. Non-traumatic coma in childhood: Clinical variables in prediction of outcome. Dev Med Child Neurol. 1983; 25(4): 493-501.
13. Singhi PD, Bansal A, Ramesh S, *et al.* Predictive value of electroencephalography and computed tomography in childhood non-traumatic coma. Indian J Pediatr 2005 ; 72(6) : 475-9.
14. Wong CP, Forsyth RJ, Kelly TP, Eyre JA. Incidence, aetiology, and outcome of non-traumatic coma: A population based study. Arch Dis Child. 2001 Mar;84(3):193-9.

In the previous edition this chapter was written by James H. McCrory, MD, FAAP, FCCM Attending Staff Pediatric Critical Care Center St. John's Regional Health Center Springfield, Missouri

Sunit Singhi and Pratibha Singhi

26 Convulsive Status Epilepticus

Status epilepticus (SE) in children is a medical emergency that requires early recognition and aggressive treatment. Any type of epileptic seizure can develop into SE but the most common ones include tonic-clonic or clonic, tonic or occasionally myoclonic that lead to convulsive SE. Non convulsive status epilepticus is a term used for ongoing prolonged EEG seizure activity without any clinical convulsion, and includes absence and complex partial SE. In this chapter, only convulsive status epilepticus will be discussed. SE may occur at any age, but is more common in children <2 years. The incidence of SE in children ranges from 18-20 per 100,000 years. It is estimated that 10-25% of children with epilepsy and up to 5% of children with febrile seizures have at least one episode of SE. Sleep deprivation or an intercurrent infection in an epileptic patient are recognized precipitating factors.

DEFINITION AND CLASSIFICATION

The International League Against Epilepsy (ILAE) defines status epilepticus as a "condition characterized by an epileptic seizure that is so frequent or so prolonged as to create a fixed and lasting condition." however, this definition is difficult for practical application. Epilepsy Foundation of America (EFA) working group on Status epilepticus defined SE in children as "seizure lasting more than 30 minutes, or recurrent seizures lasting greater than 30 minutes without full return of consciousness". This definition is generally accepted, because significant damage to the brain occurs after 30 mins of seizure activity.

A working definition for SE as 'five minutes of continuous seizure activity or successive seizures without clearing of sensorium' has been proposed because it has been observed that seizures that last for 5 minutes or more may continue for at least 30 minutes. In practice, therefore any child who continues to convulse when brought to the emergency, should be treated as a case of SE. Also a child with epilepsy should be considered in SE if the seizure persists for more than twice the usual duration of the previous seizures.

PATHOPHYSIOLOGY

Prolonged seizures cause an increased metabolic rate, cerebral oxygen extraction and consumption and subsequently neuronal injury. During the first 30 minutes of seizures there is massive sympathetic and parasympathetic over-activity, which may lead to tachycardia, hypertension, hyperglycemia, hyperthermia, excessive sweating, and salivary and tracheobronchial hypersecretion. If SE persists for more than one hour, hypotension, hyperkalemia, hypoglycemia, and respiratory acidosis may ensue(Table 1).

Treatment with benzodiazepines or barbiturates may further worsen these complications. CSF pleocytosis may occur.

ETIOLOGY

S.E may be symptomatic, wherein an underlying cause can be identified or idiopathic where no cause can be identified. Most cases are symptomatic. The causes of S.E in children are listed in table 2.

The important causes of SE may be broadly divided into:

1) *Acute:* CNS infections (meningitis, meningoencephalitis), febrile convul-

Table 1: Systemic and cerebral pathophysiological changes associated with seizures and convulsive status epilepticus

Compensation (< 30 minutes)	*Decompensation (> 30 minutes)*
Increased cardiac output Increased cerebral blood flow Increased catecholamine release Increased glucose concentration in the brain Cerebral energy requirements matched by supply of oxygen and glucose	Failure of cerebral autoregulation Hypoglycemia Hypoxia Acidosis Hypernatremia, Hypo/hyperkalaemia Disseminated intravascular coagulation Leucocytosis Falling blood pressure and cardiac output Rhabdomyolysis and renal failure

Table 2: Causes of Status epilepticus in children

Fever.	
Intracranial infections	- Meningitis. - Meningoencephalitis. - Brain Abscess.
Hypoxic Encephalopathy.	
Cerebrovascular diseases.	
Metabolic derangements	- Hypoglycemia - Hyponatremia - Hypernatremia - Hypocalcemia - Hypomagnesemia
Cerebral Tumors	- Benign. - Malignant-Primary, - Secondary
Poisonings	
Congenital abnormalities of brain	
Inborn errors of Metabolism.	
Medications e.g	- Theophylline - Tricyclic antidepressants
Drug abuse e.g.	- Cocaine or other stimulants
Epilepsy (First presentation of primary epilepsy)	

sions, vascular episodes, trauma, metabolic derangements and poisonings.

2) *Static:* SE as first manifestation of or during the course of epilepsy, with or without an underlying neurologic disorder. In children with epilepsy, non-compliance or withdrawal of anti-epileptic therapy, intercurrent infections and stress may predispose to SE.

In one study more than 80% children younger than 2 years of age had SE of febrile or acute symptomatic origin, while among children older than 2 years, 64% had a past history of seizures and 55% were known to be previously neurologically abnormal. In developing countries CNS infections are the commonest cause of SE and refractory SE (RSE).

DIFFERENTIAL DIAGNOSIS

Usually tonic-clonic seizures of SE are obvious and there are no diagnostic doubts. However, certain situations which can be confused with SE are as follows:

Tetanus- Patients suffering with tetanus may have prolonged tonic spasms of various parts of body. However, consciousness remains preserved during the attacks, there is no accompanying eye deviation, and the attacks are precipitated with the slightest of external stimuli like touch, sound or light.

Phenothiazine toxicity- Patients may have tonic upward deviation of eyes sometimes with tonic posturing of body without any loss of consciousness. History of drug ingestion, urine toxic screening may help in the diagnosis.

Peudoseizures (Psychogenic seizures)- These may sometimes be confused with SE. One should consider possibility of pseudo-status if the episode does not respond promptly to initial treatment. Following clinical features are suggestive of peudoseizure-female sex, history of psychosocial disturbance, poorly coordinated thrashing movements, back arching, pelvic thrusting, gaze aversion or eyes held shut, head rolling, vocalization, consciousness may be retained in the presence of bilateral jerking, resistance to examination, normal pupillary response during convulsion, normal tendon reflexes and plantar responses immediately after convulsion. Rarely, EEG and/or video-EEG telemetry studies are needed to rule out the above disorders.

MANAGEMENT

Of the important determinants of outcome of SE, duration of SE is the only potentially modifiable determinant. Hence, timely diagnosis and prompt and proactive treatment of SE is essential for a better outcome. The main goals of management are:

1. Supporting vital functions (stabilization of airway, breathing and circulation)
2. Termination of seizure activity as expeditiously as possible
3. Diagnosis and initial therapy of life-threatening causes of SE

A simplified management scheme is as follows:

Stabilization

Attention to airway, breathing and circulation to ensure adequate cerebral perfusion, oxygenation and glucose level is the first priority in the management. This can be achieved by maintaining optimal respiratory and hemodynamic function using PALS guideline.

Airway

Blockage of the airway may occur because of clenched jaw, poorly coordinated breathing, secretions and vomitus. Airway patency should be ensured by proper positioning of the head or by positioning the patient on the side and suctioning of the nasopharyngeal secretions. Oral or nasal airways may be used, but forced opening of the clenched jaws should be avoided. Early gastric decompression using a nasogastric tube should be done to prevent vomiting and secondary aspiration.

Breathing

To ensure adequate oxygenation, 100% oxygen using a facemask and reservoir bag should be started. Assisted ventilation with bag and mask should be started if there are signs of inadequate ventilation and oxygenation such as inadequate chest movements, poor air entry on auscultation, tachypnea, poor respiratory efforts, central cyanosis, or oxygen saturation<90%. If bag mask ventilation is unsatisfactory, intubation should be done. Bradycardia, hypotension and poor perfusion indicate severe hypoxia and an immediate need for intubation and ventilation. Endotracheal intubation is also indicated if the child has increased intracranial pressure that requires controlled oxygenation and emergency hyperventilation. Rapid sequence induction (RSI) is preferred for emergency intubation.

Circulation

A vascular access should be obtained promptly for administration of fluids to stabilize circulating volume and anticonvulsants to abort seizure. In a convulsing child, if an intravenous access cannot be established, the intraosseous (IO) route can be used. In children less than 6 years, all emergency anticonvulsants and medications and fluids that are given by IV route, may be administered by IO infusions.

Diagnostic Evaluation

Search for a cause should proceed parallel with therapeutic measures to terminate seizure. The evaluation should include a focused history, physical examination and selected investigations depending on age, suspected etiology and previous anticonvulsant therapy. The focused brief history should include the condition of the child before SE, fever, recent head injury, details of previous seizures if any, current medications, chronic diseases or allergies. A bedside blood glucose determination is helpful to detect hypoglycemia. Table 3 outlines suggested diagnostic workup in a case of SE.

Termination of Seizures

Several guidelines are available for treatment of convulsive status in children. SE but there are wide variations in selection of drugs for refractory SE.

Step1: Benzodiazepines

Intravenous benzodiazepines

Intravenous benzodiazepines are accepted as first-line treatment as they stop seizures most rapidly regardless of the etiology. Any of the three benzodiazepines can be used IV: midazolam 0.1 – 0.2 mg/kg (maximum 5 mg),

Table 3: Suggested diagnostic workup in a child in status epilepticus

Blood	Hemogram, glucose, calcium, magnesium, urea, electrolytes, blood-gases, anti-epileptic drug levels, toxicology screen, culture if febrile
Urine	Routine analysis, myoglobinuria, toxicology
CSF	In suspected meningitis
ContinuousEEG monitoring	In refractory SE and SE in neonates
Neuroimaging	In case of focal findings or in case of suspected head injury or coma

diazepam 0.3mg/kg (maximum 10mg) at a rate no greater than 2 mg/min, or lorazepam 0.05-1mg/kg (maximum 4 mg) given over 2 minutes. All the three are effective. The onset of action of these drugs is within 1-3 minutes of administration. The duration of action of diazepam is 15 –30 minutes, and that of lorazepam is 24-48 hours. Although I.V. diazepam and IV lorazepam, are equally effective in controlling SE in children, lorazepam is generally preferred as initial therapy as it has a longer duration of action and lesser incidence of respiratory depression, hypotension and need for intubation. However, the need to keep lorazepam refrigerated, and to dilute it prior to administration may make diazepam use easier in acute situations. The dose of IV benzodiazepine may be repeated after 5-10 minutes if seizure persists.

Rectal diazepam

Rectal diazepam is as effective as I.V. diazepam in aborting seizures in 96% of patients if given within 15 minutes of seizure onset. Diazepam gel (Dialstat®) in strengths of 5, 10, 15 and 20 mg has been found to be effective and is well tolerated. If diazepam gel is not available, one can use the parentral solution per rectum (0.5 mg/kg up to a maximum of 10 mg). It is used without dilution and is placed 4 cms into the rectum by using a small catheter on the end of a syringe. The anal opening should be strapped after administration for about half an hour to prevent spillage. It may be repeated after 5-10 minutes if seizures persist and then may be repeated once more.

Sublingual and Rectal Lorazepam

Sublingual Lorazepam is effective in a dose of 0.1mg/kg up to a maximum of 4mg(i.e., 40 kg patient) and may be repeated twice after every 10 minutes if a seizure persists. One has to actively look for hypotension and respiratory depression. Lorazepam is available in tablets of 0.5mg, 1 mg and 2mg.

Rectal lorazepam has not been as extensively studied as rectal diazepam. Rectal and intravenous diazepam as well as rectal and IV lorazepam, were found to be equally effective irrespective of the route of administration.

Intranasal midazolam

Intranasal midazolam is absorbed directly into the blood and cerebrospinal fluid via the nasal mucosa. It is safe, inexpensive, easy to learn by parents and paramedics, and provides better seizure control than rectal diazepam. Also, it is painless, does not require sterile technique and is socially acceptable. Intranasal midazolam (0.2mg/kg) is equally effective in control of seizures as intravenous diazepam (0.3mg/kg); moreover the overall time to cessation of seizures after arrival at hospital is faster with intranasal midazolam than with intravenous diazepam. Hence, intranasal midazolam is useful for acute control of seizures in general practice and at home.

Buccal Midazolam

Buccal Midazolam is more effective than rectal diazepam, and stops seizure in >75% of children and young people with status epilepticus. The buccal route is more socially acceptable, convenient, and has become the preferred treatment for domiciliary management of long seizures in many countries.

Intramuscular (IM) Midazolam

Midazolam being water soluble can be administered by IM route. A dose of 0.2mg/kg IM, as first line therapy, controls seizures in more than 90% of children in SE. It is as effective as intravenous diazepam for the initial therapy of SE and is particularly valuable when there is difficulty in establishing an intravenous route.

Step 2: Phenytoin and phenobarbitone

If seizure activity persists or recurs despite benzodiazepine, phenytoin, or phenobarbitone may be used.

Phenytoin

Phenytoin is given intravenously, in a loading dose of 20 mg/kg, at a rate not exceeding 1mg/kg/min (to avoid hypotension and cardiac arrhythmias). An additional loading dose up to 10 mg/kg may be used in young infants if SE persists after 10 mins. Onset of action is 10-30 minutes after infusion and duration of action is for 12-24 hours. Phenytoin should be diluted only with normal saline, and never with glucose containing solutions as it may precipitate and form microcrystals. Maintenance dose of phenytoin (5-8mg/kg/day) is given in two divided doses after 12- 24 hours of the initial loading dose to prevent seizure recurrence.

Fosphenytoin, a phenytoin prodrug, is a water-soluble phosphate ester of phenytoin that gets rapidly converted to phenytoin. In contrast to phenytoin it can be administered IM with rapid and complete absorption. The dose of fosphenytoin is 15-20mg/kg of phenytoin equivalents/kg, infused at a rate of no more than 3mg/kg/min, not to exceed 150mg/min. The cost is however a limiting factor, as it is several times more costly than phenytoin.

Phenobarbitone

Phenobarbitone is preferred over phenytoin in neonates and in SE associated with fever that has not responded to benzodiazepines. However, there is no evidence to support this preference. It is given in a loading dose of 20 mg/kg IV at a rate of 1.5 mg/kg/min. In neonates an additional dose of 5-10mg/kg may be given if seizure persists (total of 30mg/kg). The maintenance dose is 3-5 mg/kg/day, given in two divided doses 12-24 hours later. Owing to the cumulative sedative and respiratory depressant effect of benzodiazepines and barbiturates, facilities should be available for intubation and mechanical ventilation.

Summary of the important features of AEDs used in SE in shown in Table 4.

TREATMENT OF REFRACTORY STATUS EPILEPTICUS (RSE)

If seizures persist even after adequate treatment with benzodiazepine, and phenytoin and/or phenobartbitone, it is termed as refractory status epilepticus (RSE). About 10-15% of SE are refractory to conventional therapies. The commonest cause of RSE in developing countries is CNS infection, particularly meningoencephalitis, and bacterial meningitis. Structural lesions of the brain such as cerebral infarcts, developmental cortical anomalies, and malignant childhood epileptic syndromes are the other usual causes of RSE.

Although several drugs have been used in the management of refractory status epilepticus there is little consensus regarding standard protocol for management of refractory status epilepticus. Traditionally RSE is treated with barbiturate coma, continuous benzodiazepine infusion or anesthetic agents. All these are best administered in an intensive care unit, where the patient can be put on a ventilator and have a continuous EEG monitoring regardless of drug used. These modalities will not be discussed here. However, paraldehyde and newer therapies such as intravenous valproate, and intravenous levetiracetam can be given in an emergency setting. Diazepam and midazolam infusion and can also be given emergency where ICU/ventilation facilities are not readily available.

Table 4: Important features of AEDs used for control of Status Epilepticus

Drug and Route	Dose	Maximum	Rate	Repeat	Risks	Comments
Shorter term/acute cessation of seizure						
Lorazepam						
(IV,SL,I0)	0. 1 mg/kg	4 mg	<2 mg/ min	q10 min x 2	Hypotension, respiratory depression	Must be refrigerated and diluted before administration Cost more than Diazepam
Midazolam (IV/IM/Buccal)	0.1-0.2 mg/kg	5 mg	<2 mg/ min	q5-10 min	-do-	Intranasal, buccal preparations available IV prep. can also be given buccal
Diazepam (IV,IO)	0.3 mg/kg	10 mg	<2 mg/ min	q5 min x 2-3	-do-	Administer as close to vein as possible without dilution
Diazepam (PR)	0.5 mg/kg	10 mg		q5-10 min	-do-	Use gel/undiluted IV preparation 4cms deep in rectum
Paraldehyde (PR)	0.3 mL/kg	10 mL			Mucosal irritation	Dilute 1/1 in oil in glass syringe
Longer-acting anticonvulsants/acute cessation and prevention (not previously on medications)						
Phenytoin* (IV,IO)	20 mg/kg	1000 mg (30 mg/ kg)	1 mg/kg/ min	May give additional 5 mg/kg IV if unable to stop	Hypotension, arrhythmia need to be on cardiac monitor	Must be given slowly in non glucose containing seizure
Phenobarbital* (IV,I0)	20 mg/kg	600 mg (30 mg/kg)	1 mg/kg/ min		Respiratory depression, especially if Diazepam has been used	First choice in neonates

*If a patient is already on phenytoin or phenobarbital, a booster dose of 5 mg/kg may be given. Subsequent doses may be given based on anticonvulsant levels.

Drugs in boldface type is the first-choice drug; others are good alternatives or additions.

IV = intravenous; SL = sublingual; PR = per rectum; 10 = intra-osseous, IN=intranasal

Paraldehyde

Paraldehyde is given in a dose of 0.3ml/kg up to a maximum of 10 ml (i.e., 30kg patient). It is diluted with mineral oil in a glass syringe and infused per rectum about 4 cms into the rectum. The buttocks should be elevated and squeezed together for 5 minutes to avoid evacuation of rectal contents. One has to watch carefully for mucosal irritation.

Sodium Valproate

Intravenous sodium valproate has been found to be effective for the treatment of RSE. It is safe over a large range of doses, as well as various rates of administration, and also when given as a rapid bolus. It has a rapid onset of action as there is no lag time between peak serum and peak brain concentration of valproate. In a randomized trial on 40 children with RSE intravenous sodium valproate was as effective as diazepam infusion in controlling RSE and was free of adverse effects such as respiratory depression and hypotension. Sodium valproate was given as an initial loading bolus of 30mg/kg diluted 1:1 in normal saline over 2-5min, with a repeat bolus dose of 10mg/kg if the status was not controlled within 10 minutes. This was followed by infusion at rate of 5mg/kg/hr, which was continued until a seizure free period of 6 hours and then reduced at a rate of 1mg/kg/hr every 2 hourly. After discontinuation of intravenous infusion, a maintenance dose of 10mg/kg/dose 8 hourly IV was continued until the child could take oral anticonvulsants. I.V valporate should not be used in a child with suspected neuro-metabolic disorder.

Diazepam or Midazolam Infusion

Diazepam or midazolam infusion may be considered when there is an initial response to benzodiazepines and particularly when ventilator support is not readily available. Both of these drugs when used in rapidly incremental doses control RSE in about 15 minutes. Diazepam is diluted in normal saline, Ringer's lactate or dextrose water to give a strength of 0.04mg/ml. The starting dose is 0.01mg/kg/min, which is increased gradually every five minutes until the seizures are fully controlled. Most children require 0.02-0.03mg/kg/min, but can tolerate even higher doses if required. We have sometimes used up to 0.1mg/kg/min. Midazolam infusion starting with 2mg/kg/min up to 12 mg/kg/min may be used. Although higher doses up to 24 mg/kg/min been used successfully, all these patients were given mechanical ventilation. Although some units prefer midazolam, in our experience midazolam was associated with about four times higher risk of breakthrough seizures as compared to diazepam while the patient was still on the infusion. We therefore prefer diazepam infusion over midazolam infusion.

Intravenous levetiracetam

Levetiracetam is a broad spectrum anticonvulsant with various mechanisms of action. Several studies in adults and some in children have shown that it is safe and effective in children in controlling RSE. It has low risk of sedation and cardiorespiratory depression. Various doses, including a bolus of 50 mg/kg followed by 25 mg/kg over 15 minutes every 12 hours have been used. The most appropriate dose still needs to be established.

Other investigational drugs for SE include gabapentin, vigabatrin, and lamotrigine that act via GABA, felbamate that blocks NMDA receptors, and topiramate.

Role of EEG

Convulsive SE is apparent and an EEG is not needed for diagnosis. However an EEG is useful in diagnosis of SE in less obvious circumstances. More importantly an EEG is needed to confirm that an episode of SE has ended, particularly when there is a possibility of ongoing recurrent subtle seizures which can continue to occur even after clinical cessation of convulsions. EEG monitoring is required in the ICU setting in children with RSE, to ensure that a burst suppression EEG is obtained with the antiepileptic medication being used. Patients with SE who fail to recover rapidly and completely should have EEG monitoring for at least 24 hours after the last episode of seizure. EEG is also helpful in prognosis - presence of periodic lateralizing epileptic discharges (PLEDs) indicates a bad prognosis.

Complications

Uncontrolled SE is associated with several complications (Table 5). Some of these could be fatal such as cardiac arrhythmias and acute renal failure. Early recognition and appropriate management are required.

Outcome and Prognosis:

The outcome depends mainly on the age, etiology, duration of SE, and adequacy of care. In the emergency department, the outcome is primarily a function of the underlying etiology. The mortality of SE ranges from 3-10% in children and the morbidity is twice this. The mortality is higher with symptomatic SE, and in children with refractory SE it is about 20%. Neurological sequelae – motor or cognitive deficit – have been found in 9-28% and subsequent epilepsy in 23-30%. Very few children are completely normal after prolonged SE. In the absence of an acute or progressive CNS insult, morbidity and mortality are low. On the other hand mortality and morbidity are highest with SE associated with CNS infections.

In conclusion, SE is a life-threatening emergency that requires prompt and vigorous treatment. Uncontrolled seizure activity results in progressive neuronal damage. Hence all treating units should establish a time framed protocol. One such protocol being used in our PICU is shown in Table 6. Proactive approach is a prerequisite to improve the final outcome of patients with SE.

Table 5: Complications of Status epilepticus

Cardiovascular	Bradycardia, arrhythmia, cardiac failure or arrest, hypertension, hypotension, shock
Respiratory	Hyperapnea, apnea, irregular or cheyne stokes breathing, respiratory acidosis, aspiration pneumonia, pulmonary edema
Renal	Oliguria, acute renal failure, acute tubular necrosis, myoglobinuria(from rhabdomyolysis)
Autonomic	Hyperpyrexia, excessive sweating, excessive secretions with airway obstruction
Metabolic	Hyperglycemia, hypoglycemia, hyperkalemia, hyponatraemia, metabolic and lactic acidosis

Table 6: Protocol and time table for the treatment of status epilepticus

Time	Drug treatment	Supportive treatment
0		• Ensure adequate respiration • Intubation considered
2-3		• Start low flow oxygen • Start an intravenous line with D5W or normal saline • Draw blood for glucose, hepatic and renal function, CBC with DLC, electrolytes, calcium, magnesium, blood gases and toxicology screen • Obtain urine for routine examination
3-5	Diazepam: 0.3mg/kg or Lorazepam 0.1mg/kg-infused over 2 minutes	• Start second I.V. line with D5W or normal saline for simultaneous administration o a second medication and I.V. fluids.
7-8	Phenytoin- 20mg/kg dilute in saline and infuse at a rate of no more than 1 mg/kg/min	• D50W- 1ml/kg I.V. push; Thiamine-100mg-I.V. push, Pyridoxine-100-200mg of I.V. push in children < 18 months of age. • Monitor blood pressure
10	Repeat Diazepam/ Lorazepam	
15	Repeat Diazepam/ Lorazepam	
20	IV Valproate 30 mg/kg, IV, if seizure controlled 5 mg/kg/hour for 6 hours* OR	• Transfer to PICU (if possible), prepare for intubation, ventilation, get EEG
20	Diazepam or Midazolam infusion (Diazepam: 0.01mg/kg/min, max 0.1mg/kg/min, Midazolam: 2μg/kg/min up to 12 μg/kg/min in increments of 2μg/kg/min every 5 minutes till seizure control.**)	• Transfer to PICU, prepare for intubation, ventilation, get EEG.

* Start tapering 6 hours after the last seizure @1mg/kg/hr every 2 hourly.

** Continue for 6 hours after the last seizure then start tapering every hour by 1μg/kg/min.

FURTHER READING

1. Abend NS, Marsh E. Convulsive and nonconvulsive status epilepticus in children. Curr Treat Options Neurol. 2009 Jul;11(4):262-72
2. Chameides L, Hazinski MF (Eds) Pediatric Advanced Life Support. American Heart Association 2000.
3. Chin RF, Neville BG, Peckham C, Bedford H, Wade A. Incidence, cause, and short-term outcome of convulsive status epilepticus in childhood: prospective population-based study. Lancet 2006;368:222-29.
4. Choudhery V, Townend W. Best evidence topic reports. Lorazepam or diazepam in paediatric status epilepticus. Emerg Med J. 2006;23:472-3.
5. Kirmani B F, Crusp E D, Kayani S, Rajab H. Role of intravenous levetiracetam in acute seizure management of children. Pediatr neurol 2009; 41:37-39.
6. Lahat E, Goldman M, Barr J, Bistritzer T, Berkovitch M. Comparison of intranasal midazolam with intravenous diazepam for treating febrile seizures in children: prospective randomised study. BMJ. 2000;321:83-86.
7. Mahmoudian T, Zadeh MM. Comparison of intranasal midazolam with intravenous diazepam for treating acute seizures in children. Epilepsy Behav. 2004;5:253-5.
8. McIntyre J, Robertson S, Norris E et al. Safety and efficacy of buccal midazolam versus rectal diazepam for emergency treatment of seizures

in children: a randomised controlled trial. Lancet. 2005;366:205-210.

9. Mehta V, Singhi P, Singhi S . Intravenous sodium valproate versus diazepam infusion for the control of refractory status epilepticus in children-A randomised controlled trial. J Child Neurol. 2007; 22:1191-7.
10. Morrison G, Gibbons E, Whitehouse WP. High-dose midazolam therapy for refractory status epilepticus in children. Intensive Care Med. 2006;32:2070-76.
11. Proposal for revised clinical and electroencephalographic classification of commission on classification and terminology of the International League Against Epilepsy: A proposed international classification of epileptic seizures. Epilepsia 1981; 22: 489-501.
12. Saengpattrachai M, Sharma R, Hunjan A et al. Nonconvulsive seizures in the pediatric intensive care unit: etiology, EEG, and brain imaging finding. Epilepsia, 2006; 47: 1510-18.
13. Scott RC, Besag FM, Neville BG. Buccal midazolam and rectal diazepam for treatment of prolonged seizures in childhood and adolescents: a randomized trial Lancet 1999; 353:623-26.
14. Singhi S, Murthi A, Singhi P, Jayashree M, Continuous midazolam versus diazepam infusion for refractory convulsive status epilepticus. Journal of Child Neurol 2002; 17:106-10.
15. Singhi S, Singhi P, Dass R. Status epilepticus: emergency management. Indian J Pediatr. 2003 Mar;70 Suppl 1:S17-22.
16. Singhi S, Singhi PD, Banerjee S. Refractory status epilepticus- role of continuous diazepam infusion. Journal of Child Neurol 1998; 13: 23-26.
17. Walker DM, Teach SJ. Update on the acute management of status epilepticus in children. Curr Opin Pediatr 2006; 18:239-44.
18. Wolfe TR, Macfarlane TC. Intranasal midazolam therapy for pediatric status epilepticus. Am J Emerg Med. 2006; 24:343-6.
19. Working Group on Status Epilepticus: Treatment of convulsive status epilepticus: Recommendations of the epilepsy Foundation of America's Working Group on Status Epilepticus. JAMA 1993; 270: 854-9.
20. Yu KT, Mills S, Thompson N, Cunanan C. Safety and efficacy of intravenous valproate in pediatric status epilepticus and acute repetitive seizures. Epilepsia 2003;44:724-6.

Rashna Dass

27 Febrile Encephalopathy

A child or an infant presenting with an altered mental status to the pediatric emergency room presents a diagnostic challenge and poses difficult management issues to the treating pediatrician. Encephalopathy denotes a nonspecific brain insult in a patient manifesting with a combination of change in the mental status, seizures, decerebration and occasionally with ataxia, hemiplegia or cardiorespiratory arrest. Encephalopathy can be associated with fever or without fever depending on the underlying cause and pathogenetic mechanism involved. In this chapter we discuss the entity of febrile encephalopathy with regard to the etiology, pathogenesis and approach to such a child in the emergency setting.

DEFINITIONS

Any change in the mental status of a patient associated with fever or a recent history of fever qualifies for the definition of febrile encephalopathy. If the duration of fever is less than 2 weeks duration then it is termed as acute febrile encephalopathy and for those with fever > 2 weeks duration it is termed as sub-acute febrile encephalopathy. A wide spectrum of alterations in consciousness exists and therefore febrile encephalopathy can manifest in a number of ways ranging from lethargy, stupor, delirium, confusion, obtundation or frank coma. The various types of altered mental status are defined below:

***Lethargy*:** Reduced wakefulness in which the primary defect is one of attention.

Stupor: Condition of deep sleep from which the patient can be aroused only by vigorous and repeated stimuli. As soon as the stimulus disappears the patient returns to an unresponsive state.

Delirium: Floridly abnormal state characterized by disorientation, fear, irritability and hallucinations.

Confusion: A state of reduced awareness with the patient misinterpreting oncoming stimuli.

Obtundation: Mental blunting with slow responses to stimuli and often an increase in sleep time.

Coma: A state of unresponsiveness without evidence of awareness of self or environment, a state from which the patient cannot be aroused by vocal or sensory stimuli.

ETIOLOGY

A number of diseases can lead to febrile

encephalopathy both infective and non-infective (Table 1). The first and the most common cause of a patient presenting with febrile encephalopathy is infections of the central nervous system such as meningitis (both bacterial and tubercular) and encephalitis (of viral origin) [1,2]. In various studies infectious causes of febrile encephalopathy have been implicated in about one third to two third of all cases of acute encephalopathy [3-5]. This is followed by other infections of which most common in the developing countries are complicated malaria (*P. falciparum*)[6], dengue[7], enteric fever and generalized septicaemia.

Non-infective causes of febrile encephalopathy are not very common but must always be kept in mind in the occasional patient. The malignant neuroleptic syndrome, heat stroke, autoimmune thyroiditis, occasional untreated case of thyroid storm (exaggerated thyrotoxicosis) and lymphomas can present with hyperpyrexia, coma, acidosis and seizures.

PATHOGENESIS

The various etiologic agents responsible for causing febrile encephalopathy results in either a discontinuation of neurologic communication between the cerebral cortex and subcortical structures in the diencephalon, midbrain and upper pons or a transection of the reticular activating system leading to prolonged unresponsiveness. This sort of damage in febrile encephalopathy is mostly mediated by non-traumatic pathology which include anoxic damage, metabolic derangements, hormonal or electrolyte disturbances or exogenous toxins. All these results in either or all of the following:

a) Inadequate delivery of a necessary substrate required for brain function.
b) Inadequate removal of a toxin or waste product.
c) Production of a toxic metabolite.

Most organisms invade the nervous system directly and liberate bacterial cell wall constituents which in turn mediate a range of host inflammatory responses, activation of leukocytes, endothelial injury, altered vascular permeability and thrombosis which eventually lead to cerebral edema, cerebritis, encephalitis, cerebral congestion, hydrocephalus, subdural empyemas, ventriculitis, thrombophlebitis and abscesses thus resulting

Table 1: Causes of Febrile encephalopathy

Infective causes	*Non-infective causes*
Meningitis	Neuroleptic malignant syndrome or malignant hyperthermia
Bacterial	Heat stroke
Fungal	Lymphomas
Mycobacterial	Pontine hemorrhage
Encephalitis Viral (Herpes, Japanese B)	Autoimmune thyroiditis
Malaria (Cerebral-*P. falciparum*)	Thyroid storm
Enteric fever	
Cerebral abscesses	
Generalized septicemia	
Dengue	
Measles (Acute presentation of subacute sclerosing panencephalitis)	
HIV associated CNS infections	
Acute disseminated encephalomyelitis (ADEM)	

in alteration of the CNS functions. However encephalopathy may also result from the effects of extracranial infection by the syndrome of appropriate ADH secretion (SIADH), cerebral salt wasting, hyper-or hyponatraemia, inflammatory brain edema, thrombophlebitis, status epilepticus, severe endotoxemic shock and disseminated intravascular coagulation (DIC). Mycobacterial infections such as tubercular meningitis can present as an acute febrile encephalopathy with raised intracranial tension resulting from acute ventricular dilatation or multiple tuberculomata.

Viruses also cause acute febrile encephalopathy by virtue of their neurotropic nature or by attacking specific parts of the CNS such as cerebellum, temporal lobe or the aqueduct of Sylvius. They are also responsible for perivascular demyelination and invasion of neurons leading to the reversible "pyrexial convulsion syndrome".

In cerebral malaria the organism implicated is P. falciparum and the CNS effects occur because of increased cytoadherence due to formation of knobs on parasitized red blood cells leading to microvascular occlusion, cerebral anoxia, and ischaemic cerebral damage. Along with this an associated activation of the nitric oxide synthetase and complement cascade by prostaglandins and glycophosphatidil inositol results in cerebral inflammation. The other contributing factors in the encephalopathy associated with cerebral malaria are the co-existent hypoglycaemia, acidosis, electrolyte abnormalities and occasional DIC in some severely affected cases.

There are also increasing reports of measles and dengue presenting as an acute febrile encephalopathy particularly in developing countries. About 1-4% of dengue admissions are reported to have clouding of consciousness[8]. Associated hypotension, cerebral edema, cerebral hemorrhage, hyponatraemia, encephalopathy secondary to hepatic dysfunction, acute disseminated encephalomyelitis or direct invasion of the virus itself can cause the encephalopathy seen with dengue infection[9, 10].

Sepsis induced febrile encephalopathy has a wide range of manifestations from lethargy to overt coma. A number of pathogenetic mechanisms have been proposed such as bacterial invasion of brain, endotoxin injury, amino acid and neurotransmitter derangements and microvascular changes [8].

Non-infective causes lead to febrile encephalopathy by different mechanisms. In autoimmune thyroiditis there is an increase in the TNF-á concentrations[11] and this acts as an endogenous pyrogen[12] leading to an association of encephalopathy with fever in such cases. Autoimmune processes in turn by virtue of different mechanisms such as vasculitis or infarcts result in encephalopathy. Cerebral hemorrhage especially pontine hemorrhage leads to encephalopathy with fever secondary to affection of the central temperature regulating systems. Similarly reports of subacute febrile encephalopathy in Hodgkin's disease have also been described[13].

In patients who are genetically predisposed to develop the neuroleptic malignant syndrome or malignant hyperthermia, a pharmacological trigger can induce a rapid and marked increase in the metabolic rate of the individual's muscles and lead to acidosis, high grade fever and rhabdomyolysis which in turn induce cerebral edema and other systemic effects. Similarly in heat stroke, a failure of the thermoregulatory homeostasis results in a body temperature of more than 40°C and signs of severe CNS dysfunction such as delirium, coma, seizures or decerebrate rigidity. All these are secondary to cerebral edema. In both these conditions an increase in the demand on the circulatory system results in cardiac failure, hepatic ischemia and subsequent hypoglycemia which may in itself contribute to the CNS manifestations.

APPROACH TO MANAGEMENT

In any case of febrile encephalopathy the management strategy of the patient always is guided by the philosophy of "treating the treatable" and starts with the initial assessment of the ABC (airway, breathing and circulation) in the emergency room as in all emergency cases. After the initial resuscitation and stabilization of the cardiorespiratory systems the definitive management is initiated.

Management consists of:

A. Treatment of immediate problems
B. Identification of underlying cause
C. Investigations
D. Specific treatment

STABILIZATION AND EMERGENCY MANAGEMENT

Of utmost importance in any child with encephalopathy is the need to try and reverse and also to prevent ongoing neurologic damage. The initial approach should focus on the vital signs and provision of supplemental oxygen. This includes the maintenance of a patent, stable airway, thus ensuring proper breathing followed by assessment of the state of circulation by a quick examination of the pulses and blood pressure. The airway must be cleared and kept open by extension of the neck and breathing must be evaluated. All the cases of febrile encephalopathy must be evaluated by the Glasgow coma scale (GCS) or the modified Glasgow coma scale and in those whose GCS is below 8 or modified GCS below 12, endotracheal intubation must be done in the emergency area and if required assisted ventilation must be initiated. In case of evidence of circulatory collapse, efforts must be aimed at simultaneous resuscitation of the circulatory system. One must remember that the metabolic activity in the brain is relatively high and also rapidly affected by a lack of oxygen and glucose. During emergency situations the need to maintain a constant supply of these substrates and hence an adequate brain perfusion is of utmost importance and supercedes the need to treat any CNS lesion. Therefore often further damage to the brain is prevented by aggressive management of both the circulatory status and prevention of hypoxia.

One must keep in mind that most of these cases of febrile encephalopathy present with associated complications such as hypoglycaemia, seizures, fluid imbalances (dehydration, cerebral salt wasting or SIADH), acidosis and raised intracranial tension.

Hence after the first stabilization the test that must be done immediately is a bedside blood sugar estimation by Dextrostix and if the sugar is low therapy must be initiated with IV glucose in the following doses:

Neonates: Loading dose of 2ml/kg of 10% dextrose

Children: Loading dose of 5ml/kg of 10% dextrose

If hypoglycaemia is detected by dextrostix a blood sample must be sent to the laboratory. This is followed by initiation of a dextrose drip to maintain a euglycaemic state. The usual starting level of the dextrose infusion is at 3-8 mg/kg/min of glucose and depending on the weight of the child this can be achieved by using a 5, 10 or 25% dextrose solution. In majority of cases the seizures and the coma state may be completely reversed by a timely and appropriate treatment of hypoglycaemia.

In occasional cases one may encounter hypergylcaemia especially in those with severe sepsis. In such cases insulin therapy needs to be initiated and a better therapeutic effect achieved with insulin infusion than with intermittent subcutaneous doses. The advantages of an insulin drip are a good and uniform control of the blood sugar level in contrast to the erratic control by the subcutaneous route and the flexibility to taper or hike up the dose as and when required. Whether the patient has hyper or hypoglycaemia frequent monitoring of the blood sugar is required till patient achieves a sustained state of euglycaemia.

Control of seizures is initiated by an immediate administration of a bolus of diazepam (0.2-0.3mg/kg) or midazolam (0.2 mg/kg) preferably by the intravenous (IV) route. In such cases where the IV route is difficult to establish one may administer the same by the per-rectal route. If the seizures are not controlled then a loading dose of Phenobarbitone or Phenytoin (20mg/kg) diluted in about 100-200 ml normal saline is initiated. In places where IV Valproate is available it can also be used in the initial treatment of seizures. Occasional patients may present with status epilepticus not responding to the initial treatment with a benzodiazepine or phenytoin or phenobarbitone and in whom a midazolam or diazepam drip may have to be initiated.

Fluid balance is restored depending on the clinical assessment. In case of dehydration the fluid of choice for the initial replacement is normal saline or Ringer's lactate. In the initial resuscitation there is no role of restricted fluids even if there is a suspicion of SIADH.

In majority of the cases acidosis gets corrected by fluid replacement. In some cases initiation of bicarbonate therapy can be empirically done with 1 mEq/kg of Sodium bicarbonate mixed with equal amounts of distilled water slowly over 1 hour pending an arterial blood gas analysis (ABG). When ABG is available, the dose of sodium bicarbonate is calculated by the formula: 0.3 x wt. in Kg x base deficit.

Evidence of raised intracranial pressure (ICP) can be rapidly assessed in the emergency by noting the presence of bradycardia, hypertension, and abnormal pattern of breathing and pupillary changes. Treatment should be aimed at rapid control of raised ICP. It can be achieved by controlled hyperventilation to maintain a pCO_2 of 30-35 mm Hg, 20% IV mannitol (0.5 -1 gm/kg) or dexamethasone (0.15mg/kg 6 hourly). However in cases suspected of cerebral malaria steroids are contraindicated. An important aspect of management of raised ICP is the control of seizures and fever as both these can aggravate the raised ICP.

A simultaneous assessment must be done in the emergency room of the coma state of the patient by using the Glasgow coma scale or preferably the modified Glasgow coma scale in young children. This initial assessment is of importance to follow up for improvement or deterioration once the patient is shifted for more intensive care.

IDENTIFICATION OF UNDERLYING CAUSE

After the initial stabilization and management of acute complications a detailed and relevant history must be taken along with a good clinical examination. The history and clinical examination should focus on identifying the underlying etiology so that definitive investigations and therapy can be initiated at the earliest. History should focus on the type, frequency and intensity of fever, any associated features such as rash, jaundice, seizures, and focal deficits. One must also remember to take a history of any similar illness in the neighborhood in the recent. This is useful to pinpoint towards a viral illness such as Japanese encephalitis, Dengue and Measles where there would be clustering of cases around a given area and help to clinch the diagnosis even in the absence of a diagnostic test. The geographic area from which a patient comes or has traveled to in the recent past also helps to pin point towards an etiological agent for e.g. certain areas in the western regions of Uttar Pradesh and upper regions of Assam in India are known for epidemics of Japanese encephalitis. Similar is the case with Falciparum malaria, which is known to occur in epidemics in the North Eastern regions of India.

History should also be directed towards identification of exposure to any medications or surgical procedures preceding the development of encephalopathy and also towards symptoms suggestive of thyroid disease such as cold or heat intolerance.

This should be followed by a good clinical examination of the child to identify the underlying cause of febrile encephalopathy. General physical examination should be directed towards identification of the presence of jaundice, anemia, rash, peripheral edema, bleeds, positive Hess test and degree of fever (Table 2). After the initial assessment of the level of coma, further examination is directed towards reassessment of the coma state to detect any improvement or deterioration from the time of admission and treatment of immediate problems. This is followed by a detailed examination to look for signs of meningeal irritation (neck stiffness, Kernig's sign or Bruzinski's sign), focal deficits, pupillary inequality, abnormal breathing pattern, oculocephalic relex (Doll's eye movement), corneal response and motor response (decerebrate or decorticate posture, hypotonia, hypertonia). Other system examination may reveal hepatosplenomegaly, pneumonia, abscesses etc. The history and clinical examination is followed by relevant investigations.

LABORATORY INVESTIGATIONS

Investigations are directed towards:

a) Confirmation of diagnosis
b) Detection of added complications

Investigations for confirmation of diagnosis:

The first and most important investigation for confirming the diagnosis in a case of febrile

Table 2: Disease association with specific signs

Signs	*Disease implicated*
Jaundice	Hepatitis, Malaria, Enteric fever
Anemia	Malaria, Dengue
Rash:	
Maculopapular	Dengue, measles, sepsis
Purpuric /petechial	Meningococcal, peumococcal infections, dengue
Mottling	Sepsis
Edema	SIADH, dengue, sepsis
Bleeding spots	DIC (Sepsis associated), dengue
Hess test	Dengue
Hyperpyrexia (temperature > 40°C)	Neuroleptic malignant syndrome, heat stroke
Hepatosplenomegaly	Malaria, enteric fever, hepatitis, lymphomas, disseminated sepsis (e.g. Disseminated staphylococcal infection)
Abscesses	Disseminated staphylococcal disease
Meningeal signs	Meningitis, meningism
Focal deficits	Intracranial space occupying lesion (abscess, tuberculoma, infarcts)

encephalopathy is a cerebrospinal fluid (CSF) examination. A lumbar puncture must be done in all patients with febrile encephalopathy after the initial stabilization and control of seizures including in those suspected of suffering from cerebral malaria also as most of these patients may have co-existing meningitis. The only exception to this rule is the presence of focal signs or raised ICP (Table 3). In those with focal signs a cranial imaging (CAT scan/MRI) is needed to rule out any space occupying lesion before a lumbar puncture is done. CSF is sent for cell count, protein and sugar estimation and also for a gram stain, Zeihl Neelson (ZN) stain and India ink preparation and culture. Wherever possible a latex agglutination test for bacterial antigens must be done and samples preserved for viral studies.

Bacterial meningitis is defined as acute febrile encephalopathy with identification of microorganisms from the CSF, culture or latex agglutinins, or presence of 3 or more of the following abnormalities in CSF - (i) polymorphonuclear leucocytosis > 100 cells/mm^3 (ii) glucose ~ 40 mg/dl or 50% of blood sugar (iii) elevated proteins > 40 mg/dl (iv) micro-organisms seen by Gram staining. Encephalitis is defined as acute febrile encephalopathy with CSF pleocytosis with lymphocyte predominance (>5 cells/mm^3) and absence of bacteria on direct microscopy, culture or latex agglutination and where no other alternative diagnosis is identifiable and a positive viral studies wherever possible. Tubercular meningitis is defined as a febrile encephalopathy with CSF pleocytosis (> 20 cells) with lymphocyte predominance (>60%), protein > 100mg%, sugar < 60% of the corresponding blood sugar, positive ZN stain or mycobacterial culture and negative India ink studies and cytology for malignant cells (from Ahuja et al [14]). In suspected lymphomas the CSF should be examined for malignant cells. In those with suspected measles a CSF IgM for measles can also be done; if this test is available.

In all cases a good peripheral blood smear examination for malarial parasite (both thick and thin films) and a parasite index helps to establish or exclude the diagnosis of cerebral malaria. In those cases where smear examination is negative a rapid antigen test for *P. falciparum* helps to pin point towards a falciparum infection. Other tests like the Widal test, dengue serology and thyroid profile should be performed in cases where the etiology is suspected to be enteric fever, dengue or thyroid related. A complete hemogram is mandatory in all such patients where polymorphonuclear leucocytosis can be seen in septicaemic patients or very high counts with lymphocyte predominance in lymphomas.

Table 3: Contraindications of lumbar puncture
Clinical or radiological features of raised ICP
Focal signs
Status epilepticus
Coagulopathy or thrombocytopenia

Supportive Tests for Detection of Complications

Blood should also be sent for serum sodium, potassium, calcium, urea, creatinine, liver function tests and arterial blood gas analysis. A Mantoux test may be done in those with suspected tubercular etiology.

Cranial imaging (CAT scan/MRI) is done only after stabilization of the child except if there are suspected focal lesions or bleeds. Studies have shown that emergency cranial tomography in acute febrile encephalopathy in children without focal neurological signs have little influence on subsequent management[15]. Cranial imaging otherwise helps to detect hydrocephalus, cerebritis, subdural effusions or empyema, brain abscesses, basal exudates as in tubercular meningitis, intracranial bleeds, cerebral edema, fronto-temporal pathology in Herpes encephalitis or thalamic involvement in Japanese B encephalitis (Figure 1).

A plain X ray of the chest should be done be done in all cases and in occasional patients an ultrasonography of the abdomen is done to detect other foci of infection. An electro-encephalogram is helpful to detect specific findings such as periodic lateralized epileptiform discharges (PLEDS) found in cases of Herpes simplex encephalitis.

SPECIFIC TREATMENT

Prompt institution of empirical broad spectrum antimicrobials such as ceftriaxone is justified even in the absence of CSF studies in children suspected of having bacterial meningitis. Similarly institution of empiric anti-malarials (Quinine /Artesunate) is justified in cases of febrile encephalopathy where a strong suspicion of cerebral malaria exists[16]. Acyclovir is given in cases suspected of Herpes simplex encephalitis. Dantrolene is the drug of choice for treatment of the neuroleptic malignant syndrome Steroids are indicated for autoimmune thyroiditis.

Other supportive treatment such as decompression of hydrocephalus, management of SIADH, salt and water replacement in cerebral salt wasting, temperature control, correction of acidosis and electrolyte imbalance must be done actively.

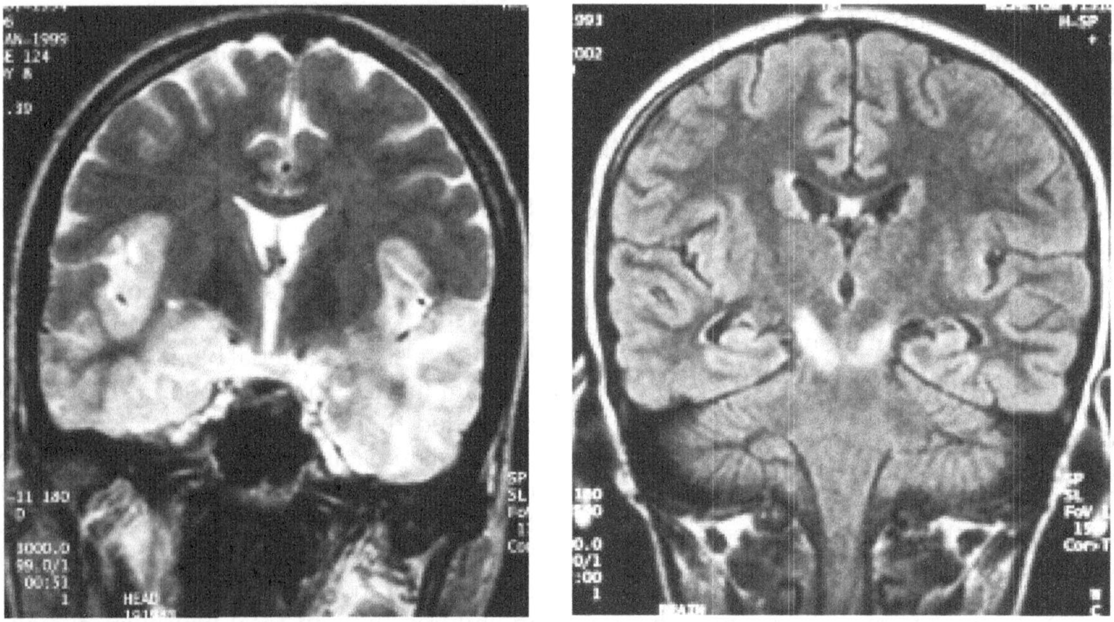

A. MRI- Herpes Simplex virus 1 Encephalitis- Early stage: Hyperintense signal on T2WI involving both gray and white matter

B. MRI - Japanese encephalitis showing increased T2W intensity in basal ganglia, thalami and midbrain

Figure 1

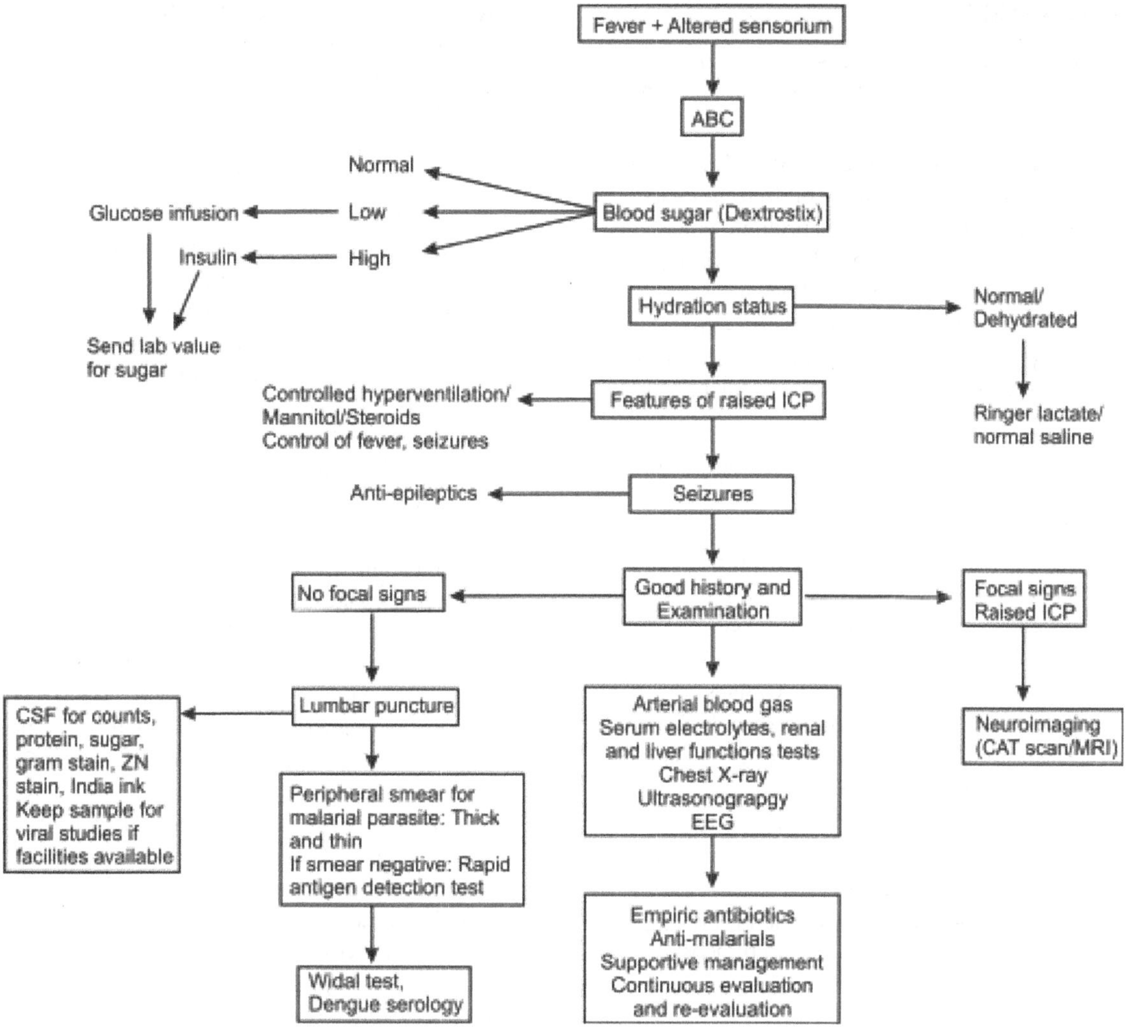

Fig. 2: Flow chart for management of febrile encephalopathy

CONCLUSION

To conclude a systematic approach as outlined in Figure 2 could be helpful in managing a child with febrile encephalopathy. A physician has to keep in mind a range of possibilities when dealing with a case of febrile encephalopathy. Factors such as the geographic area of origin or recent travel assume importance many a times. A high index of suspicion is needed in diagnosing such cases. Most patients suffering from febrile encephalopathy have a good outcome. One must remember that outcome is highly dependent on the way the patient is handled at the first contact in the emergency room. Prompt management of the immediate problems in the emergency room, close continuous monitoring of the clinical, hemodynamic and laboratory parameters and relevant neuroimaging studies subsequently, is needed for ensuring maintenance of a near normal recovery.

REFERENCES

1. Seshia SS, Seshia MMK, Sachdeva RK. Coma in childhood. Dev Med Child Neurol 1977; 19: 614-628.
2. Vannucci RC and Wasiewski WW. Diagnosis and management of coma in children. In Pellock JM and Myer EC, editors: Neurologic emergencies in infancy and childhood, 2nd Edition, Boston, Butterworth-Heinemann, 1993.
3. Minns RA. Acute encephalopathies. In Campbell AGM and McIntosh N, editors: Forfar and Arneils TB of Pediatrics, 5th Edition, Churchill Livingstone, 1998.
4. Bansal A, Singhi SC, Singhi PD, Khandelwal N, Ramesh S. Non traumatic coma. Indian J Pediatr. 2005 ; 72: 467-473.
5. Ogunmekan AO. Non-traumatic coma in childhood: etiology, clinical findings, morbidity, prognosis and mortality. J Trop Pediatr 1983; 29: 230 - 232.
6. Matuja WB, Matekere NJ. Causes and early prognosis of non-traumatic coma in Tanzania. Muhimbili Medical Centre experience. Trop Geogr Med 1987; 39: 330-335.
7. Sofiah A, Hussain HM. Childhood non-traumatic coma in Kuala Lumpur, Malaysia. Ann Trop Pediatr 1997; 17: 327-331.
8. Yeolekar ME, Trivedi TH. Febrile encephalopathy: Challenges in management. JAPI 2006; 54: 845-847.
9. Strobel M, Lamaury I, Contamin B, Jarrige B, Perez JM, Steck AJ et al. Dengue fever with neurologic expression. Three cases in adults. Ann Med Interne (Paris) 1999; 150: 79-82.
10. Kamath SR and Ranjit S. Clinical features, complications and atypical manifestations of children with severe forms of dengue hemorrhagic fever in South India. Indian J Pediatr 2006; 73 (10): 889-895.
11. Kayser L, Broholm H, Francis D, Perrild H, Olsen BE, Bendtzen Ket al. Immunocytochemical localisation of tumour necrosis factor alpha in thyroid tissues from patients with neoplastic or autoimmune thyroid disorders. *Autoimmunity* 1996; 23: 91-97.
12. Gelfand JA, Diranelo CA, Wolff SM. Fever, including fever of unknown origin. Harrison's principles of internal medicine. Chapter 16, 13th edition; 82-6.
13. Sauron B, Rancurel G, Gray F. Clinico pathologic conference at the Salpetriere. 4 November 1982. Subacute febrile encephalopathy in Hodgkin's disease. Rev Neurol (Paris). 1983; 139(10):597-604.
14. Ahuja GK, Mohan KK, Prasad K, Behari M. Diagnostic criteria for tuberculous meningitis and their validation. Tubercle and Lung Dis 1994; 75: 149-152.
15. Nadel S, Joarder R, Gibson M, Stevens J, Britto J, Habibi P et al. Emergency cranial computed tomography in the management of acute febrile encephalopathy in children.
16. Newton CR, Kirkham FJ, Johnston B, Marsh K. Inter-observer agreement of the assessment of coma scales and brainstem signs in non-traumatic coma. Dev Med Child Neurol 1995; 37: 807-813.

28 Acute Bacterial Meningitis, Acute Infectious Encephalitis

William Tsai and Robert Schafermeyer

ACUTE BACTERIAL MENINGITIS

The epidemiology of pediatric meningitis has experienced significant change in the last few decades. Vaccination and chemoprophylaxis against etiological agents have resulted in a significant decrease in the incidence of certain types of bacterial meningitis in children. Significant difficulties remain in the identification and prompt treatment of a relatively common disorder seen in the emergency department and despite advances, significant morbidity and mortality exist.

This chapter will review the pathophysiology, clinical presentation, diagnosis, and initial treatment of bacterial meningitis in children.

Pathophysiology

The symptoms and sequelae of meningitis can range from mild, self-limited disease to a fulminant bacterial process that can kill within hours. Acute bacterial meningitis most commonly results from hematogenous seeding of the meninges where surface bacterial proteins facilitate entry through the blood-brain barrier. The usual source of bacteremia is nasopharyngeal colonization or infection. Spread from contiguous sites of colonization or infection are also well-known. Such sites include the paranasal sinuses, the nasopharynx via basilar skull fracture, and meningomyelocoeles.

Bacterial virulence plays a role in the ability of certain organisms to initiate infection. The presence of specific capsular polysaccharide antigens appears to confer added virulence to these organisms[1] . After penetration of the blood-brain barrier, a cascade of inflammatory mediators[2,3] with a resulting granulocytic influx occurs and results in cytotoxic neuronal edema, proteolytic destruction, cerebral edema, and increased intracranial pressure and its ensuing complications such as brain herniation. Neuronal cell death is in part mediated by cell apoptosis.[4]

The pathologic changes of meningitis have been described since the preantibiotic era. In necropsy specimens, these consist of a widely distributed purulent meningeal exudate, thrombosis of small cortical veins, and patches of diffuse necrosis of the cerebral cortex.

Several host factors are known to predispose an individual to meningitis. Males are affected more frequently than females. Those less than four years of age are affected more often and more severely than are older children. Newborns, because of the immaturity of their immune defenses, are particularly vulnerable. Other conditions that predispose to meningitis include immuno-suppressive states such functional or anatomic asplenia or splenectomy,[5] or complement or immunoglobulin deficiencies. Cochlear implants[6] and ventriculoperitoneal shunts[7] increase the risk of meningitis. (Table 1).

Table 1: Patient risk factors for meningitis

Male
Age less than 4 years
Newborns
Group B Streptococci exposure
Crowding
Immunosuppression
Asplenia
Splenectomy
Human immunodeficiency virus
Complement deficiency
Hypogammaglobulinemia
Sickle cell disease
Malnutrition
Adrenal insufficiency
Cystic fibrosis
Adrenal insufficiency
Anatomic
Penetrating head injuries
Ventriculoperitoneal shunt
Cochlear implants
CSF fluid leak

Clinical Presentation

The clinical presentation of meningitis is protean and depends in large part on the developmental level of the patient (Table 2). The triad of fever, headache, and meningeal signs are present in only half of adult patients with bacterial meningitis and even less often in children.[8] Kernig's and Brudzinski's sign are not often seen.[9] Evidence of meningitis may be vague and nonspecific.

Table 2. Signs and Symptoms suggestive of meningitis in infants and children:

In Infants
i) Fever
ii) Refusal to feed
iii) Drowsiness and/or irritability
iv) Paradoxial irritability (dislike of being cuddled)
v) A high pitched/altered cry
vi) Photophobia, neck stiffness, Kerning's signs are unreliable in young infants. Preceding upper respiratory infections are common. Rashes may accompany.

In older children
i) Fever
ii) Photophobia
iii) Signs of meningeal irritation
iv) Convulsions

Sign of meningeal irritation may also be caused by caused tonsillitis, otitis media, upper lobe pneumonia and any of these may accompany the meningitis

Neonates may present with fever only, but in addition, may have symptoms of increased sleeping, paradoxical irritability, or difficulty feeding. Signs may include focal neurologic deficits, bulging fontanel, apnea, seizures, or an exanthem. As the symptoms and signs are nonspecific, diagnosis of meningitis should be seriously considered in any ill-appearing infant or child.

As the child becomes older, vomiting, headache, photophobia, and positive Kernig's and Brudzinski's signs may be seen. Fever is usual, but may be absent. Hypothermia may be a presenting sign, especially in neonates.[10] Response to paracetamol does not reliably distinguish sepsis or meningitis from other illnesses. Increased intracranial pressure is common and is manifested by headache or mental status change in the older child or bulging fontanel in the infant, but papilledema is not usually seen. Seizures may be the initial presentation in children and often clouds the differential diagnosis in a child presenting with seizure and fever.

Differential Diagnosis

A variety of infectious and noninfectious conditions must be differentiated from acute bacterial meningitis. These include: tuberculous, fungal, and viral meningitis; brain and epidural abscess, bacterial endocarditis with embolism, pneumonia, otitis media, pharyngitis, toxic ingestions, adrenal hypoplasia, and heart disease. Finally, children with simple febrile seizures often present a diagnostic dilemma for the clinician. Most clinicians agree that fever and a seizure in a child less than twelve months of age requires the careful consideration of meningitis.[11]

Laboratory Evaluation

The lumbar puncture is the essential diagnostic test if bacterial meningitis is suspected. If there is the possibility of increased intracranial pressure, a computerized tomographic scan of the head may be performed prior to lumbar puncture, but treatment should not be withheld during this time.[12,13,14] Table 3 outlines the usual diagnostic tests performed on the cerebrospinal fluid (CSF) and their interpretation[15].

Early in the course of disease, the CSF WBC count may be normal and have a predominance of lymphocytes. Typically as disease progresses, CSF leukocytosis follows with a neutrophilic predominance. Typically WBC counts will rise to > 1000 WBC/HPF.

Table 3: Cerebrospinal fluid values

(Table adapted from Lipton JD, Schafermeyer RW. Evolving concepts in pediatric bacterial meningitis – part I: Pathophysiology and diagnosis. Ann Emerg Med 1993;22:119-132 Table 3)

	Color	*Cell count*	*Glucose*	*Protein*	*Gram stain*
Normal	Clear	0-5 wbc/mm^3 Lymphocytic Neonate: 0-30 wbc/mm^{3a} Up to 60% PMNs	50-80 mg/dl	15-45 mg/dl	No organisms
Bacterial	Cloudy	>1000 wbc/mm^3 <20% PMNs	<40 mg/dl <60% serum value	>500 mg/dl	Positive, may be gram-negative diplococci, gram-negative bacilli, gram-positive cocci
Viral	Cloudy	10-1000 wbc/mm^3	Normal to low	Normal to mildly elevated	No organisms
Fungal	Clear	10-1000 wbc/mm^3	Normal to low	Normal to mildly elevated	No organisms
Viral Encephalitis	Clear	0-1000 wbc/mm^{3,b} elevated	Normal	Normal to mildly	No organisms

[a]Sarff LD, Platt LH, McCracken GH, *et al.* Cerebrospinal fluid evaluation in neonates: Comparison of high-risk infants with and without meningitis. J Pediatr 1976;88:473-477.

[b]Herpes simplex encephalitis may show red blood cells on CSF study.

CSF gram stain is positive in 80% of patients with untreated bacterial meningitis and CSF hypoglycoracchia is an independent risk factor for bacterial disease. In patients with CSF pleocytosis, clinical prediction rules may be useful in identifying patients at very low risk for bacterial disease.[16]

Patients who have received antibiotics prior to lumbar puncture will have sterile CSF cultures.[17] However, other CSF abnormalities such as leukocytosis, hypoglycoracchia, and increased protein will persist for several days after the appropriate antibiotics are started.

Past techniques such as bacterial antigen testing in CSF, blood, or urine seldom offer benefits in patient management and are hampered by poor sensitivity and specificity.[18] However, rapid detection and identification of organisms causing bacterial meningitis remain important. PCR amplification of bacterial genome sequences are currently under development to help provide rapid and accurate diagnosis especially in patients who have been pretreated with antibiotics.[19,20] PCR detection of enterovirus and HSV infection are widely used and may offer benefits in management.

Traumatic lumbar puncture complicates the diagnostic picture. Attempts at using WBC to RBC ratios or other techniques should be used with great caution in the diagnosis of bacterial meningitis, especially if the child appears ill.[21, 22]

Antibiotic Therapy

Prompt empiric therapy for bacterial meningitis should take into account the age of the patient, the presence of any predisposing or high risk factors, and the local antibiotic resistance pattern (Table 4).

The early (0-7 days) presenting neonate is typically started on ampicillin and an aminoglycoside or 3rd generation cephalosporin. The late (7-28 days) presenting neonate is generally treated with vancomycin or antistaphylococcal penicillin and a 3rd generation cephalosporin[23]. Older children

Table 4 : Recommendations for initial antimicrobial therapy in children
(Table adapted from IDSA Tunkel AR, Hartman BJ, Kaplan SL, et al. Practice Guidelines for the Management of Bacterial Meningitis. Clin Infect Dis 2004;39:1267-1284, Table 4)

Factor	*Common bacterial pathogens*	*Antimicrobial therapy*
< 1 month	Streptococcus agalactiae, Escherichia coli, Listeria monocytogenes, gram negative enteric bacilli	Ampicillin plus cefotaxime or ampicillin plus an aminoglycoside
1-23 months	Streptococcus pneumoniae, Neisseria meningitidis, S. agalactiae, Haemophilus influenzae, E. coli	A third-generation cephalosporin*
2 years through adolescent	N. menengitidis, S.pneumonia	A third-generation cephalosporin*
CSF shunt	Coagulase-negative staphylococci, S. aureus, pseudomonas aeruginosa, erobic gram-negative bacilli, propionibacterium acnes	Vancomycin plus cefepime, vancomycin plus ceftazidime, vancomycin plus meropenem**
Post-Neurosurgery	Pseudomonas aeruginosa, aerobic gram-negative bacilli, S. aureus, coagulase-negative staphylococci	Vancomycin plus cefepime, vancomycin plus ceftazidime, vancomycin plus meropenem

* Vancomycin is added in places with high level of resistance to ceftriaxone.

** Vancomycin alone is reasonable unless gram stain reveals gram-negative bacilli.

may start a 3rd generation cephalosporin (with vancomycin in places with high level of ceftriaxone resistant pheumococcus) until initial therapy can be narrowed based on cultures.[24]

Patients with risk factors such as ventriculoperitoneal shunt or those with risk factors for nosocomial flora may start on vancomycin and a 4th generation cephalosporin or carbanepenem.

Supportive Care

Fifteen percent of patients with bacterial meningitis present with septic shock.[25] As with any life-threatening condition, initial priorities should include management of the airway, breathing, and circulation. While prompt diagnosis and early appropriate antibiotic therapy are important, management of the ABC's are paramount. Resuscitative measures to reverse shock, control seizures, to manage cerebral edema, and to recognize and treat increased intracranial pressure are commonly necessary.

Patients with a high risk of clinical deterioration should be admitted to an intensive care unit to anticipate and manage complications. Risk factors for deterioration, and which also predict poor neurologic outcome and mortality, include depressed mental status, early or persisent seizures, severe depression of CSF glucose, and presence of shock.[26]

Dexamethasone

A randomized, double blind placebo controlled trial in adult patients found that the administration of dexamethasone along with the first dose of antibiotics improved neurologic sequelae, including mortality, in a subgroup of patients with pneumococcal meningitis.[27] Smaller pediatric studies also show improvement in patients with H. influenzae meningitis and incremental improvements in patients with pneumococcal meningitis.[28] There is no current evidence to support the use of dexamethasone in children less than 6 weeks of age and in developing countries. The use of dexamethasone in older children should take into account the etiologic agent and the possibility of reduced antimicrobial penetration into the CNS due to decreased permeability of the blood brain barrier.[29]

Prevention and Chemoprophylaxis

The epidemiology of bacterial meningitis has changed dramatically during the past few decades due to active immunization efforts and antimicrobial chemoprophlaxis. The advent of H. influenzae, type B vaccine (Hib) has resulted in a marked decrease in H. influenza meningitis in areas where Hib is used. In areas where 7-valent pneu-mococcal vaccine is used, a marked decrease in invasive streptococcal infection, including meningitis, has occurred. In California, since use of pneumococcal vaccine, there has been a 90% reduction in invasive pnemococcal disease.[30] In England, meningococcal vaccine against serogroup C has reduced meningococcal infection by 80%.[31] Finally, chemoprophylaxis of maternal group B streptococcal infection in the peripartum period has reduced the incidence of early invasive group B streptococcal disease in neonates.

In cases of H. influenza and N. meningitidis meningitis, chemoprophylaxis of close contacts with antimicrobials such as rifampin is recommended.

ACUTE ENCEPHALITIS

Encephalitis is an inflammation of the brain parenchyma that may involve all areas of the central nervous system including the spinal cord. Infectious and parainfectious etiologies occur in children. Infectious etiologies are dominated by the viral encephalitides. The clinical spectrum of encephalitis is quite varied in presentation and depends heavily on the area of the CNS involved. Specific viral organisms display tropism to specific areas of the CNS. Japnese encephalitis remains the most important form of encephalitis globally. West Nile virus (WNV) has recently emerged as an important pathogen. Herpes simplex encephalitis (HSE) deserves special attention because of the importance of prompt diagnosis and the prompt institution of specific and effective antiviral therapy.

Pathophysiology

Encephalitis may be subdivided into two categories – infectious and parainfectious—based on disease pathophysiology. The infectious encephalitides involve entry into the CNS via hematogenous spread via the choroid plexus or, in the case of rabies virus, direct transport to the CNS through peripheral neurons. Once in neuronal tissue, viral replication continues, cell to cell spread occurs, resulting in direct cytotoxic injury, neuronal edema, and neuronal cell death. Clinical manifestations depend in large part on the pattern of CNS spread and the extent of CNS cell injury and death. Parainfectious etiologies such as acute disseminated encephalomyelitis (ADEM) are autoimmune in nature and will not be discussed further.

Clusters of encephalitis often occur concurrent with arbovirus and enterovirus epidemics in late summer or early fall. Thus, the diagnosis is usually presumptive and based on the clinical picture and current epidemiology (Tables 5 and .6).

The mode of entry into humans differs among the viral etiologies. Arbovirus infections are transmitted by an arthropod vector, usually a mosquito. The rabies virus in contrast is transmitted in the saliva of infected mammals and travels up sensory nerves into the CNS. Herpes simplex virus (HSV) may reach the CNS from hematogenous routes, retrograde from ganglia, or across the cribiform plate from the nasopharynx. Naegleria fowleri is a free-living ameba that causes lethal amebic encephalitis by entering the body through the nasopharynx and crossing the cribiform plate. It has been identified in recent outbreaks in the southeast United States.[32]

Table 5: Infectious causes of encephalitis

Agents	*Season*
Herpes Viruses	
Herpes Simplex 1 and 2	Any
Cytomegalovirus	Winter/spring
Varicella-zoster virus	Winter/spring
Epstein-Barr virus	Winter/spring
Simian herpes B virus	
Arboviruses	
California encephalitis virus	Summer/fall
St Louis encephalitis virus	Summer/fall
Eastern encephalitis virus	Summer/fall
Western encephalitis virus	Summer/fall
West Nile virus	Summer/fall
Other Viruses	
Human immunodeficiency virus	Any
Rabies virus	Any
Lymphocytic choriomeningitis virus	
Influenza virus	Winter/spring
Mumps virus	Winter/spring
Measles virus	Winter/spring
Other Agents	
Mycoplasma pneumoniae	Any
Rickettsia rickettsii	Summer/fall
Naegleria fowleri	Summer/fall

Clinical Picture

There is considerable variation in the clinical presentation depending on age, pathogen, host immunocompetence, and area of the CNS involved. Children may present with a non-specific viral illness, fever, headache,

Table 6: Likely etiology of viral encephalistis based on assoicated signs and symptoms

Symptoms and signs	*Probable causative Virus*
Summar Colds/Diarrhea/ Pharyngitis/abdominal pain/rash Respiratory symptoms/ Herpangina/pleurodynia/	Enterovirus
Preceding epidemics of Conjuctivitis	Enterovirus 70
Smell/Teste/Behaviroal Abnormalities	Herpes Simplex
Respiratory Symptoms/Epidemics of cold	Adenorivus
Rash	Enterovirus, Adenovirus, Measles
Conjuctivits	Adenovirus, Enterovirus 70 Measles
Parotitis	Mumps, Enterovirus, Epstein-Barr Virus, HIV
Pharyngitis	Adenovirus, Enterovirus, Epstein-Barr Virus, other respiratory viruses
Adenopathy	Epstein-Bar Virus, Cytomegalovirus
Croup	Measles, Adenovirus, Influenza
Bronchiolitis	Adenovirus, Influenza
Pneumonia	Adenovirus, Measles, Varicella, Cytomegalovirus, Dengue
Enteritis	Enterovirus
Hepatitis	

neck stiffness, mental status changes, or seizures. Subtler symptoms may mimic psychiatric disorders and may include hallucinations or behavioral change. Involvement of specific areas of the CNS may manifest as cerebellitis, optic neuritis, other cranial nerve palsies, or movement disorders.

Differential Diagnosis

The differential diagnosis of encephalitis should include five major categories of illness. These include disease or injury causing increased intracranial pressure, infectious diseases, metabolic derangement, demyelinating disease and toxins (Table 5).

History

A detailed history is invaluable and may suggest the diagnosis. The patient or family must be questioned about any exposure in the preceding three to four weeks to viral illnesses, animals (especially horses), ticks, exposure to fresh water lakes or streams, and travel outside the United States. The child's maternal, perinatal, and immunization history should be reviewed, and the possibility

Table 7: Differential diagnosis of encephalitis

Category	*Diagnoses*
Increased ICP	Tumor, trauma, CNS bleed, hydocephalus
Infectious Disorders	Viral, bacterial, fungal, mycoplasma, chlamydia, parasites
Metabolic Disorders	Hepatic encephalopathy, uremia, hypoglycemia, electrolyte cerbral malaria disorders
Demyelinating Disease	Acute demyelinating encephalomyelitis (ADEM), multiple sclerosis, postinfectious encephalomyelitis
Toxic Encephalopathy	Lead, drugs, Reye's syndrome

of toxic exposure must be addressed. The child's immune status and any risk for human immunodeficiency virus (HIV) infection must be considered. Regional epidemiology must also be considered.

Physical Examination

The physical examination should be thorough and all inclusive with particular attention to the neurologic exam and assessment of mental status. Findings suggesting viral etiologies such as fever, lymphadenopathy, exanthem, and splenomegaly should be noted document the presence or absence of papilledema, venous pulsations, or nuchal rigidity.

In a suspected case of viral enceptalitis associated other signs may provide a clue to etiologic diagnosis (Table 6).

Laboratory Examination

Hematologic testing provides evidence of a nonspecific infection and a metabolic profile may identify electrolyte abnormalities. CSF studies may show a leukocytosis with a lymphocytic predominance but may also be normal. Typical CSF studies are shown in Table 2. Additional CSF studies may include PCR for enterovirus, PCR for HSV, or specific testing for West Nile virus. Serum, urine, and nasal aspirates may be helpful in viral diagnosis. Acute and convalescent titers may eventually yield a diagnosis. CSF viral cultures are frequently unhelpful.

Head CT may be normal or demonstrate a mass, demyelination, edema, or vasculitis. MRI findings are non-specific and typically do not point to a specific viral etiology but are characterized by signal defects consistent with inflammation, hemorrhage, or edema.

Management

Most patients with encephalitis have an undiagnosed viral etiology and require only supportive care. As with any life-threatening condition, initial priorities should include management of the airway, breathing, and circulation. While prompt diagnosis and early appropriate antimicrobial therapy are important, management of the ABC's are paramount. Resuscitative measures to reverse shock, control seizures, to manage cerebral edema, and to recognize and treat increased intracranial pressure are commonly necessary. Empiric antibiotics should be started if bacterial etiology is suspected. Antiviral therapy with acyclovir is started early until HSE can be eliminated from the differential diagnosis.

Other encephalitides may respond to other specific therapies. Children with varicella zoster encephalitis may respond to a combination of acyclovir and steroids.

Other agents used in immunocompromised hosts include foscarnet, ganciclovir, and cidofovir on a risk-benefit basis. Children with amebic encephalitis should be treated with appropriate amebicidal agents such as amphotericin B.

HERPES SIMPLEX ENCEPHALITIS

Because specific, effective therapy exists for HSE, it is critical to consider this disease promptly and to institute early appropriate therapy with acyclovir. The neonate is born normal but transmission occurs at, or just preceding birth. In the first two weeks, more than half of infants will develop a vesicular rash.[33] The illness begins with poor feeding, jaundice, irritability and subtle CNS changes. Seizures, conjunctivitis, fever and pneumonia are also part of the clinical presentation.

HSE presents with a CSF pleocytosis ranging from 0 to 200 WBC with PMNs predominating early and monocytes predominating late in the course. Because HSE causes hemorrhagic encephalitis, red blood cells (RBC's) are expected on LP. The CSF glucose is normal and protein is normal to modestly elevated. Viral cultures of CSF, blood, nasopharynx, urine and stool should be sent. Vesicular skin lesions should be properly cultured and sent for HSV direct fluorescent antigen. MRI is frequently nonspecific but may show bilateral hemorrhagic involvement of the sylvian fissure and temporal lobes.[34] An electroencephalogram (EEG) will be abnormal initially in 80 to 90 percent of patients with encephalitis, especially those with HSE. The finding of paroxysmal lateral epileptiform discharges (PLEDs) though not pathognomonic, is typical of HSE.

Intravenous acyclovir should be started promptly in any patient with suspected HSE. Early diagnosis and therapy has been associated with improved outcomes.[35,36]

JAPNESE ENCEPHALITIS

Japanese encephalitis (JE) is numerically the most important causes of viral encephalitis worldwide, causing an estimated 50000 cases and 15000 deaths annually. Even among the survivors 50% have severe neuropshychiatric sequalae. The prevalence of JE is highest in Asia and Pacific rim regions.

Epidemiology

JE virus is a small (50nm) lipoprotein envelope surrounding a nucleocapsid with at least five genotypes. Pigs are the most important natural host of the virus and reservoir of infection. It is transmitted naturally between wild and domestic birds and pigs by *Culex tritareorrhynchus*, which breeds in pools of stagnant water (such as paddy fields). Transmission to humans occurs from bite of infected culex mosquito. Huge epidemics occur during the summer months, corresponding with a rise in temperature above 20°C. At cooler temperature, rate of virus transmission is slow. Most case occurs in rural areas after the monsoon rains when mosquitoes breed prolifically. Humans are dead end hosts.

Clinical Features

It is a disease of children and young adults. Incubation period is 5-16 days. Most infections are asymptomatic or result in a non-specific flu-like illness; estimates of the ratio of symptomatic infection vary between 1 in 25 and 1 in 1000. Typically patients present after a few, days of non-specific febrile illness (which may include coryza, malaise, diarrhea, and rigors) with headache, vomiting, and a reduced level of consciousness, often heralded by a convulsion.

Sometimes abnormal behavior may be presenting features resulting in an initial diagnosis of a mental illness. A proportion of patients make a rapid spontaneous recovery (abortive encephalitis), while some patients have aseptic meningitis and have no encephalopathic features.

Convulsions occur often in 85% of children and 10% of adults. Generalized tonic-clonic seizures occur more often than focal motor seizures. Multiple or prolonged seizures or and status epilepticus are associated with a poor outcome. In some children subtle motor seizures (twitching of digit, eye or mouth, eye deviation, nystagmLis, excess salivation, irregular respiration) are difficult to identify without EEG.

Extrapyramidal features are characteristically seen with JE. Dull flat mask-like facies with wide unblinking eyes, tremor, generalized hypertonia, and congwheel rigidity is seen in 20-40% children. Opisthotonus and rigidity spasms, particularly on stimulation indicate poor prognosis. Other extrapyramidal features include head nodding and pill rolling movements, opsoclonus myoclonus, choreoathatosis, and bizarre facial grimacing, and lip smaking.

Upper motor neuron facial nerve palsies occur in around 10%. Rarely patient may present with rapid onset of flaccid paralysis after a short febrile illness.

Changes of respiratory pattern, flexor and extensor posturing, abnormalities of the papillary and occulocephalic reflexes indicate brain-stem involvement and are poor prognostic suns.

Radioimaging and EEG

In about 50% patients CT scan shows characteristic bilateral non-enhancing low density areas in one or more of the thalamus, basal ganglia, midbram, pons, and medulla. Magnetic resonance imaging is more sensitive and shows more extensive lesions. (typically high signal intensity on T2 weighted images) of the thalamus cerebral hemispheres, and cerebellum. Imaging studies may be useful in distinguishing Japanese encephalitis from herpes simplex encephalitis. SPECT-shows hyperperfusion in the thalamus and putamen.

EEG may show a range of findings from theta and delta coma, to burst suppression. epileptiform activity, and occasionally alpha coma. Diffuse slowing may be useful in distinguishing Japanese encephalitis from herpes virus.

Diagnosis

For all practical purposes Japanese encephalitis is diagnosed serologically. The haemaglutination inhibition test was used for may years. However, it required paired serum, and could not give an early diagnosis. IgM and IgG capture enzyme linked (ELISAs) has a sensitivity and specificity of >95%.

Virus may be isolated sometimes from CSF or from brain tissue either at necropsy or postmortem or needle biopsy. Immunohisto-chemical staining of CSF cells or necropsy tissue with anti JE virus polyclonal antibodies may be positive.

WEST NILE NEUROINVASIVE DISEASE

West Nile virus (WNV) is an arbovirus that has gained prominence in the western hemisphere. From an outbreak of cases first seen in New York City in 1999, it has spread westward and been reported in 43 states including the District of Columbia, encompassing over 4000 cases/year, including 177 fatalities in 2006.[37]

WNV is transmitted to humans primarily from mosquitoes that have acquired the infection from infected birds. WNV has also been acquired through blood transfusion, organ transplants, transplacentally, and possibly through breast milk.[38] Clinical symptoms range from asymptomatic infection to West Nile fever, which is symptomatic infection that does not affect the CNS. West Nile neuroinvasive disease (WNND) may cause meningitis, encephalitis, or acute flaccid paralysis. While both the incidence and mortality rise with increasing age, 105 cases of WNND were identified in pediatric patients in 2002.[39]

Clinical symptoms of WNND in children may be clinically indistinguishable from other encephalitides. Non-specific rash may be reported more frequently in pediatric than adult patients.[40]

Diagnosis in suspected cases is established by identifying serum and CSF WNV IgM and IgG antibody by ELISA of IFA or by identifying CSF WNV nucleic acid[41]. Treatment is symptomatic. Ribavirin inhibits WNV replication in vitro, but clinical use is based on no controlled clinical trials.

SUMMARY

The diagnosis of encephalitis in the acute care setting requires a careful consideration of patient history, clinical findings, and local epidemiology. Care for patients with encephalitis remains mainly symptomatic, how-ever, prompt consideration, identification, and empiric treatment of HSE is critical.

REFERENCES

1. Huang SH, Jong AY. Cellular mechanisms of microbial proteins contributing to invasion of the blood-brain barrier. Cell Microbiol 2001;3:277-287.
2. Ramilo O, Saez-Llorens X, Mertosola J, *et al.* Tumor necrosis factor alpha/cachectin and interleukin 1 beta intiate meningeal inflammation. J Exp Med 1990;172:497-507.
3. Leib SL, Tauber MG. Pathogenesis of bacterial meningitis. Infect Dis Clin North Am 1999;13:527-548.
4. Mitchell L, Smith SH, *et al.* Dual phases of apoptosis in pneumococcal meningitis. J Infect Dis 2004;190:2039-2046.
5. Schutze GE, Mason EO, *et al.* Invasive pneumococcal infections in children with asplenia. Pediatr Inect Dis J 2002;21:278-282.
6. Reefhuis J, Honein MA, Whitney CG, *et al.* Risk of bacterial meningitis in children with cochlear implants. N Engl J Med 2003;349:435-445.
7. Odio C, McCracken GH, Nelson JD. CSF shunt infections in pediatrics: A seven-year experience. Am J Dis Child 1984;138:1103-1108
8. Van de Beek D, de Gans J, Spanjaard L, *et al.* Clinical features and prognostic factors in adults with bacterial meningitis. N Engl J Med 2004;351:1849-1859.
9. El Bashir H, Laundy M, Booy T. Diagnosis and treatment of bacterial meningitis. Arch Dis Child 2003;88:615-620.
10. Lipton JD, Schafermeyer RW. Evolving concepts in pediatric bacterial meningitis – part I: pathophysiology and diagnosis. Ann Emerg Med 1993;22:1602-1615.
11. AAP Practive Parameter: The neurodiagnostic evaluation of the child with a first simple febrile seizure. Pediatrics 1996;97:769-772.
12. Rennick G, Shann F, de Campo J. Cerebral herniation during bacterial meningitis in children. BMJ 1993;306:953-955.
13. Shett AK, Deselle BC, Craver RD, Steele RW. Fatal cerebral herniation after lumbar puncture in a patient with a normal computed tomography scan. Pedaitrics 1999;103:1284-1287.
14. Hasbun R, Abrahams J, Jekel J, *et al.* Computed tomography of the head before lumbar puncture in adults with suspected meningitis. N Engl J Med 2000;345:1727-1733.
15. Lipton JD, Schafermeyer RW. Evolving concepts in pediatric bacterial meningitis – part I: Pathophysiology and diagnosis. Ann Emerg Med 1993;22:1602-1615.
16. Nigrovic LE, Kuppermann N, Macias CG, *et al.* Clinical prediction rule for identifying children with cerebrospinal fluid pleocytosis at very low risk of bacterial meningitis. JAMA 2007;297:52-60.

17. Kanegaye JT, Soliemanzadeh P, Bradley JS. Lumbar puncture in pediatric bacterial meningitis: Defining the time interval for recovery of cerebrospinal fluid pathogens after parenteral antibiotic pretreatment. Pediatrics 2001;108:1169-1174.
18. Nigrovic LE, Kuppermann N, McAdam AJ, *et al.* Cerebrospinal latex agglutination fails to contribute to the microbiologic diagnosis of pretreated children with meningitis. Pediatr Infect Dis J 2004;23:786-788.
19. Schuurman T, de Boer RF, Kooistra-Smid AM, *et al.* Prospective study of use of PCR amplification and sequencing of 16S ribosomal DNA from cerebrospinal fluid for diagnosis of bacterial meningitis in a clinical setting. J Clin Microbiol 2004;42:734-740.
20. Bryant PA, Li HY, Zaia A, *et al.* Prospective study of a real-time PCR that is highly sensitive, specific and clinically useful for diagnosis of meningococcal disease in children. J Clin Microbiol 2004;42:2919-2925.
21. Bonadio WA, Smith DS, Goddard S, *et al.* Distinguishing cerebrospinal fluid abnormalities in children with bacterial meningitis and traumatic lumbar puncture. J Infect Dis 1990;162:251-254.
22. Mazor SS, McNulty JE, Roosevelt GE. Interpretation of traumatic lumbar punctures: Who can go home? Pediatrics 2003;111:525-528
23. Chavez-Bueno S, McCracken GH. Bacterial meningitis in children. Pediatr Clin N Am 2005;52:795-810.
24. Tunkel AR, Hartman BJ, Kaplan SL, *et al.* Practice guidelines for the management of bacterial meningitis. Clin Infect Dis 2004;39:1267-1284.
25. Kornelisse RF, Westerbeek CM, Spoor AB, *et al.* Pneumococcal meningitis in children: Prognostic indicators and outcome. Clin Infect Dis 1995;21:1390-1397.
26. Arditi M, Mason EO, Bradley JS, Tan TQ, Barson WJ, *et al.* Three-year multicenter surveillance of pneumococcal meningitis in children; clinical characteristics, and outcome related to penicillin susceptibility and dexamethasone use. Pediatrics 1998;102:1087-1097.
27. De Gans J, va de Beek D, *et al.* Dexamethasone in adults with bacterial meningitis. N Engl J Med 2002;347:1549-1556
28. Committee on Infectious Diseases. Dexamethasone therapy for bacterial meningitis in infants and children. Pediatrics 1990;86:130-133.
29. Martinez-Lacasa J, Cabellos C, Martos A, *et al.* Experimental study of the efficacy of vancomycin, rifampicin and dexamethasone in the therapy of pneumococcal meningitis. J Antimicrob Chemother 2002;49:507-513.
30. Black S, Shinefield, Baxter R, *et al.* Postlicensure surveillance for pneumococcal invasive disease after use of heptavalent pneumococcal conjugate vaccine in Northern California Kaiser Permanente. Pediatr Infect Dis J 2004;23:485-489.
31. Miller E, Salisbury D, Ramsay M. Planning, registration, and implementation of an immunisation campaign against meningococcal serogroup C disease in the UK: a success story. Vaccine 2001;20(suppl 1):S58-67.
32. CDC. Primary amebic meningoencephalitis – Georgia, 2002;MMWR 2003;52:962-964.
33. Silvia MT, Licht DJ. Pediatric central nervous system infections and inflammatory white matter disease. Pediatr Clin N Am 2005;52:1107-1126.
34. Silvia MT, Licht DJ. Pediatric central nervous system infections and inflammatory white matter disease. Pediatr Clin N Am 2005;52:1107-1126.
35. Kimberlin DW, Lin CY, Jacobs RF, *et al.* Natural history of neonatal herpes simplex virus infections in the acyclovir era. Pediatrics 2001;108:223-229.
36. Kimberlin DW, Lin CY, Jacobs RF, *et al.* Safety and efficacy of high-dose intravenous acyclovir in the management of neonatal herpes simplex virus infections. Pediatrics 2001;108:230-238.
37. CDC. West Nile virus activity – United States. 2006.2007;56(22)556-559.
38. Hayes EB, O'Leary DR. West nile virus infection: A pediatric perspective. Pediatrics 2004;113:1375-1381.
39. Hayes EB, O'Leary DR. West nile virus infection: A pediatric perspective. Pediatrics 2004;113:1375-1381.
40. Civen R, Villacorte F, Robles DT, *et al.* West nile virus infection in the pediatric population. Pediatr Infect Dis J 2006;25:75-78.
41. Hayes EB, O'Leary DR. West nile virus infection: A pediatric perspective. Pediatrics 2004;113:1375-1381.

Alka Khadwal

29 Reye Syndrome

A condition characterized by an acute non inflammatory encephalopathy and hepatic failure. It was first described in 1963 by RDK Reye. There are no specific clinical manifestations suggesting a diagnosis of Reye syndrome. It should be considered in any afebrile child presenting with acute onset protracted vomiting and altered state of consciousness. Early recognition and treatment are keys to prevent mortality and morbidity associated with this condition. Centres for Disease Control and Prevention have provided criteria for establishing the diagnosis of Reye syndrome (Table 1).

INCIDENCE

Over the last thirty years the frequency of Reye syndrome has shown a declining trend. Incidence may vary with the viral epidemics associated with seasonal changes. In children younger than 18 years, it is estimated to be < 1 per 100000 people. Early diagnosis and aggressive management has brought down the mortality from 50% to < 20%. Cerebral edema and/or increased intracranial pressure (most commonly), myocardial dysfunction, cardiovascular collapse, respiratory failure, renal failure, GI bleeding, status epilepticus or sepsis are the usual causes of mortality in such cases. Out come in survivors can vary from complete recovery to some neurological impairment.

Table 1: Centres for Disease Control and Prevention Criteria for diagnosis of Reye syndrome

- Acute non inflammatory encephalopathy with an altered level of consciousness.
- Hepatic dysfunction with a liver biopsy showing fatty metamorphosis or a more than 3-fold increase in alanine aminotransferase (ALT), aspartate aminotransferase (AST), and/or ammonia levels.
- No other explanation for cerebral edema or hepatic abnormality
- CSF with 8 or fewer WBCs per cubic millimeter ($8X\,10^9/L$ or fewer)
- Brain biopsy with cerebral edema without inflammation

ETIOLOGY AND PATHOGENESIS

It is one of those conditions where etiology is still unknown, but it is thought to occur most commonly after a viral upper respiratory or gastroenteric illness especially if aspirin was used during the illness. Many other conditions can mimic Reye syndrome. Common conditions associated with / mimicking the syndrome is listed in Table 2. Like etiology the pathophysiology is also unclear but it has been postulated that in a virus-infected or in a predisposed host there is mitochondria dysfunction resulting in inhibition of oxidative phosphorylation and fatty acid beta-oxidation. Histologically there is minimal tissue inflammatory response, hepatocytes show cytoplasmic fatty vacuolization, in brain there is astrocyte edema and neuronal loss, and in kidneys there is fatty degeneration of proximal tubular cells. At cellular level, mitochondria are pleomorphic in shape, reduced in number and appear swollen, and there is depletion of glycogen.

Table 2: Reye syndrome-Etiological associations

- Viral Illnesess- Influenzae A & D ,Varicella Zoster, less commonly parainfluenza, Adenovirus, Coxsackie viruses A and B, Echovirus, Epstein-Barr virus, Cytomegalovirus, Herpes simplex virus and Poliovirus.
- Drugs-Salicylates, Valproic acid, paracetamol, Antiretroviral drugs viz., zidovudine,didanosine, Antiemetics viz., phenothiazines.
- Toxins-Pesticides, herbicides, paint, certain hepatotoxins mushrooms, oil (margosa), hypoglycin (in akee fruit)
- Inborn errors of metabolism-Fatty acid oxidation defects (MCAD), Urea cycle defects, certain aminoacidopathies, organic acidaemia and disorders of carbohydrate metabolism.
- Post vaccination (live virus vaccination)

Pathophysiology of CNS manifestation in Reye syndrome is depicted in following flow diagram:

Mitochondria dysfunction in hepatocytes
↓
Hyperammonemia
↓
Astrocyte edema
↓
Cerebral edema
↓
Increased intracranial pressure

CLINICAL FEATURES

Although children of 5-14 years of age group seem to be most commonly affected, it can rarely be seen in newborns or in persons older than 18 years. There is no sex predilection. Usual history is that of abrupt onset of protracted vomiting occurring 12 hours – 21 days (mean 72 hours) following a viral illness. 24-48 hours after the onset of vomiting, neurologic dysfunction ensues with lethargy being the earliest symptom. Other neurological features include irritability, restlessness, delirium, seizures and coma. In very young children (< 2 years), diarrhea and hyperventilation may be the initial symptoms. Examination may show afebrile child with or without dehydration, minimal or no icterus and in half of the cases there is associated hepatomegaly. Various systems of staging encephalopathy are available in literature. CDC describes encephalopathy in 6 stages (Table 3).

Table 3: Stages of encephalopathy in Reye syndrome

Stage	*Manifestation*
1	Vomiting, sleepiness, lethargy
2	Restlessness,irritability, combativeiiess, disorientation, delirium, tachycardia, hyperventilation, dilated pupils with sluggish response, hyperreflexia, positive Babinski sign, and appropriate response to noxious stimuli.
3	Obtunded, comatose, decorticate rigidity, and inappropriate response to noxious stimuli.
4	Deep coma, decerebrate rigidity, fixed and dilated pupils, loss of oculovestibular reflexes, and dysconjugate gaze with caloric stimulation.
5	Seizures, flaccid paralysis, absent deep tendon reflexes, no pupillary response, and respiratory arrest.
6	Patient who cannot be classified because they have been treated with curare or other medication that alters level of consciousness.

Investigations

Laboratory studies show transient abnormalities in blood biochemical para-meters to support the diagnosis:

- Liver functions- Serum bilirubin may be mildly raised (usually not more than 3mg/dl) in some cases. Serum levels of transaminases (AST and ALT) are increased beyond three times of upper limit of normal values. Ammonia levels are raised as much as 1.5 times normal especially within 48 hours of onset of alteration in sensorium. Arterial blood sampling should be done for measuring ammonia levels as venous samples are not reliable. Cooled specimen should be promptly measured for accurate results.
- Coagulation profile- the prothrombin time (PT) and activated partial thromboplastin (aPTT) time are prolonged in majority of the patients. Specific factor assays show decreased levels of factor II, VII, IX and X and fibrinogen due to compromised liver synthesis.
- Blood sugar levels- Hypoglycemia is frequently encountered in extremely sick and children younger than 2 years.
- Others- there may be presence of metabolic acidosis, increased levels of lipase, amylase, blood urea nitrogen and creatinine. Free fatty acids and amino-acids (especially glutamine, alanine lysine) are elevated.

Radiological Studies

CT scan or MRI findings are usually normal but may reveal cerebral edema of variable extent.

CSF Studies

Lumber puncture may be needed at times to exclude other causes but it should only be undertaken if there are no evidences of raised intracranial pressure. Analysis of CSF may not show any significant findings except hypoglycorrhachia and/ or cell count less than 8 cells/mm^3.

Liver Biopsy

It should be done only after the coagulation parameters are normalized. This procedure can aid in histological diagnosis and may provide enzymatic as well as ultra structural features specific for this entity. Histologically there is presence of pan lobular micro vesicular steatosis without any evidence of hepatic necrosis or inflammation. Histo-chemical staining reveal marked reduction in mitochondrial enzymes viz., succinic dehydrogenase and cytochrome oxidase. Most characteristic feature of this entity is seen under electron microscopy in the form of swollen mitochondria showing pleomo-rphism with fragmented cristas and flocculation of intramatricial protein. Besides the mitochondrial changes there is loss of glycogen, accumulation of lipids and increase in peroxisomes. These findings revert to normal within a month if patient survives.

DIFFERENTIAL DIAGNOSIS

Children presenting with vomiting, alteration in sensorium and abnormalities of liver transaminase levels can cause diagnostic dilemma. One need to consider a wide differential diagnosis of conditions which can mimic Reye syndrome and the most important of them are inborn errors of metabolism especially in infants. Hypoxic liver and brain damage, shock with severe sepsis, generalized viral illnesses causing hepatitis and encephalopathy, glycogen storage disease, fulminant hepatitis before the onset of jaundice and various toxin/drug induced hepatitis are other conditions with similar presentation.

TREATMENT

Reye syndrome is a rare disease affecting

predominantly previously well children and is lethal if not recognized early and managed aggressively. No specific treatment is available except providing best possible supportive care. The therapy is mainly directed towards prevention of progression of encephalopathy and treating cerebral edema in an intensive care setting, correction of liver dysfunction, maintenance of fluid and electrolyte balance and to identify possible etiopathogenic factors.

Basic care involves maintaining airway, avoiding hypoxia, and prevention of dehydration as well as hyperammonemia, monitoring for hypoglycemia and its management. Correction of any electrolyte abnormalities and maintenance of acid-base balance, if detected in blood biochemical studies. Care of cases would depend on the stage of the disease.

Mild Disease (Stage 1)

Provide basic supportive care by maintaining airway, breathing and circulation. Keeping patient quiet as far as possible. Continuous and careful monitoring of vitals and blood studies would guide further course of treatment. Prevention and correction of fluid-electrolyte and acid-base abnormalities is mandatory. On detection of hypoglycemia, an IV bolus of 10% dextrose at the dose of 2-4 ml/kg should be administered and child should be maintained on IV dextrose infusion with frequent monitoring to prevent further such episodes. Tight euglycemic state should be maintained and if hyperglycemia occurs, insulin can be used. Some people advocate use of bicarbonate in the dose of 1 mmol/kg/hour if pH is less than 7.2 but this is not an accepted standard treatment modality. Over hydration or under hydration is detrimental for brain as over hydration can precipitate cerebral edema whereas under hydration may decrease intravascular volume and reduce cerebral perfusion causing worsening of encephalopathy.

Advanced Disease (Stage 2 or More of Encephalopathy)

These patients would need referral to a tertiary pediatric intensive care unit.

General supportive measures: Apart from all above measures needed for care of stage 1 patients, continuous vital monitoring, urine output measurement and EEG monitoring are accepted standard of care in advanced disease. Hyperthermia should be prevented/promptly treated. Avoidance of hypo- or hyperglycemia is the rule.

Fluid therapy can be guided by establishing central venous line and measurement of CVP. Overload can be controlled by using furosemide and colloids can be used to maintain normal intravascular volume.

Hyperammonemia: There is no specific recommendation to use any medical therapy like Sodiumphenylacetate/sodiumbenzoate as recommended for treatment of acute hyperammonemia with encephalopathy in patients with inborn errors of metabolism involving urea cycle enzymes though their use have been mentioned in literature. If ammonia levels are >500mcg/dl hemodialysis can be used to treat nonresponsive hyperammonemia. Medications can be used before or in conjunction during dialysis. Benzoate works by combining with glycine forming hippuric acid which is excreted in urine. In children weighing < 20 kg the recommended IV loading dose is 250 mg/kg over 2 hours followed by maintenance dose of 250 mg/kg/day over 24 hours (through central line) and those weighing more than 20 kg should be loaded with 5.5 gm/m^2 over 2 hours and 5.5 gm/m^2/day over 24 hour infusion through central line. Increase in intracranial pressure should be prevented by elevating the head end of bed by 30°and avoiding over hydration and use of hypotonic fluids.

Management of Encephalopathy: The degree of encephalopathy largely determines the outcome, hence current treatment consists of using aggressive measures to reduce brain edema in combination with direct intracranial pressure (ICP) monitoring where facilities for such monitoring is available. Patient with severe encephalopathy should be sedated with short acting agents like propofol and should be intubated and mechanically ventilated. Reduction of cerebral blood flow can be achieved emergently with intermittent hyperventilation in cases of intermittent surges in ICP. Cerebral edema in Reye syndrome is of cytotoxic variety where blood-brain barrier is intact rather than vasogenic type where blood-brain barrier is damaged. Hyperosmolor therapy with mannitol in bolus dose of 0.5g/kg can help in reducing the intracranial pressure but frequent repeated dosing may not be helpful. Mannitol acts by increasing serum osmolality, drawing fluid along an osmotic gradient from brain to intravascular compartment. In patients with associated renal failure absence of osmotic diuresis may cause increment in intravascular and in turn increase in intracranial blood volume to counteract any removal of fluid from cerebral tissue. Using hypertonic saline to induce hypernatremia (up to 150mmol/L) has been found especially useful to control early increases in ICP. For uncontrollable rise in ICP mild hypothermia and use of cerebral vasoconstrictor like Indomethacin, have been found to be useful.

Convulsions: If patient is convulsing, phenytoin should be administered intravenously at loading dose of 10-20 mg/kg followed by maintenance dose of 5-8 mg/kg/day in divided doses.

Coagulopathy: This should be corrected with the use of vitamin K and fresh frozen plasma especially if one is contemplating ICP monitoring with the use of subarachnoid screws and/or liver biopsy.

Complications can be encountered in the form of sepsis, bleeding, pancreatitis, shock, ARDS, pneumonia, status epilepticus, acute renal failure, brain herniation and death.

OUTCOME

A very strong association has been found between the timing of diagnosis and referral to pediatric intensive care setting and overall outcome. As there is no specific therapy for the condition till date, prompt and aggressive supportive care have been fundamental in survival. The decrease in the mortality from 50% to 15% can be attributed to the advancement in intensive care in recent years. Children less than 5 years of age and those presenting in stage 4 or 5 or with rapid progression from stage 1 to 3 have been associated with poor outcome and those who survive have a risk of long term neurological sequalae of variable extent.

PREVENTION

Avoiding use of salicylate or its derivatives for trivial febrile illnesses. Where aspirin is needed for therapeutic indication viz., acute rheumatic fever and as an anti- platelet measures in Kawasaki disease, one should be very vigilant about development of this condition and the drugs should be stopped and alternatives should be used after consultation with the experts.

FURTHER READING

1. Canalese J, Gimson AES, Davis C, Mellon PJ, Davis M and Williams R. Controlled trial of dexamethasone and mannitol for the cerebral oedema of fulminant hepatic failure. Gut 1982;23: 625-9.
2. Dezateux, Dinwiddie R, Helms P and Mathew DJ. Recognition and early management of Reye's syndrome. Arch Dis Child 1984;59:230-5.
3. Jenkins JG, Glasgow JFT, Black GW, Fannin TF, Hicks EM, Keily SR and Crean PM. Reye's syndrome : assessment of intracranial monitoring. BMJ 1987;294:337-8.

4. CDC : From the Centers for Disease Control . Reye syndrome surveillance-United States, 1989. JAMA1991;265(8):960.
5. Thabet F, Durand P,Chevert L, Fabre M, DebrayM, Brivet M and Devictor D. Severe Reye syndrome : report of 14 cases managed in a pediatric intensive care unit over 11 years. Arch Pediatr 2002;9(6) : 581-6.
6. Blei AT. Brain Edema in Acute Liver Failure. Crit Care Clin 2008;24:99-114.

Pratibha Singhi

30 Acute Paralysis

Acute paralysis is a common neurologic emergency in children. It may involve one limb-monoplegia, both lower limbs-paraplegia, all four limbs-quadriplegia, or one side of the body-hemiplegia. At times it may be multifocal, or generalized –involving the whole body. In cases with bilateral involvement, the limbs may often show asymmetric involvement; paralysis of three limbs – triplegia is generally clubbed with quadriplegia for practical purposes. Acute hemiplegia is generally secondary to stroke and will be discussed in a separate chapter. The paralysis may be in the form of a sudden onset, one time event with maximum deficit at onset, or may be progressive over hours or few days. Early appropriate intervention can often be curative or can minimize residual neuromorbidity. Basic understanding of the pathogenesis of acute paralysis secondary to various causes is essential for directed appropriate investigations and management. In this chapter, an approach and management of acute non-traumatic paralysis in children, requiring emergency care are discussed.

PATHOGENESIS

Acute paralysis can result from a lesion in the brain, brainstem, spinal cord, anterior horn cells, nerve roots, peripheral nerves, neuromuscular junction or the muscle. All of these present with motor weakness and either areflexia or diminished tendon reflexes in the acute stage. Other associated signs or symptoms depend on the site of involvement. Most cases of acute paraplegia and quadriplegia are because of involvement of the spinal cord or of the peripheral nerves.

Cord involvement: may occur because of inflammation of the cord, i.e. myelitis or because of compression, or secondary to vascular compromise, i.e. ischemic. Inflammation may involve the cord completely (complete transverse myelitis-CTM) or partially (partial transverse myelitis-PTM). The resultant deficits depend on the site and extent of involvement, and are associated with sensory loss. The dermatomal level of the sensory loss is generally 2-3 segments lower than the actual level of cord involvement as the first order neuron synapses in the cord, cross to the other side over 2-3 segments and form the spinothalamic tract. This is most prominently observed in the cervical spinal cord. Compression of the cord can occur because of any mass lesion, which may be intramedullary or extramedullary, intradural or extradural. The most important clinical condition is extradural abscess which can spread rapidly as pus traverses easily in the loose extradural space and can be associated with significant morbidity if left untreated even for a few hours.

The arterial supply of the spinal cord comes from one anterior spinal artery, that lies in the anterior median fissure, two posterior spinal arteries and radicular arteries (mainly anterior) at certain segmental levels of the cord. One of the radicular artery – the arteria radicularis magna arises from the descending thoracic aorta at around 8th thoracic segmental level. Thus an aortic dissection spreading lower down may occlude these arteries and may present as cord infarct. The corticospinal tract is located at the watershed zone of the spinal cord, hence it is the earliest to be affected if there is an extradural intraspinal lesion causing vascular compromise.

Involvement of peripheral nerves and radicles is most commonly seen with acute inflammatory demyelinating polyradiculoneuropathy (AIDP). This occurs because of an immunologic attack directed against myelin components. The inflammation and demyelination is generally multifocal and is often associated with axonal degeneration which may be primary or secondary.

Paralysis due to **neuromuscular junction involvement** that is seen in pediatric emergency is in children with myesthenia gravis (MG), or rarely botulism or other toxins.

Involvement of anterior horn cells occurs characteristically with polio virus and may cause flaccid asymmetric paralysis of one or more limbs simultaneously. Other viruses such as enteroviruses, echoviruses and Coxsackie viruses and recently documented West Nile Virus can also cause a polio like illness.

Cerebral causes for paraplegia are rare, and may be due to involvement of paracentral lobules, on either side of the midline that lie on the anterior and posterior side of the central sulcus. This area contains corticospinal neurons that supply both lower limbs and is also the highest centre for bladder and bowel control. In case of a rare anatomic variation wherein a single anterior cerebral artery supplies both halves of cerebral hemisphere, occlusion of that single artery by thrombosis, embolism or vasculitis may manifest as acute paraplegia.

Knowledge of basic neuroanatomy is essential for localization.

CLINICAL APPROACH

Acute paraplegia or quadriplegia in a child can be because of various causes. A detailed history and a proper clinical examination help in distinguishing the site of lesion and the type of injury. The common causes of acute paralysis in children are listed in Table 1.

History

The important points in history include:

1. Onset and progression of weakness - sudden catastrophic (transverse myelitis) or acute, progressive – (AIDP), mode of progression (ascending - AIDP or descending botulism).
2. History of viral prodrome or immunization a few days before onset of paralysis indicates an immune mediated problem such as AIDP or ADEM.
3. Fever and malaise at the time of paralysis indicate either a viral etiology such as polio, or a bacterial one such as epidural abscess.
4. Sensory symptoms such as numbness, tingling, pain, indicate peripheral nerve involvement (AIDP).
5. A history of prolonged low grade fever, weight loss, malaise, followed by acute paralysis could be suggestive of spinal TB with acute vertebral collapse.
6. Bladder or bowel involvement-early in myelitis, late in AIDP.
7. Precipitating factors such as exertion (periodic paralysis).

Table 1: Causes of acute nontraumatic paralysis in children (neuroanatomical)

- **Cranial**
  - Acute disseminated encephalomyelitis (ADEM)
  - Sagittal sinus thrombosis
  - Brain stem lesions
  - Posterior fossa lesions
- **Spinal**
  Non compressive
  - Acute transverse myelitis: complete (CTM), partial (PTM)
  - Cysticercus granuloma
  - Cord infarction

  Compressive
  - Epidural abscess
  - Spinal abscess/ tuberculoma/cysticercus granuloma
  - Vertebral tuberculosis with acute cord compression
  - Atlantoaxial dislocation
  - Spinal AVM with bleed (uncommon)
  - Vertebral metastasis - rare (lymphoma/neuroblastoma and eosinophilic granuloma)
- **Anterior horn cell disease**
  - Acute poliomyelitis
  - Other viruses (enterovirus 71, Coxsackie, West Nile virus)
- **Radiculoneuropathy**
  - Acute inflammatory demyelinating polyradiculoneuropaathy (AIDP)
  - Paralytic rabies
  - Snake bite
  - Toxins
  - Porphyria
- **Neuromuscular junction**
  - Acute presentation of myaesthenia gravis (MG), myesthemic crisis
  - Botulism
- **Muscle** – membrane
  - Periodic paralysis

8. Extra-ocular muscle involvement (ptosis) and sudden paralysis precipitated by infection (myesthenic crisis).
9. History of dog bite – paralytic rabies
10. Ingestion of canned/contaminated food (botulism), toxins (organophosphates)

A detailed history provides an etiological clue which is further reinforced by a proper examination.

Physical and Neurological Examination

A thorough examination as for any child presenting to the pediatric emergency with emphasis on the ABCs (airway, breathing, circulation) needs to be done, and the child stabilized. The points of particular interest include:

- Tone, power and reflexes to characterize the type, extent and degree of weakness.
- Any alteration in sensorium (ADEM), and if so the degree of coma.
- Any Cranial nerve involvement (Brainstem lesion).
- Ptosis, Fatiguability, bulbar involvement (MG).

- Opthalmoplegia with muscle weakness (MG, Miller Fisher variant of AIDP), botulism).
- Sensory system – level of sensory loss.
- Bladder bowel involvement (myelitis).
- Autonomic involvement (heart rate/BP-postural variations) sweat test, pupillary responses (AIDP).
- Spinal tenderness (epidural abscess).
- Paravertebral fullness (tubercular cold abscess).
- Pain during straight leg raising (radiculopathy).
- Systemic involvement –fever (viral-illness polio, entero viruses, bacterial – epidural abscess), dehydration (saggital sinus thrombosis).

Differential Diagnosis

In the emergency, if a child presents with acute paraplegia or quadriplegia with intact higher mental functions and no cranial nerve involvement, it is usually because of a spinal cord lesion or peripheral nerve involvement. In rare cases, if there are associated symptoms and signs such as seizures, altered sensorium, or cranial nerve involvement, the lesion may be in the brain or brainstem. Acute onset ascending paralysis is most often due to AIDP, or at times secondary to transverse myelitis. Presence of sensory symptoms just before or associated with paralysis indicate AIDP, whereas a definite dermatome level of sensory loss indicates transverse/ascending myelitis. Some of the differentiating features of the two are shown in Table 2. At times it may not be easy to distinguish the two clinically, particularly in very young children. Acute flaccid monoplegia is often due to anterior horn cell disease caused by polio or polio like viruses.

INVESTIGATIONS

These have to be decided according to the suspected site of lesion and cause of paralysis.

Table 2: Clinical differentiation between transverse myelitis and AIDP

Features	*Transverse Myelitis*	*AIDP*
• Motor weakness	• Usually acute, complete (may progress rapidly over few hours) • Often no upper limb involvement; if involved, weakness is equal in upper and lower limbs	Starts with lower limbs, 'ascends' to involve upper limbs Upper limbs often involved, generally less than lower limbs
• Sensory loss	A dermatomal level of sensory loss; arms not usually involved	No level of sensory loss
• Bladder/bowel involvement	Usually present early	Uncommon, late
• Cardiovascular autonomic dysfunction	Not present (only rarely seen with cervical involvement)	Common
• Cranial nerve involvement	Nil	May be involved (facial/extra ocular muscles)

1. **Electrophysiological Studies** such as nerve condition velocity are indicated in cases with suspected AIDP.
2. **MRI Spine:** (often gadolinium enhanced) is indicated in all cases of suspected myelopahty. *The first priority is to exclude a compressive lesion particularly an epidural abscess* and others such as a tubercular abscess, hematoma, vertebral compre-ssion etc. In case of myelitis MRI helps in determining the site and extent of myelitis.
3. **Lumbar Puncture:** in suspected AIDP, CSF examination helps in confirming the diagnosis. It also helps in differentiating inflammatory (pleocytosis) from non inflammatory causes of myelopathy. In cases of inflammatory CSF, viral studies (PCR) are indicated.
4. **MRI Brain:** is indicated rarely in cases where a lesion in the brain - (ADEM, saggital sinus thrombosis), brain stem (infarction) or in the posterior fossa (tumor) is suspected. It is also helpful in differentiating cases of paralytic rabies from AIDP.
5. **X-ray spine:** craniovertebral junction is done in suspected Atlanto Axial Dislocation (special views are done), vertebral tuberculosis.
6. **Others:** according to the cause, such as CT head, MRV for saggital sinus thrombosis, for infection - hemogram, blood culture and pus culture sensitivity from the source of infection, if identified, in cases with epidural abscess, investigations for evidence of tuber-culosis elsewhere in the body, including X-ray chest, Mantoux test, gastric aspirate for acid fast bacillus (AFB) etc. in cases with spinal TB, spinal angiography for vascular malformations of the cord, demonstration of Negri bodies from scraping of skin from nape of neck in cases with rabies, metabolic profile for suspected metabolic causes such as potassium levels for periodic paralysis, toxicology studies for suspected toxic paralysis, urine for porpho-bilinogens in suspected porphyria.

SPECIFIC CAUSES

Acute Inflammatory Demyelinating Polyra-diculoneuropathy (AIDP)

Also known as Landry Guillain Barre syndrome, is an autoimmune process characterized by acute progressive weakness of the limbs with areflexia. The weakness generally starts symmetrically in both lower limbs and ascends over a few days to involve the upper limbs and in a quarter of cases may also involve the respiratory muscles, resulting in severe respiratory insufficiency requiring ventilator care. The progression generally plataeus by 2 weeks and improvement starts by 4 weeks in most cases. Cranial nerves may be involved in a few cases. In about two third cases there is a history of upper respiratory infection or diarrhea or immunization, 1-4 weeks preceding the onset of weakness. However, generally the child is afebrile, when the weakness sets in. (Presence of fever at the time of paralysis must raise suspicion about other active infective processes like epidural abscess). Some children have sensory symptoms particularly pain before or with the onset of motor weakness. However sensory loss is not a prominent feature of AIDP. Autonomic dysfunction with changes in heart rate, orthostatic hypotension, anhidrosis may at times be present. Bladder involvement in AIDP is less common and occurs later in the course of the illness. There are several variations that may be occasionally seen. These include:

1. The Miller Fisher Syndrome (MFS) characterized by opthalmoplegia, ataxia and areflexia.
2. Fulminant acute motor sensory axonal neuropathy (AMSAN) with poor prognosis.

3. Acute motor axonal neuropathy (AMAN) with no sensory component.

CSF characteristically shows albumino cytologic dissociation after the first week of illness. Diagnostic confirmation is by electrophysiological studies suggestive of multifocal demyelination with secondary axonal degeneration. Common abnormalities include prolonged distal and F wave latencies, absent F waves, slowing of motor conduction velocities, reduction in distal CMAP amplitudes, and conduction block. Contrast MRI of spine may show gadolinium enhancement of lumbar roots, but is not routinely indicated.

Transverse Myelitis (TM)

Transverse Myelitis (TM) is a clinical syndrome in which an immune-mediated process causes neural injury to the spinal cord resulting in varying degrees of weakness, sensory alterations and autonomic dysfunction. The child presents with acute bilateral lower limb weakness, which is flaccid with areflexia in the acute phase, although later pyramidal signs appear. Generally there is a dermatomal level of sensory dysfunction. In adults this is mostly at the thoracic level; however, children have a higher frequency of cervical spinal cord involvement and a cervical sensory level. Often there is associated bladder/bowel dysfunction, and some cases may have sensory symptoms such as numbness, or paresthesias. However, paresthesias are unusual for children

Autonomic symptoms such as urinary urgency, bowel or bladder incontinence and difficulty or inability to void may occur. In half the cases, there is a preceding illness including nonspecific symptoms such as fever, nausea, and muscle pain or of immunization within one month of the onset of symptoms.

Spinal MRI shows T2 signal abnormality that can range from one vertebral segment to several segments (Figure 1). The lesion also enhances with gadolinium. CSF shows pleocytosis with elevated protein.

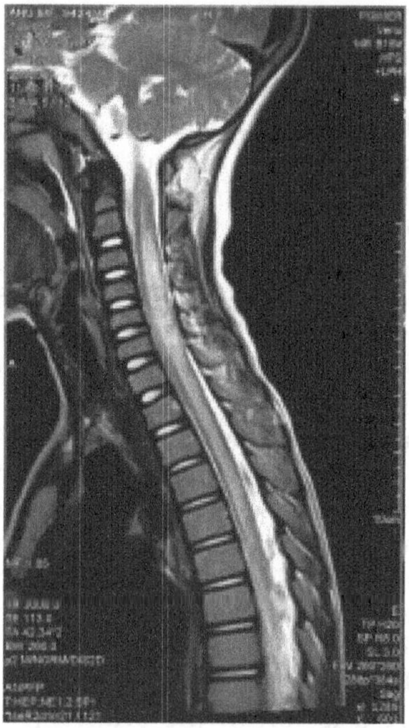

Fig. 1: MRI spine, T2 weighted, showing extensive swelling and hyperintensity of the cord in a child with transverse ascending myelitis.

Atlantoaxial dislocation (AAD): Atlantoaxial dislocation is one of the common causes of acute onset quadriplegia in children. A high index of suspicion is very important as prompt diagnosis and management can be life saving. Any child with quadriplegia of acute onset wherein the etiology is not clear, must have an X-ray craniovertebral junction in neutral position (lateral view) with immobilization of the neck to exclude atlantoaxial dislocation. AAD is often not thought of if the presentation is somewhat atypical such as paraparesis or triparesis or very rarely monoparesis.

The child with AAD often has an underlying craniovertebral junction abnormality which stays asymptomatic for several years and then may present acutely because of a mobile atlantoaxial dislocation. An acute presentation may represent one of the repeated attacks. Hence a past history of similar quadriparesis is important. The dislocation may occur denovo secondary to a viral infection of the upper respiratory tract or bacterial tonsillopharyngitis, or rarely there may be a prevertebral pyogenic or tuberculous abscess. Precipitating features include short hypoplastic odontoid process, connective tissue diseases, mucopolysaccharidoses (particularly Morquio). Down's syndrome, Paget's disease etc. AAD can be life threatening if the odontoid hits against the medulla and compresses the vital centres. Tuberculosis of the atlanto axial region is rare accounting for less than 1% of all cases of Pott's spine.

The presentation may be very acute, occurring suddenly during flexion of the neck or it may manifest in hours following a faulty posture during sleep. In addition to acute onset of weakness, the child may complain of neck pain especially on movement. In the acute phase the tone and reflexes may be diminished or absent because of spinal shock. Often there is associated urinary retention and sensory loss below the level of neck, and up going plantars. Examination may reveal a low neck: body ratio (1: 13), short neck associated with Klippel Feil anomaly pointing to underlying craniovertebral junction anomaly. X-ray of craniovertebral junction or MRI, with special views, establishes the diagnosis.

Spinal Epidural Abscess

In children with acute paraplegia, this is one of the most important diagnosis to be considered because early diagnosis and surgical intervention is life saving or at least prevents permanent disability. The presentation is usually that of a febrile, sick child who complains of low backache, radiating along the lumbosacral radicles with weakness of both lower limbs. The patient may develop urinary hesitancy and later retention, as well as constipation. There may be history of rapidly ascending radicular symptoms or weakness. A source of infection such as pyoderma or infected wound is often identified.

Clinical features depend on the duration of illness before presentation. Early cases may have only features of radiculopathy such as radicular pain, sensory loss and motor deficit in radicular distribution, and straight leg raising (SLR) sign is positive. The weakness is more proximal than distal. If the child presents later, there may be features of rapidly ascending myelopathy with a sensory loss-dermatome upper level depending on the site of myelopathy. Deep tendon jerks and superficial reflexes are diminished or absent in the acute stage. However, plantar response is usually extensor if muscle power is somewhat preserved. There may be asymmetric compression because of loculation of pus. A spinal MRI defines the site and extent of the abscess. A search for a source of infection, particularly staphylococcal infection, or an open wound is warranted in all such cases.

Any child with fever and features of myelopathy, myeloradiculopathy or even AIDP must get a spinal MRI to rule out spinal epidural abscess.

Spinal Tuberculosis

Vertebral tuberculosis is not uncommon in countries where TB is endemic. Acute paraplegia or quadriplegia may occur because of a cold abscess compressing the cord, pathological compression collapse of vertebra leading to cord compression, bony spur or fragment of damaged vertebral portion pressing on the cord, ischemia of cord due to strangulation by thick exudates, or vasculitis, or compression of blood vessels by cold abscess. There may be associated arachnoiditis, and features of myelopathy. The child often has a history of weight loss, anorexia, and low grade fever, for several days before presentation. On examination, there may be local spinal deformity like gibbus, kyphosis, spinal tenderness, or a palpable paraspinal cold abscess. A search for a family contact with tuberculosis must be made. MRI spine shows destruction of veretebra, often with collapse compression and accumulation of caseous material.

Paralytic Rabies

Rabies continues to be a problem in developing countries. It is caused by the transmission of the virus by infected saliva through the bite of a rabid animal-usually a dog. The incubation period varies from 1 to 3 months. Most (>80%) cases are of the furious type with classic hydrophobia, aerophobia, hyperexcitability and autonomic dysfunction. Some cases present with the paralytic type which is characterized by flaccid paralysis that starts in the bitten limb and ascends rapidly symmetrically or asymmetrically, and finally involves all the limbs. Respiratory and bulbar paralysis along with urinary and fecal incontinence occur within a few days followed by cardiac arrhythmias, coma and death. Paralytic rabies can resemble AIDP; a history of dog bite gives the clue. Confusion may arise in a case where after the dog bite, the child received anti rabies vaccine (ARV) and a possibility of post ARV, poly-radiculoneuropathy may be considered. Certain points that distinguish the two include (i) post ARV AIDP has a shorter incubation period of about 2 weeks (ii) bladder bowel involvement are usually seen in paralytic rabies but are rare in post ARV AIDP (iii) paralytic rabies progresses rapidly and death ensues within 2 weeks whereas AIDP does not have such a fulminant course and has a better prognosis.

The MRI in post ARV AIDP is normal whereas in rabies it shows T2 hyper-intensities in the basal ganglia, thalami, pontine and midbrain nuclei. Diagnosis of rabies is confirmed antemorterm by demonstration of rabies by PCR in the saliva, or by full thickness nuchal skin biopsy. Rabies virus antibodies in the CSF supports the diagnosis. Rabies virus can be cultured from the saliva or brain biopsy.

Acute Myesthenic Crisis

This may occur in a child already diagnosed with myasthenia gravis, in which case it is easy to diagnose. However in a child without a previous diagnosis, who presents for the first time in myesthenic crisis, it may not be thought about and may therefore be potentially life threatening. A history of weakness exacerbated by stress, presence of ptosis or opthalmoplegia and respiratory weakness should alert the clinician.

Botulism

Classic botulism occurs after ingestion of food contaminated by preformed toxin. It is characterized by bulbar symptoms such as blurred vision, diplopia, ptosis, dysphagia and dysarthria within 12-36 hours after ingestion of contaminated food. The weakness has a 'descending' pattern and respiratory paralysis may occur. Ventilatory support is life saving in such cases.

Infantile botulism occurs after ingestion of spores of C. botulinum that multiply in the gastrointestinal tract to produce the toxin in vivo. Ingestion of honey and corn syrup have been associated with infantile botulism, but no cause may be found in many cases.

The infant is constipated and develops descending paralysis, with a weak cry, feeding difficulty, cranial nerve involvement, followed by limb weakness with reduced tendon reflexes. Respiratory weakness may occur. Electrophysiologic studies including repetitive nerve stimulation are helpful. Diagnosis is confirmed by isolation of the organism or toxin in stool.

Acute Disseminated Encephalomyelitis (ADEM)

This is an immunologic illness that generally presents a few days after a viral infection with altered sensorium, seizures and multifocal neurodeficitis including limb weakness with variable reflexes. The presentation may resemble meningoence-phalitis – presence of multifocal deficits gives a clue. Associated myelitis and optic neuritis may be seen.

MRI head characteristically shows patchy white matter involvement; deep gray matter may be involved in a third of cases. CSF may show mild pleocytosis and at times oliogoclonal bands.

Sagittal Sinus Thrombosis

This can occur in child who has diarrhea with dehydration, or underlying anemia, infection, polycythemia, or procoagulant state. It generally presents with headache, vomiting, altered sensorium, focal or generalized seizure and acute lower limb weakness with urinary and/or fecal incontinence. On examination there may be features of raised intracranial pressure. The tone and reflexes in both lower limbs may be diminished or absent in the acute stage. The plantar reflexes may show an extensor response. This along with the presence of seizures and altered sensorium indicates that the lesion is in the brain.

A non contrast CT scan of the head may show areas of hemorrhagic infarct involving both paracentral lobules. Signs of cortical venous thrombosis with cord like hyper-density in the affected area (cord or string sign) may be seen. A positive delta sign with central triangular hyperdense area may diagnose sagittal sinus thrombosis in the early stage (upto a week). Thereafter the thrombus density decreases and it becomes isodense and later hypodense. In contrast CT scan, the area of hemorrhagic infarct may be better visualized and one may see an "empty delta sign" sometime during the evolution of the thrombus because the contrast appears as a thin rim of enhancement around the hypo or isodense area of the thrombus. MRI and magnetic resonance venography (MRV) characterize the abnormal flow of blood along the venous sinuses and the thrombosis in detail. The gold standard for diagnosis used to be cerebral angiography (venous phase) but this is hardly ever needed, once the MRI/MRV are diagnostic.

Posterior Fossa Lesion

Very rarely, a child may present with acute quadriplegia and cranial nerve palsies (depending on the site and extent of involvement) secondary to brainstem infarction. The underlying causes for such infarct may vary and include hyper-coagulation disorders, single vertebral artery with compression by craniovertebral junction anomalies. An MRI detects the infarcts, and management depends upon the etiology of the infarct.

Brainstem Space Occupying Lesion

Rarely, lesions in the brain stem such as tuberculomas or tumors with sudden bleed, may present with acute onset quadriparesis with cranial nerve palsies, with or without bladder or bowel and sensory tract involvement. MRI brain delineates the lesion.

MANAGEMENT

General

Any child who comes to the emergency with paralysis needs to be managed just like any other acutely ill child, with attention to:

- ABCs (airway, breathing and circulation). Timely ventilatory support can be life saving in many situations such as myesthenic crisis.
- Close monitoring of progression such as in AIDP, to particularly watch for respiratory involvement that may warrant ventilatory support, and for cardiovascular autonomic dysfunction that may require pharmacologic intervention.
- Supportive care such as posturing of the paralytic limbs in appropriate neutral position, catheterization in cases with

urinary retention, pain relief in children with associated significant pain.

Specific

Acute inflammatory demyelinating polyradiculoneuropathy (AIDP): Specific therapy consists of intravenous immune globulin (IVIG) 0.4g/kg/day for 5 days or 1g/kg/day for 2 days. Plasma exchange has also been found effective. However corticosteroids have not been found to be of any benefit.

Transverse myelitis: The usual treatment consists of intravenous methylprednisolone or dexamethasone for 3-5 days followed by oral prednisone for 14 days. However, there are no randomized, placebo-controlled trials to support this approach.

Plasma exchange has been used in patients with severe (though incomplete) TM, who have not significantly improved with intravenous steroids.

In non responsive cases, intravenous cyclophosphamide and other immunomodulatory treatments have been tried.

Atlantoaxial dislocation (AAD): Prevention of neck movement by appropriate neck traction or cervical collar. Immediate neurosurgical consultation and surgical management.

Spinal Epidural Abscess: Urgent removal of pus. As the commonest organism is staphylococcus aureus, the antibiotics should include Cloxacillin (100 mg/kg/day) intravenously in four divided doses along with amikacin 15 mg/kg intravenously in two divided doses. Once the report of pus culture sensitivity is available, antibiotics can be changed appropriately. Epidural abscess in children can be associated with disseminated staphylococcal disease, hence chest X-ray to detect pneumonia and search for staphylococcal infection else where in the body must be done.

Spinal Tuberculosis: Management is surgical, along with appropriate antitubercular therapy.

Acute Myesthenic Crisis: An early diagnosis with immediate ventilatory support are life saving. High dose corticosteroids with IVIG or plasma exchange are the mainstay of management. The precipitating factor(s) such as sepsis need to be treated.

Acute disseminated Encephalomyelitis: Intravenous methylprednisolone for 3-5 days followed by oral steroids has shown good results with near complete recovery in about half the cases.

Saggittal sinus thrombosis: control of seizures, proper hydration, and management of raised intracranial pressure. Search and treatment of underlying factors needs to be done after the child is stable.

FURTHER READING

1. Bershad EM, Feen ES, Suarez JI. Myasthenia gravis crisis. South Med J. 2008, 1:63-9.
2. Brinar VV, HAbek M, Zardo I, *et al.* Current concepts in the diagnosis of transverse myelopahties. Clin Neurol Neurosurg 2008, 9:919-27.
3. Chitra Krishnan 1, Adam I. Kaplin 2, Deepa M. et al. Transverse myelitis: pathogenesis, diagnosis and treatment. Frontiers in Bioscience 9, 1483-1499, May 1, 2004.
4. Hemachudha T, Wacharapluesadee S, Laothamatas J, *et al.* Wild Rabies. Curr Neurol Neurosci Rep. 2006, 6:460-8.
5. Jacob A, Weinshenker BG, *et al.* An approach to the diagnosis of acute transverse myelitis. Semin Neurol 2008, 1:105-20.
6. Jani-Acsadi A, Lisak RP. Myasthenic crisis: guidelines for prevention and treatment J Neurol Sci. 2007, 261(1-2):127-33.
7. Krishnan C, Kaplin AI, Deshpande *et al.* Transverse Myelitis: pathogenesis, diagnosis and treatment. Fronto Biosci 2004, 9:1483-99.
8. Kumar S. Differentiating paralytic rabies from post antirabies vaccine polyradiculoneuropathy Neurol India 2004, 52:270.
9. Leung AK, Davies HD, Hon KL *et al.* Rabies: epidemiology, pathogenesis, and prophylaxis. Adv Ther. 2007, 6:1340-7.
10. Pittock SJ, Lucchinetti CF. Inflammatory transverse myelitis: evolving concepts Current Opinion in Neurology 2006, 19:362–368.

Sunit Singhi and Pratibha Singhi

31 Headache: Approach in Emergency Room

Headache is the most frequent neurological symptom. About 60-70% of children experience headache by the age of 7-9 years. It continues to be a frequent cause of emergency department (ED) use but is relatively unusual as an isolated complaint (0.7% to 1.3.% of visits) in United States EDs. The most commonly diagnosed headaches are the primary headache disorders, most often migraine or tension-type headache. The overall prevalence of non-migraine headache is 10-25%. In ED it is essential to rule out life-threatening causes.

EVALUATION

Headache can be caused by primary entities (as in migraine or tension-type headache) or the pain may result from secondary causes, such as brain tumors, raised ICP, hypertension or acute febrile illnesses (e,g,,CNS infections, influenza).

The cornerstones of ED management are (1) to determine the correct headache diagnosis, (2) to exclude secondary causes of headache, such as infection, mass lession, or hemorrhage, (3) to initiate appropriate therapy to relieve headache (4) to give prompt referral for definitive management, if needed. Diagnosing or classifying the individual headache can be challenging. Providing a diagnosis for every patient is easier said than done. Up to one third of patients who present to an ED with headache cannot be assigned a specific diagnosis.

To determine the nature and cause of a child's headache, the evaluation begins with a thorough medical history, followed by meticulous physical examination.

History should include in particular the following details:

1. Mode of onset, duration, frequency, location of headache (unilateral or bilateral, frontal or temporal), and character (pulsating, pressing).
2. Severity of pain (unable to carry out daily activity, school studies), aggravating and relieving factors: any worsening with bending over or coughing (sinusitis or raised intracranial pressure).
3. Time and circumstances of headache: early morning headache or the one that awakens a child from sleep indicating increased intracranial pressure.
4. Associated symptoms such as (fever, vomiting, neck pain, phono and photophobia, visual change, confusion,

disorientation etc.). Vomiting is often associated with intracranial pathology.
5. In chronic or recurrent headache any change from previous headache pattern, history of projectile vomiting, focal weakness.
6. Recent or remote trauma, exposure to medication or toxin
7. Preexisting/co-existing medical problems, immunocompromised patients, social and emotional factors.

On Examination Patient's appearance (sick or well looking), vital signs including blood pressure (to rule out hypertension) and temperature should be noted. Presence of sinus or dental tenderness, nuchal rigidity, lymphadenopathy, signs of trauma, cutaneous lesions (café-au-lait lesions and others suggestive of neurocutaneons syndromes), heart murmur, cranial bruits, and visual acuity should be looked for.

Complete neurological examination including fundoscopy (for papilloedema) must be performed in all cases to look for evidence of an organic cause.

Based on above, five temporal patterns of headache may be identified: acute, acute recurrent, chronic progressive, chronic nonprogressive, and mixed pattern.

DIFFERENTIAL DIAGNOSIS

Acute Headache

Fever caused by infections is probably the most common cause of headache in children. Single episode without prior history is usually secondary to an upper respiratory febrile illness such as sinusitis and otitis media. In toxic-appearing patient with fever and headache, meningitis and encephalitis should be ruled out. Sudden severe unilateral headaches correlate with carotid or vertebral dissection; suspect subarachnoid hemorrhage if the onset is sudden and headache very intense. In children, bleeds due to rupture of aneurysms or AV malformations are more common.

Acute Recurrent Headache

Recurrent episodes of headache with symptom-free intervals are usually caused by migraine and its variants, tension headache and cluster headache. Neuralgias are very uncommon in children.

Chronic Progressive Headache

It is characterized by gradual increase in frequency and severity of headache. The differential diagnosis often includes serious causes such as brain tumor, hydrocephalus, chronic meningitis, brain abscess, vasculitis, AV malformation, subdural hematoma, hypertension etc. History and examination should focus on features suggestive of intracranial pathology and increased intracranial pressure.

A headache is more likely to be caused by a tumor or other intracranial mass if following characteristics are associated with it: occipital headaches or headaches localized to the nape of the neck, headache worsening with sneezing, coughing, straining or bending forward, headaches that awaken the child from sleep or that are worse in the morning and headaches associated with blurred vision.

Chronic Nonprogressive Headache

Frequent or constant headache without change in frequency or severity is most often caused by chronic sinusitis, post traumatic headache and stress-related headache.

The diagnosis of primary headache disorders such as migraine and tension-type rests principally on clinical criteria as set forth by the International Headache Society. Clues to secondary causes of headache are uncovered through history and physical examination and ancillary diagnostic testing.

In some cases, diagnostic testing may be necessary to **exclude primary from secondary causes.**

INVESTIGATIONS

Majority of patients with normal physical examination do not require investigation in the emergency department. CBC and blood culture should be sent for suspected infection.

Lumbar puncture should be done for suspected meningitis. CT scan should be obtained prior to LP if there is evidence of increased ICP, altered level of consciousness, focal findings, or papilledema.

Table 1: Indications for neuroimaging in Children with Headache

1. Persistent headaches of > 6-month duration, not responding to medical treatment.
2. Headache associated with abnormal neurologic findings, especially papille-dema, nystagmus, or gait or motor abnormalities.
3. Persistent headaches not associated with a family history of migraine.
4. Early morning headache or the headache that awakens a child from sleep.
5. Persistent headache associated with episodes of confusion, disorientation, or vomiting.
6. Clinical or laboratory findings suggestive of CNS involvement.

Children with underlying immunocompromised state, known neoplasm, sickle cell disease, coagulopathy etc are predisposed to intracranial pathology. In this group, presence of severe headache should have a low threshold for neuroimaging.

(From: Medina S, Pinter JD, Zurakowski D, et al. Children with headache: clinical predictors of surgical space-occupying lesions and the role of neuroimaging. Radiology 1997;202:819-24).

Emergent neuroimaging in children

Quality Standards Subcommittee of the AAN and the Practice Committee of the Child Neurology Society does not recommend neuroimaging study on a routine basis in children who have migraine (with or without aura), recurrent headaches and a normal neurologic examination. Recently published guidelines of American College of Radiology also rate need for neuroimaging very low in isolated headache, unaccompanied by neurologic signs and symptoms. In essence, those guidelines underline essentiality of neuroimaging in identifying children with space-occupying or surgical lesions. Neuroimaging should be considered in children with headache who have an abnormal neurologic examination (eg. focal findings, signs of increased intracranial pressure, significant alteration of consciousness), coexistence of seizures or both, and having acute severe incapacitating headache of recent onset in absence of family history of migraine, a change in the type of headache (increasing frequency, duration and intensity) or if there are associated features that suggest neurologic dysfunction. In one study, 94% of children with brain tumors had abnormal neurological findings and 60% had papilloedema.

CT scan versus MRI

CT detects most of the abnormalities that may cause headaches. CT generally is preferred to MRI for evaluation of acute subarachnoid hemorrhage, acute head trauma and bony abnormalities. MRI is more sensitive than CT in the detection of posterior fossa and cervicomedullary lesions, ischemia, white matter abnormalities, cerebral venous thrombosis, subdural and epidural hematomas, neoplasms, and CNS infections including cerebritis and brain abscess.

Contrast enhancement can increase the visibility of a subtle collection.

Electroencephalography

Practice Committee of the Child Neurology Society does not recommend EEG in the routine evaluation of a child with recurrent headaches, as it is unlikely to provide an etiology, improve diagnostic yield, or distinguish migraine from other types of headaches.

Lumbar Puncture

After neuroimaging is performed, lumbar puncture often is indicated in children having headache with fever or other symptoms or signs suggestive of meningitis, a subacute or progressive headache and an atypical chronic headache.There are many potential complications of lumbar puncture, the most common of which is low CSF pressure headache, which occurs in approximately 30% children.

MIGRAINE

Migraine is one of the most common causes of acute and recurrent headache in children. By 15 years of age, 3-10% of children experience migraine headache. Migraine incidence begins to peak in early adolescence and may be a concern in children as young as 5 or 6 years of age. In general, children may present with bilateral headache of shorter duration and without the combination of photo- and phonophobia. In 17% of patients, headache had an accompanying aura. (Table: Criteria for diagnosis of migraine). There are limitations to present diagnostic criteria for migraine. Modifications to these criteria have been proposed. Children are prone to have unusual headache pattern, most notable as manifestation of migraine with aura, basilar artery migraine and hemiplegic migraine. Ophthalmic migraine may present with focal neurologic symptoms of ptosis or complete third-nerve palsy. Stress, fatigue including lack of sleep, hunger, glare, head trauma, and certain foods containing nitrates, caffeine, tyramine, glutamate, or salt are common triggers. Eye strain, cold foods, and high altitude are less common triggers.

Table 2: International Headache Society (IHS) criteria for the diagnosis of migraine

Criteria for pediatric migraine without aura

A. At least 5 attacks fulfilling B-D
B. Duration of 1-48 hours
C. Headache has at least two of the following:
- Bilateral (frontal/temporal) or unilateral location
- Pulsatile quality
- Headache intensity moderate or severe
- Aggravation by routine physical activity

D. During headache at least one of the following occurs:
- Nausea and/or vomiting
- Photophobia and/or phonophobia

Criteria for pediatric migraine with aura

A. At least 2 attacks fulfilling B-D
B. At least 3 of the following :
- One or more fully reversible aura symptoms including focal cortical and/or brain stem dysfunction.
- At least 1 aura developing gradually over more than 4 minutes, or 2 or more symptoms occurring in succession
- No auras lasting more than 60 minutes
- Headache follows less than 60 minutes

TENSION TYPE HEADACHE

Tension-type headache is rarely severe and only infrequently causes an ED visit. The pain is typically bilateral, pressing or tightening in quality, and of mild to moderate intensity without migraine's characteristic features, such as nausea, vomiting, severe intensity. Traditional management of tension-type headache calls for nonsteroidal analgesics.

Cluster Headache

Cluster headache is a rare and infrequent cause of ED presentation, particularly when compared with migraine or tension-type headache.

TREATMENT

Early identification and appropriate treatment of underlying conditions causing headache can result in complete headache resolution.

Acute Recurrent Headache (Migraine)

First line management of pediatric migraine often consists of simple analgesics, such as ibuprofen (10 mg/kg orally) or acetaminophen (15 mg/kg orally). Both are safe and effective in children. Triptans may be used if needed. Sumatripan nasal spray is easy to use and provides faster initial relief; oral is not so effective. Other triptans : Rizatriptan (5mg orally) and Zolmitriptan (2.5-5mg orally) have been evaluated in adolescents, but without much benefit. Prochlorperazine (0.15 mg/kg IV, maximum 10mg) is effective in reducing symptoms in severe acute migraine attack in emergency room; it is superior to ketorolac (0.5mg/kg IV). The antiemetic dopamine antagonists are commonly used.

Identification and removal of triggers such as sleep disturbance, stress and fatigue and rest in quiet dark room is effective at onset of migraine. Caffeine should be avoided, it can precipitate headache in adolescents and may be associated with rebound headache.

Migraine recurrence is common in first 24-48 hours, particularly if the patient is discharged from emergency without complete relief of pain.

DISPOSITION AND REFERRAL

Admit serious secondary causes for further treatment. Outpatient follow-up with neurology referral is needed in chronic progressive headache, in children < 3 years and recurrent migraine headache.

FURTHER READING

1. Brenner M, Oakley C, Lewis D. The evaluation of children and adolescents with headache. Curr Pain Headache Rep. 2008 Oct;12(5):361-6.
2. Ahad R,Kossoff EH. Secondary intracranial causes for headaches in children. Curr pain Headache Rep. 2008 Oct;12(5):373-8.
3. Evans RW Diagnostic testing for migraine and other primary headaches. Neurol Chin 2009:27:393-415.
4. Friedman BW, Grosberg BM. Diagnosis and management of primary headache disorders in emergency department setting. Emerg Med Clin N Am 2009;27: 71-87.
5. Sliver S,Gano D, Gerresten P. Acute treatment of paediatric migraine: a meta-analysis of efficacy. 6: J Paediatr Child Health.2008 Jan;44(1-2):3-9.
6. Walker DM, Teach SJ. Emergency department treatment of primary headaches in children and adolescents. Curr Opin Pediatr.2008 Jun;20(3):248-54.
7. Winner P. Pediatric headache. Curr Opin Neurol.2008 Jun;21(3):316-22.
8. Expert panel on Pediatric imaging. Headache-child. American College of Radiology (ACR) http://www.acr.org.

Puneet Jain

32 Acute Dystonia

Dystonia is the second most common movement disorder in children after tics. It may be defined as a movement disorder in which involuntary sustained or intermittent muscle contractions cause twisting and repetitive movements, abnormal postures or both. The appearance is one of an abnormal posture rather than an involuntary movement. Table 1 summarizes the differential diagnosis of abnormal posturing.

Table 1 : Differential diagnosis of abnormal posturing

Dystonia
Hysteria
Muscular dystrophy
Myotonia
Neuromyotonia
Rigidity
Spasticity
Stiffman syndrome

CLASSIFICATION AND CAUSES

Dystonia may be classified by location as *focal*(involving a single part of the body), *segmental*(involving muscles of two contiguous body parts), *hemidystonia* (involving all or most muscles on one side of the body), *multifocal* (involving two or more non contiguous body regions) or *generalized*. It may be classified by etiology as *primary*, when dystonia is the predominant or the only clinical feature, or *secondary*, when there is a history of prior CNS insult as in asphyxia, neonatal jaundice, stroke, etc (symptomatic dystonias) or it is a part of heredodegenerative disease. It may also be classified by the onset of symptoms as *acute* or *chronic*.

Acute dystonias in children are usually seen with the use dopamine antagonists (anti-emetics and anti-psychotics) as an acute idiosyncratic reaction. Certain paroxysmal movement disorders such as paroxysmal kinesigenic dykinesia (PKD) and paroxysmal non-kinesigenic dyskinesia (PNKD) may also present acutely for the first time. Their paroxysmal nature, classical precipitating factors and normal neurological examination in between these episodes helps in the diagnosis.

Acute CNS insult/injury/infections may also present with acute dystonias (Table 2). Certain poisonings (carbon monoxide, cyanide) and even wasp sting has been associated with acute dystonias. Sometimes hypocalcemia may cause features resembling those of acute dystonia.

Acute onset of symptoms is also known in patients with primary and secondary dystonias. Occasionally these patients develop severe episodes of generalized dystonias and rigidity which may be refractory to standard drug therapy. This has been termed as 'status dystonicus' or '*dystonic storm*'.

Dystonia in the context of the emergency room has been under-recognized and underestimated, despite the disabling features of the disorder. This chapter will cover the various etiologies, clinical presentation and management of acute dystonia.

Table 2 : Etiology of Acute Dystonia

Drug induced
Anti-psychotics
Anti-emetics
Anti-depressants
CNS insults/injuries
Hypoxia
Head trauma
Stroke
Intracranial hemorrhage
Central pontine myelinolysis
Infectious/Post-infectious/Inflammatory
Viral encephalitis
Tuberculosis
ADEM
Reye's syndrome
Lupus
Neurotoxins
Manganese
Carbon monoxide
Cyanide
Methanol
Wasp sting
Metabolic disorders
Hypoparathyroidism
Status dystonicus
Seen in primary and secondary dystonias
Paroxysmal dyskinesias
Kinesigenic
Non-Kinesigenic
Exercise induced

DRUG INDUCED DYSTONIA

There is a higher rate of acute dystonic reactions to medications in children than in adults. This has been reported to be as high as 10-20% in some series. This is most commonly seen with neuroleptic medications. Acute dystonias may be very frightening for the parents. Hence the physician should be familiar with the prevalence of and the risk factors for acute dystonia and should know how to prevent and treat the condition.

Drugs that are commonly associated with acute dystonia include anti-psychotics, anti-depressants (esp SSRIs) and anti-emetics (metoclopramide, domperidone and prochlorperazine). Atypical anti-psychotic drugs such as olanzapine and risperidone are associated with low risk of dystonia. Clozapine is the only known atypical antipsychotic drug that does not induce acute dystonia. There have been several case reports of acute dystonia in patients being treated with other drugs such as anti-vertigo agents (cinnarizine, flunarizine), anti-epileptics (phenytoin, carbamazepine), anti-malarials (chloroquine, hydroxychloroquine) and cocaine. Anecdotal case reports of acute dystonia have been reported during the use of buspirone, diazepam, sumatriptan, phenylpropanolamine, *ecstasy*, cetrizine, tiagabine, felbamate and etoposide. Acute dystonic reaction has also been reported with the use of aripiprazole, a dopamine agonist although the drug's suggested mode of action largely precludes occurrence of such reaction.

The *pathogenesis* of acute dystonic reactions is still debatable. It has been postulated that blockade of D1 receptors in basal ganglia is partly responsible for such reactions. The delay between receptor blockade and onset of the clinical symptomatology suggests involvement of additional mechanisms, possibly a secondary dopamine-receptor hypersensitivity. The differential rates of dystonia which occur with different antipsychotic drugs might be explained by the receptor blocking ratio between dopamine and acetylcholine in the basal ganglia. The higher the ratio of dopamine-acetylcholine antagonism, higher is the risk of acute dystonia. Risk factors for acute drug induced dystonia include young age, male sex and a history of acute dystonia.

In 90-95% cases, acute dystonic reaction occurs within 96 hours of initiation of anti-psychotic therapy or after a large increase in the dose. Cranial, pharyngeal, cervical and axial muscles are most commonly affected. Possible reactions include trismus, grimacing, blepharospasm, uncontrollable tongue movements, torticollis, retrocollis, oculogyric crisis, dysarthria, swallowing difficulties and opisthotonus. The oculogyric crisis is the only form of acute dystonia that may occur while the patient is receiving a stable dose of an antipsychotic drug; it may be provoked by alcohol, emotional stress or fatigue. Life threatening dystonias may occur rarely. The acute reactions are usually self limited or respond to treatment but they may be prolonged and resistant to therapy.

The *treatment* of acute dystonic reactions is usually easy and nearly always effective. Intravenous diphenhydramine, 1-2 mg/kg/dose rapidly reverses drug induced dystonias. Alternatives include promethazine, benztropine or biperiden. Rarely second or third dose may be required; these should be administered at half hour intervals. If the patient has an oculogyric crisis that does not reverse with anti-cholinergic drugs, a trial of diazepam may be given. Following resolution of the acute dystonic reaction, anti-cholinergics are usually continued for atleast 48 hours, along with anti-psychotics, to prevent a recurrence.

Prophylactic use of anti-cholinergics along with anti-psychotics is highly controversial. Patient's risk factor profile for development of acute dystonic reactions, pharmacological properties of anti-psychotic being used (dose, potency, intrinsic cholinergic activity) and tolerability of anti-cholinergic may aid the physician to decide regarding the prophylactic use of anti-cholinergics.

STATUS DYSTONICUS

Status dystonicus or *'dystonic storm'* is a life threatening disorder that may occur in patients with primary or secondary dystonia. Following an apparently unremarkable disease such as respiratory illness or introduction/withdrawal of a drug, child may develop severe and intractable hyperkinetic dystonia with flinging movements of arms, legs or head. This may be associated with opisthotonic posturing or severe limb extension. The most severe cases may develop bulbar and ventilation complications.These arise from dystonia affecting the lingual, masseter and pterygoid muscles. Dystonic spasms of upper airway and respiratory muscles result in alveolar hypoventilation and hypoxemia. Rarely, adductor spasm of the vocal cords may cause inspiratory stridor. Metabolic complications such as rhabdomyolysis and renal failure may ensue secondary to intense muscle activity. Indeed, status dystonicus represents a *medical emergency*.

Treatment is extremely difficult and may require general anesthesia to abate the movement. A trial of levodopa is necessary in all early onset cases. Anti-cholinergic agents like benzhexol may be added. Tetrabenazine, which depletes all three monoamine neurotransmitters, may be used in more severe cases. Post-synaptic dopamine blockade may be achieved with haloperidol or pimozide.

Paralysis, ventilation and sedation may be required in severe cases of status dystonicus in order to prevent bulbar and respiratory complications and obtain 'muscles/brain resting'. Intravenous midazolam has been used as first line agent, in an ICU setting, for management of status dystonicus. Low dose propofol (iv) may be added if midazolam alone fails to control the dystonic storm. Intrathecal baclofen infusion may be required in resistant cases especially those with underlying neurodegenerative disorder. Surgical procedures like bilateral thalamotomy and deep brain stimulation may be warranted only in drug refractory cases (Figure 1).

Dystonic storm can continue for months and can be life threatening, usually requiring intensive care monitoring. It can recur in the context of a subsequent illness. The course and outcome of status dystonicus is highly variable. The prognosis is guarded and partly depends on underlying etiology.

CONCLUSIONS

Majority of acute dystonias in childhood are related to drugs and their treatment is usually straightforward. An acute CNS insult should be ruled out in an appropriate setting. In a patient with a pre-existing primary or secondary dystonia, status dystonicus is a life threatening condition and its management can be an arduous task. An approach to acute dystonias in childhood is summarized in Figure 2.

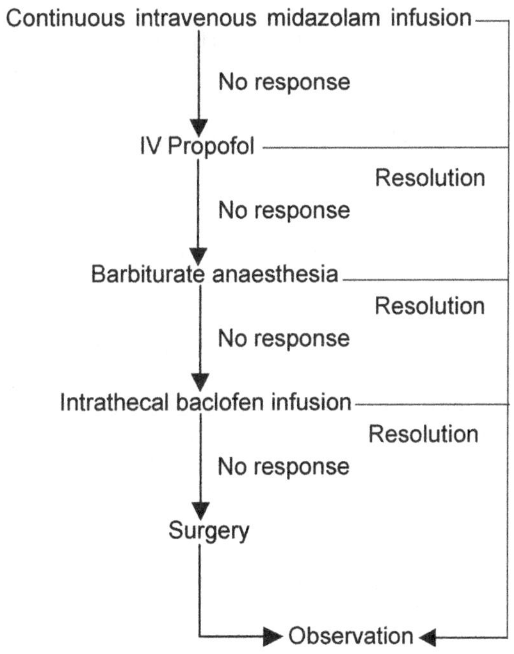

Fig. 1 : Management of status dystonicus in an ICU setting. (Serial neurological assessment is required; Monitor cardiorespiratory and renal status, fever, myoglobulinuria, CK).

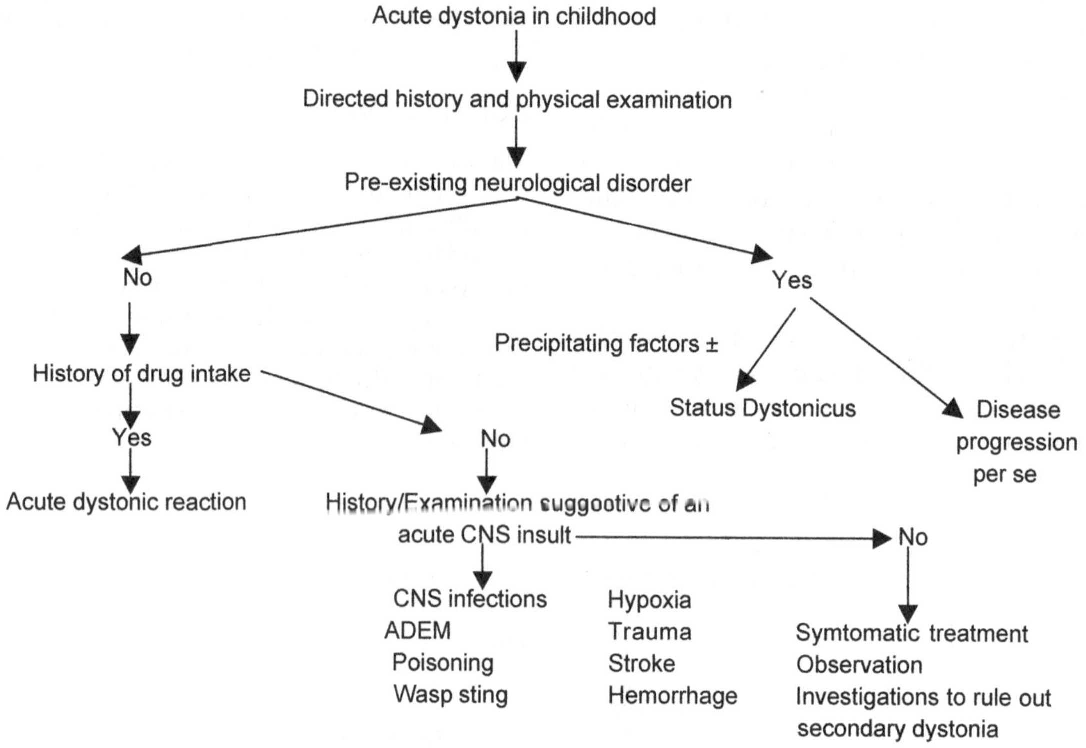

Fig. 2 : Approach to a child with acute dystonia

FURTHER READING

1. Sanger T, Mink JW. Movement disorders. In:Pediatric Neurology, Principles and Practice, Fourth edition. Elsevier 2006. p1271.
2. Fenichel GM. Movement disorders. In: Clinical Pediatric Neurology, A signs and symptoms approach, Fifth edition. Elsevier 2005. p281.
3. van Harten PN, Hoek HW, Kahn RS. Acute dystonia induced by drug treatment. Brit Med J 1999;319:623-626.
4. Manji H, Howard RS, Miller DH, et al. Status dystonicus : the syndrome and its management. Brain 1998;121:243-252.
5. Mariotti P, Fasano A, Contarino MF, et al. Management of status dystonicus : Our experience and review of the literature. Mov Ds 2007; 22:963-968.

Sunit Singhi and Pratibha Singhi

33 Syncope

Syncope is defined as sudden, brief and temporary loss of consciousness and postural tone due to an abrupt, transient, and diffuse reversible disturbance of cerebral perfusion or substrate delivery. It is usually a benign isolated event. Unconsciousness usually lasts for 1-2 minutes. The overall incidence is 0.1-0.5% in children and adolescents and 1-3% of emergency visits. The incidence peaks in adolescents. Up to 25% of pediatric and adolescent patients with sudden death have had at least one prior episode of syncope.

COMMON CAUSES

In true syncope, there is transient, acute loss of consciousness caused by a decreased cerebral blood flow secondary to vasodilation or decreased cardiac output. Neurological events such as seizures and migraine, and hysterical (pseudoloss of consciousness) may mimic syncope.

Common causes of true syncope are shown in Table. Most cases of true syncope in children are due to benign etiologies requiring minimal investigations. One-third to one-half of cases are simple vasodepressor (vasovagal) episodes. Even so, syncope may be due to a life-threatening condition in children and adolescents. Other disorders of autonomic control, including ***orthostatic hypotension, breath-holding spells, situational syncope*** (e.g. tussive syncope, micturition syncope), and ***hyperventilation*** are also common. Hysterical faints (pseudosyncope) are common in adolescents.

Table 1 : Common causes of True Syncope (Potentially life-threatening causes)

Neural-mediated syncope (NMS)	Vasovagal syncope, Autonomic mediated reflex syncope (breath-holding, coughing, micturition, defecation)
Orthostatic	Blood or fluid loss
Cardiovascular	Arrhythmias, Long QT syndrome
Congenital heart disease	
Cardiomyopathy	
Metabolic	Hypoglycemia
Hypoxic	Carbon monoxide
Neurologic	Syncopal migraine (rare; basilar artery most common), seizure

EVALUATION

The goal of the ED evaluation is to identify the rare, pediatric patient with a serious underlying disorder, while realizing that the majority of patients have probably suffered a vasovagal (vasodepressor) episode. Extensive work-ups are rarely required.

The history and physical exam are enough to suggest the most likely cause of syncope in vast majority of patients.

History

A detailed history of event is critical. This should include precipitating factors such as time of last meal, activities, environmental conditions, patient position, length of episode, seizure-like activity and details of recovery. History of recent medications, past medical history (cardiac conditions, seizures, syncope), metabolic abnormalities, and intercurrent illness is helpful. A syncopal attack is likely to be due to a serious, underlying disorder if it is associated with fall and bodily injuries, seizure-like activity; incontinence; occurs in infancy or if it is recurrent.

Patients with vasodepressor syncope usually experience a prodrome and often faint after a precipitating event. The patient is usually unconscious for only a matter of seconds, and incontinence is rare. Once awake, there may be some mild fatigue, but a true post-ictal period with decreased responsiveness and marked confusion is absent. Tonic-clonic movements if seen, usually are near the end of a syncopal episode and last for only a few seconds, while they often are more persistent and last for at least a few minutes in patients with seizures.

The history that suggests a cardiac cause includes occurrence of syncope during exertion, palpitations and/or chest pain preceding syncope, absence of prodromal warning symptoms, need for cardiopulmonary resuscitation or if the event occurred while supine. Recent onset fatigue, exercise intolerance or known structural heart disease also favour a cardiac cause. These patients may have a family history of syncope, premature or unexplained sudden death in young adults, unexplained accidents (single motor vehicle accidents, drowning), known arrhythmia, long QT syndrome, implanted cardiac device, early myocardial infarction or a seizure disorder.

On Examination

Detailed focused examination should include vitals signs, postural changes in heart rate and blood pressure, hydration, pallor, cardiac and pulmonary assessment, neurologic examination and concurrent injuries.

Patients presenting with evidence of cardiovascular disease (congestive failure, abnormal ECG), chest pain, cyanotic spells, apnea or bradycardia requiring vigorous stimulation, or focal neurologic signs, status epilepticus or meningeal irritation are at risk of life. Acute toxic ingestions, orthostatic hypotension (resistant to fluid therapy) are also indicator of a life threatening syncope.

In an unexplained syncope a Head-up Tilt (HUT) test should be done. In postural orthostatic tachycardia syndrome an increase of > 30 and ≤ 120 beats/min occur during the first 10 min of HUT. Orthostatic hypotension is diagnosed if there is a persistent decrease of more than 20mmHg systolic blood pressure or decrease of more than 10 mmHg diastolic blood pressure within 3 min after the start of HUT or standing test.

Investigation

Routine investigations have low yield. However, a 12-lead ECG is indicated in all patients. Consider chest X-ray, CBC, glucose, carboxyhemoglobin, toxicology screen, and βHCG depending on clinical evaluation. Consider neurology referral for EEG, CT, or

MRI head if patient has atypical episodes, seizures and focal CNS findings. If there is history suggestive of recurrent refractory episodes or a cardiac cause, cardiology consultation is needed for Doppler echocardiogram

Recently Zhang *et al.* (2009) have suggested a Diagnostic Protocol (Figure), by using which they were able to arrive at a diagnosis in 81% of cases while optimizing the laboratory investigations. Briefly, Step-1 of the protocol entails detailed history taking, physical examination, standing test and a standard ECG. Step-2 includes a focused clinical evaluation and laboratory investigations in patients for whom a cause of syncope is strongly suspected from initial history and examination. These tests are guided by a diagnostic hypothesis, which is based on the abnormalities found in the initial clinical assessment. Patients for whom a cause of syncope remained undertermined, after step-2 should undergo a *head-up tilt testing*.

The above diagnostic protocol of syncope developed for children and adolescents was effective and economical. Initial evaluation gave a definitive diagnosis in 59 (12.4%) and a possible diagnosis in 54 (11.4%) of 474 patients. After the first step of the diagnostic protocol, 382 patients with unexplained syncope underwent HUT testing. It revealed Vasovagal syncope in 203 (43%) cases,

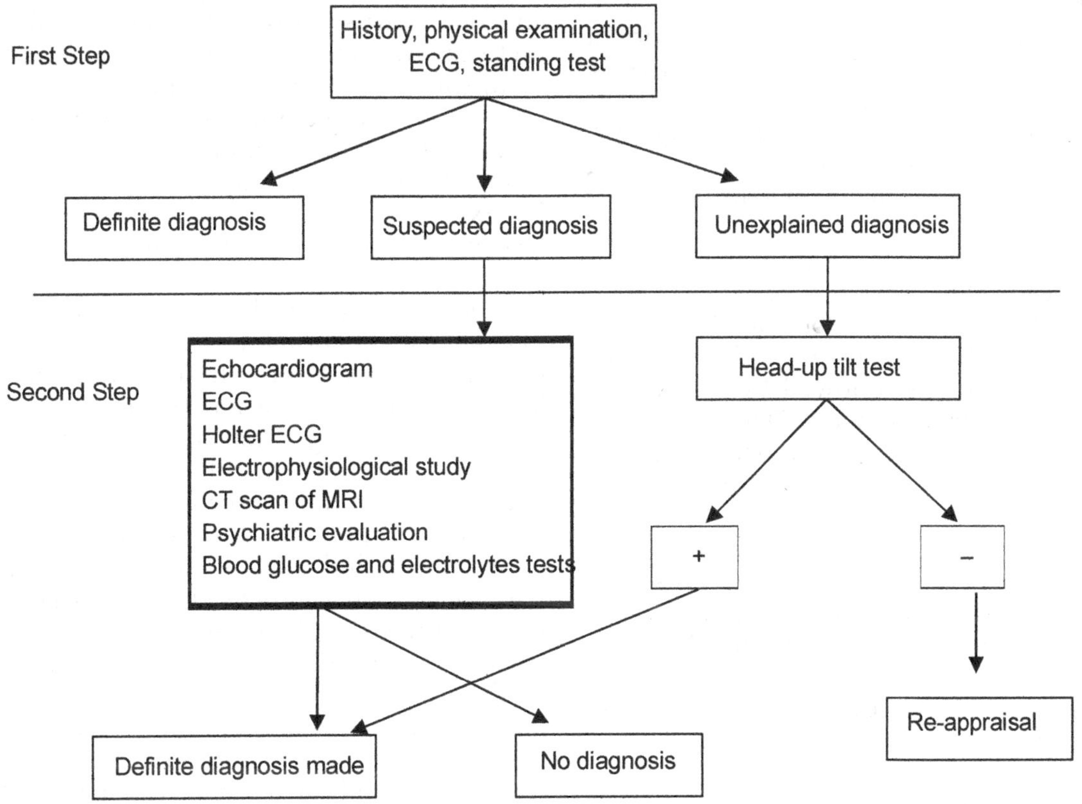

Fig. 1: Diagnostic approach suggested in a case of syncope (adapted from Zhang Q *et al.* 2009)

postural orthostatic tachycardia syndrome in 87 (27%) cases and orthostatic hypotension in three cases. A final diagnosis could not be made in 89 patients.

Vasovagal syncope (Vasodepressor syncope)

Vasovagal syncope is common in teenage females, and accounts for about 50% of childhood syncope. These patients have abnormality of reflex, which is responsible for maintaining blood pressure on standing. This results in vasodilation and vagally mediated bradycardia manifesting as rapid drop in BP and bradycardia, nausea, vomiting, sweating, pallor, numbness, blurred vision, and weakness.

The usual triggers are prolonged upright posture, warm/humid environment (crowds, hot tub, shower), intercurrent illness, over-the-counter medications, painful, emotional, fearful, or noxious stimuli such as coughing paroxysms, hair combing, micturition.

In the *prodromal phase* (lasting for seconds to minutes) the patient feels dizziness or lightheadedness, visual or hearing changes, headache, nausea or abdominal pain, warm, hot, or cold sensation and excessive sweating. This is followed by *brief loss of consciousness* (5-20 seconds). During this stage patients have a pale or ashen appearance, cold skin, profuse sweating, dilated pupils, and rarely seizure-like activity near the time of termination of the attack, The patient has no recall of the event. *Recovery period* lasts from (5-30 minutes). The patient complains of fatigue, dizziness, weakness, headache, or nausea.

Management is directed at preventing triggers.

Cardiac Syncope

Cardiac syncope is often life threatening and can lead to sudden death. It is important to rule out cardiac causes during evaluation of syncope in the emergency room. It should include consideration of following conditions:

Structurally Abnormal Heart: Cardiomyopathy (hypertrophy, restrictive, dilated), postoperative, congenital heart disease, myocarditis, congenital coronary abnormality, aortic stenosis, and pulmonary hypertension. An aberrant coronary artery that courses between the aorta and pulmonary artery can be associated with exertional syncope, due to ischemia and resulting arrhythmias.

Primary Electrical Disorder: Long QT syndrome, Wolff-Parkinson-White (WPW) syndrome, atrioventricular fibrillation, ventricular tachycardia, complete heart block, and sick sinus syndrome. Supraventricular tachycarida may cause presyncopal symptoms, and rarely true syncope. Congenital complete heart block may not become symptomatic until later childhood. Complete heart block may also be acquired. Paroxysmal episodes of ventricular tachycardia may occur in the setting of a long QT interval.

Holter monitoring should be considered in cases with abnormal ECG or echocardiographic findings. Electrophysiological study is indicated by abnormal findings from noninvasive testing. Transthoracic echocardiography findings may be diagnostic in hypertrophic cardiomyopathy with outflow obstruction, primary pulmonary artery hypertension and dilated cardiomyopathy with dilated left ventricle. Prolonged ECG monitoring using 24-h Holter monitor is useful in diagnosis of sinus pause $\geq$3s, sinus bradycardia $\leq$45 beats/min, second-degree atrioventricular block, complete atrioventricular block, nonsustained ventricular tachycardia > 5 beats/min, congenital long-QT syndrome with prolonged QT interval, relative bradycardia, T-wave abnormalities and episodic ventricular tachycardia, particularly torsades de pointes and superventricular tachycardia $\geq$ 180 beats/min

Long QT Syndrome

Long QT syndrome is diagnosed by finding a long QT interval on the patient's ECG. The QT interval must be corrected (QTc) for the patient's heart rate using Bazett's formula: QTc = (QT/ RR').

The QTc should be < 0.45 seconds in infants under 6 months of age, <0.44 seconds in children, and <0.425 seconds in adolescents. Occasionally, a patient's QTc may only become long with exertion, and exercise testing may be required to make the diagnosis.

Long QT syndrome is associated with sensorineural hearing loss and autosomal recessive inheritance in the Jervell Lange-Nielsen syndrome, and with autosomal dominant inheritance and normal hearing in the Romano-Ward syndrome. Family history of recurrent syncope, tachyarrhythmias, seizures, sudden death, and hearing loss should be ascertained.

Patients with long QT have a mortality rate of up to 70% if not treated. Immediate cardiology consultation is required. Management includes Beta-blockers for the disease, admission for further monitoring and the ECGs of family members to investigate for the familial forms. A long QT interval may be acquired in the setting of electrolyte abnormalities such as hypocalcemia.

Breath Holding Spells

Breath holding spells are a common cause of syncope in infants and toddlers. It is probably related to developmental differences in autonomic control. In cyanotic breath-holding spells, some provocation produces crying. The child develops a sustained expiration and becomes silent followed by deepening cyanosis, a loss of muscle tone, and often opisthotonus. There may be a brief period of tonic-clonic movement near the end. The child then makes an inspiratory gasp, resumes breathing and slowly awakens.

With **pallid** breath-holding spells, there is usually the abrupt onset of pallor and loss of consciousness after one to two cries. Opisthotonus is followed by relaxation and gradual awakening. Children with pallid breath-holding spells are known to develop vasodepressor syncope in later life.

Breath-holding spells associated with unconsciousness are seen in up to 5% of all children. Onset of spells is usually in the first year of life and almost always by age 2. These are benign events that resolve spontaneously, and the spells cease occurring in 50% of children by age 4, 90% by age 6, and >99% by age 8.

Micturition syncope, syncope with defecation, and syncope occurring during menses are all related to orthostatic changes. Several medications may cause orthostasis: these include antihypertensives, antidepressants, phenothiazines, sedatives, and diuretics. Tussive syncope seen in patients with pertussis and severe asthma results when coughing—respiratory spasm, and valsalva cause increased intrapleural pressure, decreased venous return, and decreased left ventricular filling.

Medications and other drugs associated with tachyarrhythmias

Nonsedating antihistamines (terfenadine and astemizole)

Cisapride

Tricyclic antidepressants

Carbamazepine (usually in overdose only)

Drug abuse- Amphetamines, Cocaine (including crack)

Syncope may be a presenting symptom of **atypical migraine**. Often there is a history of an aura and headaches. Nausea and vomiting are common. Pain is frequently unilateral and may be throbbing in nature. A family history of migraines can help make the diagnosis.

Metabolic Derangements

Hypoglycemia can cause syncope. This is rare in children after infancy, except those on insulin. A decreased level of conscious-ness due to hypoglycemia usually does not resolve spontaneously.

Pseudosyncope (hysterical faints)

Psychiatric illness considered as a potential cause of syncope includes generalized anxiety disorder, panic and somatization disorder and major depression. These are usually seen in adolescents. They typically occur in front of an audience, with an absence of physical findings. There is often eye fluttering behind half-closed eye lids. Self-protective behaviors are preserved (e.g. patients will not allow their own hand to fall and hit their face). Social history often reveals marked stress at home, in school, or in other social situations.

TREATMENT

The most effective treatment for vasovagal and orthostatic syncope is to prevent triggering events and ensure adequate fluid intake. Older children and adolescents should drink about 2 litres water and fluids daily. The patient should drink enough so that their urine remains pale and clear. Small amounts of salty food may also help to maintain intravascular volume. Counsel patients to sit or lie down when they have prodromal symptoms to prevent episodes of syncope. Cardiac syncope requires treatment of the cause.

Syncope is an uncommon emergency. The major goal in ER is to differentiate life threatening underlying syncope from the more common vasovogal syncope. History and physical examination including HUT test generally are enough to suggest the most likely cause.

FURTHER READING

- Steinberg LA, Knilans TK. Syncope in children: diagnostic tests have a high cost and low yield. J Pediatr.2005;146(3):355-358.
- Strieper M. Disinguishing benign synocope from life-threatening cardiac causes of syncope. Semin Pediatr Neurol. 2005;12(1): 32-38.
- Zhang Q , Du J ,Wang C,Du Z,Wang L,Tang C. The diagnostic protocol in children and adolescents with syncope: a multi-centre prospective study. Acta Pediatrica 2009;98:879-884.

Wayne Rutledge

34 Gastrointestinal Bleeding

Gastrointestinal bleeding can occur anywhere along the GI tract which is a highly vascularized organ that covers a large surface area. Seeing blood in the child's stool or emesis may cause significant anxiety in the parent which must be tempered to gain control of the situation. There are many causes of GI bleeding in infants and children ranging from benign disorders such as ingestion of maternal blood during birthing which require little or no treatment at all, to serious diseases such as esophageal varices that may require emergent intervention. This chapter will discuss a variety of disorders that may produce GI bleeding in infants and children.

ETIOLOGY OF BLEEDING

Acute gastrointestinal bleeding can occur from a variety of sources in pediatric patients. They can be further characterized by dividing them into 4 age groups the neonate (0 to 30 days), the infant (30 days to 2 years), the preschool child (2 to 5 years), and the school-age period (older than 5 years). This separation of age groups combined with differentiation of upper and lower bleeding sources allow better prediction of clinical course and care requirements.

Neonate

A common cause of hematemesis or passage of bloody stools in a healthy newborn is from swallowing maternal blood during delivery or while nursing.[1] One method with which to distinguish maternal blood from fetal blood is by using the Apt-alkali test. In this test, the stool is mixed with sodium hydroxide. Because fetal blood is alkaline resistant, a color change signifies the presence of maternal blood.[2] Necrotizing enterocolitis is the most important diagnosis to exclude in the neonate with rectal bleeding. This usually begins with poor feeding, diarrhea, followed by blood in the stool and the appearance of abdominal distention and pneumatosis intestinalis. Other considerations are gastric and peptic stress ulcers, hemorrhagic gastritis, Hirschsprung enterocolitis, midgut volvulus and coagulopathies such as hemorrhagic disease of the newborn and hemophilia.

Infant

Anorectal fissures are one of the most common causes of rectal bleeding in patients younger than 1 year. They are diagnosed easily by spreading the perineal skin to evert the anal canal. The history is consistent with painful defecation, constipation, grunting and streaks of blood on the stool. In addition, food allergy may lead to gastrointestinal bleeding by one of the following mechanisms: food-induced enterocolitis syndrome, food-induced colitis, and allergic eosinophilic gastroenteritis. Classic symptoms of food-induced enterocolitis syndrome include protracted vomiting and bloody diarrhea, frequently resulting in dehydration in infants younger than 3 months. Some infants may exhibit malabsorption, protein-losing enteropathy, and failure to thrive. Cow's milk and soy protein are most often the responsible agents.[3] Gastroesophageal reflux is a very common occurrence in infants and occasionally will cause reflux esophagitis with blood loss. Bowel obstruction with ischemic injury should be suspected in an infant or young child with vomiting, pain, and small amounts of blood in the stool. Intestinal volvulus and ileocolic intussusception are the most important diagnoses. Intussusception in infants is usually idiopathic or associated with lymphoid hyperplasia of the terminal ileum. Older children with intussusception should be investigated to exclude a mass lesion, such as a polyp, intestinal duplication, or Meckel's diverticulum.[4] The child with intussusception typically presents with colicky abdominal pain, vomiting, palpable sausage-shaped abdominal mass, and passage of "currant jelly stool" Volvulus is characterized by bilious vomiting, abdominal distension, and sometimes melena; the latter results from mucosal injury secondary to ischemia of the volvulized bowel.[5] Meckel's diverticulum, a congenital remnant of the vitellointestinal duct described by Meckel in 1809, is the most important source of small bowel hemorrhage in children. It obeys the rule of 2s: present in 2% of the population, located 2 feet from the ileocecal valve, and bleeding in children younger than 2 years of age. The diverticulum arises on the antimesenteric border of the ileum and is lined by ileal mucosa that frequently contains ectopic gastric or pancreatic tissue. Bleeding occurs because of peptic ulceration of ectopic gastric tissue within the diverticulum or adjacent ileum or because of ischemic injury accompanying intussusception. Diagnosis is by radionuclide scan (technetium 99m-pertechnetate) or surgical exploration. Treatment is surgical resection.[4] Other causes of GI bleeding in this age group include lymphonodular hyperplasia of the colon, intestinal arteriovenous malformations, and hemangiomas.

Preschool Child

Beyond infancy the most common cause of GI bleeding is juvenile polyps and infectious enterocolitis, however infectious enterocolitis can present with bloody stool at any age.[6] Important bacterial pathogens include Salmonella, Shigella, Campylobacter, Yersinia enterocolitica, Clostridium difficile, and Escherichia coli (0157:H7).[7] Entamoeba histolytica is the most important parasitic pathogen. One of the most serious complications and causes of GI bleeding from E. coli enterocolitis is Hemolytic Uremic Syndrome. Hemolytic-uremic syndrome is characterized by a triad of microangiopathic hemolytic anemia, thrombocytopenia, and acute renal failure.[8] Abdominal pain, vomiting, and bloody diarrhea frequently precede the illness. Lower gastrointestinal hemorrhage can result from small-vessel occlusion and mucosal ischemia of the intestine.[5] Henoch-Schönlein purpura is an immunologically mediated systemic vasculitis of small blood vessels that primarily involves the skin, gastrointestinal tract, joints, and kidneys. Gastrointestinal manifestations occur in 45 to 75% of cases and include vomiting, colicky abdominal pain, and melena or bloody stools. Bloody stools often result from diffuse mucosal hemorrhage. Intussusception associated with Henoch-Schönlein purpura can also cause gastrointestinal bleeding. Gastrointestinal symptoms precede the appearance of the purpura in upto 15% of patients.[9] Beyond infancy, juvenile polyps are the most common source of significant rectal bleeding and typically present with intermittent painless hematochezia in children 2 to 5 years of age.[4] Most of these polyps are solitary and located within 30 cm of the anus. The diagnosis is made by digital rectal examination, barium enema, sigmoidoscopy or colonoscopy.[10] Variceal bleeding caused by portal hypertension is a serious complication of chronic liver disease. Bleeding from esophageal varices usually is brisk and associated with significant hematemesis. Portal hypertension may occur from liver cirrhosis or other extrahepatic causes. Endoscopy is the treatment of choice for diagnosis and treatment.

School-aged Child

The range of disorders in school-aged children with lower gastrointestinal bleeding is similar to that of the preschool children with the addition of inflammatory bowel disease. Mild limited colitis in a child can present with minor amounts of rectal bleeding without a history of diarrhea, urgency, pain, or other clinical signs of colitis. Severe hemorrhage may ensue with progression to severe diffuse disease and transmural extension into deeper vascularized layers of the bowel wall or focal deep ulceration.[4] Diarrhea, abdominal pain, weight loss, and fever are common presenting symptoms. The diagnosis is confirmed with colonoscopy and biopsy. Although rare in this age group, colon cancer may present as unexplained rectal bleeding and should be considered as part of the differential.[11]

CLINICAL PRESENTATION

The clinical history is very important and should include information concerning the time course, estimated blood loss, and any associated symptoms such as dyspepsia, heartburn, abdominal pain and weight loss. In infants, these features may be evidenced by poor feeding and irritability. The history should include organ system function information, such as recent onset of jaundice, easy bruising, and change in stool color, which may suggest underlying liver disease. The age of the child is also important as certain causes of GI bleeding are seen more commonly in specific age groups, but considerable overlap exists. At all ages, stress (burns, central nervous system trauma) and ingestion of aspirin or nonsteroidal anti-inflammatory drugs (NSAIDs) may lead to gastric or duodenal stress erosions and ulcerations.[10] The physician must then determine if the patient has bled. Many substances ingested by children that can mimic blood include red food coloring, fruit juices and beets. Stools may become black following ingestion of iron, bismuth containing products, spinach or blueberries. The vomitus or gastric aspirate can be tested for blood using gastroccult and the stool by guiac or hemoccult.

It is then important to determine the location of the bleeding into either upper GI bleeding or lower GI bleeding. Upper GI bleeding is defined as bleeding above the ligament of treitz, whereas, lower GI bleeding is defined as bleeding below the ligament of treitz. Hematemesis can be seen with bright red blood indicating a high flow rate bleed or as coffee ground emesis indicating a slow bleed or bleeding that has stopped. This also may result from the placement of a nasogastric tube resulting in localized trauma which can cause a small amount of blood in the gastric aspirate. Melena and hematochezia can be seen in either upper or lower GI tract bleeds. Melena refers to the passage of black tarry stools from the rectum, which usually indicates upper GI bleed or bleeding from the proximal small bowel. Hematochezia refers to the passage of bright red blood per rectum. It usually suggests lower gastrointestinal bleed (typically from the colon or rectum) but can occur rarely with a massive upper GI bleed.

Once a focused history is taken it is important to obtain a good physical exam to determine if the child needs immediate stabilization and to investigate potential sites of bleeding. In a child, age adjusted tachycardia is the most sensitive indicator of acute, severe blood loss.[4] Hypotension, delayed capillary refill and lethargy are ominous signs of severe hypovolemia and shock.[4] The evaluation should include a nasopharyngeal exam to look for inflamed tonsils or excoriated nasal mucosa from nose picking. Jaundice or scleral icterus may indicate a chronic or acute liver disease. The skin should be examined for purpura, telangiectasias or petechiae. The abdominal exam is of particular significance whereas a distended abdomen may indicate organome-galy or ascites as seen in liver disease or portal hypertension. The rectal exam can indicate presence of melena or hematochezia, fissures or polyps and to obtain stool for guiac testing.

ANCILLARY EVALUATION

Measuring hemoglobin and hematocrit levels will assist the clinician in determining the severity of bleeding and in deciding when or whether the patient will require transfusion. If the bleeding is profuse then a type and cross-match would be required. A low platelet count may indicate chronic liver disease with portal hypertension, sepsis or hemolytic-uremic syndrome.[5] Prolonged prothrombin and partial thromboplastin times may be seen in liver disease, hemophilia, disseminated intravascular coagulation and vitamin K deficiency (seen in cystic fibrosis). Eosinophilia may signify milk allergy or parasitic infestation.[12] An increase in the blood urea nitrogen in the absence of kidney disease would indicate an upper GI bleed rather than a lower GI bleed where the blood has more time to be absorbed. Liver function tests confirm hepatocellular disease and billiary dysfunction. Stool evaluation for leukocytes, bacterial culture, viral culture, ova and parasites, and clostridium difficile toxin should be considered in patients with bloody diarrhea. A urinalysis should be performed if Henoch-Schönlein purpura or hemolytic-uremic syndrome is suspected. Supine and upright abdominal radiographs may identify signs of intestinal obstruction or air outside the GI tract. Pneumatosis intestinalis is characteristically seen in necrotizing enterocolitis.[5]

TREATMENT

The treatment is outlined in Fig. 1. Treatment should begin with airway protec-tion. If the patient is vomiting uncontrollably and unable to protect the airway then intubation should be considered as this will help prevent aspiration and also to help facilitate upper endoscopy should it be necessary for bleeding control. Adequate oxygen delivery with supplemental oxygen and large bore venous access should be obtained to restore blood volume. Peripheral venous access may be difficult to achieve in a small child or a child in hypovolemic shock due to peripheral vasoconstriction, therefore, central venous

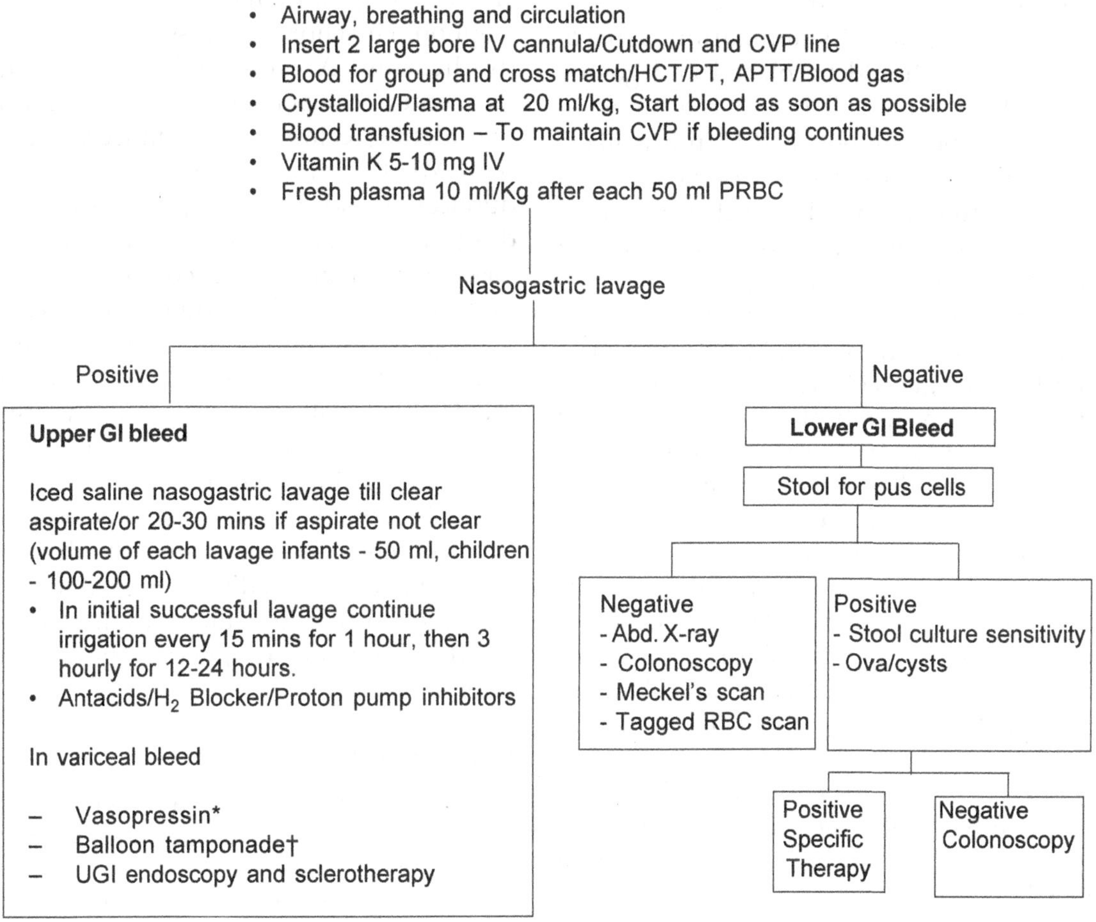

* Dose – infusion in 5% dextrose 0.1 unit/minute – Increase by 0.05 unit/minute hourly upto maximum 0.2 Unit/min upto 5 years, 0.3 Unit/min 6-12 years, 0.6 Unit/min in adolescents.
Side effect – Myocardial ischemia, arrhythmia, limb vasoconstriction, sodium and water retention.

† Only in endoscopically confirmed varices, indicated in: (1) Massive life-threatening blood, and (2) Continued bleeding despite 4-6 hours of vasopressin.

Fig. 1: Outline of treatment of GI bleed in a child

access, venous cut-downs or intraosseus access should be considered for large volume resuscitation. Correction of coagulopathies and any life-threatening electrolyte or metabolic disturbances is vital in initial stabilization. If the child is in profound shock then uncross-matched blood O-negative should be considered, especially if patient shows signs of active bleeding.

Following initial stabilization, a nasogastric tube should be placed and gastric contents aspirated. If bright red blood or coffee-grounds are obtained then it is likely an upper GI bleed, however, absence of blood does not rule out bleeding just distal to the pyloris.[10] A saline lavaged may be carried out if fresh blood is present.

If an upper GI source is found then acid suppression therapy should be initiated to neutralize gastric acid secretion. An intravenous infusion of a histamine 2 (H_2) receptor antagonist or a proton pump inhibitor is used to decrease gastric acidity.[13] Medications that induce visceral vasoconstriction, such octreotide[14] or vasopressin,[15] may be useful for suspected active variceal bleeding. Both are tolerated well by children, but octreotide may be the drug of choice because of equal efficacy and lack of significant side effects.[4] If bleeding is severe then a gastroenterologist and a surgeon should be consulted. Endoscopic therapy is the treatment of choice for children with active bleeding and high risk of recurrent bleeding. After stabilization of the patient's condition, endoscopic evaluation remains the most rapid and accurate method to identify the origin of acute bleeding in the majority of lesions in the pediatric age group.[16] In addition, it allows for risk stratification regarding the likelihood of continued bleeding, and permits therapeutic intervention.

If a lower GI source is found, the same stabilization measures apply. Rectosigmoidoscopy or colonoscopy is the procedure of choice if the cause is still obscure and the bleeding is not brisk. Colonoscopy is helpful in the diagnosis of colitis or inflammatory bowel disease, polyps, lymphonodular hyperplasia and arteriovenous malformations. Barium enema is helpful in the diagnosis of intussusception, Hirschprung's disease and colonic duplication. A radionuclide scan using technetium-99m pertechnetate (Meckel scan), will identify ectopic gastric mucosa located in a Meckel diverticulum or intestinal duplication and should be performed if such diagnosis is suspected.[17] Patients with vascular anomalies may require excision of focal lesions (e.g., blue rubber bleb nevus) or surgical resection or exclusion of a larger segment of involved bowel (e.g., rectosigmoid venous malformation)[18] Surgery is most often indicated for bleeding resulting from nonreducible intussusception or a vascular anomaly.[19] Stool cultures should be obtained as infectious causes are frequently identified with a lower GI bleeding source. Antibiotic therapy can then be guided by the culture results for a more specific therapeutic intervention.[20]

REFERENCES

1. Bulstrode NW Cuckow PM, Spitz LS. Neonatal gastrointestinal pseudo-haemorrhage. J R Coll Surg Edinb 1998; 43: 355.
2. Silber G. Lower gastrointestinal bleeding. Pediatr Rev 1990; 12: 85–93.
3. Leung AK. Food allergy: a clinical approach. Adv Pediatr 1998; 45: 145–177.
4. Fox, Victor L. Gastrointestinal Bleeding in Infancy and Childhood. Gastroenterology Clinics - Volume 29, Issue 1 (March 2000), W. B. Saunders Company.
5. Leung, Alexander K.C.; Wong, Andrew L. Lower gastrointestinal bleeding in children.

Special Features: CME Review Article. Lippincott Williams & Wilkins, Inc. 2002 Volume 18(4), pp 319- 323.
6. Chhabra RS, Glaser JH: Salmonella infection presenting as hematochezia on the first day of life. Pediatrics 1994; 94: 739-741.
7. Philpott DJ, Ismaili A, Sherman PM: Enterohemorrhagic Escherichia coli O157:H7 infection and colitis in children. J Pediatr Gastroenterol Nutr 1997; 24: 623-625.
8. Robson WL, Leung AK, Kaplan BS. Hemolytic-uremic syndrome. Curr Probl Pediatr 1993; 23:16–33.
9. Robson WL, Leung AK. Henoch-Schönlein purpura. Adv Pediatr 1994; 41 : 163–194.
10. Brown Marilyn R., Oski's Pediatrics : Principles & Practice, Lippincott Williams & Wilkins, editor-in-chief, Julia A. McMillan; editors, Ralph D. Feigin, Catherine D. DeAngelis, M. Douglas Jones, JR.— 4th ed. Section VII 2006; 346:1928-32.
11. Kravarusic D, Feigin E, Dlugy; E, *et al.* Colorectal carcinoma in childhood: A retrospec-tive multicenter study. J Pediatr Gastroenterol Nutr 2007; 44 : 209.
12. Hill SM, Milia PJ. Colitis caused by food allergy in infants. Arch Dis Child 1990; 65:132–133.
13. Kelly DA: Do H_2 receptor antagonists have a therapeutic role in childhood? J Pediatr Gastroenterol Nutr; 1994 19:270-276.
14. Siafakas C, Fox VL, Nurko S: Use of octreotide for the treatment of severe gastrointestinal bleeding in children. J Pediatr Gastroenterol Nutr 1998; 26:356-359.
15. Tuggle DW, Bennett KG, Scott J, *et al*: Intravenous vasopressin and gastrointestinal hemorrhage in children. J Pediatr Surg 1988; 23:627-629.
16. Kay Marsha H; Wyllie Robert: Therapeutic Endoscopy for Nonvariceal Gastrointestinal Bleeding. Lippincott Williams & Wilkins, Inc. Volume 2007;45(2), August 2007, p 157–171.
17. Kester RR, Welch JP, Sziklas JP. The 99m Tc-labelled RBC scan. A diagnostic method for lower gastrointestinal bleeding. Dis Colon Rectum 1984; 27:47–52.
18. Fishman SJ, Burrows PE, Leichtner AM, *et al*: Gastrointestinal manifestations of vascular anomalies in childhood: Varied etiologies require multiple therapeutic modalities. J Pediatr Surg 1998; 33:1163-1167.
19. Ein SH, Alton D, Palder SB, *et al.*: Intussusception in the 1990's: Has 25 years made a difference? Pediatr Surg Int 1997; 12:374-376.
20. Fisher David, Synopsis of Pediatric Emergency Care: Part VI Chapter 20, 179-183.

In the previous edition this chapter was written by David Fisher, MD
Clinical Assistant Professor Surgery/Emergency Medicine Staff Physician
Deaconess Hospital Emergency Department, Oklahoma City, Oklahoma

John J. Fraser and Edwsin Ide Smith

35 Acute Abdominal Pain

Twenty percent of all children will seek medical help for abdominal pain by the age of 15 years. It is estimated that 5 percent of the group will require hospitalization or surgical intervention. A study of patients 2 to 16 years of age, seen in a pediatric emergency facility for acute abdominal pain, found that nine diagnoses accounted for 84 percent of the patients seen. Medical conditions accounted for 56.5 percent, surgical 8.5 percent, and non-specific abdominal pain 35 percent. Appendicitis was the only surgical condition to appear in more than 1 percent of the patients. Patients with severe pain lasting more than six hours have a high probability of having a condition requiring surgical therapy.

Appropriate diagnosis depends on the basic tools—clinical history and physical examination aided or confirmed by appropriate laboratory and radiological studies. Early diagnosis is reflected in lessened morbidity and mortality. In the appropriate management of the pediatric patient with acute abdominal pain, it is necessary that an attempt be made to make a defensible tentative. diagnosis and that operation is not considered on the basis that the abdomen represents a "surgical abdomen" with the disease and site unspecified. Early surgical consultation is of value in order that several examinations over time are possible. Progression of the disease can be appreciated at an earlier stage.

PATHOPHYSIOLOGY

Acute abdominal pain arises from three nervous pathways: parietal, referred, and visceral. Parietal pain is the "first pain" which is carried by somatic nerves. This somatic pain can be cutaneous, superficial, or deep pain from muscles or tendons. The retroperitoneal, retroileal area beneath the mesentery and the pelvic areas do not generate parietal pain, and are "silent areas". Referred pain occurs when pain fibers converge on a spinal tract or higher with resultant pain in the referred area. An example is the shoulder pain with diaphragmatic irritation. Visceral pain is carried by sympathetic and parasympathetic fibers and is poorly localized. Visceral pain may be caused by ischemia, some chemical mediators as in inflammation or trauma, stretching and distension, and extremes of thermal change.

While the pathophysiology of the various conditions causing acute abdominal pain varies, several generalizations are present. Organs inflamed either primarily or secondarily by contact tend first to hyperfunction and then to hypofunction. Trauma or inflammation within the free peritoneal cavity tends to produce gastrointestinal symptoms and signs. Obstruction of a tubular organ causes hypertrophy and enlargement proximally and usually results in emptying distally. Colicky pain is usually associated with obstruction, while constant pain is associated with ischemia and necrosis.

The anatomy of the peritoneal cavity and its organs is important in the interpretation of signs and symptoms. In general the pain representation of the stomach and small intestine tend to be supraumbilical, with the appendix and the large bowel being infraumbilical.

CLINICAL PRESENTATION

The clinical presentations of the common conditions causing acute abdominal pain in infants and children are shown in Figure 1. The first three considerations for the clinician are (1) the age of the patient; (2) the duration and the severity of the pain; and (3) the presence of other gastrointestinal, urinary, respiratory, and genitourinary signs and symptoms.

DIFFERENTIAL DIAGNOSIS

Infants (Newborn to Two Years of Age)

The major differential diagnosis in the infant (not the neonate) includes medical conditions such as acute viral or bacterial (Shigella, Salmonella) gastroenteritis, pneumonia, colic, milk allergy, and constipation with a localized impaction. The primary surgical conditions to rule out are midgut volvulus associated with incomplete rotation and intussusception.

Acute volvulus usually presents in the first year of life with over half of the patients being under 30 days of life. The onset is usually sudden with bilious vomiting, apparent pain, and abdominal distension. With vascular compromise, a bloody stool may be passed. The patient can progress rapidly to hypovolemia and shock. Babies with midgut volvulus tend to appear ill. The abdomen is distended and firm. Anemia from intraluminal bleeding is common. Usually a contrast study from below delineates the volvulus and incomplete rotation.

Intussusception usually occurs in a previously well infant who is a good eater and often has the history of a recent viral infection. Fifty percent of patients with intussusception are 6 to 12 months of age, and 85 percent are seen before the age of 2 years. Characteristically the infant begins with intermittent colicky pain during which the legs are drawn up. The intermittent episodes of pain become more frequent and severe. A bloody or "currant jelly" stool may be passed. On examination, a sausage-shaped mass may be palpated in the right side or upper abdomen. Listlessness and lethargy are also frequent in babies with intussusception. The majority of intussusceptions are ileocolic and idiopathic. Lead points such as a Meckel's diverticulum or ileocecal lymphoma are more common in older children. A contrast study is necessary for the diagnosis and may achieve therapeutic reduction. Contraindications for a contrast study are pneumatosis, signs of peritoneal irritation, and possibly symptoms lasting longer than 48 hours.

Incarcerated inguinal hernia is also common, and often difficult to see immediately in well-nourished infants.

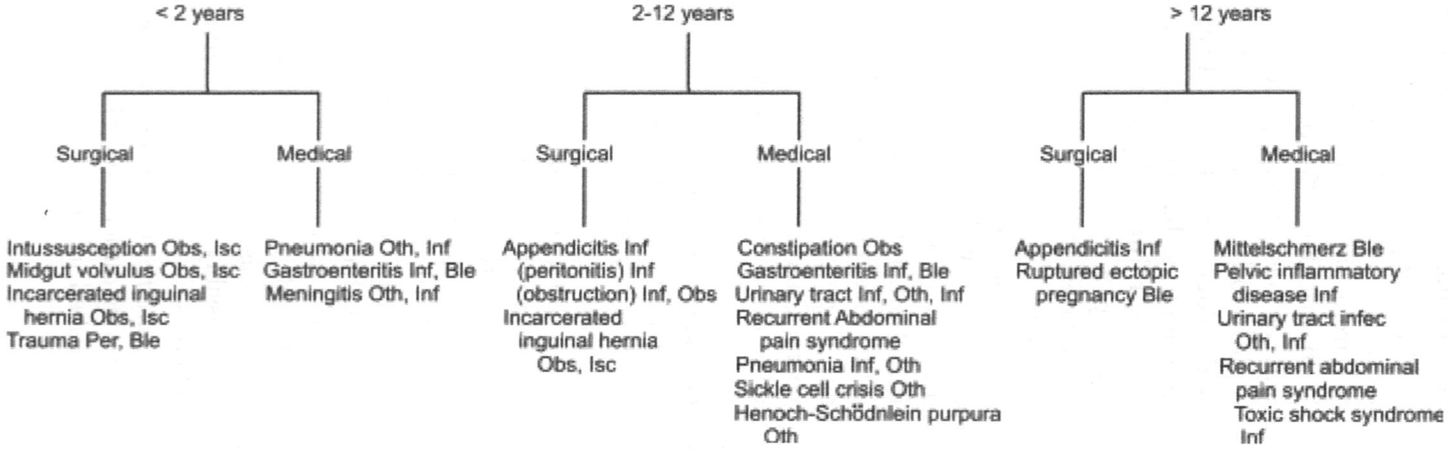

Fig. 1: Acute abdominal pain, clinical presentation by age (Inf = Inflammation [pain, hyperfunction-hypofunction, fever], Obs = Obstruction [pain, vomiting, absence stools], Oth = Other [respiratory, urinary], Isc = Ischemia [pain, blood GI tract], Ble = Bleeding [pain, anemia, hypovolemia], Per = Perforation [pain, fever])

Children (2 to 12 Years of Age)

In this age group, acute appendicitis is the chief surgical condition to be ruled out. Trauma in childhood is very often occult and should be considered even in the absence of a positive history. Medical conditions include constipation, acute viral or bacterial enteritis, urinary tract infections, recurrent abdominal pain syndrome, pneumonia, sickle cell disease, and Henoch-Schönlein purpura. Apley has pointed out that 10 percent of all children have recurrent abdominal pain.

In *acute appendicitis* in childhood, the classic time sequence of abdominal pain followed by vomiting may be altered. Twenty percent of children with acute appendicitis have been found to have a history of recent respiratory or gastrointestinal infection in the two previous weeks, and 24 percent had symptoms on admission. The physical examination is the key to the diagnosis of acute appendicitis.

Adolescents (More Than 12 Years of Age)

Appendicitis remains a major consideration, but with the onset of puberty, gynecological considerations become important in the adolescent female and include mittelschmerz or bleeding from a follicle cyst, pelvic inflammatory disease with tubo-ovarian abscess, and ectopic pregnancy. Biliary tract disease and inflammatory bowel disease must also be included in the differential diagnosis.

HISTORY AND PHYSICAL EXAMINATION

Taking the history from the child depends considerably on age. Many times the second hand history of the parent must be relied upon, a history that varies in accuracy. The onset of the present illness begins with the change from a well to a different child. The nature of the abdominal pain and its onset are important as is any means of relief. Sudden pain with a bump in the road is a good sign of peritoneal irritation. Disturbances of gastrointestinal (GI) function such as anorexia, vomiting, and alteration of bowel function are common in acute appendicitis.

Small children have no significant omentum, and they may have diarrhea or dysuria with an inflamed appendix that is adherent to the ileum (high-output diarrhea), the sigmoid (low-output diarrhea), or the bladder (dysuria, retention). Localization of pain in the small child is often not exact. Midline and even left-sided symptoms can be seen.

The physical examination should be complete. The critical examinations should be performed first and the troublesome examinations such as the pharyngeal and rectal last. It helps to sit down as one examines a small child, thus removing some of the scariness. Inspection of the child is valuable-sick or not, moving actively or lying quite still. Combative and hyperactive children rarely have peritonitis in which case they are more likely to remain still and to resist movement. Inspection of the conjunctivae, the skin, and the mucous membranes is very helpful with the viral infections, Henoch-Schönlein purpura, and streptococcal disease. The abdomen is examined for distension, for visible loops of bowel, and for an incarcerated inguinal hernia. Palpation should be very gentle, and the avoidance of pain is critical to a successful examination. It often helps to start with the child pointing to the area of greatest pain. Very light palpation is performed using the two sides of the abdomen as controls. Eight points, upper and lower rectus bilaterally, upper outer muscle groups, and lower outer muscle groups, are palpated. The degree of rigidity and/or spasm on one side is compared with the other side. Guarding and abdominal tenderness are the most important findings in acute appendicitis (2). Percussion is used in preference to rebound tenderness to elicit peritoneal irritation. While palpating or percussing the child, the eyes and face are carefully observed as indicative of a positive response. Bowel sounds are of limited value.

There are three rules for the diagnosis of appendicitis: (1) The abdominal examination in acute appendicitis should equal the vital signs of pulse, respiration, and blood pressure (rule of relativity). (2) Peritonitis in the child is acute appendicitis until it is proven otherwise. (3) Intestinal obstruction in the child without a history of an abdominal operation is acute appendicitis until it is proven otherwise.

The rectal examination is of greatest importance in demonstration of a mass or a fecal impaction and of less importance in determining tenderness. The male genitalia should be carefully examined. Both testis should be carefully palpated as torsion of an undescended testis may present with abdominal pain.

LABORATORY EVALUATION

Blood studies should include a routine complete blood count (CBC) with a differential and a sickle cell preparation when one is indicated. Although extremes in the leukocyte count may be helpful, this count is often not helpful in the difficult diagnostic situation. White blood cell counts (WBC) of 15,000 to 18,000/mm^3 are not uncommon with gastroenteritis. A routine urinalysis is necessary to look for ketonuria, glycosuria, bacturia and pyuria. Routine electrolytes and a blood urea nitrogen (BUN) should be performed in patients who have had significant vomiting or who are dehydrated. A pregnancy test is advised for all female patients past puberty.

Radiological and Other Special Studies

The radiological examination is quite helpful, particularly in the smaller child; however, it is not necessary in every case. Specific abdominal findings in appendicitis are an appendiceal fecolith and intraluminal appendiceal air. Non-specific signs are a generalized or localized ileus, scoliosis concave to the right, masses, and extraluminal air in an abscess. The abdominal roentgenogram also gives information concerning the location of the cecum. If a fecal impaction is suspected in the absence of acute peritoneal irritation, a low saline or hypertonic enema can be given. Pneumonia in a dehydrated child may show little X-ray evidence of consolidation until rehydration has occurred.

Ultrasonography is used increasingly in the diagnosis of acute abdominal pain in children and adolescents. It had a sensitivity of 89 percent and a specificity of 92 percent in one study. It proves most helpful in the patient with an unclear diagnosis, particularly in the adolescent female where there is high accuracy in delineating gynecological disease.

Barium enema examination of the child with abdominal pain may also be employed where the diagnosis is not clear. Complete filling of the appendix should exclude acute appendicitis, but it is often difficult to determine the entire extent of the appendix.

MANAGEMENT

The management of the patients with abdominal pain depends on the urgency of treatment, particularly that involving an operation (Figure 2). In some patients, the diagnosis can be made readily and a treatment plan formulated. An example of this would be a midgut volvulus where an emergency operation would be clearly indicated. A second group of patients will have a tentative diagnosis but will need stabilization and observation prior to surgical correction. The major areas that may need correction are fluid deficits, infection and pain. A third group of patients remain with an unclear diagnosis and require observation within the emergency department or in the hospital. These patients require several points

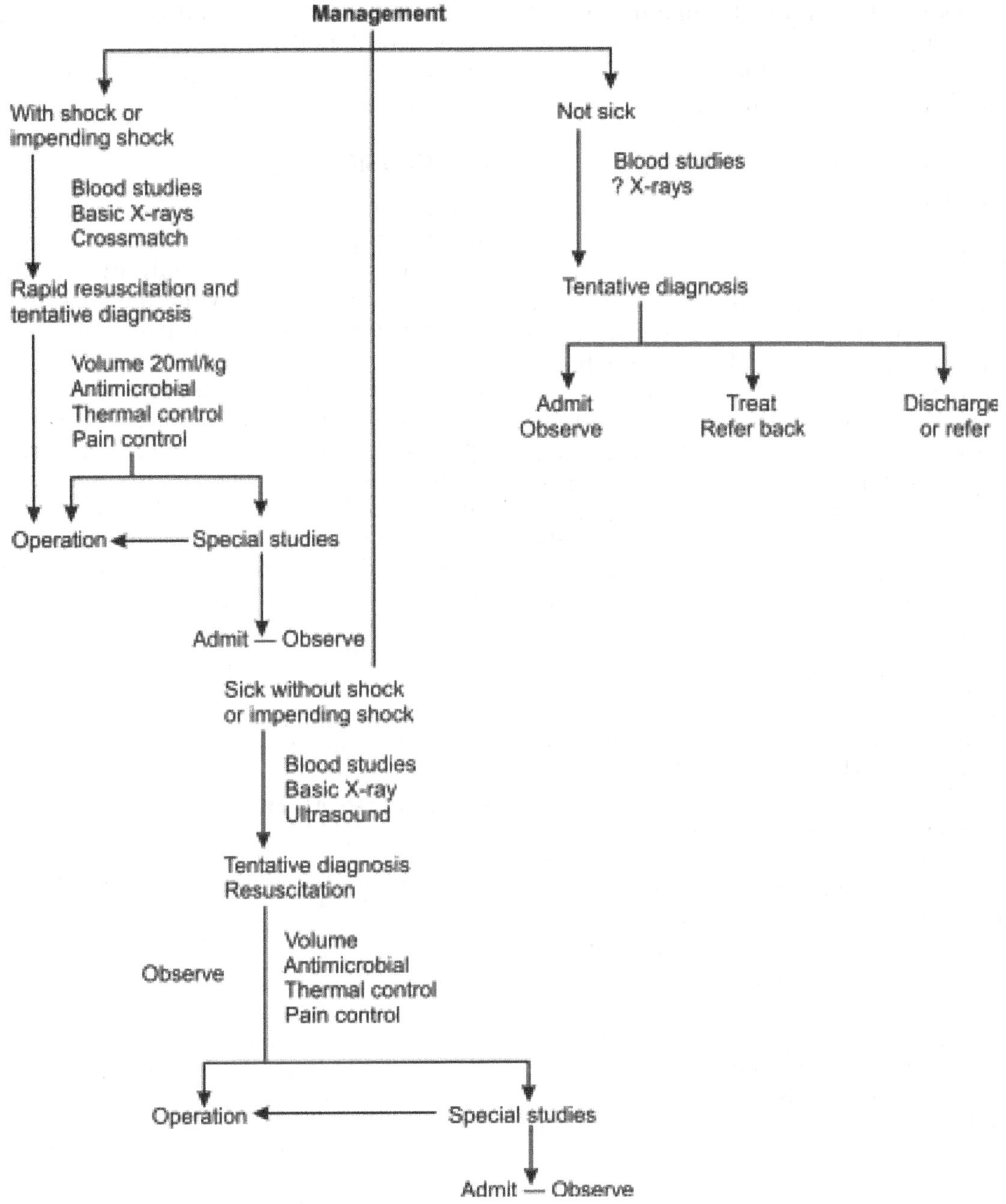

Fig. 2: Acute abdominal pain

on their "illness curve" to clarify their probable diagnosis.

Resuscitation should proceed concomitant with diagnosis. When the patient is dehydrated and perhaps hypovolemic, initial resuscitation with intravenous fluids either

Ringer's lactate or normal saline dependent on site of lossor with colloid is begun early, usually 20ml/kg as a bolus. Analgesia should be withheld until a tentative working diagnosis is established. Temperature elevation is controlled with rectal or oral acetaminophen.

Infant

Resuscitation of the infant is doubly important as fluid losses and hypovolemia can produce hypovolemic shock. These should be initiated prior to special studies. Observation of some infants may be necessary to rule out an intraperitoneal process. Sedation of the infant will often make demonstration of the abdominal mass possible. If hospitalization is planned, the earlier the patient can be transferred to the nursing unit the more desirable it is for the infant.

Child

Resuscitation again should be started promptly. Short periods of observation to assist in diagnosis are important. Where exploration for possible appendicitis has been decided on, antibiotics should begun. Choice of drugs should provide both gram negative and positive coverage. Addition of a drug effective against anaerobic infection is necessary where an abscess or diffuse peritonitis exists.

The patient should be made NPO *(nil per os)*, have a nasogastric tube inserted and have intravenous (IV) fluids begun. Temperatures should be taken axillarily or orally if there is a pelvic abscess.

Adolescent

In management of the adolescent, appropriate attention should be given to the special needs. Often sedation and observation are very helpful. In the adolescent, female use of ultrasonography to examine the adnexae can be particularly helpful.

CONCLUSIONS

The diagnosis and management of acute abdominal pain in children and adolescents continues to pose a challenge to the emergency physician. While the majority of the patients seen will probably have nonsurgical disease, often self-limited, the identification of patients with surgical or probably surgical disease, particularly acute appendicitis, is critical. One hundred percent accuracy is not possible, and one should err on the side of inclusion into the surgical group. Ancillary laboratory and diagnostic technological examinations are adjunctive and should be used to support or to rule out tentative diagnoses that have been made on the basis of the history and physical findings. Age is a major determinant of the probable cause of the symptom sign complex with which the patient presents.

FURTHER READING

1. Buchert GS. Abdominal pain in children: An emergency practitioner's guide. Emer Med Clin NA 1989;7:497-517.
2. Apley J. The child with abdominal pains. Springfield, Ill.: Charles C Thomas, 1959.
3. Scholer SJ, Pituch K, Orr DP, Dittus RS. Clinical outcomes of children with acute abdominal pain. Pediatrics 1996; 98 (4 Pt 1) : 680-5.
4. Carrico CW, Fenton LZ, Taylor GA, *et al.* Impact of sonography on the diagnosis and treatment of acute lower abdominal pain in children and young adults. AJR Am J Roentgenol 1999 Feb; 172(2): 513-6.
5. Erkan T, Cam H, Ozkan HC, Kiray E, *et al.* Clinical spectrum of acute abdominal pain in Turkish pediatric patients: A prospective study. Pediatr Int 2004; 46(3): 325-9.

6. Loening-Baucke V, Swidsinski A. Constipation as cause of acute abdominal pain in children. J Pediatr 2007 Dec; 151 (6): 666-9. Epub 2007 Jul 30.
7. Tseng YC, Lee MS, Chang YJ, Wu HP. Acute abdomen in pediatric patients admitted to pediatric emergency department. Pediatr neonatol 2008; 49(4): 126-34.
8. Bundy DG, Byerley JS, Liles EA, *et al.* Does this child have appendicitis? JAMA 2007 Jul 25; 298 (4): 438 -51.
9. Waseem M, Rosenberg HK. Intussusception. Pediatr Emerg Care 2008; 24 (11): 793-800.

In the previous edition this chapter was written by Edwin Ide Smith, MD Professor of Surgery, Chairman–Division of Pediatric Surgery, University of Texas Southwestern Medical Center Dallas, Texas

Puneet Jain and Alka Khadwal

36 Excessive Crying and Irritability

Excessive crying is the most common reason for seeking medical attention in the first three months of life. Although the prevalence of excessive crying varies by definition employed, the peak nevertheless occurs during the second month of life with a prevalence of 1.5% to 11.9%. The epidemiology of serious illness in infants who present to the emergency department with a chief complaint of excessive crying is unknown. Parental misconception may account for some complaints of excessive crying.

Infants communicate and express discomfort by crying. Crying, by stimulating and distressing the parents or caretakers, assures survival of the helpless infant. As demands of crying are met, conditioning occurs and infant-parent bonding is established. Healthy children cry on average nearly 3 hours per day at 6 weeks of age with the peak occurring between 3 PM and 11 PM. By the time parents present to the emergency department with their crying child, caregivers are often anxious, frustrated, and sleep deprived. These emotions contribute to making the evaluation of the nonverbal, crying infant very difficult. Many clinicians feel pressured by anxious parents to do something and this may lead to overdiagnosis and over treatment.

DEFINITION

No consensus has been reached on the definition of excessive crying. The available definitions mostly concern the duration of infant crying or its effects on the parents. Regarding duration, the widely accepted definition is that of Wessel which distinguishes between "fussy" and "seriously fussy" children. A 'fussy' infant was defined as one who, otherwise healthy and well-fed, had paroxysms of irritability, fussing or crying lasting for a total of more than three hours a day and occurring on more than three days in any one week. A 'Seriously fussy'infant is the one whose paroxysms continued to recur for more than 3 weeks, or became so severe that the pediatrician felt that medication was indicated.

A variety of definitions has been used regarding the effect of infant crying on parents, , such as to what extent parents are able to console their child, think that their child is colicky or cries a lot, seek professional help or experience the crying of their infant as problematic.

COMMON CAUSES

Crying in infants is most commonly due to hunger, thirst, discomfort and even boredom. Typically, parents are able to identify accurately the cause of crying, but if it takes longer than usual or there are deviations in characteristics of cry, they seek medical attention The etiology of crying ranges from benign to life-threatening (Table 1). Differentiating children at high risk for harbouring a serious illness from others is a key task for emergency physicians.

Table 1: Differential diagnosis of excessive crying

GI Causes: Aphthous stomatitis, evening colic, milk allergy, anal fissure, pinworms, appendicitis, malrotation, midgut volvulus, intussusceptions, incarcerated/strangulated hernia, peritonitis, cholelithiasis, pancreatitis, intestinal obstruction.

Cardiac: Myocarditis, congestive cardiac failure, supraventricular tachycardia.

Chest: Hypoxia, hypercarbia, pneumonia, bronchiolitis, acute airway obstruction (croup, foreign body, asthma).

Genitourinary: Testicular/ovarian torsion, urinary tract infection, nephrolithiasis.

Head and Neck: Trauma, Foreign body, blocked nose, acute suppurative otitis media, corneal abrasion.

Hematologic: Sickle cell disease, malignancy, anemia, neutropenia, thrombocytopenia.

Skin/Musculoskeletal: Septic arthritis, osteomyelitis, digital tourniquet, fracture, dislocation, subluxation, non accidental trauma, scurvy, cellulitis.

Neurologic: Meningitis, encephalitis, intracranial hemorrhage, hydrocephalus, cerebral edema, epilepsy, degenerative disorders.

Toxic/metabolic: Prenatal drug use, toxin ingestion, electrolyte abnormality, inborn error of metabolism, hyperthyroidism.

General: Bacteremia, sepsis, hypovolemia, hyperbilirubinemia.

Miscellaneous: Insect bites, DPT vaccine, temper tantrums, poisonings, perinatal cocaine exposure.

EVALUATION

Although the differential diagnosis is extensive and involves every organ system, a meticulous history and a detailed physical examination often helps physician to arrive at a diagnosis. However, excessive crying, especially in the absence of any predisposing conditions and localizing features, poses a great diagnostic challenge to a physician.

History

Detailed history should be elicited to identify preceding events and associated symptoms. Episodes of inconsolable cry in the late afternoon or evening in infants 2-8 weeks of age with characteristic flushing of face and drawing up of legs with termination of episode with passage of flatus/feces is highly suggestive of evening colic.

Episodes of crying with arching of back and poor feeding may indicate underlying GERD. Crying or fussiness while feeding may suggest the possibility of nose block or aphthous stomatitis. Other causes of crying related to feeding are hunger, air swallowing and food intolerance. History of progressive abdominal distension, vomiting and constipation may alert the pediatrician to the possibility of underlying obstruction. When an infant with acute gastroenteritis develops sudden constipation with passage of currant jelly stools and episodes of inconsolable crying, it is highly suggestive of acute intussusception. Chronic constipation and crying while defecating are suggestive of anal fissure.

Poking fingers or pulling at ears may point towards an underlying otitis media. Cough, rapid breathing and feeding difficulty may suggest a respiratory or cardiovascular illness.

Some infants with adverse perinatal events may have increased incidence of unexplained crying. Head banging, vomiting, lethargy or photophobia may indicate a CNS disorder. Crying during micturition, frequency, urinary retention or abnormality in urinary stream suggest underlying abnormality of genitourinary system.

Excessive crying and restlessness may also occur due to a painful condition originating in any of the body systems. The site of pain may be suggested by certain gestures like flexion of thighs over abdomen (intestinal colic), head banging (headache), inability to move a limb (pseudoparalysis; scurvy, osteomyelitis, arthritis, fracture-dislocation, congenital syphilis), blinking/rubbing/watering of eyes (foreign body), pulling at ears (earache), touching and rubbing genitals (UTI). Unexplained episodes of severe abdominal pain and bone pains may occur due to vaso-occlusive crises of sickle cell disease and in children with acute leukemia.

Presence of fever usually suggests an underlying infective etiology. In these cases, the cause of crying can be usually established. One should look for symptoms referable to various systems of the body.

Breast feeding mothers may be unaware that medications they are taking might be transmitted to their infants during feeds. Special effort is required to elicit such history. High index of suspicion is required to diagnose cases of non-accidental and intentional trauma.

Persistent inconsolable crying is a well known complication of DPT vaccine. Changes in the emotional milieu of infants are also important causes of fussiness and excessive crying.

The history may identify "red flags" suggesting an increased likelihood of an underlying serious condition (Table 2).

Table 2 : Red flags for serious etiologies presenting with excessive crying

Premature rupture of membranes
Perinatal maternal fever or infections
History of fever (particularly in first two months of life)
Vomitting (particularly if billous)
History of bloody stools
Decreased feeding or activity
Increased somnolence
Abnormal behavior or 'spells'
Difficulty in feeding, diaphoresis during feeding, poor weight gain
Recent antibiotic use
Recent trauma, unexplained brusing or inconsistent history
Delay in seeking care
Caregiver intoxication
Caregiver mental illness
Maternal drug use

Table 3 : Nature of cry as an important clue

High pitched/shrill cry: Raised intracranial pressure, meningitis, hydrocephalus, kernicterus.
Hoarse gruff cry : Hypothyroidism
Grunting cry: Pneumonia
Hoarse cry: Laryngitis
Weak cry: Myasthenia gravis, Werdnig Hoffman disease.
Cat like cry: Cri du chat syndrome
Bleating lamb cry: Cornelia de Lange syndrome
Whimper cry: Seriously ill child

Physical Examination

The physical examination may reveal the diagnosis or provide clues to the diagnosis of the etiology of excessive crying. The pediatrician should take note of the infant's overall appearance, mental status and parental interaction. The quality of cry should be noted as it may give clue about the underlying disease (Table 3).

Observe whether the child is consolable or not. The child should be observed for paradoxical irritability. Normally the infants are soothed and calmed by being held and rocked gently in a caregiver's arm. Paradoxical irritability is present when an infant appears to be comfortable when lying still than when gently rocked. Conditions causing raised intracranial pressure such as meningitis may present as paradoxical irritability.

Watch for range and strength of spontaneous movements of all the extremities. In case of pseudoparalysis of an extremity, an infant will fail to move that affected extremity. Infants with 'pulled elbow' are unable to move the arm which is kept semiflexed and supinated. The skin should be examined for insect bites, abscesses, bruises, abrasions, burns and scars. Bruising in young infants is uncommon and more likely to be a manifestation of abuse than in older children.

Infant weight should be measured and compared to birth weight. Vital signs should be recorded which may reveal fever, hypothermia, tachycardia, tachypnea or hypotension.

Physical examination must be thorough, with the baby completely undressed. The head should be explored for evidence of trauma. The fontanelles should be evaluated for size and fullness. Oral examination should be performed to look for aphthous ulcers, swelling of gums, etc. Infants have rapidly growing fingernails and poor hand control, putting them at risk for corneal abrasions. Fluorescin staining of eyes may reveal such lesions. The eyelids must be everted to look for any evidence of a foreign body. Fundoscopy should be attempted (retinal hemorrhages may be seen in shaken baby syndrome). Otoscopy is mandatory to visualize tympanic membrane to exclude acute otitis media. The neck should be examined for evidence of trauma, adenopathy, masses and for range of motion.

Each finger and toe should be inspected closely to rule out strangulation by hair or thread. Careful palpation of all long bones should be done to look for evidence of any trauma. The diaper must be removed and careful search should be made for incarcerated hernia or testicular torsion. When indicated, rectal examination should be done to exclude intussusceptions.

Systemic examination should be conducted to exclude potentially life threatening conditions. The pediatrician should assess infant's work of breathing and auscultate the lungs. Abnormal breath sounds may be suggestive of pneumonia, bronchiolitis or congestive heart failure. History of sudden choking, stridor and unilateral wheezing are diagnostic of a foreign body in the air passages. The heart should be auscultated for abnormal tones. The presence of a murmur, ventricular heave or thrill suggests congenital heart disease. Examination of the abdomen of the crying infant is exceedingly difficult and may require repeated assessments over time. Look for abdominal distension and peristaltic movements to exclude intestinal obstruction. Look for a distended bladder. Rectal examination should be performed to look for signs of anal fissure and intussusception. Crying may be the sole symptom of an occult urinary infection so a specimen of urine must be obtained for analysis.

However, many children will have a completely normal examination.

Investigations

In a study by Poole *et al,* the history provided clues to the diagnosis in 20% of infants, physical examination revealed the diagnosis in 41% of cases and provided clues to the diagnosis in another 13%. Thus, a detailed history, complete physical examination and close observation are most important to identify the cause of inconsolable crying in a child.As previously discussed, the differential diagnosis is extremely broad and to evaluate each child for all of these conditions is not intuitively appealing. Therefore, investigations should be guided by the clues obtained on clinical assessment.

When tachypnea/dyspnea are associated, a detailed cardiorespiratory work up is indicated including CXR, ECG and a blood gas analysis. When abdominal distension is present, abdominal X-ray along with an ultrasonography is warranted. A lumber puncture with neuroimaging (if indicated) may be required in infants with lethargy, poor feeding abnormal cry or bulging fontanel. If non accidental trauma is suspected, a skeletal survey and a head CT should be included in the work up.

In absence of any clues from history and examination, a prudent approach is to perform a septic work up including complete blood count, blood culture, urine examination and culture, electrolytes including a glucose measurement and an ECG. An extensive laboratory work up is rarely indicated.

DIFFRENTIAL DIAGNOSIS IN YOUNG INFANTS

Infant Colic Syndrome

Cyclic discrete periods of intractable crying, usually on a daily basis, with onset at 1 to 4 weeks of age lasting longer than "normal" suggest infantile colic syndrome. Usually there is a dramatic spontaneous improvement by 3 to 4 months of age. The "classic" definition of infantile colic was first described by Wessel in 1954 as: "crying lasting more than 3 hours per day, 3 days per week, and continuing more than 3 weeks in infants less than 3 months of age." The crying is not relieved by normal parental interven-tions such as feeding, burping, changing diapers, providing a pacifier, and/or rocking. Vomiting, diarrhea, or poor weight gain are not features of the infant colic syndrome. Providing the family with accurate information on "normal" amounts of inconsolable crying and when they can expect improvement is helpful.

Esophagitis secondary to gastro-esophageal reflux in young infants may mimic colic. It presents in the first few months of life with intractable crying as the chief complaint. There is often a history of frequent, non-forceful, non-bilious regurgitation follwing feedings. On attempt to feed the infant may take the first few sips avidly, but then turns away, crying in pain. Occasionally the infant with esophagitis exhibits a torticollis-like positioning of the neck. A trial of anti-reflux treatment drugs can be given where no other organic cause for excessive crying is identified and for a limited duration, and if no improvement is seen, these should be discontinued. Antireflux measures used for treatment of GER include thickening of feeds, propped up posture during and after feeding, and use of medications like antacids (eg. ranitidine) and prokinetics (e.g., cisapride) in combination or alone. Surgical management in the form of fundoplication may be needed in extreme cases.

Corneal abrasion should be considered in any afebrile infants less than 6 months of age presenting with a chief complaint of crying and whose general examination is normal. Redness of eye or discharge is usually absent. A corneal exam with fluorescein staining will reveal the diagnosis. The baby should be treated with topical antibiotics and medication for pupillary dialation. Eye patch may be provided to avoid discomfort. Superficial corneal abrasions heal within 4-5 days.

A **hair tourniquet** could also present like this but a meticulous physical exam (of digits penis, clitoris and vulva) should make that diagnosis obvious.

Septic arthritis of hip should be considered in a febrile infant presenting with excessive crying. It is a surgical emergency with devastating consequences if not recognized in time. The crying increases when changing the diaper. The infant may exhibit "pseudo-paralysis" of the limb, with a preference for abduction and external rotation of the hip.

Urinary tract infection should also be considered in any infant with excessive crying, especially in a female infant. This condition is suspected in a febrile infant with vomiting, frequency, discomfort while micturition, or smelly urine. UTI can occur in the absence of fever especially in babies < 1 month of age and the physical examination may be normal. Leukocytosis, abnormal urinanalysis and positive urine cultures clinch the diagnosis. However, less than 50% of febrile infants below 2 months of age with positive urine cultures have abnormalities in routine urine examination.

Intussusception has a peak incidence between 6-9 months of age. Classically it presents with paroxysmal irritability and crying, vomiting and bloody diarrhea in a febrile infant. It may be misdiagnosed as sepsis, a toxic ingestion, or a closed head injury. Palpation of abdomen reveals a sausage shaped mass. Triad of vomiting, screaming episodes and lethargy is present in < 40% patients. A high index of suspicion should be there whenever confronted with an infant with unexplained crying having vomiting with or without lethargy. If the diagnosis is in doubt a per rectal examination may be helpful. Barium enema can be both diagnostic as well as therapeutic and is considered as the investigation of choice. Ultra-sonography by an experienced radiologist can be diagnostic. Reduction of intussusception during barium studies under fluoroscopy or more recently air or saline hydrostatic reduction can relieve the obstruction without resorting to surgical intervention.

Midgut volvulus may present with excessive crying. Eighty percent cases present in the first 4 weeks of life and the cardinal diagnostic sign is bilious vomiting. Most infants presenting are non-toxic and calm in appearance, with a benign abdominal examination until the gut begins to infarct.

Supraventricular tachycardia is another condition where an afebrile infant may present only with excessive crying or fussiness. The heart rate will be >220/minutes or too fast to count. ECG tracing can provide the diagnosis.

Battered baby syndrome may present with unexplained excessive crying and irritability. A history of listlessness or lethargy may be there. Generally there is no external sign of trauma; any facial bruising or unexplained tenderness over extremeties should be major "red flag signs". Retinal hemorrhage is generally the only physical finding. It is often misdiagnosed. Threshold for radio- and neuro-imaging should be low if this diagnosis is suspected.

Shaken baby syndrome is a distinct entity. It is a triad of subdural bleed, retinal hemorrhage and brain damage resulting from non-accidental injury to an infant resulting from sudden acceleration - deceleration injury to the brain. It should be suspected if there is inappropriate or inconsistent history given by parents or caretakers and baby is having features of acute encephalopathy with subdural and retinal hemorrhages or tears accompanied by presence of gripping injuries, or extra cranial injuries like damage to neck or spine. Besides, the supportive care for acute encephalopathy including management of raised intracranial pressure, involvement of social services and local legal authorities is needed as the baby may need care in foster home. Counseling of the family regarding the rearing practices and if the baby is sent back to the family after treatment then regular follow-up home visits by a social worker or a nurse is required to ensure well being of the baby.

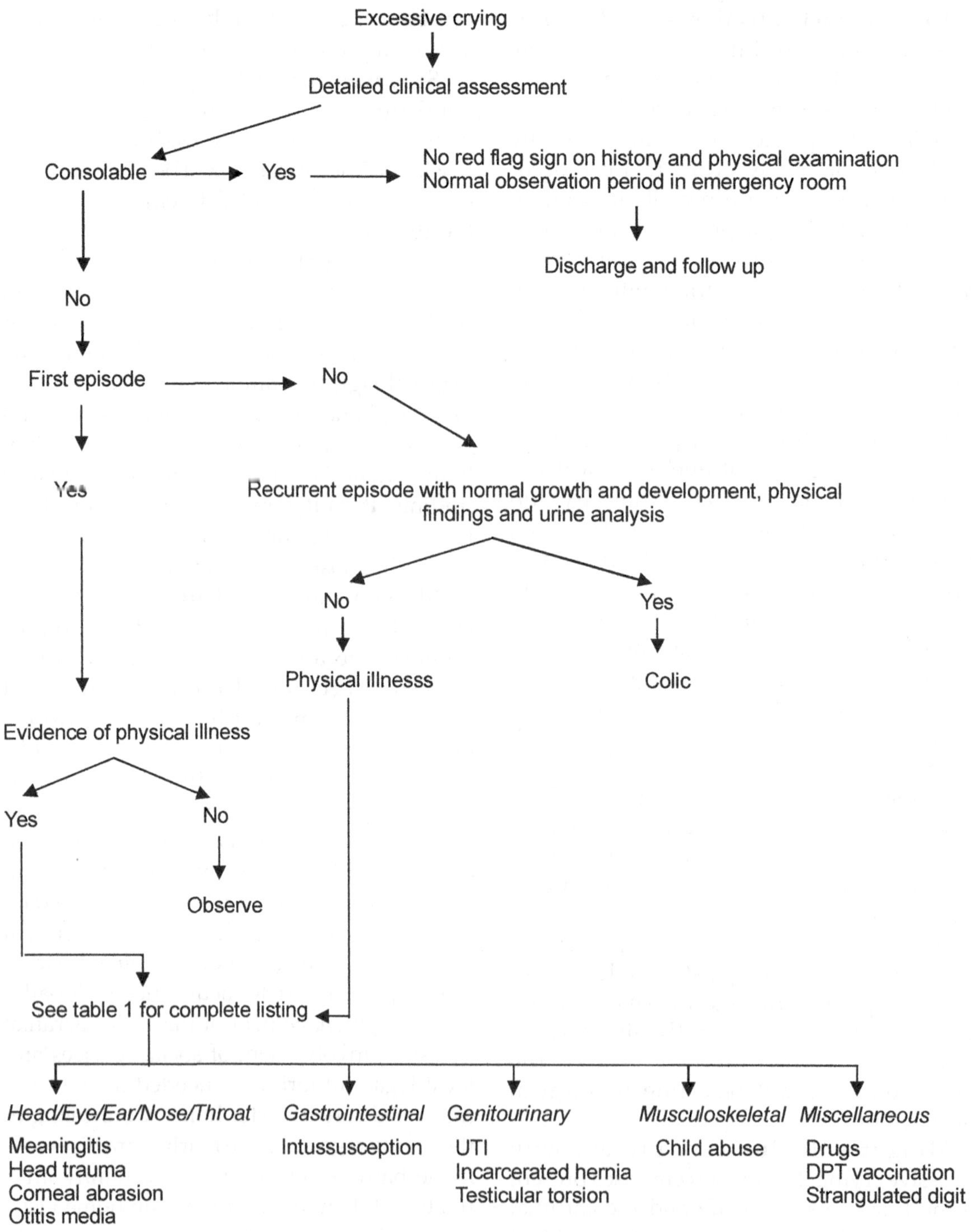

Fig. 1: Approach to a child with excessive crying

MANAGEMENT

There is no specific treatment for excessive crying. Although the main objective of the emergency visit for the child with excessive crying is to identify serious underlying illnesses, there are several benign causes amenable to treatment in the emergency room. These include corneal abrasions, hair tourniquets, oral thrush, nasal congestion, anal fissure, eczema, diaper dermatitis, constricting clothing and overbundling. If a simple cause has been identified, and the child is calm after the simple cause has been addressed, it is acceptable to discharge the child if follow up is assured.

Although relatively common, colic is a diagnosis of exclusion. Management is difficult as there is no immediate cure. Rocking, car rides, cuddling, swaddling, producing a dull continuous background noise and pacifiers may all reduce crying. Use of medications is controversial. Although drugs like simethicone, dicyclomine, cimetropium, etc have been tried, none has shown to be effective. Herbal medications like fennel seed oil emulsion, asfoetida, carom seeds, aesculus, acismelsica and anethi seeds have been used with limited success.

Often parents require more special handling than the infants. The most effective treatment appears to be counseling and empathy. The pediatrician should acknowledge the difficulty in caring for such an infant, identify and offer help for parental stresses, emphasize the overall good health of the infant, reassure that crying is not harmful for the infant and encourage time away from the infant for the parent. The infant colic gradually resolves and spontaneously disappears by age of 3 months.

Children who persist to have excessive inconsolable crying after benign causes have been ruled out are at relatively high risk for harboring a serious illness. A detailed clinical assessment and guided investigations are warranted for such children. An approach to a child with excessive crying has been briefly summarized in Figure 1.

CONCLUSIONS

There are no evidence based guidelines specific to a child with excessive crying. Crying episodes may resolve without any specific intervention on part of the parents or health care providers. Establishing an orderly approach to a child with unexplained crying is important to rule out the occasional physical illness and to provide preliminary guidance to the family.

FURTHER READING

1. Brazelton TB. Crying in infancy. *Pediatrics* 1962;29:579-588.
2. Wessel MA, Cobb JC, Jackson EB *et al*. Paroxysmal fussing in infancy, sometimes called "colic". *Pediatrics* 1954;14:421-434.
3. Illingworth RS. Crying in infants and children. *Brit Med J* 1955;1:75.
4. Poole SR. The infant with acute unexplained excessive crying. *Pediatrics* 1991;88:450-455.
5. Ronald GB, Brian H, James AG. Crying as a sign, a symptom and a signal. Cambridge University Press 2000;p96.
6. Sijmen AR, Emily B, Remy AH. Excessive infant crying : The impact of varying definitions. *Pediatrics* 2001;108:893-897.
7. Metcalf TJ, Irons TG, Sher LD, Young PC: Simethicone in the treatment of infant colic: A randomized, placebo-controlled, multicenter trail. Pediatrics 1994; 94:29-34.
8. Rittichier KK, Roback MG,Bassett KE: Are signs and symptoms associated with persistent corneal abrasions in children? Arch Pediatr Adolesc Med 2000; 154:370-374.

Joseph H. Chang, MD, MBA and Monira Vakil, DO

37 Intussusception

Intussussception is the telescoping of a proximal segment of small bowel into the distal segment or the intussuscipien. This results in bowel wall venous congestion and edema, and often bowel obstruction. Severe cases result in bowel infarction, perforation and death. Timely diagnosis and treatment has greatly reduced mortality in developed countries.

Intussusception is one of the most common causes of intestinal obstruction in children less than 2 years old. Some authors suggest that it is common up to 6 years of age. Incidence is greatest between the ages of 5-12 months old with 60% less than one year and 80% less than 2 years old.[1,2] Intussusception occurs in 1-4 in 1,000 live births with a 4:1 male predominance.[3] Intussusception occurs when a proximal segment of small bowel (intussusceptum) is telescoped into the distal segment of bowel (intussuscipiens), resulting in venous congestion, edematous bowel wall, bowel obstruction, and in severe cases, infarction and perforation of bowel wall. If not treated properly, it can lead to fatality. In developed countries, timely diagnosis and treatment t has greatly reduced mortality caused by intussusceptions.[4]

ETIOLOGY

The cause of intussusceptions remains unknown. The seasonal incidence of disease has lead to speculation that adenovirus infections may be the cause. Other diseases such as otitis media, gastroenteritis, Henoch-Shönlein purpura, Meckel's diverticulum, lymphoma, polyps, postsurgical scars, celiac disease, cystic fibrosis, and upper respiratory tract infection, are also known to be associated with intussusceptions.[5,6,7,8] Additionally, a rotavirus vaccine, RotaShiled, was found to have association with intussusceptions that results in its' withdrawal from the market in 1999. Two additional vaccines, RotaTeq and Rotarix were licensed in 2006; so far, surveillance has not revealed any increased risk of intussusceptions.[9, 10]

The most popular theory suggests a lead point such as enlarged Peyer's patches after a recent viral infection that causes mucosal prolapse of the ileum into the colon, however, these recognizable lead points are only found in 2-8% of patients.[11, 12] Intussusceptions may occur at any point along the gastrointestinal tract, but greater than 95% of intussusceptions occur near the ileocecal junction but may occur at any point along the gastrointestinal tract. Ileojejunal, jejuno-, appendico-, and colocolic intussusceptions are also possible.

SIGNS AND SYMPTOMS

The classic triad of symptoms in intussusceptions include acute abdominal pain, vomiting (some authors use palpable abdominal mass), and currant-jelly stool. These symptoms are present in only about one third of patient.[13,14] Three quarter of patients has two symptoms, and 13% have either one or none of the symptoms.

Typical presentations of patients with intussusceptions include sudden onset of severe colicky abdominal pain that recur in cycles lasting 10 to 15 minutes. These episodes are accompanied by straining efforts, demonstrated by knees and legs flexed towards the abdomen, and inconsolable crying. The patient may initially be comfortable and behave normally between the episodes of pain; but as the disease progresses, the patient becomes progressively more weak and lethargic. Past medical history may reveal a recent viral illness. The patient may have constipation, vomiting and/or diarrhea on presentation. Blood may be present in either the stool or the emesis. On physical exam a palpable abdominal mass or rectal mass may be found. During later stages, the patients may have altered mental status ranging from lethargy to frank coma. Some authors suggested the late appearance of lethargy may be related to development of shock.[15,16] Yet recently several authors have suggested that altered mental status may be an early sign. Emergency practitioner should be aware of variations in signs and symptoms and maintain a high index of suspicion to prevent diagnostic delay.[17,18,19]

Physical Examination

Due to cyclic nature of the pain, the general appearance and vital signs may vary significantly. Patients may be cheerful and interactive or lethargic to comatose, normotensive or hypotensive, febrile or afebrile. As stated by Hess in 1905 "the tumor of invagination is the most important physical sign from the diagnostic standpoint" Palpation of the abdomen may reveal a sausage-like mass located in the right upper abdomen that may change in size and firmness during the pain episode (60-95% of cases)[20]. The pathognomonic sign, although relatively uncommon, for intussusceptions is Dances' sign. This is an empty space was found in the right lower quadrant representing the movement of the cecum out of its normal position. Rectal exam may show bleeding, although thought to be a late sign. Rectal bleeding is found more frequently than an abdominal mass.[21,22] Losek noted that 75% of cases with intussusceptions had stool that was guaiac-positive.[23] Other findings may less frequent but possible are abdominal distension, hypoactive bowel sounds, and abdominal tenderness.

DIFFERENTIAL DIAGNOSIS

The differential diagnosis of abdominal pain is very broad; patients' presentation can complicate the differential diagnoses. However, physician should know what differentiates intussusceptions from other diagnoses. For example, if the patient presents with abdominal pain and vomiting, differentials should include volvulus, Henoch-Schönlein Purpura (HSP), incarcerated hernia, acute gastroenteritis, bowel obstruction. GI bleed should lead a physician to consider HSP or Meckel's , a painless source of painless rectal bleeding. If fever and lethargy is presenting complaint, infection etiologies must also be considered.

Other differential diagnosis to consider:

	Infant	*Child*
Mechanical	• Malrotation with midgut volvulus • Intussusception • Incarcerated inguinal hernia • Meckel's diverticulum (painless rectal bleed) • Hirschsprung's disease	• Constipation • Incarcerated inguinal hernia • Meckel's diverticulum (painless rectal bleed) • Bowel obstruction
Infectious	• Necrotizing enterocolitis	• Gastroenteritis (less pain, less regular, diarrhea) • Appendicitis • Henoch-Schönlein Purpura (join symptoms) • Pancreatitis • Gastritis • Biliary tract disease
Genitourinary Misc.	• Urinary tract infection • Colic • Child abuse • Toxic Ingestion • Munchausen by proxy	• Urinary tract infection • Pneumonia • Metabolic disorder • Tumor • Ulcer • Diabetic ketoacidosis • Sickle cell • Toxic ingestions • Child abuse • Munchausen by proxy

Adapted from Marx, John, Robert Hockberger, and Ron Walls. *Rosen's Emergency Medicine, Concepts and Clinical Practice*. St. Louis: Mosby, 2001.

DIAGNOSIS

The key to making the diagnosis is obtaining a detailed and careful conducted history and physical examination and maintaining a high level index of suspicion. The presentation of intussusceptions is varied and therefore difficult to diagnose. However, diagnosis by signs and symptoms has only been correct in 50% of the time at an Emergency Department.[24] Imaging and laboratories results become an important tool in making the diagnosis.

Laboratory Studies

No particular laboratory studies are helpful in making diagnosis of intussusceptions, but they could be used to aid in excluding other diagnosis. Basic electrolyte could be used to assess the status of hypovolemia, complete blood count (CBC) could be used to assess the status of infection/anemia. Other studies such as urine analysis, toxicology screen, bedside blood glucose strip, liver function test, ammonia, arterial blood gas and culture of blood, urine, and cerebrospinal fluids

(CSF) could also be used if diagnosis is unclear.

X-ray

Abdominal X-ray with a minimum of 2 views is the first step is the radiologic assessment. The entire colon and the cecum should be visualized. Some degree of intestinal obstruction is seen in 23-50 % of cases. [25, 26], The signs of a soft tissue mass, mass effect, obstruction, little or no gas in the bowel, and free air should be carefully examined. The most common radiographic finding is a soft-tissue mass in the right upper quadrant, effacing the adjacent hepatic contour. Other signs specific to intussusception include reduced air in the small bowel or a gasless abdomen, air in a displaced appendix, and obstruction of the small bowel.

The most specific radiographic findings are the target sign and meniscus sign. The target sign consists of a soft-tissue mass that contains concentric circular lucency due to the mesenteric fat. The meniscus sign, consists of a crescent of gas within the colonic lumen that outlines the apex of the intussusceptions. "Identification of a cecum filled with gas or feces in the normal location is the finding that allows exclusion of intussusceptions with the most confidence"[27]. Nonspecific or indeterminate films required additional imaging.

Barium Enema

Historically, barium enema has been the gold standard as both diagnostic and therapeutic method. On the X-ray, a sharp filling defect can be seen at the point where barium contrast meets the intussuseptum in the obstruction (Figures. 1, 2a, and 2b). The classic signs of intussusceptions are the "meniscus signs" (analogous to X-ray "meniscus sign", produced when the rounded apex of the intussusceptum protruding into the column of contrast material) and "coiled spring sign" (produced when the edematous mucosal folds of the telescoping limb of the intussusceptum are outlined by contrast material in the lumen of the colon). However, due the potential sequel of perforation and chemical peritonitis, 28 other contrasts such as water-soluble contrast are being considered. The pathological changes in the peritoneum such as granulomas, adhesion, and loculated ascites seem to be less significant when water soluble contrast was used.[29] However, several randomized studies have not shown statistically significant differences in reduction and perforation rates between barium and liquid enema. [30,31,32]

Air Enema

Alternatively, air enema could also be used to reduce intussusceptions with a success rate greater than 60%. The advantages of air enema are less time consuming and a high reduction rate of 73-95%. Air enemas also have the advantage of less radiation exposure to the child compared to barium enemas. This is due to shortened time required achieving reduction and technique. Some physicians preferred air enema over barium contrast studies. [33,34,35,36] However, it was reported that air enema was associated with higher perforation rate of 2.8%. [37] In both barium and air enema, a pediatric surgeon back up is necessary in case of failure to reduce the intussusceptions or perforation.

Ultrasound

Ultrasound has many advantages over barium enema. It has higher level of patient comfort and safety, ability to arrive an alternative diagnosis, and a high sensitivity for the diagnosis of intussusceptions (98%-100%).[38, 39,40] Ultrasound is least invasive and most commonly available in most Emergency Department. The intussusceptions mass is a

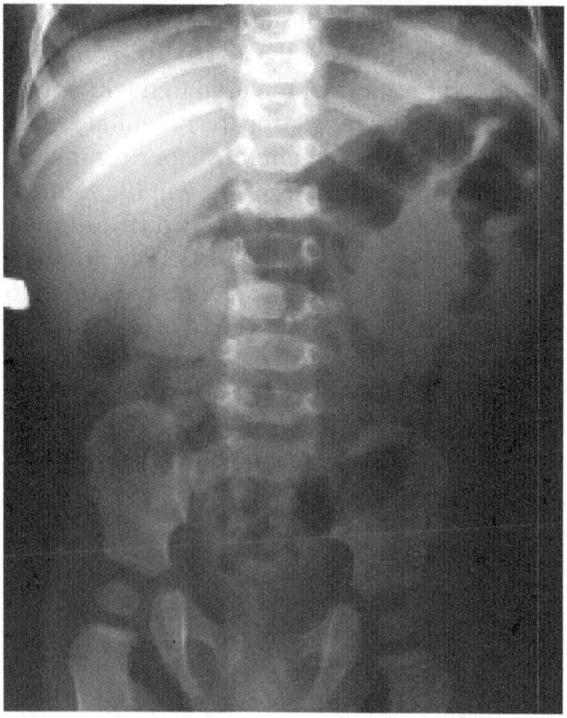

Fig. 1: The KUB demonstrates a round density of the right lower quadrant. There is however no evidence of intestinal obstruction. The bowel gas pattern is normal

Picture courtesy of Dr. Leonard Swischuk, University of Texas Medical Branch

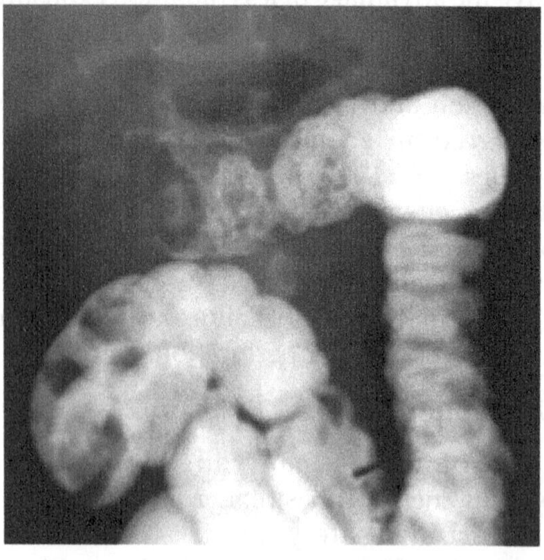

Fig. 2a: Barium enema. Image from a barium enema study shows the contrast material filled distal colon but has a clear filling defect

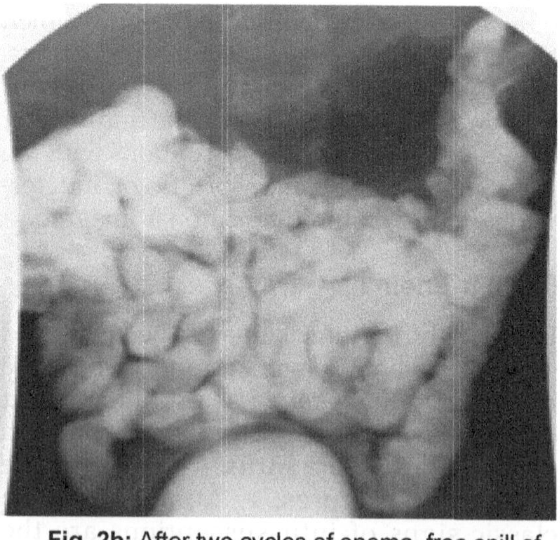

Fig. 2b: After two cycles of enema, free spill of contrast material into the ileum was seen and total reduction of the intussusception was achieved

Pictures courtesy of Dr. Leonard Swischuk, University of Texas Medical Branch

large in size greater than 5 x 2.5 cm that is easily identified, even by inexperienced operators.[41] Appearance that are characteristic of intussusceptions are; multiple concentric ring sign[42], crescent-in-doughnut sign [43] on axial scan, the sandwich signs[44] and hayfork sign[45] on longitudinal scan. Ultrasound is also useful in demonstrating reduction of the intussusceptions by hydrostatic or air enema.

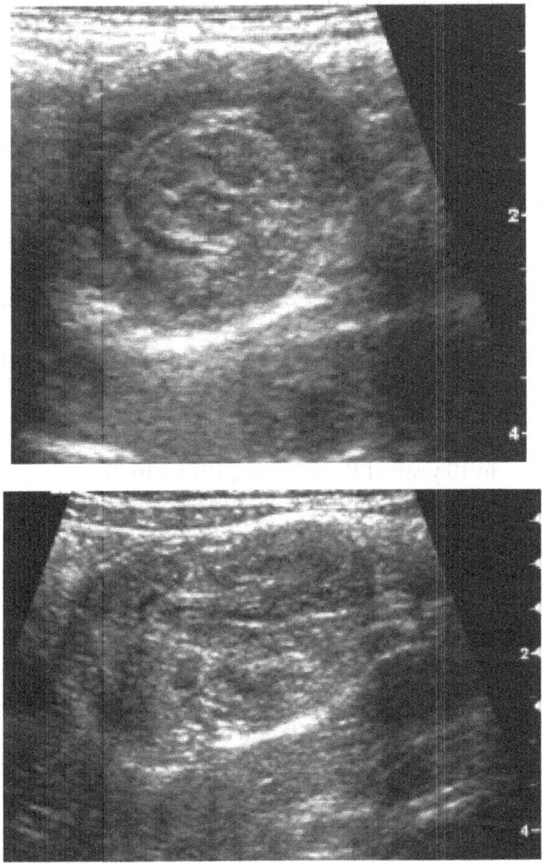

Figi. 3 a & b: Ultrasound. There is evidence of a mass in the epigastric region measuring about 3 cm x 3 cm in cross section. There is evidence of a hyperechoic center. On longitudinal section that is a sausage appea-rance. There is increased flow within the lesion. Findings are suggestive of a colo-colic intussusception.

Pictures courtesy of Dr. Leonard Swischuk, University of Texas Medical Branch.

TREATMENT

1. As in any emergency setting, attention should be Airway, Breathing, Circulation (ABCs).
2. Bolus intravenous fluids of 20 mL/kg normal saline should be given till adequate volume status is achieved.
3. Patients should be nothing by mouth (NPO).
4. Nasogastric tube decompression when there is evidence of significant obstruction with severe gaseous distention
5. Broad-spectrum, triple-antibiotics coverage with ampicillin, gentamicin and either clindamycin or metronidazole when child is febrile or toxic appearing.
6. Prompt surgical consult. Surgical intervention maybe required if the barium or air enema fails to reduce or if perforation occurs. Other indications for surgical treatments are: shock that cannot be corrected, lead points necrosis, pneumatosis intestinalis.[46]
7. Reduction is an emergency procedure and should be performed immediately after diagnosis in a stable patient, regardless of age and duration of symptoms. [47]
   - Radiologic reduction under fluoroscopic or ultrasonic guidance success rate when performed within 48 hours of presentation: 70-90%
   - Radiologic reduction under fluoroscopic or ultrasonic guidance success rate when performed greater than 48 hours of presentation: 50%
   - Ileoileal intussusceptions are best diagnosed by ultrasonography, Reduction by barium, saline, or air enema may not be possible.
8. Admission for observation is recommended for all patients after reduction.[48] In 24 hour time period, intussusceptions may recur in 7-10% of patients who undergo radiologic reduction and 2-5% of patients who undergo surgical reductions. [49]

DISPOSITION

Definitive imaging is required with all children presenting to Emergency Department when considering intussusceptions. Children with radiological finding consistent with intussusceptions should be reduced by either barium/air enema or surgery. Admission is recommended for all patients after reduction.

SUMMARY

Intussusception is a clinically severe and potentially lethal disease. Emergency physician should keep the diagnosis of intussusceptions in the differential diagnosis for all children presenting to Emergency Department with abdominal pain, vomiting, or for those who present with altered mental status. Careful history, abdominal and rectal examination, judicial use of abdominal radiography with facilitates timely diagnosis. Along with early diagnosis, stabilization of the critically ill child with prompt consultation of radiologist and pediatric surgeon are the primary roles of an emergency physician.

REFERENCES

1. Felter RA: Nontraumatic surgical emergencies in children. *Emerg Med Clin North Am* 1991; 9:589.
2. Bonadio WA, Clarkson T, Naus J: The clinical features of children with malrotation of the intestine. *Pediatr Emerg Care* 1991; 7:348.
3. Buchert GS: Abdominal pain in children: An emergency practitioner's guide. *Emerg Med Clin North Am* 1989; 7:497.
4. World Health Organization. Initiative for Vaccine Research Department of Vaccine and Biologicals. Acute intussusceptions in infants and children. Incidence, clinical presentation and management: A global perspective. WHO/V&B/02.19/2002.
5. Friman S, Svanvik J, Radberg G: Intussusception at four separate locations in the small intestine: Case report. *Acta Chir Scand* 1988; 154:485.
6. Ravikumar K, Khope S, Rao P: Idiopathic colo-colic Intussusception *J Postgrad Med* 1988; 34:246.
7. McCombe AW, Orr JD: Gastric lipoma and Intussusception in a child. *Scott Med J* 1988; 33:310.
8. Kim YS, Ruh JH: Intussusception in infancy and childhood: Analysis of 385 cases. *Int Surg* 1989; 74:114.
9. Dennehy PH, Goveia MG, Dallas MJ. Heaton PM. The integrated phase III safety profile of the pentavalent human-bovine (WC3) reassortant rotavirus vaccine. Int J Infect Dis. 2007 Nov;11 Suppl 2:S36-42.
10. Dennehy PH. "Rotavirus vaccines: an overview" Clin Microbiol Rev. 2008 Jan: 21(1):198-208.
11. Dennison WM, Shaker M. Intussusception in infancy and childhood. Br. J Surg 1970:57679-684.
12. Mulcahy DL. A two-part study of the etiological role of rotavirus in intussusceptions. J Med Virology 1982:9:51-55.
13. World Health Organization. Initiative for Vaccine Research Department of Vaccine and Biologicals. Acute intussusceptions in infants and children. Incidence, clinical presentation and management: A global perspective. WHO/V&B/02.19/2002.
14. Kim YS, Ruh JH: Intussusception in infancy and childhood: Analysis of 385 cases. *Int Surg* 1989; 74:114.
15. Ein SH, Stephesn CA. Intussusception: 354 cases in 10 years. J Pediatr Surg 1974;6:16-27.
16. Gross RE, Ware PF. Intussusception in childhood. NEJM 1948;239:645-652.
17. Singer J. Alterted Consciousness as an early manifestation of intussusceptions. Pediatrics 1979; 64:93-95.
18. Swischuk LE. Lethargy and vomiting in an infant. Pediatr Emerg Care 1991;7:97-98.
19. Rachmel A, Rosenbaum Y, Amir J, *et al.* Apathy as an early manifestation of intussusception.
20. Losek JD, Fiete RL: Intussusceptions and the diagnostic value of testing stool for occult blood. AM J Em Med 1991;9:1-3.
21. Ein S.H., Stephens C.A.: Intussusception: 354 cases in 10 years. *J Pediatr Surg* 6. 16-27.1971.
22. Pollack E.S.: Pediatric abdominal surgical emergencies. *Pediatr Ann* 25. 448-457: 1996.
23. Losek J.D., Fiete R.L.: Intussusception and the diagnostic value of testing stool for occult blood. *Am J Emerg Med* 9. 1-3.1991.
24. Beasley SW. Auldist AW. Sokes KB. The diagnostically difficult intussusceptions: Its characteristics and consequences. Pediatr Surg Int. 1988; 3:135-138.

25. Fanconi S, Berger D, Aldose PP. Intussusception: A classic clinical picture? Helv Paediat Acta 1982;37:345-352.
26. Gierup J, Jorulf H, Livaditis A. Managmeent of intussusceptions in infants and children: A survey based on 288 consecutive cases. Pediatric 1972; 50: 535-545.
27. Sargent MA, Babyn P. Alton DJ. Plain abdominal radiography in suspected intussusceptions: A reassessement. Pediatri Radiol 1994: 24: 17-20.
28. Hadidi AT, El Shal N: Childhood intussusception: A comparative study of nonsurgical management. *J Pediatr Surg* 1999; 34:304.
29. Ginai AZ. Experimentation evaluation of various available contrast agents for use in the gastrointestinal tract in case of suspected leakage: Effects on peritoneum. Br J Radiol 1985; 58:969-978.
30. Meyer JS, Dangman BC, Buonomo C, Berlin JA. Air and liquid contrast agents in the management of intussusception: a controlled, randomized trial. Radiology 1993; 188:507-511.
31. Palder SB, Ein SH, Stringer DA, Alton D. Intussusception: Barium or air? J Pediatr Surg 1991; 26:271-275.
32. Poznansky AK. Why I still use barium for intussusception. Pediatr Radiol 1995; 25:92-93.
33. Bhisitkul DM, *et al*: Clinical application of ultrasonography in the diagnosis of intussusception. *J Pediatr* 1992; 121:182.
34. Del-Pozo G, Albillos J, Tejedor D: Intussusception: US findings with pathologic correlation—the crescent in doughnut sign. *Radiology* 1996; 121:182.
35. Hadidi AT, El Shal N: Childhood intussusception: A comparative study of nonsurgical management. *J Pediatr Surg* 1999; 34:304.
36. Meyer JS, Dangman BC, Buonomo C, Berlin JA: Air and liquid contrast agents in the management of intussusception: A controlled, randomized trial. *Radiology* 1993; 188:507.
37. Stein M, Alton DJ, Daneman A. Pneumatic reduction of intussusception: 5-year experience. Radiology 1992; 183:681-684.
38. Pracros JP. Tran-Mihn VA. Morin de Finfe CH, Defrenne-Pracros P. Louis D, Basset T. Acute intestinal intussusceptions in children contribution of ultrasonography. Ann Radio 1987, 30:525-530.
39. Verschelden P, Filiatrault D, Garel I, *et al.* Intussusception in children: Reliability of US in diagnosis—a prospective study. Radiology 1992; 184: 741-744.
40. Woo SK, Kim JS, Suh Sj, Paik TW, Choi SO. Childhood intussusceptions: US guided hydrostatic reduction. Radiology 1992:182:77-80.
41. Daneman A, Alton DJ, Intussusception: Issues and controversies related to diagnosis and reduction. Radiol Clin North AM 1996;34:743-756.
42. Hold S, Samue E. Multiple concentric ring signs in the ultrasonographic diagnosis of intussusceptions. Gastrointest Radiol 1978; 3:307-309.
43. Del-Pozo G, Albillos JC, Tejedor D. Intussusception: US findings with pathologic correlation the cresent-in-doughnut sign. Radiology 1996; 199:688-692.
44. Montali G, Croce F, de Pra L. Solbiati L. Intussusception of the bowel: A new sonographi pattern. Br J Radiol 1983: 56:621-623.
45. Alessi V, Salerno G. The "hay-fork" sign in the ultrasonographic diagnosis of intussusceptions. Gastrointest Radiol 1985;10:177-179.
46. Stringer MD, Pablot SM, Brereton RJ. Paediatric intussusception. Br J Surg 1992; 79:867-876.
47. Gierup J, Jorulf H, Livaditis A. Management of intussusceptions in infants and children: A survey based on 288 aconsecutive cases. Pediatrics 1972: 50:535-545.
48. Hadidi AT, El Shal N: Childhood intussusception: A comparative study of nonsurgical management. *J Pediatr Surg* 1999; 34:304.
49. Hadidi AT, El Shal N: Childhood intussusception: A comparative study of nonsurgical management. *J Pediatr Surg* 1999; 34:304.

In the previous edition this chapter was written by Phyllis T. Doerger, MD Chief Resident Wright State University School of Medicine Department of Emergency Medicine Dayton, Ohio

and

Jonathan Singer, MD Professor of Emergency Medicine and Pediatrics Wright State University School of Medicine Vice-Chair and Program Director Department of Emergency Medicine Dayton, Ohio

Shiva Kalidindi

38 Acute Appendicitis

Appendicitis is acute inflammation and infection of the vermiform appendix. Appendectomy for acute appendicitis is one of the most common surgical procedures in the North American continent.[1] Approximately 250,000 cases of appendicitis occur annually, accounting for 1,000,000 hospital days per year.[1] The lifetime risk of appendicitis is 8.6 percent for males and 6.7 percent for females. In males, the incidence of non perforating appendicitis rises from 44 per 100,000 population in the 0 to 9 years of age group, to a peak of 170 cases per 100,000 in the 10 to 19 years of age group.[2] Yet the etiology and epidemiology of appendicitis remain poorly understood. The evaluation of abdominal pain where appendicitis is a consideration is without doubt one of the most common problems encountered in emergency departments today.

PATHOPHYSIOLOGY

In most instances, obstruction of the lumen of the appendix is the event that leads to appendicitis. It has been recognized that chronic and recurrent appendicitis does occur.[3] In the usual case, however, the appendiceal lumen becomes acutely obstructed by a fecalith. Less common causes are lymphoid tissue hypertrophy, bacterial infections, inspissated barium, seeds, intestinal worms, edema, or foreign bodies. As obstruction progresses, the appendix becomes distended, leading to periumbilical pain. The appendiceal mucosa may suffer ischemic damage with increasing luminal pressure. When the integrity of the appendiceal wall has been compromised, bacteria invade the wall, and infection contributes to continued appendiceal damage. Ultimately gangrene or perforation may occur, allowing spill of grossly contaminated material.

When the appendiceal wall becomes inflamed, the nearby peritoneum is irritated, and pain is localized to the right lower quadrant (McBurney's point). If perforation occurs and is not well contained, diffuse peritonitis ensues.

CLINICAL PRESENTATION

Appendicitis in children presents with a widely varying clinical spectrum. In preschool children, the classic triad of pain, vomiting, and fever is not always readily apparent. Older children tend to have a more obvious presentation, but younger children may have a more confusing picture that necessitates more extensive evaluation (Figure 1).

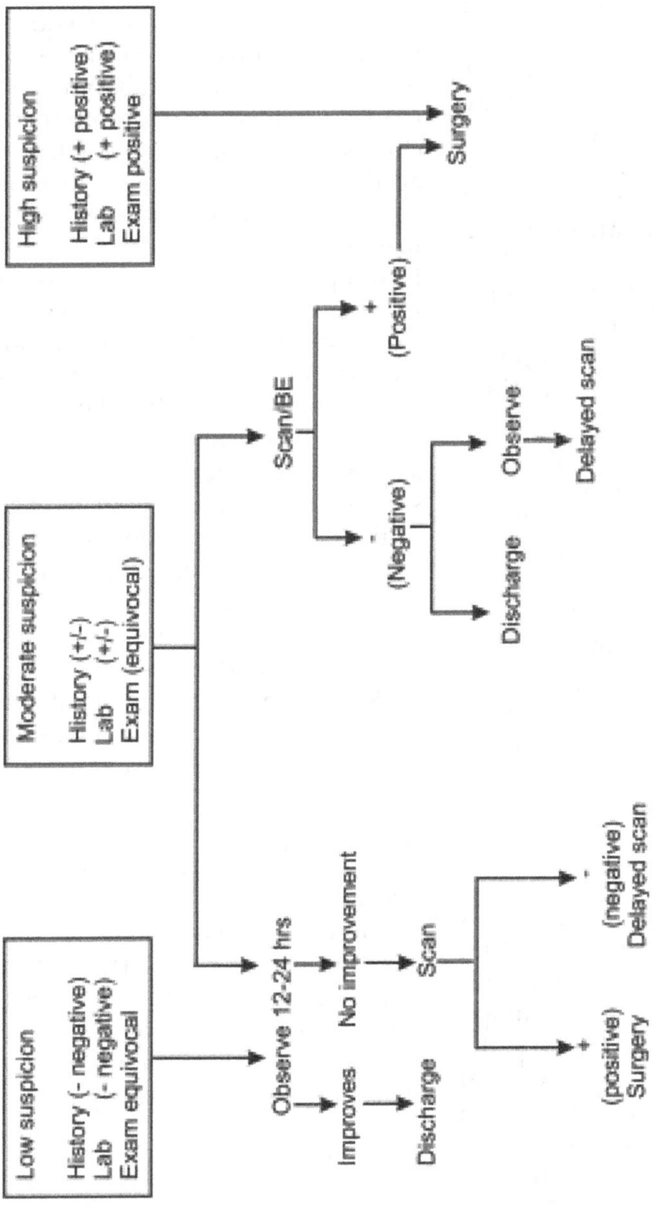

Fig. 1: Abdominal pain

HISTORY

Abdominal pain is the predominant symptom of appendicitis. In a classic case, pain begins as a vague discomfort in the periumbilical region, relocating to the right lower quadrant 1 to 12 hours later. This pain may persist for 24 to 48 hours. Occasionally the pain may subside then reappear with a more diffuse pattern consistent with perforation. Delays in diagnosis, however, are not uncommon due to variations in the location of the appendix[4] such as retrocecal or pelvic locations or coexistent malrotation. This may occur in up to one-third of cases.

Anorexia commonly accompanies appendicitis. It is more often variable in children than in adults, however. In otherwise healthy teenagers, appetite may not be negatively influenced so that close question-ing is vital. Vomiting occurs in 75 percent of patients but rarely more than once or twice prior to surgery unless bowel obstruction is present. Obstipation or diarrhea may accompany other symptoms but are not reliable enough to offer help in the differential diagnosis. In older patients, the typical sequence of symptoms is anorexia, followed by pain and nausea or vomiting. In younger patients, this sequence of events is more variable.

Physical Examination

Observation of the child with appendicitis will more often be revealing than actual physical examination. The typical child with appendicitis is reluctant to move. A bumpy ride to the hospital is painful. Tapping the heels or rocking the bed elicits abdominal pain. The child may limp while ambulating or be unable to extend the right leg.

Bowel sounds may be normal with acute appendicitis. Bowel sounds with perforation may suggest bowel obstruction with high-pitched tinkles or be completely silent with an ileus. The chest should be carefully auscultated to rule out pneumonia mimicking appendicitis.

Gentle abdominal examination will be more rewarding than vigorous evaluation. It is best to start the exam in a quadrant away from the source of pain. A very light percussive tap on the abdomen is all that is required to identify peritonitis because of the child's abdominal wall being thinner than an adult's. Obese children will require more aggressive evaluation since their body habitus may mask many of the signs of appendicitis. If the appendix lies in proximity to the psoas muscle, the psoas sign will be positive. The sign is elicited by having the child lie on the left side and hyperextending the right thigh. This maneuver stretches the psoas muscle; a positive response suggests an inflamed appendix overlying the muscle. The *obturator sign* maneuver consists of internal rotation of the flexed right thigh while the child lies in the supine position. A positive result occurs when this maneuver produces hypogastric pain. Rectal examination may demonstrate right-sided tenderness.

Rectal examination is of value in about 50 percent of children with abdominal pain. It is more likely to be helpful in the adolescent female who presents with right lower quadrant pain. A positive psoas or obturator sign suggests a retrocecal inflammatory process.

Signs of trauma or abuse should be looked for. Occult or overt trauma can mimic appendicitis. Evidence for other causes of abdominal pain such as petechiae (Henoch-Schönlein purpura), abdominal masses, or insect bites should be sought.

Complications

Rupture of the appendix is the major complication of the disease and occurs more commonly when diagnosis and surgery is delayed. As compared with uncomplicated cases, rupture typically produces tenderness that is more diffuse, a higher fever, and a greater degree of leukocytosis. As peritonitis progresses, the child typically lies quietly supine because the slightest movement causes pain. The child will often complain of pain over the entire abdomen rather than just in the right lower quadrant. In older children, the perforation may wall off to form an appendiceal abscess. If this abscess ruptures or progresses to severe peritonitis, the child will show signs of extreme toxicity and sepsis.

Laboratory and X-ray

The white blood cell count (WBC) may or may not be elevated in early appendicitis. As many as 20 percent of patients may have a normal WBC upon presentation. Frequently a high band count or a left shift will be noted. Urinary examination may reveal a few white or red blood cells per high-powered field. Other laboratory determinations have not been routinely helpful.

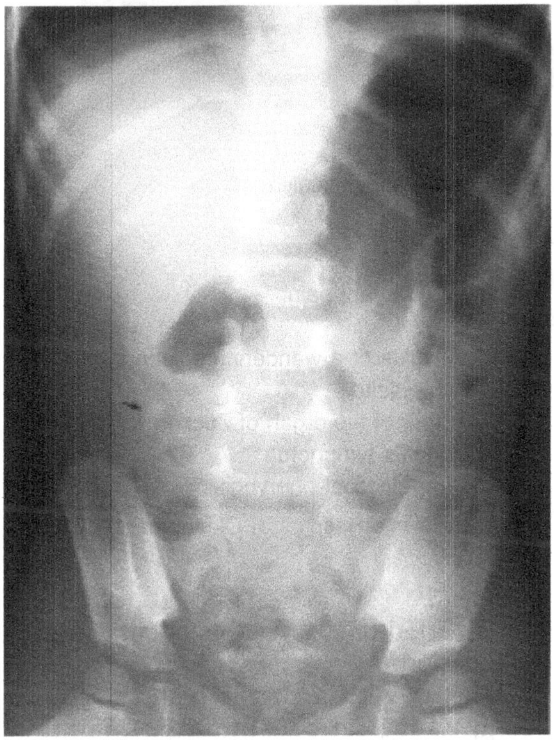

Fig. 2: A child with fever and acute abdominal pain. Plain film abdomen showing (arrow) "appendicolith"

If the diagnosis is in doubt, then imaging studies can provide important information. Abdominal radiographs are occasionally helpful. Radiological signs suggestive of appendicitis include a fecalith (Figure 2), right lower quadrant ileus, scoliosis, a psoas shadow, and small bowel obstruction. Ultrasonography has been widely used to evaluate the child with abdominal pain (Figure 3)[8,9]. The advantages of ultrasonography include its noninvasiveness, lack of radiation, no contrast medium, and minimal pain. The downside of ultrasonography is that the examination is operator dependent. In experienced hands, ultrasonography has an overall sensitivity of 85% and a specificity of 94% in pediatric patients. CT scans have become the modality of choice for diagnosing appendicitis in children. Although radiation exposure is a concern, CT scans have been shown to have an accuracy of 97% in diagnosing appendicitis.

DIFFERENTIAL DIAGNOSIS

Many other illnesses can mimic appendicitis in children. Specific facets of the history or physical examination may lead the physician to a different diagnosis. Common illnesses that mimic appendicitis include pneumonia, bacterial or viral gastroenteritis, acute pharyngitis, urinary tract infections, and gynecologic disorders in adolescent females. Unusual causes of abdominal pain may also mimic appendicitis (Table 1).

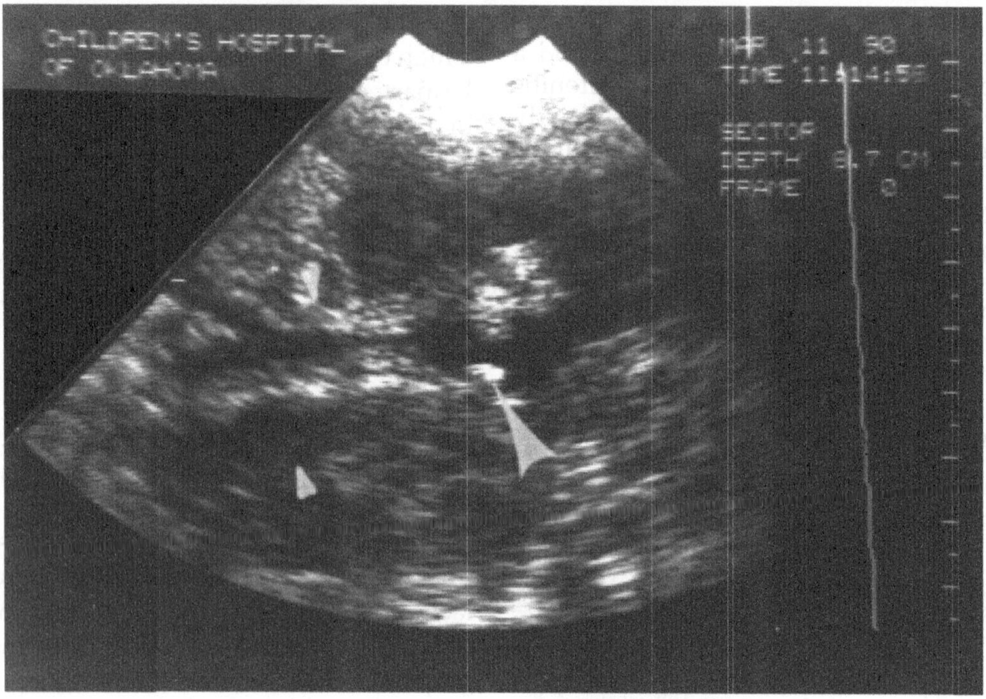

Fig. 3: Ultrasound: Large arrows showing appendicolith

Table 1: Unusual causes of right lower quadrant pain

Hirschsprung's enterocolitis	Volvulus of a wandering spleen
Foreign body bowel perforation	Acute ileitis
Internal hernia with volvulus	Tumor of the organ of Zucker-Kandl
Acalculus cholecystitis	Burkitt's lymphoma
Torsion of the ovary	Streptococcal pharyngitis

A partial list of other illness mimicking appendicitis at the Children's Hospital of Oklahoma 1987-1991.

MANAGEMENT

The definitive treatment for appendicitis is appendectomy. However if the diagnosis of appendicitis is unclear, consider obtaining a double-contrast abdominal CT scan. Serial examinations and test results may also help to clarify the diagnosis. If uncertainty persists after a period of observation, obtain surgical consultation.

Patients with a classic history require prompt surgical consultation. Maintain nothing-by-mouth status in patients with suspected appendicitis and start intravenous fluids to restore intravascular volume and ensure adequate hydration. Antibiotic therapy with broad-spectrum antibiotics (eg, ampicillin, gentamicin, and clindamycin or a cephalosporin) directed against gram-negative and anaerobic organisms should be considered before surgery. Antibiotics have been shown to reduce morbidity even in nonperforated cases[13]. Fever may be controlled with acetaminophen given by rectum. An appendectomy is performed as soon as the patient's condition has been stabilized. Open and Laparoscopic appendectomy are equally safe and acceptable in children[14]. For patients who have symptoms for 5 days or longer and a palpable mass consistent with an appendiceal abscess, many surgeons initially prefer nonsurgical management with braod spectrum antibiotics followed by an elective appendectomy in 6 to 8 weeks[15] (Figure 4).

PROGNOSIS

Generally, prognosis is good for uncomplicated appendicitis treated with prompt surgical intervention. The the mortality is less than 1%, and long-term morbidity is primarily the risk of adhesive small-bowel obstruction. The average hospital stay is approximately 2 days [16]. Despite increasing use of radiographic imaging, the incidence of perforated appendicitis exceeds 30%[17]. Therefore it is

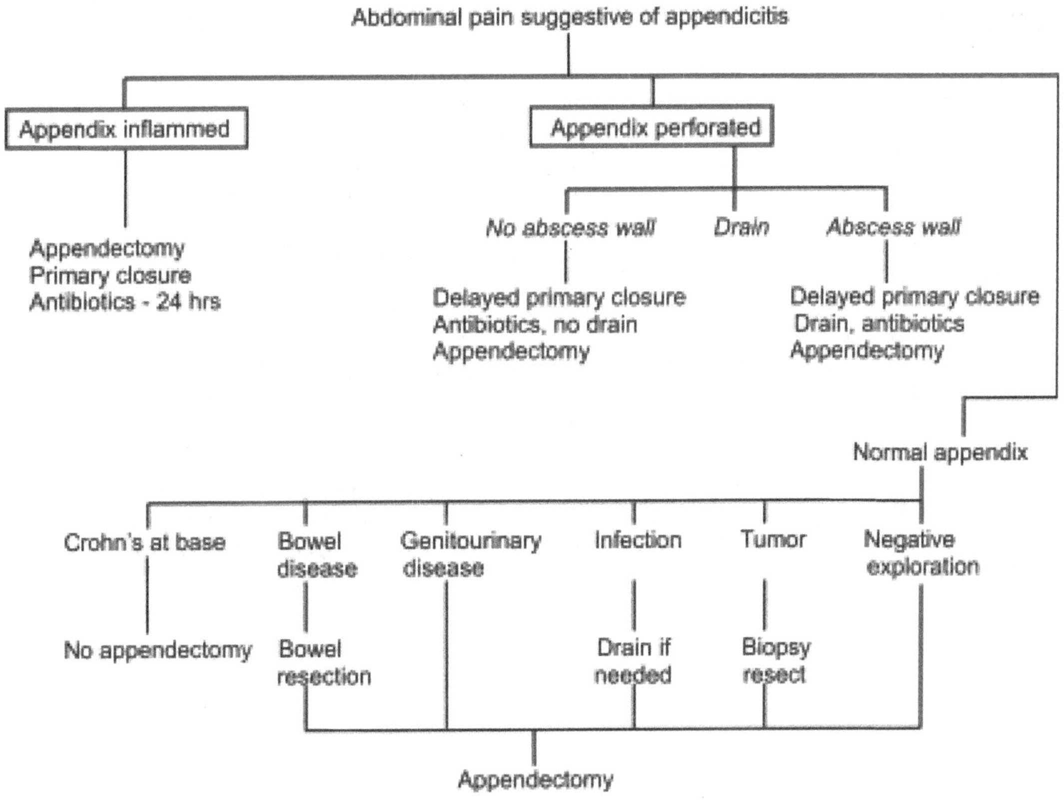

Fig. 4: Algorithm

important to maintain a high index of suspicion for appendicitis as early diagnosis is the key for a successful outcome.

CONCLUSION

The identification of appendicitis in childhood requires a thorough knowledge of abdominal physiology and diagnostic probabilities. Even in this era of sophisticated radiologic evaluation of patients with abdominal pain, a negative exploration rate of 10 to 20 percent is still appropriate because of the high incidence of perforation in children. Selective use of imaging modalities may lower this rate slightly, but the morbidity of a missed appendicitis mandates the removal of an occasional normal appendix.

REFERENCES

1. Sivit, CJ. Imaging the child with right lower quadrant pain and suspected appendicitis: current concepts. Pediatr Radiol 2004; 34:447.
2. Addiss DG, Shaffer N, Fowler BS, et al. The epidemiology of appendicitis and appendec tomy in the United States. Am J Epidemiology 1990;132:910-925.
3. Crabbe MM, Norwood SH, Robertson HD, et al. Recurrent and chronic appendicitis. Surg Gynecol Obstet 1986;163:11-13.
4. Bennion, RS, Baron, EJ, Thompson, JE Jr, et al. The bacteriology of gangrenous and perforated appendicitis—revisited. Ann Surg 1990; 211:165.
5. Poole GV. Anatomic basis for delayed diagnosis of appendicitis. South Med J 1990;83(7):771-773.
6. Graham, JM, Pokorny, WJ, Harberg, FJ. Acute appendicitis in preschool age children. Am J Surg 1980; 139:247.
7. Paulson, EK, Kalady, MF, Pappas, TN. Clinical practice. Suspected appendicitis. N Engl J Med 2003; 348:236.
8. Puylaert JB, Rutgers PH, Lalisang RI, et al. A prospective study of ultrasono-graphy in the diagnosis of appendicitis. NEJM 1987;317:666-669.
9. Rubin SZ, Martin DJ. Ultrasonography in the management of possible appendicitis in childhood. J Pediatr Surg 1990;25(7): 737-740.
10. Kosloske AM, Love CL, Rohrer JE, et al. The diagnosis of appendicitis in children: outcomes of a strategy based on pediatric surgical evaluation. Pediatrics. 2004;113: 29-34.
11. van den Broek WT, van der Ende ED, Bijnen AB, et al. Which children could benefit from additional diagnostic tools in case of suspected appendicitis ? J Pediatr Surg. 2004;39:570-574.
12. Kharbanda AB, Taylor GA, Fishman SJ, et al. A clinical decision rule to identify children at low risk for appendicitis. Pediatrics. 2005;116:709-716.
13. Busuttil RW, Davidson RK, Fine M, et al. Effect of prophylactic antibiotics in acute nonperforated appendicitis: a prospective, randomized, double-blind clinical study. Ann Surg. 1981;194:502-509.
14. Oka T, Kurkchubasche AG, Bussey JG, et al. Open and laparoscopic appendectomy are equally safe and acceptable in children. Surg Endosc. 2004;18:242-245.
15. Weber TR, Keller MA, Bower RJ, et al. Is delayed operative treatment worth the trouble with perforated appendicitis in children? Am J Surg. 2003;186:685-688.
16. Newman K, Ponsky T, Kittle K, et al. Appendicitis 2000: variability in practice, outcomes, and resource utilization at thirty pediatric hospitals. J Pediatr Surg. 2003;38:372-379.
17. Smink DS, Fishman SJ, Kleinman K, et al. Effects of race, insurance status, and hospital volume on perforated appendicitis in children. Pediatrics. 2005;115:920-925.

39 Hypertrophic Pyloric Stenosis

Hee-Kwang Yoo, D.O.

An extensive literature review of publications over the past 10 years was conducted to write this chapter. This chapter will focus on the history and physical exam needed to make the diagnosis of HPS, currently accepted imaging modalities, and preoperative management of infants diagnosed with this condition.

Hypertrophic Pyloric Stenosis (HPS) is a condition affecting young infants, in which the antropyloric portion of the stomach becomes abnormally thickened and manifests as gastric outlet obstruction[1]. HPS is one of the most common gastrointestinal conditions affecting infants in the first six months of life. It is also the most common condition requiring surgery in infants. Although many theories have been postulated, a clear etiology still remains unknown. Typically, infants with HPS are clinically normal at birth, and manifest symptoms about the first three to sixth weeks of life. It is rare for symptoms to occur before the second week or after five months of age. Symptoms manifest as nonbilious "projectile" vomiting. Accurate clinical diagnosis rests on a detailed history and physical exam. On physical exam, palpation of a thickened pylorus or "olive" along with a corroborating history clinches the diagnosis. Many times patients may go to the operating room without the need for imaging if the "olive" can be palpated.

If the hypertrophied pylorus cannot be palpated, current imaging techniques, particularly ultrasonography, are noninvasive and accurate for identification of HPS. Infants with a delay in diagnosis or prolonged periods of illness can present with extensive weight loss, lethargy, and dehydration with severe electrolyte abnormalities. The emergency physician's role is not only to correctly make the diagnosis but to preoperatively correct the patient's acid-base status, fluid deficit, and electrolyte abnor-malities.

EPIDEMIOLOGY

The incidence of HPS has been reported to be in the range of two to five cases per 1,000 births per year among the white population. The reported incidence does vary among studies from different geographic regions and the time period when these studies were conducted. HPS is less common in India and among black and Asian populations, with a frequency approximately one third to one fifth that of the white population[2]. The male to female ratio is approximately 4:1, with reported ratios ranging from 2.5:1 to 5.5:1 [3]. Male and female offspring of affected mothers carry a 20% and 7% risk of developing the condition, whereas male and female offspring of affected fathers carry a 5% and 2.5% risk respectively[1]. One can conclude that there is a greater likelihood of occurrence in an offspring of a mother affected with HPS compared with that of an affected father.

ETIOLOGY

The true etiology of this condition remains unknown despite HPS being a well-known condition. Over the past decade or two, researchers have applied much of their efforts on examination of the hypertrophied muscle in HPS, with some interesting findings. It has been found that when compared with control specimens, the muscular layer is deficient in the number of nerve terminals, markers for nerve-supporting cells, nitric oxide synthase activitiy, and interstitial cells of Cajal and that it contains increased insulin-like and platelet derived growth factors along with an increased expression of insulin-like growth factor-I messenger RNA[1]. Researchers believe that this abnormal innervation of the muscular layers leads to failure of relaxation of the pyloric muscle, increased synthesis of growth factors, and subsequent hypertrophy, hyperplasia and obstruction[4].

From a congenital standpoint, the hypergastrinemia hypothesis proposes that an inherited increase in the number of parietal cells initiates a cycle of increased acid production, repeated pyloric contraction, and delayed gastric emptying. Development of HPS after initiation of feedings, increased postprandial gastrin levels, and markedly increased gastric acid secretion in infants with HPS support this hypothesis[5].

HPS is almost never present at birth and develops within the first 2-12 weeks of life, when feedings have already been initiated. Relief of the obstruction by incision of the muscular layers leads to a relatively rapid involution of the muscle and return of the anatomy to normal. It is difficult to make the argument that the abnormalities of the muscular layer of HPS is congenital, given their rapid resolution after relief of the obstruction and the absence of functional or anatomic abnormalities at birth. These facts suggest that an obstructing event at the gastric outlet may initiate a feedback cycle, resulting in obstruction that resolves once the obstruction is relieved and normal gastric activity resumes[1].

PATHOPHYSIOLOGY

Hypertrophy of the antropyloris eventally leads to obstruction at the gastric outlet. The affected infant develops gastric distention, regurgitation and eventual projectile vomiting. Vomiting of gastric contents lead to a wide range of metabolic disturbances which includes depletion of sodium, potassium, and hydrochloric acid which results in a chloride/saline responsive, hypochloremic, hypokalemic metabolic alkalosis. Initially, the urine is alkaline with a pH > 7.0 as a result of bicarbonate losses, with little or no chloride loss in the urine[6]. In an effort to maintain intravascular volume, the renin-angiotensin-aldosterone pathway is activated, in which the kidney conserves sodium and bicarbonate at the expense of hydrogen and potassium ions, leading to the urine becoming more acidic. Although a portion of potassium is lost in gastric contents, the majority of potassium is lost in the urine.

Along with considerable hydrogen ion loss from the gastric secretions, chloride is also lost. The resulting hypochloremia results in maximal chloride conservation, with urinary chloride < 20 mEq/L. The urine chloride is usually similar to that of sodium in hypovolemic states since sodium and chloride are reabsorbed together. The findings of low urinary urine sodium and/or chloride concentrations indicates extracellular fluid volume (ECFV) contraction and that severe metabolic alkalosis is present. These patients respond well to sodium, potassium and chloride replacement. A urine chloride > 20 mEq/L suggests volume status has been corrected[6].

CLINICAL PRESENTATION

The classic child is a 2-12 weeks male infant who presents with persistent "nonbilious" projectile vomiting, lethargy and dehydration. Initially vomiting is intermittent in frequency and increases to follow all feedings. Since the child is unable to achieve adequate nutrition, he or she will have a insatiable appetite despite vomiting with feeds. Starvation will result in diminished hepatic glucoronyl transferase activity creating a mild jaundice in 1-2% of affected infants. A classic case will also demonstrate a palpable epigastric mass or "olive". The "olive" may be palpated at the lateral margin of the right rectus abdominus muscle or in the midline of the abdomen. Success in palpating the pyloric mass varies from 40-100%. Successful palpation usually requires a calm and healthy infant without a distended abdomen. Weight loss can be significant, and the infant may be below birth weight at the time of presentation. A differential diagnosis for a vomiting infant includes pylorospasm, pyloric duplication, antral web, volvulus, intussuseption, hiatal hernia, malrotation, preampullary duodenal stenosis, gastroenteritis, and gastroeso-phageal reflux among others.

RADIOLOGIC IMAGING/DIAGNOSIS

Plain films although nonspecific for HPS will often show a distended abdomen (Figure 1). Presently, there are two main imaging modalities used to diagnose HPS, the upper GI series and ultrasound. In the upper GI series, barium is swallowed by the child drinking from the bottle. Insertion of an NG tube may be necessary if the child is vomiting or the stomach is overdistended. The diagnosis is made by demonstrating obstruction of contrast flow beyond the stomach. If barium fills the entire elongated and compressed pyloric canal, the resultant image of linear contrast is known as the "string sign" (Figure 2).

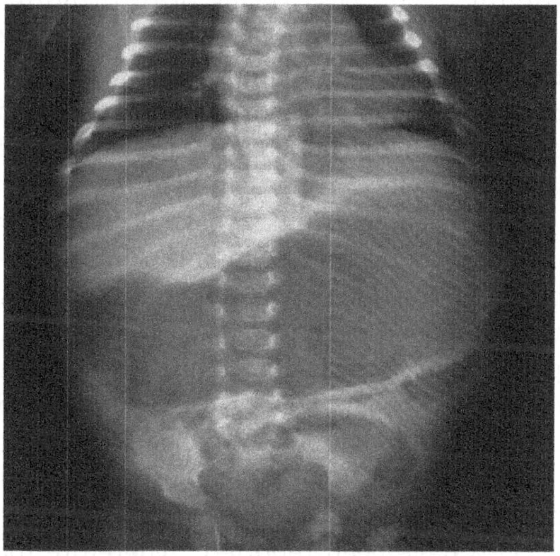

Fig. 1: Plain film showing dilated stomach

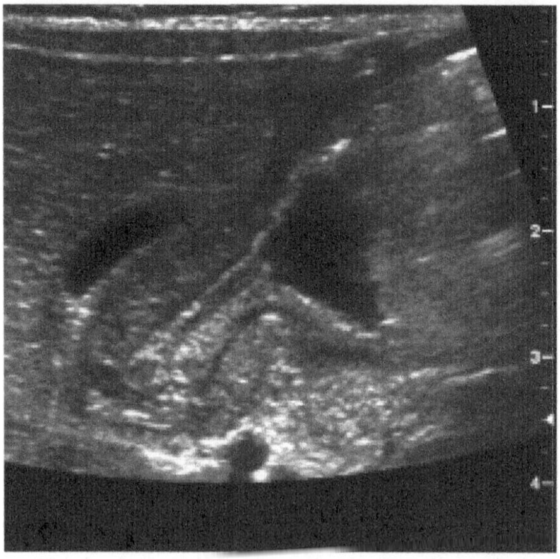

Fig. 2: String sign of HPS

In comparison, a normal upper GI series shows the prepyloric antrum to be widely distensible and quick normal egress of barium through the pyloroduodenal junction without obstruction[8].

The upper GI series does have its shortcomings. The UGI series only provides indirect information regarding the status of the antropyloric canal based on the morphology of the canal lumen as outlined by contrast material. Failure of relaxation of the antropyloric canal can also be seen in pylorospasm, which may make it difficult to differentiate from HPS. Infants with a high-grade obstruction may require more imaging time because it requires waiting for the passage of contrast material through the obstructed canal. This results in increased exposure to radiation[8]. The sensitivity of the upper GI series for the diagnosis of HPS is approximately 95%, but error rates as high as 11% have been reported[9]. Therefore the quality and accuracy of the exam largely depends on the skill and experience of the examiner.

The use of ultrasound (US) to diagnose HPS was introduced by Teele and Smith in 1977 [10]. They showed the classic pyloric olive of HPS in the transverse plane as a "doughnut" or "bagel" with an echogenic center representing mucosa and mucus surrounded by circumferential, thickened pyloric muscle (Figure 3). Ultrasound has since become the mainstay diagnostic imaging tool in the diagnosis of HPS. The unequivocal diagnosis of HPS is made by identifying the hypertrophied and elongated pylorus. The US diagnosis of HPS is made using measure-ment and imaging criteria. Widely accepted measurement criteria for a reliable diagnosis of HPS are a pyloric length of 18 mm or greater and an individual wall thickness of 3-4 mm or greater[11]. A wall thickness of 3 mm or greater should be seen throughout the examination. Measurements that change from abnormal to normal during the US study suggest the diagnosis of pylorospasm. The major advantages of ultrasound is the fact that it can be performed on sicker children at the bedside and without any radiation exposure. The quality and accuracy of ultrasound is also largely operator dependent.

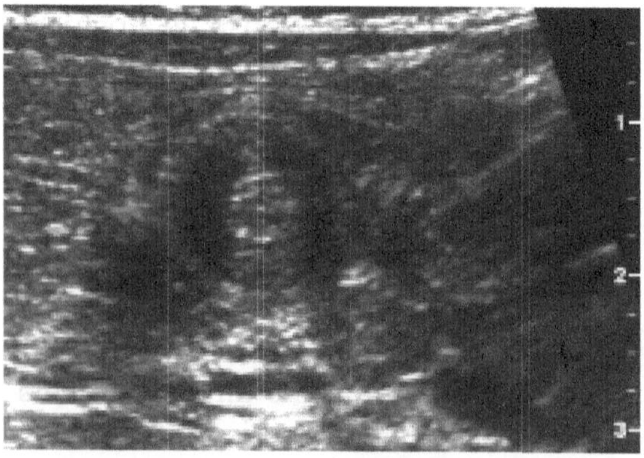

Fig. 3: Doughnut sign of hypertrophic pyloric stenosis

TREATMENT

Although surgical intervention is the definitive treatment for HPS, nonsurgical medical management prior to surgery is of paramount importance for a favorable intraoperative and postoperative outcome. It is the emergency physician's role to identify and correct the child's acid-base status, fluid deficit, and electrolyte disturbances preoperatively. The emergency physician in conjunction with radiology and surgical specialists must work together to effectively diagnose and treat a child with HPS in a timely fashion.

The typical metabolic disturbance as described earlier is a hypochloremic, hypokalemic metabolic alkalosis with elevated plasma bicarbonate associated with various degrees of dehydration. Blood gas determination and measurement of urine chloride is the most effective way to assess the severity of the alkalosis and contraction of the ECFV. Uncorrected alkalosis may delay recovery from anesthetic agents and cause postanesthetic apnea, therefore effective preoperative rehydration is imperative [6].

Correction of the metabolic alkalosis and hypochloremia in infant's with HPS depends on restoring ECFV, replacing sodium and chloride to enable the kidney to excrete bicarbonate and correct the alkalosis, and maintaining urine chloride > 20 mEq/L.

For mild to moderate dehydration corresponding to 5-15% loss of body weight or a fluid deficit of 50-100 mL/kg and moderate alkalemia (HCO_3 32-42 mEq/L), replacement is achieved preferably with normal saline with half the estimated deficit given over the first six to eight hours.

For severe degrees of dehydration corresponding to a loss of body weight of >15% or a fluid deficit > 150 mL/kg with severe alkalemia (HCO_3 > 42 mEq/L), fluid resuscitation is achieved initially with 20 mL/kg of normal saline. Once urine output is established, potassium chloride is added with a maximum replacement of 3 mEq/L/day.

Once the deficit is restored, maintenance fluid (2/3, 1/3 or D5W-0.2N saline and potassium supplementation) is given at a rate of 4mL/kg/hr. The plasma chloride concentration is used as a reliable marker for the assessment and correction of alkalosis during resuscitation in HPS and recommended that an appropriate target plasma chloride concentration be at least 106 mEq/L. A plasma chloride concentration > 105 mEq/L corresponds to a urine chloride concentration > 20 mEq/L and the latter may be used to confirm that ECFV is restored[6].

In 1911, Conrad Ramstedt performed his first operation for HPS. The surgical standard of treatment remains the Ramstedt Pyloromyotomy. The Ramstedt procedure divides the hypertrophied muscle, leaving the intact mucosa bulging through the incision. The procedure can be performed via abdominal incision or by laparoscopy. The surgery is considered a "cure" for HPS. Today, Ramstedt's procedure has a complication rate well under 8 percent and a mortality rate well below 2%. Current research on HPS is focused on finding a definitive etiology for this condition in order to prevent HPS from ever developing in children altogether.

REFERENCES

1. Hernanz-Schulman M. Infantile Hypertrophic Pyloric Stenosis. Radiology. 2003; 227: 319-331.
2. Schechter R, Torfs CP, Bateson TF. The epidemiology of infantile hypertrophic pyloric stenosis. Paediatric Perinatal Epidemiology. 1997; 11: 407-427.

3. Mitchell LE, Risch N. The genetics of infantile hypertrophic pyloric stenosis. Am J Dis Child 1993; 147: 1203-1211.
4. Oue T, Puri P. Smooth muscle cell hypertrophy versus hyperplasia in infantile hypertrophic pyloric stenosis. Pediatr Res 1999; 45: 853-857.
5. Rogers IM. The enigma of pyloric stenosis: Some thoughts on the aetiology. Acta Paediatr 1997; 86: 6-9.
6. Bissonnette B, Sullivan PJ. Continuing Medical Education: Pyloric Stenosis. Can J Anaesthesia 1991; 38:5 p. 668-676.
7. Haran PJ, Darling DB, Sciammas F. The value of the double-track sign as a differentiating factor between pylorospasm and hypertrophic pyloric stenosis in infants. Radiology 1966; 86: 723-725.
8. Blumer SL, Zucconi WB, Cohen HL, Scriven RJ, Lee TK. The vomiting neonate: A review of the ACR Appropriateness Criteria and Ultrasound's Role in the workup of such Patients. Ultrasound Quarterly 2004; 20: 79-89.
9. Hernanz-Schulman M, Sells LL, Ambrosino MM, *et al.* Hypertrophic pyloric stenosis in the infant without a palpable olive: Accuracy of sonographic diagnosis. Radiology 1994; 193: 771-776.
10. Teele RL, Smith EH. Ultrasound in the diagnosis of idiopathic hypertrophic pyloric stenosis. N Eng J Med. 1977; 296: 1149-1150.
11. Cohen HL, Zinn H, Haller J, *et al.* Ultrasonography of pylorospasm: Findings may simulate hypertrophic pyloric stenosis. J Ultrasound Med. 1998; 17: 705-711.

* Images in chapter courtesy of Leonard E. Swischuk, MD, Faculty Pediatric Radiologist at UTMB Galveston.

**In the previous edition this chapter was written by David Fisher, MD
Clinical Assistant Professor Surgery/Emergency Medicine Staff Physician
Deaconess Hospital Emergency Department, Oklahoma City, Oklahoma**

Sunit Singhi

40 Acute Diarrhea

Acute infectious diarrhea in childhood represents a common symptom in young children and is associated with significant morbidity and mortality. It is an important concomitant of malnutrition, and causes death. In our emergency unit, about 20% of all patient visits every year are for acute diarrheal illness.

DEFINITION

Diarrhea is passage of liquid or watery stools, > 3 per day. It is the recent change in consistency of stool that is important.

Dysentery is presence of blood and pus is stools, often with abdominal cramps and fever.

Following is not diarrhea:

i) Passage of frequent formed stools.
ii) Passage of pasty stools in exclusively breast fed infant.
iii) Stool passed immediately after feeds- gastrocolic reflex.
iv) Transitional stools between day 3 to 5 of life.

ETIOLOGY

In general, rotavirus (15-20%) and toxigenic Echerichia coli (10-25%) are the two most important agents causing acute diarrhea in India. Shigella accounts for 5-15% and Cholera accounts only for 5-10 percent of illnesses of acute diarrhea but these diseases continue to occur as outbreaks in different parts of India. Shigella and salmonella, the two main causes of acute dysenteric illness, are important in view of the emergence of multiple antibiotic resistances and the substantial risk of complications.

Table 1 : Common agents causing acute diarrhea in infants and young children

DIAGNOSTIC EVALUATION/ASSESSMENT

It should focus on assessment of dehydration, presence of dysentey, serious non-intestinal infection and malnutrition.

History

- Define the length of illness and stooling pattern.
- Establish that an abnormal pattern exists. Focus on frequency, consistency (watery, mushy etc.) presence of blood, response to change in the diet.
- Associated symptoms: vomiting and its frequency, fever, convulsions.

Table 1 : Common agents causing acute diarrhea in infants and young children

Agents	*Incidence*	*Pathogenesis*
1. Rotavirus	Responsible for upto 50% of diarrheas associated with clinical dehydration in children aged 6-24 months. Causes 15-20% of all diarrheas.	Cytopathic to small intestinal epithelial cells
2. Entero-toxigenic *Escherichia coli* (EREC)	Causes upto 25% of all diarrheas in all age groups	Produces heat labile (LT) and /or heat-stable (ST) entero-toxins causing secretory diarrhea of small intestine
3. Shigella	Causes upto 5-10% of acute diarrheas in all age group	Dysentery syndrome by invasion of large bowel. Enterotoxin-mediated small bowel diarrhea
4. *Vibrio cholera*	In cholera-endemic areas: commonly in children 2-10 years of age. Accounts for only 5-10% of hospitalized patients in all age groups in non-epidemic situations.	Secretory diarrhea of small bowel origin due to an enterotoxin
5. Non-typhoid	In developing countries 2-10% diarrheas in children can be due to salmonellae	Intracellular invasion of ileal epithelium.
6. Campylobacter jejeuni	Causes 5-15% of all diarrheas Disease is a zoonosis like salmonellosis.	May be invasive and/or produce an enterotoxin

- Hydration indicators: Define the amount of fluids intake and stool and urine output. Urine output may be assessed from number of times urine was passed in last 6 hours, and when was the last urine passed.

Physical Examination

- Adequacy of airway and ventilation
- Hydration status (Table 2).
- Vital signs, skin turgor, moisture of buccal mucosa.
- Signs of toxicity
- Measurement of weight changes.

Laboratory Studies

Examination of Stool

Microscopy for fecal leukocytes and protozoa is a reliable test to determine etiologic agents. A small amount of mucus is placed on a clear glass slide and mixed with two drops of methylene blue. A coverslip is placed on the slide. Staining takes about 2 mins. On microscopy, presence of polymorphs in several fields suggest infections caused by invasive bacterial agents viz. shigella, salmonella, compylobacter, etc.

Table 2 : Assessment of Dehydration

Signs	Mild (0-5%)	Moderate (5-10%)	Severe (>10%)
Watery stools	<4/day	4-10/day	>10/day
Vomiting	Some/None	Some/None	Very frequent
Thirst (Cry)	Some	Marked	Unable to drink
General condition	Well	Irritable/sleepy	Sleepy/sick/comatose
Eyes	Normal/depressed	Depressed	Sunken &dry
Fontanel	Normal/depressed	Depressed	Very sunken
Mouth &Tongue	Wet/dry	Dry	Very dry/parched
Skin turgor	Normal	Poor (slow return)	Very slow return (>2 sec.)
Respiratory rate	Normal	Fast	Fast,deep,acidotic
Pulse rate	Normal	Fast	Very fast
Pulse volume	Normal	Normal	Weak, theady
Blood pressure	Normal	Normal	May be low
Urine flow	Normal	Less, dark	Very scanty/anuria >6 hrs.

Note : Some of the above signs may not be reliable in malnourished children. Marásimic children may have sunken eyes, diminished skin turgor without dehydration. Skin turgor may be masked by edema in children with kwashiorkor; irritability and apathy may be present in both the types. In such children thirst, dry tongue and mouth, and signs of hemodynamic compromise are most reliable indicators of dehydration.

Microbiologic Studies

Culture of stool should be reserved for those patients in whom results will be of therapeutic value.

Following categories of patients should be cultured if facilities permit:

a. Toxic tooking infant<1 year who has polymorphs (pus cells) in stool.
b. Children with immunocompromised states, or hemoglobinopathies

Blood Counts

TLC, DLC may be useful in distinguishing salmonella from Shigella infections, Shigella having a marked shift to the left.

Blood Biochemistry

Blood for electrolytes, urea and glucose must be obtained in all seriously ill patients requiring IV fluid therapy, and in those with severe dehydration.

Septic workup: Blood counts, stool culture, blood culture is indicated in following groups of patients:-

1. Neonates with acute diarrhea
2. Infants < 3 months, with fever > 38.5^o C
3. Older infants and children with fever, seizure and altered consciousness level.

MANAGEMENT

Objectives

1. Prevention of dehydration if it has not occurred.
2. Correction of dehydration (deficit replacement) and maintenance fluid therapy.
3. Maintenance of normal nutrition, and
4. Identification of small number of patients requiring antimicrobial therapy.

Children With no Sign of Dehyration

They need extra fluids and salt to replace

their continuing water and electrolyte losses, and to provide for their daily fluid requirement. In general any fluid which contains some carrier (cereals, pulses, vegetables, sugar etc.) with some salt in form of a drink is acceptable. Easily available home made/home available fluids such as rice water or kanji, dal-water, lassi or butter milk, coconut water, lemon water or sugar-salt solution are appropriate. A simple sugar-salt (2 pinch salt + 1 heaped tea-spoon sugar/ 200ml) or rice-salt solution can be prepared at home.

Breast-feeding in infants and food and cereals in older children must be continued even during diarrhea uninterrupted. The aim is to give as much nutrient rich food as the child will accept.

Treatment of a Child With Dehydration

Oral rehydration therapy using WHO-formula containing 90mEq/L sodium is the best way of treating dehydration.

Reported success rates of WHO-ORS exceed 95%, failure is most of time due to extremely rapid purging. WHO-ORS has been studied in thousands of children and found to be safe and effective in diarrhea of all etiologies, dehydration of all degrees of severity up to the point of shock, and electrolyte disturbances including both hypo- and hypernatremia. It may be administered by the parent using bottle or cup and spoon and may be given by nasogastric tube. In randomized controlled trials in which ORT was compared with standard intravenous therapy, both in the developed and developing countries. ORT was found to be more rapid in correcting dehydration and acidosis while being devoid of the complications associated with intravenous therapy. Furthermore, the use of ORT appears to reduce the risk of seizure during correction of hypernatremic dehydration in children.

Commercial ORS resembling WHO formulation containing citrate are Punarjal, Electrobion, Winhydran, Electral and Emlyte. Mothers must be advised about the correct method of preparing ORS solution and the adequate quantities of ORS solution to be given to prevent diarrhea associated dehydration. Guidelines for rehydration therapy are given in Table 3.

Modified from "A manual for the treatment of acute diarrhea".

When using the table consider all of the following points:

i) Rehydration must be assessed by clinical examination, not by fluid–volume given.

Table 3 : Guidelines for rehydration

Degree of Dehydration	*Age group*	*Type of fluid*	*Volume of fluid (per kg body wt)*	*Rate of administration*
Mild	All	ORS	50 ml/kg*	Within 4 hours
Moderate	All	ORS	70 ml/kg	Within 4 hours
Severe	All	Ringer's Lactate**	100 ml/kg*	Within 3 hours. Initially as fast as possible until radial pulse is palpable
If signs of dehydration are still present, follow by:				
		ORS	20 ml/kg	Every hour

ii) The volumes can be increased to achieve rehydration.
iii) Puffiness around the eyes suggest over hydration.
iv) Maintenance therapy should be started as soon as the signs of dehydration have gone, not before it.
v) Intravenous fluids are required only for those children who are severely dehydrated, have paralytic ileus or are unable to drink.

Guidelines for Oral Rehydration Therapy (ORT)

1. Indications for ORT:
i. All children with mild and moderate dehydration.
ii. Children with severe dehydration after expansion of intravascular volume and passage of urine.

2. Amount of ORS required:

	Mild dehydration	Moderate dehydration
Total amount in ml/kg*	50	80-100 ml
Duration of administration	4 hrs	4 hrs
Amount given each time	2 ml/kg	4 ml/kg
Frequency of administration	10 min	10 min

*Ongoing losses are calcultated as 50-100 ml/ diarrheal stool and given concurrently with deficit correction. ORS should be given after each large loose motion as follows: Below 2 years 50-100 ml, 2-10 years 100-200ml, and above 10 years as much as child is able to drink.

More recent WHO guidelines have removed the differentiation between mild and moderate dehydration and has used the term "some dehydration". Oral fluid therapy is recommended in all such patients at a rate of 75 ml/kg over 4 hours.

Newer Forms of ORS: Newer forms of ORS are aimed at providing nutrition with rehydration, and if possible to reduce duration and volume of diarrhea. Rice based ORS is prepared by cooking rice instead of cooked rice may be used. It does reduce stool output by 35% in cholera patients and about 15% in non-cholera diarrhea. Amino acid fortified ORS and maltodextrin ORS are also available.

Oral rehydration therapy is ineffective if there is:
1. Increased rate of purging >10 stools/day; >15 ml/kg/h.
2. Persistent vomiting >3/hour.
3. Severe dehydration.

Treatment of Severe Dehydration

Intravenous fluids are required for these patients (look for details in the Chapter on Dehydration). *If IV or intraosseous fluids cannot be given in a remote area* within next 30 minutes.

A. Start put in a nasogastric tube and starts rehydration with ORS solution by NG tube at rate of 20 ml/kg/hour over 6 hours.
   Reassess the patient every 1-2 hours, if hydration is not improving after 3 hours send patient for IV therapy.
B. Start oral rehydration at 20 ml/kg/hour, and send patient urgently for IV therapy to the nearest suitable place.

Food

Food should never be withheld. Feeding must continue during diarrhea and increased thereafter. Breast-feeding should always be continued without interruption. Other foods including undiluted milk, cereals and vegetables should also be continued if the baby is more than 4 months of age. The aim is to give as much nutrient rich food as the child will accept.

Antibiotics

Antibiotics have only limited value in the treatment of acute diarrheal illness. Selected antimicrobials have an established role in the treatment of shigellosis (to decrease the symptomatic period and reducing the length of excretion), suspected cholera and suspected systemic infections.

Antibiotics prolong the carriage of salmonellae. Febrile, toxic children under 1 year of age in whom salmonella bacteremia is a consideration as well as those with a hemoglobinopathy or immunodeficiency should be treated presumptively depending upon blood and stool culture results. Table 4 gives details of antimicrobial therapy in diarrhea.

Antidiarrheal Agents

There is little place for these medications in pediatrics. Kaolin and Pectin suspensions have little value in altering the clinical course.

Parental Education

For the patient with mild diarrhea who is sent home from the emergency department for ongoing management by the parent of caretaker, very specific and detailed instructions are imperative. An instruction sheet containing fluid management, instructions for advancing the diet, and signs and symptoms requiring re-evaluation should be included.

Parental Instrucition Sheet for Child with Diarrhea

- Give only clear liquids – as much as your child wants-use one or more of the following during the first 24 hours: rice-water, dal-ka-pani, salted lassi etc.

Table 4: Antimicrobials in acute diarrhea

Causes	*Drug(s) of choice*	*Alternative*
Cholera	Tetracycline 12.5 mg/Kg/four doses a day for 3 days Doxycycline 5 mg/Kg single dose for 2-3 days	Erythromycin 12.5 mg/Kg four doses a day for 3 days Co-trimoxazole (trimethoprim 5 mg/Kg or sulphamethoxazole 25 mg/Kg) two doses a day for 3 days
Shigella dysentry	Ciprofloxacin 15 mg/Kg two doses a day for 3 days	Ceftriaxone 50-100 mg/Kg single dose IM/IV for 2-5 days Azithromycin 6-20 mg/Kg/single dose for 1-5 days Cefixime 8 mg/Kg/day single or twice daily dose for 5 days
Acute intestinal amoebiasis	Metronidazole 30mg/kg/day in 3 doses for 5-10days	
Acute giardiasis	Metronidazole 15 mg/kg/day in 3 doses for 5-10days	Furazolidine 6 mg/Kg/day 3 doses for 5 days

- If child is vomiting, give clear liquids slowly: in younger children, start with a teaspoon full and slowly increase the amount.
- After 24 hours your child's diet may be advanced if the diarrhea has improved. Give him normal diet with cereals.
- If the child has had a prolonged course, do not use boiled skim milk.
- Consult if:-
- The diarrhea or vomiting is increasing in frequency or amount.
- The diarrhea does not improve after 24 hours of clear liquids.
- Vomiting continues for more than 24 hours.
- The stool has blood or the vomited material contains blood or turns green.
- Signs of dehydration develop including decreased urination, dry mouth, weight loss, lethargy or irritability.

FURTHER READING

1. World Health Organization, new formula for oral rehydration salts will save millions of lives. Press release WHO/35, May 2002.
2. World Health Organization. Integrated management of childhood illness WHO/CHD.97.3A, WHO, Geneva, 1997.
3. Guidelines for management of diarrhea in children report of task force on diarrheal disease, Indian academy of pediatrics and government of India, 2000; 1-62.
4. World Health Organization, Integrated management of childhood illness: Assess and classify the sick child age 2 months up to 5 years WHO/CHD/97.3B, WHO, Geneva, 1997.
5. Choice study group. Multicentre randomized double blind clinical trial to evaluated the efficacy and safety of a reduced osmolarity oral rehydration solution in children with acute watery diarrhea. Pediatrics 2001;107:613-618.
6. WHO/UNICEF Statement. Oral rehydration salts (ORS): A New Reduced Osmolarity Formulation. World Health Assembly, New York, May 2002.
7. Bhan MK. Current concepts in management of acute diarrhea. Indian Pediatr 2003;40:463-476.
8. Brown KH, Gastanaduy AS, Saavedra JM. Effect of continued oral feeding on clinical and nutritional outcome of acute diarrhea in children. J Pediatr 1988;112:191-200.
9. Jelliffe DB, Jelliffe EFP. Dietary management of young children with acute diarrhea, 2nd edn. Geneva, WHO/UNICEF, 1991.

Mickery J. Viator, MD. FAAP

41 Dehydration and Electrolyte Problems

Dehydration, the condition of a decrease in body water, is a common illness that occurs in children. Several factors predispose infants and children to develop dehydration. Firstly, infants and children have a larger ratio of surface area to body mass because of their smaller size and disproportionate increase in head and trunk as compared to adults, resulting in increased insensible water losses through the skin. Secondly, children are at increased risk for developing acute febrile illness with infections, also increasing water needs. Lastly, vomiting and diarrhea, occur more frequently in the pediatric population compared to the adult population.

The purpose of this chapter is to review the pathophysiology, clinical presentation, differential diagnosis, laboratory evaluation and treatment of dehydration. We will also explore together the recent advances and review the literature to see what if anything is new, in the management of dehydration. Even though the world has seen marked improvements in public health and preventive care, dehydration continues to be a major cause of mortality, especially in the underdeveloped world. Even in developed countries with better access to preventive health and advanced medical care, dehydration remains a significant cause of morbidity and a major depleter of health care resources.

Let us begin with a review of the pathophysiology of dehydration. To fully understand how dehydration occurs and the effects on the patient, one must be familiar with how shifts in the water balance and electrolytes occur in the body fluid compartmentments. One must also be aware of how the body responds to these shifts, and the reasoning behind and the limitations to medical correction of these changes in body fluid composition.

PATHOPHYSIOLOGY

Water is the largest single component of the human body, comprising 60 to 80 percent of total body weight depending on the age of the child. During fetal development and early infancy water accounts for 80% of the body weight, but falls falls progressively from 6 months to 12 months of age to 60 to 65 percent, after which it remains constant. The distribution of water in body compartments is very complex, but simplification to the two major compartments of intracellular and extracellular compartments will make understanding a bit easier. Intracellular water is the total amount of water contained in the various cells in the body, while extracellular fluid is the water contained in interstial spaces and in plasma. The ratio of intracellular fluid and extracellular fluids also varies with age. With advancing age there is a gradual increase in the intracellular fluid with a corresponding decrease in the extracellular fluid component.

There are also differences in the electrolyte composition between the intracellular and extracellular fluid compartments. These become important during treatment and rehydration. The most notable are the differences in sodium (Na) and potassium (K) ions. The intracellular concentration of Na is 20 mEq/L while the K concentration is 150 mEq/L. In the extracellular fluid the reverse is true, with the concentration of Na being 150 mEq/L and the K concentration being between 3 to 5 mEq/L. Intracellular fluid contains the bulk of the phosphate and protein concentrations while the extracellular fluid contains nearly all of the chloride ions (98-110 mEq/L) and bicarbonate ions (20-25 mEq/L). In early dehydration, most of the losses are from the extracellular fluid compartment, which guides us in the selection of replacement fluid components. With prolonged dehydration, losses from the intracellular fluid compartment become progressively more important as the duration of dehydration increases.

Dehydration occurs when water intake plus the water produced by the process of oxidation in bodily metabolism fails to equal fluid losses. Distribution of water between the intracellular and extra cellular fluid compartments is regulated by forces of osmotic differences between the two compartments. As dehydration evolves, compensatory mechanisms, primary by the kidney, come into play. Antidiuretic hormones (ADHs) produced by the body causes reductions in the volume of free water in the urine that is excreted by the kidneys. The renin-angiotension-aldosterone system then acts to intiate the process of retention of Na in the kidneys. Measurements of the blood urea nitrogen (BUN), the serum creatinine (Cr), and urine sodium concentration are laboratory tests that can help the medical provider assess the effects of these compensatory mechanisms. As the limits of these compensatory mechanisms are approached, the onset of renal failure will force adjustments to fluid management and therapy.

There are multiple causes for disruption of water and electrolyte imbalances. (See Figure 1)

Dehydration can in three different ways dependent upon the relative losses of water and electrolytes, isotonic, hypotonic, or hypertonic. Isotonic dehydration is defined as a loss of total body water with the maintenance of normal serum sodium concentrations (Na 135 to 145 mEq/L). Most patient's present with this form of dehydration. The serum sodium is a function of the electrolyte concentration of abnormal body fluid loss, what resuscitation fluids were used prior to presentation for rehydration and the trans compartment shifts that have occurred during the body's attempt at compensation for losses.

Hypotonic dehydration (serum Na less than 130 mEq/L) most commonly is caused by losses that are replaced by hypotonic solutions at home. Water and juices do not contain enough sodium to replace electrolyte losses. Extrarenal losses of Na and water

Total Body Water	*Decreased*					*Normal or Increased*			
Serum Sodium Concentration	*Decreased*		*Normal*	*Increased*		*Decreased*		*Increassed*	
Physiologic Derangement	*Hypotonic Dehydraton*		*Isotonic Dehydraton*	*Hypertonic Dehydraton*		*Water with Sodium Retention*		*Sodium with water Retention*	
Urine Sodium	*<10mEq/L*	*>20mEq/L*	*Variable*	*<10mEq/L*	*>20mEq/L*	*<10mEq/L*	*>20mEq/L*	*<10mEq/L*	*>20mEq/L*
Causes	GI Loss-ess Vomitting Diarrhea Fleatue Third Space Lossess Burns Peritonitis CSF Drainage	Adrenal Insufficiency Sodium Loaling Nephropathy Blcarbonaturia Motabolic Alkalosis Rnal Tubolaz Acidosis Diureitic Excesa Post Obstructive Opresis		Diabetes insipidus Sweating Diarrhea Vomitting Fever Thyrotoxico-sis Cystic Fibrosis	Ornotic Dluresis	Nepbrotic Syndrome Cardiac Failure Hepatic Failure Acute Water Loading	Excess ADM SIADM Renal Failure Hypothyroi-dism Glucocorti-cold Deficiency	Carrdiac Cirrhosis Nephrosis	Primary Hyper Aldostero-nism Cushing Syndrome Sail Ingestion $NaHCO_3$ Excess Chronic Renal Failure
Treatment	Isotonic Saline		1/2 NS	1/3 NS		Water Restriction		Sodium Restriction Divreticss Dislysis	

Figure 1

leads to activation of the negative Na balance and hypovolemia in the extracellular fluid compartment. The body responds by increasing the production of antidiuretic hormone (ADH) resulting in maximal reabsorption of water, concentration of the urine, and hyponatremia

Hypernatremic dehydration (serum Na greater than 145 to 150 mEq/L) occurs when there is a loss of free water in excess of sodium losses. This results in a hyperosmolar state in the ECF with movement of water from the ECF to the ICF spaces. In this scenario, clinical signs of dehydration, such as tachycardia, diminished skin turgor, and dry mucus membranes are less pronounced. The neurons in the brain compensate for this hyperosmolar state by generating "idiogenic" osmoles. Therefore in the case of hypertonic dehydration rapid correction of fluid losses is to be avoided, as this may result in cerebral edema.

The diagnosis of dehydration is made on clinical grounds. Clinical signs and symptoms can help the clinician assess the severity of the dehydration guiding the planning of rehydration therapy. Using clinical parameters such as appearance, presence of tears, capillary refill, heart rate, estimation of urinary output, etc. dehydration can be classified as mild (< 5%), moderate (5 to 10%) and severe (> 10%).

Clinical estimations of fluid deficits are helpful and dependable in the face of isotonic or hypotonic dehydration. However due to the fluid and electrolyte shifts that occur in hypertonic dehydration, clinical signs may be masked in hypertonic dehydration.

A more accurate method of assessment of degree of dehydration is weight based method. If pre-illness weights are available, the percent dehydration can be calculated directly using the formula:

Fluid deficit (L) = pre-illness weight (kg) – illness weight (kg) % dehydration = (pre-illness weight – illness weight)/pre-illness weight X 100%

CLINICAL PRESENTATION

As the body water composition is lost, there are clinical signs that can be evaluated by the clinician. There may be a decrease in production of tears, sweat, and saliva resulting in dry mucus membranes. There is also a decreased resilience of subcutaneous tissues with water loss in the integumentary system resulting in sunken eyes, decreased skin turgor (tenting on pinching of the skin), and infants may have a sunken anterior fontanelle.

As fluid loss passes the 5% mark, the body's defenses attempt to correct for the decreased volume by increasing the heart rate, and increasing peripheral vascular resistance to adjust for the decreased intravascular volume. This results in tachycardia, a narrowed pulse pressure, and prolongation of capillary refill time past 2 to 3 seconds.

With continued losses of 15 % or greater, clinical signs of shock develop. Blood pressure falls and metabolic acidosis develops to inadequate tissue perfusion. Skin is cold and clammy and urine output is decreased leading to renal failure initially followed by multisystem organ failure due to tissue hypoxemia.

DIFFERENTIAL DIAGNOSIS

Even though decrease in body water from any of a multitude of causes, careful history and review of systems should be take to help identify the type of dehydration that is present as this will guide the fluid rehydration therapy plan. Firstly, we must determine if the total body water is decreased, normal, or increased? Are the systems caused by a redistribution of body water within the intravascular, extracellular, or intracellular spaces? We must determine the osmolality of the extracellular fluids, which will guide our choice of rehydration solutions. Also, as we have alluded to before, hypernatremic dehydration poses special problems and will require correction of fluid losses at a slower rate to avoid complications.

Lastly, we also need to assess the functionality of the renal system to determine whether the kidneys are compensating for the fluid loss, or if malfunction of the kidneys are the cause of, or a contributing factor to the fluid losses. Finally, we must determine if dehydration has been present for a time period long enough to have damaged the kidneys and whether this damage needs to be taken into account in planning fluid resuscitation measures

Laboratory Evaluation

In mild to moderated dehydration, in which the etiology is clear by history of present illness in previously well children, the laboratory usually is normal and does not contribute significantly to initial management. In cases where dehydration is severe or if the etiology is unclear or if pre-existing complex medical problems exist, then laboratory assessment will help guide management and therapy. The following laboratory studies should be measured::

1. Serum: pH, Na, K, Cl, CO2, BUN, Cr, and glucose.
2. Urine: specific gravity, osmolality, Cr, Na, Cl, and K.
3. Continuous measurement of urine output ml/kg/hr.

The electrolytes in the serum will be useful in assessing the osmolality of the extracellular fluid and in evaluation of the distribution of fluids in the fluid compartments. Renal function is assessed with the BUN and Creatine. Serum pH and CO_2 will help to assess the etiology of the dehydration. Losses from the lower gastrointestinal tract (distal to pylorous) result in a metabolic acidosis, while losses from the stomach or from excessive sweating will cause a metabolic alkalosis. The metabolic acidosis that occurs from uncomplicated dehydration has a normal anion gap (Normal range: 16 [+ or -] 4 or 12 to 20 mEq/L). An increase in the anion gap suggests an underlying problem such as drug ingestion, metabolic disease, or renal failure. The anion gap can be calculated using the following formula:

Anion gap = serum [Na] mEq/L – [Cl-HCO_3] mEq/L

In uncomplicated metabolic acidosis with normal respiratory compensation, the digits to the right of the decimal point in the pH, approximates the value of the total CO_2. For example, total CO_2 of 18 will be found in dehydrated patient with a pH of 7.18 with no mitigating factors present.

Potassium losses cannot be assessed from the measurement of serum K alone due to the intracellular shift of potassium with decreases in pH. Potassium will shift into the cellular space at a rate of 1 mEq/L for each 0.2 increase in pH. Measuring the spot urine K in the urine will help determine the status of total body potassium needs. If urinary excretion of K is low (less than 10 mEq/L) the body is conserving potassium and IV fluids containing K should be administered in the rehydration regimen.

MANAGEMENT

There are as many management strategies as they have authors and textbooks. Fluid deficits can be calculated by a variety of methods. Calculations of electrolyte deficits and maintenance requirements can be calculated to be replaced mEq by mEq, but one of the simplest management strategy for uncomplicated dehydration that I have seen was proposed by A. Eugene Osborne, the author of this section in the first edition of this book. I will reproduce it here.

Management of dehydration can be divided into six stages (Figure 2):

1. Assessment of the need to treat shock or significant intravascular volume depletion.

Resuscitation Fuitds	D_5 Normal Saline or D_5 Lactated Ringers			20 cc/Kg over 30 minutes May repeat x2		
				Volume	Composition	Plate
Maintenance Requirement	3 - 10 Kg → 100.00 Kg 11 - 20 Kg → 1000.00 + 50.00 Kg over 10 Kg > 20 Kg → 1500.00 + 20.00 Kg over 20 Kg					
	24 hour Maintenence requirements 00					
Estimated Volume deficit	HYPOTONIC DEHYDRATION	ISOTONIC DEHYDRATION	HYPERTONIC DEHYDRATION			
MILD	< 5 %	< 5 %	10 %			
MODERATE	5 %	10 %	15 %			
SEVERE	10 %	15 %	> 15 %			
	Deficlt extimate → Wt (Kg) x Deficit 00					
	Total Volume Requirement → Maintenance + deficit x					
Sodium Concenttration of Repair Solution	80 - 100 mEq/L	50 - 80 mEq/L	30 - 40 mEq/L			
	0.45%NoC0.5% (27 mEq/L)	0.33%NoC0.5% (54 mEq/L)	0.2%NoC0.5% (34 mEq/L)			
	Satine concentration • KCL HCO_3 • Inducted →				Solution	
Rate of Deficit Replacement	4 - 6 hours	6 - 8 hours	24 - 8 hours			
	1/2 Total Volume Requirement / hours for replacement •					
	10 - 20 hours	15 hours	24 - 35 hours			
	1/2 Total Volume Requirement / hours for replacement •					

Theraputic End Points

- Adequate Urine Volume
- Urine Spacific Gravity = 1.010
- Normal Electrolysis
- Denrated BUN decreased by one half every 15 - 30 hours
- Normal Acid-Base Status
- Urine Potassium > 40 mEq/L

2. Calculation of the amount of calories, water, and electrolytes needed to maintain normal cellular metabolism.
3. Estimation of the degree of volume deficit that has occurred.
4. Selection of a fluid composition that should correct accrued deficits and provide ongoing maintenance needs.
5. Estimation of the optimal time necessary to correct the fluid and electrolyte imbalance most safely.
6. Use of therapeutic endpoints to monitor needs to alter the initial plan.

Stage 1: Assessment of The Need to Treat Shock or Significant Intravascular Volume Depletion

If shock is present, immediate replacement of a minimum of 20 cc. per kilogram of crystalloid solution (9 NS or Lactated Ringers) given rapidly as a bolus intravenously should be administered. Assessments of pulse rate, capillary refill, mental status and blood pressure should be performed after the bolus. If signs of hypovolemia are still present, repeat boluses of 10 to 20 ml per kg should be administered until hemodynamic stability is achieved, with clinical reassessments performed between each bolus. It is also important at this stage to assess glucose via capillary blood assessment (dextrostick or accucheck) as large boluses of glucose poor IV fluids may result in hypoglycemia.

Stage 2: Calculation of The Amount of Calories, Water and Electrolytes Needed to Maintain Cellular Metabolism

Once hypovolemia has been corrected with isotonic solutions, the clinician should calculate the amount of fluids and electrolytes that will be needed to maintain normal metabolic demands. This will be added to the estimates of deficits and be replaced over the next 24 to 48 hours. This can be done using either the weight method or the surface area method using normograms. In the clinical setting, the weight method is easily calculated.

Maintenance water requirement calculation by weight:

100 ml/kg for the first 10 kg = 1000 mls
plus
50 ml/kg for each kg between 10 to 20 kg = 500 mls
plus
20 ml/kg for each kg over 20 kg

Electrolyte requirements can also be calculated:

Na requirements = 2 to 3 mEq per 100 mls of maintenance H_2O per day.

K requirements = 2 mEq per 100 mls of maintenance H_2O per day.

Stage 3: Estimation of The Degree of Volume Deficit That Has Occurred

Clinical signs of dehydration need to interpreted with the acknowledgement of the type of dehydration present since hypertonic dehydration will require more water replacement than isotonic or hypotonic dehydration (See Table 2).

Based on your clinical assessment of dehydration by percentage, the volume deficit to be replaced can be calculated using the equation:

Deficit estimate = weight (kg) X percent deficit = ml deficit.

Stage 4: Selection of A Fluid Composition That Should Correct Accrued Deficits, Replace Ongoing Losses, and Provide Maintenance Needs

In the emergency department setting, it is not necessary to carefully calculate the fluid and electrolyte replacement fluid composition. Discussions of the details of replacement fluid compositions can be found in any Pediatric text.

A simplification of intravenous fluid replacement recommendations are as follows:

For hypotonic dehydration use D5 ½ to ¼ NS
For Isotonic dehydration use D5 1/3 to ½ NS
For Hypertonic dehydration use D5 ¼ NS

These solutions given over the time periods recommended for the type of dehydration should safely replace both maintenance and deficits present. Detailed calculations can be performed but once all the components of electrolytes and water requirements calculated are combined, the final fluid composition will closely resemble the simplified recommendations above.

Note

Total fluid resuscitation fluid volumes will be the sum of maintenance fluid requirements plus estimated fluid deficits plus ongoing fluid losses (by diarrhea, vomiting, sweating, fever, etc). Estimated ongoing losses are replaced on a ml by ml basis based on measured output or estimated requirements.

Stage 5: Estimation of the optimal time necessary to correct the fluid and electrolyte deficits

After the initial replacement of intravascular volume with isotonic crystalloids to correct hypovolemia and correct or stabilize hypovolemic shock, we need to determine how quickly to correct the residual fluid and electrolyte deficits present. Isotonic and hypotonic dehydration can be corrected rapidly over a period of hours safely, while the hypertonic (hypernatremic) dehydration needs to be corrected slowly, over a period of 1 to 2 days to allow the body to adjust to the changes in the fluid compartment osmolalities. Correcting hypertonic dehydration too rapidly can lead to rapid shift of water across the blood-brain barrier resulting in cerebral edema, seizures, and even brainstem herniation.

The fluid volumes that need to be administered are then halved, the first half of calculated volume will then be administered at a more rapid rate while the second half of the calculated volume replacement more slowly, as follows:

Type of Dehydration	*First ½*	*Second ½*
Hypotonic	4-6 hours	20-18 hours
Isotonic	6-8 hours	18-16 hours
Hypertonic	24 hours	24 hours

Stage 6: Use of therapeutic endpoints to monitor needs to alter the initial plan

During the rehydration process the patient should be carefully monitored for changes in sensorium (cerebral edema), vital signs (intravascular fluid volume dynamics), and repeat blood chemistry determinations (electrolyte and osmolality). Urine output should be maintained at a minimum of 1 ml per kg per hour. When normal renal function is confirmed the BUN should drop by 50% every 15 to 20 hours as a measure of response to therapy. The metabolic acidosis will take 1 to 2 days to completely resolve. To completely replace total body potassium losses, potassium supplementation will need to continue for several days.

The above treatment guidelines will work for most cases of dehydration, however, extremes of hyponatremia or hypernatremia may require modification to treatment regimen. For example, serum sodium less than 120 mEq/L will require more rapid replacement of Na. In this case, 3% NaCl (0.5 mEq/ml) can be added to the first few hours of IVF replacement in a dose of 10 to 12 mls per kg to rapidly raise the serum sodium by 10 mEq/L. Severely hypernatremic children may require dialysis as well as fluid resuscitation.

ORAL VS. INTRAVENOUS REHYDRATION

Oral rehydration solutions have been a mainstay of therapy in underdeveloped countries for many years. The Morbidity and Mortality Weekly Report (MMWR Nov. 21, 2003/vol.52/No. RR-16) published guidelines for the management of acute gastroenteritis. In this report, emphasis was placed on the use of oral rehydration solutions to replace losses. See Table 1 for the composition and electrolyte concentrations of commercially available.

Table 1: Composition of commercial oral rehydration solutions (ORS) and commonly consumed beverages

Solution	*Carbohydrate (gm/L)*	*Sodium (mmol/L)*	*Potassium (mmol/L)*	*Chloride (mmol/L)*	*Base* (mmol/L)*	*Osmolarity (mOsm/L)*
ORS						
World Health Organization (WHO) (2062)	13.5	75	20	65	30	245
WHO (1975)	20	90	20	80	30	311
Europeon Society of Paediatric Gastroenterology, Hepatology and Nutrition	16	60	20	60	30	240
Enfalyte	30	50	25	45	34	200
Pedialyte	25	45	20	35	30	250
Rehydralyte	25	75	20	65	30	305
Ceralyte	40	50-90	20	N/A	30	220
Commonly used beverages (not appropriate for diarrhea treatment)						
Apple juice	120	0.4	44	45	NA	730
Coca-Cola Classic	112	10.6	N/A	N/A	13.4	650

Actual or potential bicabonate (e.g. lactate, citrate, or acetate)

Mead-Johnson Laboratories, Princeton, New Jersey. Additional information is available at http://www.meadjohnson.com/products/cons-infant/entalyte html

Ross Laboratories (Abbott laboratories), Columbus, Ohio. Data regarding Flavored and Freezer Pop Pedialyte are identical. Additional information is avaiable at http:/pedialyte.com

Ross Liaboratories (Abbott laboratories), Columbus, Ohio. Additional information is availabel at http:/rpdcon4D ross.com/print/PediatricProducts NSF/web_Ross.com_XML_PediatricNutrition/96A5745811839473856AB0007546ES?OpenDocument.

Cera Product LL.C. Jessup. Maryland. Additional information is avaitable at http://www.ceralyte.com/index.htm.

Not applicable.

Meeting U.S. department of agriculture minimum requirements.

Coca-Cola Corporation Atianta, Georgia. Figures do not include electrolytes that might be present in local water used for bottling. Base a phosphate.

CHOICE OF REHYDRATION SOLUTIONS

The choice of rehydration fluids can be guided by the WHO trials started in 1975 whereby the WHO and United Nations Children's Fund (UNICEF) promoted a single oral rehydration solution (WHO-ORS) containing the following concentrations in mmol/L:

Sodium	90
Potassium	20
Base	30
Glucose	111 (2 %)

This solution has proven to safe and effective after a quarter century of experience. Later studies have supported the use of a lower osmolality solution with proportionally reduced concentrations of sodium and glucose. The lower osmolality has been associated with less vomiting, less stool output, and a reduced need for unscheduled intravenous infusions compared with standard ORS. As a result of these studies, WHO and UNICEF, revised their recommendations in May 2002, recommending ORS containing the following concentrations (in mm/L):

Sodium	75
Glucose	75
Potassium	20
Chloride	65
Base	30

DIETARY THERAPY

Traditional lore in pediatric literature used to recommend formula dilutions and progressive diets, including the BRAT diet (Banana, Rice, Apple sauce, Toast). Meta-analyses and controlled studies have failed to show significant benefit from progressive dilution of formula during recovery, in fact have been associated with prolongation of studies. Studies have also shown that lactose intolerance as a result of viral gastroenteritis, in non-lactose intolerant individuals, is very rare supporting the reintroduction of milk based formulas during recovery. The practice of withholding food for greater than 24 hours has no basis in fact and may lead to delay in recovery. Early feeding decreases changes in intestinal permeability, reduces duration of illness, and improves nutritional outcomes.

Regular diets can be resumed as soon as vomiting resolves keeping some specific principles in mind. Soy formulas have been shown to reduce liquid stools without changing overall stool output, perhaps cosmetically decreasing diaper rash development. Liquids and foods with high simple carbohydrate concentrations are to be avoided (fruits, juices, carbonated drinks) as the osmolality will worsen diarrheal stools.

SUPPLEMENTAL ZINC THERAPY

Zinc deficiency (Acrodermatis enteropathica) is associated with diarrhea and multiple studies have linked diarrhea, increased stool zinc loss, negative zinc balance, and reduced tissue levels of zinc. Several studies in underdeveloped countries have been published in recent literature showing some benefit of zinc supplementation in chronic prolonged diarrhea or in those patients with pre-existing nutritional zinc deficiency. Existing evidence does not in my opinion support the use of zinc supplementation in the acute infections gastroenteris treatment regiments in developed countries.

ANTIEMETIC THERAPY

The recent decade in the United States has seen a change in the practice of prescribing antiemetic therapy in children. Reports in the literature of adverse effects of the phenothiazine derivatives (dystonic reactions, respiratory depression, sudden death, hyperexcitable paradoxical reactions, and akathiasia), led to the issuance of a "black box" warning by Wyeth laboratories declaring promethazine (Phenergan) to be:

"Contraindicated for use in Pediatric patients less than 2 years of age": as well as, "Caution should be exercised when administering phenergan tablets and suppositories to pediatric patients 2 years of age and older because of the potential for fatal respiratory depression and apnea..."

Due to concerns for patient safety and medicolegal concerns, antiemetic therapy for acute gastroenteritis decreased precipitously. This was supported by the lack of clear evidence-based proof that antiemetic therapy improved outcomes in rehydration therapy for acute gastrenteritis.

The development of newer antiemetic drugs, namely serotonin 5-HT3 Receptor Antagonists have resulted in renewed interest and studies using these drugs in the treatment of AGE. This class of drugs have proved to be more effective with a more favorable safety profile than other classes of antiemetics (Histamine H1 Receptor Antagonists, Domamine Receptor Antagonist, Trimethobenzamide, etc.)

Ondansetron has been the most used and studied serotonin 5-HT3 receptor antagonist and several studies have shown benefits in the treatment of acute gastroenteritis induced vomiting in both its parenteral and oral forms. It has been shown to have a beneficial role in those AGE patients who are unable to tolerated oral fluids and decreasing the time when oral rehydration therapy can be re-instituted.

SUMMARY

The purpose of this chapter is to review the etiology and pathophysiology of the common pediatric problem of dehydration. This problem has plaqued the physician for centuries as this is a common pediatric illness with significant morbidity and mortality. In developed countries with good access to medical care, mortality has improved, but morbidity in the sense of utilization of medical resources, lost work days for the parent who have to remain and home for the care of the child, and absence from the school setting adversely affecting the child's educational experience.

Despite the safety, efficacy, and cost effectiveness of oral rehydration therapy, surveys of emergency medicine practices continue to show that this method of rehydration is underutilized in this setting. This may be because IV access for laboratory sampling is commonly done routinely, allowing IV fluid hydration to be the simplest and surest wall to assure rehydration is performed in a timely manner. Oral rehydration is labor intensive if done by ED personnel. Even if the parents are engaged in assisting with the small frequent oral challenges, this requires persistence, full understanding, and compliance by both the parent and the child to facilitate the oral rehydration process.

The risks associated with older antiemetic therapy had effectively removed this from the armentarium of the clinician for the routine treatment of gastroenteritis. Recent literature has confirmed the safety profile and effectiveness of the serotonin 5-HT3 receptor antagonist, ondansetron, making this drug an adjunct to those patients who have intractable vomiting and who are unable to tolerate the oral rehydration regimens without resolving the nausea and vomiting.

Sandhu, BK published guidelines in 2001 which are summarized by the MMWR recommendations into seven principles of appropriate treatment for children with diarrhea and dehydration. See below:

Box: Seven principles of appropriate treatment for children with diarrhea and dehydration

1. Oral rehydration solution (ORS) should be used for rehydration.
2. Oral rehydration should be performed repidly (i.e., within 3-4 hours).
3. For rapid realimentation, an age-appropriate, unrestricted diet is recommended as soon as dehydration is corrected.
4. For breastfed infants, nursing should be continued.
5. If formula-fed, diluted formula is not recommended, and special formula usually is not necessary.
6. Additional ORS should e administered for ongoing losses through diarrhea.
7. No unnecessary laboratory tests or medications should be administered.

Source: Adapted from Sandhu B.K. practical guidelines for the management of gastroenteritis in children. J Pediatr Gastroenterol Nutt 2001; 33(Suppl 2); S 36—9).

These seven principles serve as a excellent summarizations of the established recommendations for the effective treatment of children with diarrhea and dehydration. Approaching this common pediatric medical problem in a structured manner will greatly standardize treatment options and facilitate the effective use of Emergency Department resources.

FURTHER READING

1. Osborne, E. O. Dehydration and Electrolyte Problems. Synopsis of Pediatric Emergency Care. Andover Medical Publishers 1993; pp. 285-92.
2. Managing Acute Gastroenteritis Among Children. MMWR 11/21/2003: Vol. 52, no.RR-16.
3. Practice Parameter: The Management of Acute Gastroenteritis in Young Children. Pediatrics. Vol. 97, No.3, March 1996, pp.424-435.
4. Sandhu BK. Practical Guidelines for the Management of Gastroenteritis in Children. J Pediatr Gastroenterol Nutr 2001: 33(Suppl 2): S36-9.
5. http://drugs.com/pro/phenergan-injection.html

In the previous edition this chapter was written by A. Eugene Osburn, DO, FAAP, FACEP Associate Professor of Pediatrics Children's Hospital of Oklahoma University of Oklahoma Health Sciences Center Oklahoma City, Oklahoma

Deepti Suri and Sunit Singhi

42 Dysuria, Urinary Frequency and Hematuria

Renal or urologic disorders are frequently encountered in emergency practice presenting with urinary symptoms. A disordered pattern of micturation or change in volume or composition of urine definitely indicates 'a' renal pathology, however it must be remembered that renal diseases may present without any symptoms or present with symptoms which do not directly point towards renal etiology.

DYSURIA AND FREQUENCY OF URINATION

Pain during micturation is termed as dysuria. It is caused by irritation of mucosa of the bladder or urethra. Voiding of small volume of urine frequently is referred as "frequency". Children between 5-14 years of age pass urine 4-8 times per day. Increased frequency is seldom a complaint in pediatrics but is usually significant if associated with urgency. Increase in frequency occurs either because of polyuria, reduced capacity or incomplete emptying of bladder or bladder irritation due to inflammation or infection or a neurogenic cause.

Causes

The single most important cause of frequency and dysuria is urinary tract infections.The other causes include the following:

1. Cystitis/Pyelonepheritis.
2. Vulvovaginitis in girls, Balanitis in boys.
3. Urinary calculus.
4. Trauma Foreign body.
5. Chemical irritation: (Detergents, bubble bath, perfumed soaps).

Polyuria manifesting as increased frequency without urgency or dysuria can occur with excessive water drinking, diabetes insipidius, diabetes mellitus and renal tubular dysfunction.

History and Examination

A detailed history with respect to onset and progression of dysuria and change in frequency of micturation must be taken. History of systemic features like fever, irritability, abdominal pain, trauma as well as symptoms suggestive of systemic diseases like diabetes and renal disease must be sought. Past history of urinary tract infections and breach in uroprophylaxis, may suggest urinary tract infection. Family history of renal disease especially calculi may indicate crystaluria. Examination is directed towards abdomen and genitalia for tenderness, costovertebral angle discomfort, and other findings. Spine and nervous system should be examined in all children with micturation difficulty to exclude spina bifida and neurogenic bladde.

Laboratory Evaluation

Laboratory analysis includes complete urine examination for WBC's, RBC's, castes and crystals. Appropriate urine cultures must be sent and processed fast in the laboratory for better results. Ultrasonography of the kidneys and bladder may be performed in these children.

HEMATURIA

Hematuria is presence of blood in urine. It may be transient phenomenon of little significance or sign of a serious renal disorder. It may be macroscopic (gross), urine is pink, red or cola colored to naked eye or microscopic. Normal individuals may excrete as many as 10^4 to 10^5 RBCs in the urine during a 12-hour period, corresponding to several RBCs in the sediment of a randomly collected, centrifuged urine specimen examined with a high-power objective.

Thus, a working definition of microscopic hematuria is the presence of at least five red blood cells (RBCs) per mm^3 in the urine. On the basis of presence of symptoms hematuria could also be classified as symptomatic or asymptomatic and persistent or transient.

Etiology

Microscopic hematuria is often asymptomatic, and can be present during a variety of unrelated conditions; for example viral or bacterial respiratory infections, after febrile illness, gastroenteritis with dehydration and exercise. Urine may also occasionally get contaminated from blood from external genitalia, urethral meatus. Screening of healthy children for urinary abnormalities revealed that transient microscopic hematuria is common. The cumulative incidence of microscopic haematuria is estimated to be 32 per 1000 girls and 14 per 1000 boys in a large school based study. The evaluation of pediatric patients with persistent, isolated microhematuria is often not fruitful, and no identifiable cause is found in approximately 80% of cases. The most common cause identified is hypercalciuria (22%–30%).

Gross hematuria, on the other hand is usually a sign of serious underlying disorder. It accounts for 1.3/1000 visits to the emergency. In a two-year retrospective review of 150 patients presenting to a tertiary pediatric emergency center with gross hematuria urinary tract infection (UTI) was the underlying diagnosis in half of the patients. Other causes being perineal or urethral irritation (18%), trauma (7 %), acute nephritis (4 %), coagulopathy (3%), stone (2 %). In 10 percent of patients, no etiology was found. While in a recent retrospective review of 100 consecutive patients with gross hematuria, glomerular gross hematuria was found in approximately 25% patients, with most common cause being immunoglobulin A (IgA) nephropathy. Nonglomerular gross hematuria was found in 56% patients, and the most common etiologies were hypercalciuria, urethrorrhagia and hemorrhagic cystitis. No etiology was found in 26% patients with nonglomerular gross hematuria.

The important and common causes of hematuria in various age groups are listed in the table below:

Table 1: Age wise common causes of hematuria in children

Newborn	*Infancy*	*Children*
Vascular injury: Hypoxia Renal vein thrombosis	Renal vein thrombosis Infection	Acute glomerulonephritis UTI, Cystitis
Cystic disease	Hemolytic uremic syndrome	Hypercalciuria
External	Wilm's tumor	Nephrotic syndrome
		Benign recurrent hematuria

Clinical Evaluation of Hematuria

Microscopic confirmation of red cells is necessary as red urine *without RBCs* is seen in a number of conditions. Heme-positive urine on dip stick test without RBCs is caused by the presence of either hemoglobin or myoglobin. Heme-negative urine may appear red, cola colored, or burgundy, owing to ingestion of various drugs or food dyes, whereas dark brown (or black) urine may result from various urinary metabolites. Urate crystals appear red or reddish brown and may be confused with blood especially when present on nappy of a newborn. Bright red urine with or without clot is most likely from external or lower urinary tract source.

It is important to distinguish the children with "glomerular hematuria" from extra golmerular causes. This can be carefully identified by a good urine examination and is characterized by deformed red cells. Red cell casts and proteinuria also point towards glomerular origin. The Table 2 summarizes the important differences between glomerular and nonglomerular hematuria. Extra glomerular hematuria is seen in infection, trauma, malformation, bleeding disorder, cystic diseases, drugs, tumor, calculi, sickle cell disease. A careful ultrasonographic evaluation is therefore necessary to rule out the urologic abnormalities.

Blood in the initial part of the urinary stream suggests a urethral origin of bleeding while terminal hematuria especially associated with suprapubic pain points towards bladder as the cause. Recurrent episodes of isolated gross hematuria with normal urine in between is seen in Immunoglobulin. A nephropathy, hypercalciuria, Alport syndrome, thin basement memberane disease and benign recurrent hematuria.

Acute Glomerulonepheritis

Acute glomerulonephritis is characterized by hematuria, oliguria, azotemia and periorbital puffiness and edema. Post infectious acute glomerulonephritis is the most common cause in children and is usually sudden in onset with history of preceding skin or upper respiratory infection in last 2-3 week. Urine examination reveals proteinuria, granular and red cell casts.

Immediate assessment in emergency is targeted towards the degree of fluid overload, blood pressure due to risk of cardiac failure, hypertensive encephalopathy, hyperkalemia, metabolic acidosis, and uremia (acute renal failure).

Immediate Management

In case of mild disease without any abnormality of blood pressure or renal

Table 2: Summarizing the differences between glomerular and extra glomerular hematuria

Urinary finding	*Glomerular*	*Extraglomerular*
Red cell casts	May be present	Absent
Red cell morphology	Dysmorphic	Uniform
Proteinuria	Present	Absent
Clots	Absent	May be present
Red cell casts	May be present	Absent
Color	May be red or brown	May be red

function test no specific therapy is required. Hypertension is usually transient needs to be controlled using a diuretic; furosemide 1-2 mg/kd /day or oral nifedepine 0.25-0.5 mg/kg /dose every 4-6 hourly. Intravenous anti hypertensive, sodium nitroprusside is required if signs of hypertensive encephalopathy are present. Hyperkalemia and acidosis need immediate treatment. Dialysis may be needed for correction of fluid overload, hyperkalemia, acidosis and uremic encephalopathy.

Urinary Tract Infection

Urinary tract infection should be suspected if hematuria is associated with fever, urinary frequency, burning, dysuria, pyuria and bacteriurea. Gross hematuria with UTI is uncommon; generally suggests acute cystitis. Urine examination and cultures are required for confirmation. Oral antibiotics (like trimethoprim-sulfamethoxazole, nitrofurantoin, amoxicillin, cefexime) can be used pending the culture report. Treat symptomatically as well. If the child is acutely ill or infants, risk of pyelonephritis is high and hence parentral antibiotics (IV ceftriazone 50-75 mg/kg/24 hours) is required.

Wilm's Tumour

In a child with hematuria, an abdominal mass may suggest a tumor, hydronephrosis or polycystic kidney disease. The most common malignant renal tumor in childhood is Wilm's tumor which usually presents as painless gross hematuria. It can be easily confirmed by an ultra sonography of the kidney.

Benign Recurrent Hematuria

Benign recurrent hematuria is a diagnosis of exclusion in a child with recurrent attacks of painless hematuria, with no evidence of urinary tract infection, mass, and a normal ultrasound and normal laboratory tests.

Trauma

Direct abdominal or pelvic trauma leading to hematuria usually has suggestive history. It may be associated with dysuria. An ultrasonography of the abdomino-pelvic region may be helpful in localizing the renal injury but the helical computed tomography is the best. Management in the emergency is mainly targeted 'towards' stabilizing the hemo-dynamics, followed by surgery.

Calculi

Stones are associated with pain in the back and abdomen along with gross or microscopic hematuria. A family history of renal calculi may be obtained. X-ray and ultrasonography may be helpful. A noncontrast helical computed tomography is the imaging modality of choice.

Hematologic Diseases

Gross or microscopic hematuria may be associated with inherited or acquired causes of disorders of coagulation, (hemophilia, idiopathic thrombocytopenic purpura, disseminated intravascular coagulation, or exogenous intake of anticoagulant drugs or therapy) though this is rarely the sole manifestation.

CONCLUSIONS

In conclusion, hematuria although an alarming symptom mandates a careful and systematic clinical evaluation as summarized in Figure 1. Evaluation of pediatric patients with persistent, isolated microhematuria may not identify a cause in many patients. Gross hematuria may suggest a serious systemic disorder.

Care must be take to recognize the life threatening condition which may arise and early optimum therapy instituted.

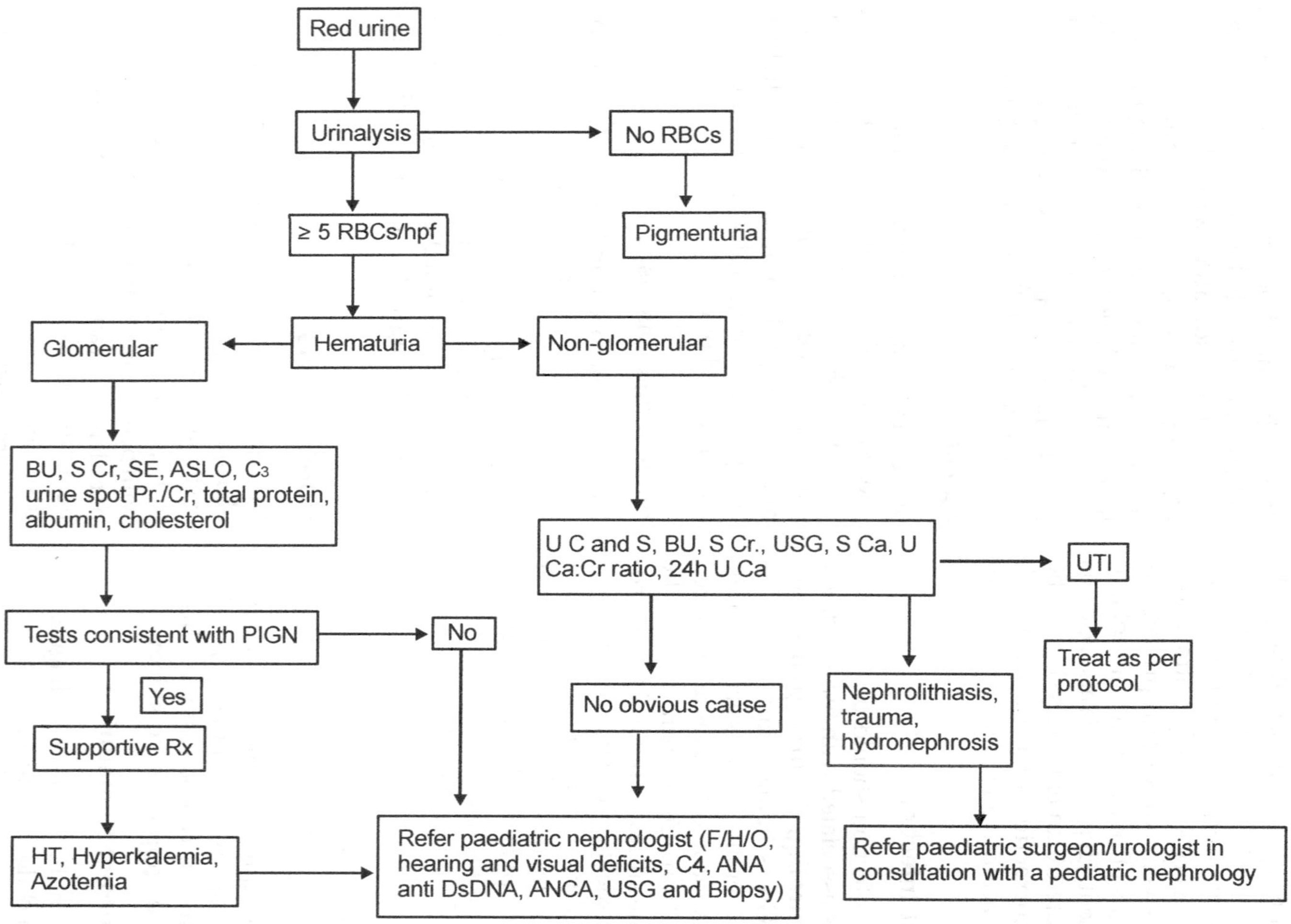

Fig. 1: Stepwise approach to a child with hematuria. (Adapted from Consensus Statement on Evaluation of Hematuria Indian Pediatric Nephrology Group, Indian Academy of Pediatrics, Indian Pediatr. 2006)

FURTHER READING

1. Pan CG.Evaluation of gross hematuria. Pediatr Clin N Am. 2006:53; 401– 412.
2. Dodge WF, West EF, Smith EH, *et al.* Proteinuria and hematuria in schoolchildren: epidemiology and early natural history. J Pediatr 1976;88:327–47.
3. Phadke KD, Vijayakumar M, Sharma J, Iyengar A; Indian Pediatric Nephrology Group. Consensus statement on evaluation of gross hematuria. Indian Pediatr. 2006 Nov;43(11): 965-73.
4. HoppeB, Kemper MJ .Diagnostic examination of the child with urolithiasis or nephrocalcinosis. Pediatr Nephrol. 2008 Dec 23(epub).
5. Cohen RA, Brown RS. Microscopic hematuria. N Engl J Med 2003;348:2330–8.
6. Patel HP, Bissler JJ. Hematuria in children. Pediatr Clin North Am 2001;48(6):1519–37.

Deepti Suri

43 Acute Renal Failure

Acute Renal Failure (ARF) is a common pediatric emergency, the diagnosis of which may be made in the outpatient clinic, in the emergency department, or in an inpatient setting. ARF is actually an outcome of various conditions and it may occur in otherwise healthy children, may complicate underlying chronic kidney disease, or may result from multiorgan disorders. The therapy is tedious, costly and carries high morbidity and mortality. Acute renal failure is often preventable, and hence identification of patients at risk and institution of appropriate preventive measures is crucial. In established acute renal failure, rapid recognition and treatment may prevent irreversible loss of nephrons. It is therefore mandatory for all clinicians to be able to recognize the symptoms and signs of acute renal failure, request and interpret initial investigations, initiate appropriate treatment, and know when, and how urgently, to consult a specialist.

DEFINITION

Acute renal failure (ARF) is characterized by an abrupt decline in glomerular filtration rate and an inability of the kidneys to appropriately regulate fluid, electrolytes, and acid-base homeostasis.

In pediatrics, this is evidenced by an increase in serum concentration of creatinine from baseline of more than 50% and an increase of nitrogenous waste products. This is usually associated with decrease in urine output, however it may be increased or may remain within normal

Oliguric: Urine output < 1 ml/kg/h or < 300 ml/m^2/day

Non oliguric : GFR 5-15 ml/min/ 1.73m^2, through urine output is maintained

Oliguia occurs in approximately 30% of ARF patients, leaving 70% with normal or increased urine output. Nonoliguric ARF may more commonly follow nephrotoxic insults, whereas ischemic injury is more likely to result in oliguria, depending in part on the severity of the insult.

The loss of renal function may occur over hours to days, leading to inability of the kidneys to excrete sufficient quantity or adequate composition of urine to maintain body fluid homeostasis. This result in life threatening consequences like volume overload, hyperkalaemia, and metabolic acidosis which need immediate attention and therapy.

The Acute Dialysis Quality Initiative (ADQI) recently proposed changing the terminology from acute renal failure to acute kidney injury (AKI) in an effort to focus attention on the early recognition of renal insult and interventions to prevent or mitigate the effects of significant renal failure.

Acute kidney injury (AKI) is abrupt reduction in kidney function within 48 hours associated with increase in serum creatinine and reduction in urine output. Staging of acute kidney injury is shown in Table 1.

A multi-dimensional system termed the RIFLE criteria [risk, injury, failure, loss and end stage renal disease (ESRD)] that classify the degree of renal insult by changes in serum creatinine and/or the duration of oliguria. RIFLE is an empiric classification system which has only recently undergone clinical validation and is merely a first step in addressing the lack of a uniform AKI definition.

Several urinary biomarkers are being studied which may herald AKI before the serum creatinine rises. A few important ones are neutrophil gelatinase-associated lipocalin (NGAL), kidney injury molecule 1 (KIM-1),serum cystatin C assay. These biomarkers may prove as assets in the emergency room for early recognition of renal injury in future.

EPIDEMOLOGY

The two most common causes of ARF in children are the hemolytic uremic syndrome (HUS) and volume depletion from diarrhea-induced ARF.

From a hospital-based perspective, the leading causes of ARF in children in developing countries are hemolytic-uremic syndrome (31%), glomerulonephritis (23%), and postoperative sepsis or prerenal ischemia (18%). These statistics contrast with the three most common causes of pediatric ARF in industrialized countries: intrinsic renal disease (44%), postoperative septic shock, especially after open-heart surgery (34%), and organ or bone marrow transplantation (13%). Previously unrecognized congenital renal disease presenting as renal failure is a distinct entity in pediatric patients and must always be kept in mind. Children with septicemia and shock, acute renal failure as a part of multi organ dysfunction also form important cohort of children who require renal replacement therapy.

ETIOPATHOGENESIS

The causes of renal failure are conventionally categorized into three pre-renal, intrinsic or renal and post-renal. The causes of renal failure have been summarized in the (Table 2) below.

Table 1: Staging of Acute Kidney Injury

Stage	*Serum creatinine*	*Urine Output*
Stage1	Increase of >0.3mg/dl or >150-200% from base line	<0.5 ml/kg/hour> 6 hours
Stage2	Increase of> 200-300% from base line	<0.5% ml/kg/hour for> 12 hours
Stage 3	Increase of >300% from baseline	<0.3% ml/kg/hour for> 24 hours or anuria for 12 hours

Table 2 . Causes of acute renal failure in infants and children

Pre-renal failure

Intravascular volume depletion

Hemorrhage/bleeding

Severe dehydration

Diarrhea/vomiting/gastrointestinal losses

Nasogastric drainage

Third-space losses

Sepsis, burns, trauma, nephrotic syndrome, capillary leak syndrome

Central or nephrogenic diabetes insipidus

Salt wasting (renal or adrenal disorders)

Diuresis (drug-induced or osmotic)

Decreased effective intravascular blood volume

Congestive heart failure

Cardiac tamponade

Pericarditis

Liver failure

Renal hypoperfusion

Non-steroidal anti-inflammatory drugs

Angiotensin converting enzyme inhibitors

Abdominal aortic aneurysm

Renal artery stenosis/occlusion

Hepatorenal syndrome

Intra-renal/renal parenchymal disease

Glomerular disease

Acute glomerulonephritis

Post-infectious glomerulonephritis, cryoglobulinaemia, Henoch-Schonlein purpura, systemic lupus erythematosus, antineutrophil cytoplasmic antibody associated glomerulonephritis, anti-glomerular basement membrane disease

Hemolytic uremic syndrome

Thrombotic—disseminated intravascular coagulopathy, thrombotic microangiopathy

Tubular injury

Acute tubular necrosis

Hypoxic/ischemic injury-prolonged renal hypoperfusion

Drug-induced/exogenous toxins

Nephrotoxic antibiotics (aminoglycosides, amphotericin B)

Nephrotoxic anticancer compounds (cisplatin)

Nonsteroidal antiinflammatory drugs

Angiotensin-converting enzyme inhibitors

Angiotensin II receptor antagonists

Radiocontrast agents

Heavy metals (lead, mercury)

Envenomations

Endogenous toxins

Rhabdomyolysis (myoglobinuria)

Hemolysis (hemoglobinuria)

Tumor lysis syndrome

Interstitial nephritis

Drug induced—non-steroidal anti-inflammatory-drugs, antibiotics

Infiltrative—lymphoma

Granulomatous—sarcoidosis, tuberculosis

Infection related—post-infective, pyelonephritis

Vascular

Cortical necrosis

Renal vein/artery thrombosis

Malignant hypertension

Vascuitis, cryoglobulinemia

Congenital renal diseases

Renal dysplasia/hypoplasia

Cystic renal diseases (polycystic kidney disease, cystic dysplasia)

Postrenal/obstructive

Urethral obstruction (posterior urethral valves)

Obstruction of solitary kidney

Bilateral ureteral obstruction: bilateral stone, stricture

WHEN TO SUSPECT RENAL FAILURE?

- Non specific sign and symptoms suggestive of uremia nausea, anorexia, drowsiness or convulsions
- Oliguria or anemia especially in children with predisposing illness such as diarrhea
- Hyperventilation due to acidosis, dehydration
- History of nephrotoxic drugs
- Edema
- Hypertension
- Hematuria or proteinuria
- Sign of urinary obstruction such as poor stream, dribbling and abdominal mass

CLINICAL EVALUATION

A thorough history and careful physical examination remains the mainstay of evaluation of the patient with suspected ARF. In emergency setting, a child may present with vague complaints of fatigue, headache, or other nonspecific constitutional symptoms or may complain of dark urine, gross hematuria, reduced urine output or edema. Hyperventilation due to acidosis must prompt the care taker towards renal dysfunction. A complete medical history, including recent infections especially diarrhoeal illness, trauma, joint pains, skin rashes, and fevers, should be sought. Information concerning intake and output and use of prescription drugs, over-the-counter medications may be important clues towards the clinical condition. The physical evaluation should focus specifically on volume status, dehydration, blood pressure, weight changes, and skin and joint findings, in addition to the full head-to-toe examination. Signs of acute renal compromise may not be evident without a high degree of clinical suspicion. Hypertension with or without other findings often constitutes an indication for prompt hospital admission while the rest of the evaluation takes place.

Step 1: Is it acute or chronic renal failure?

- Features suggesting chronic renal disease include
- History renal disease and associated symptoms
- Family history of hereditary nephritis e.g. Alport's syndrome. cystinosis, polysystic disease.
- Significant growth failure and anemia.
- Bony changes of rickets
- Chronic hypertension retinopathy, left ventricular hypertrophy
- Previous creatinine measurements
- Small kidneys on ultrasound (except diabetes)

Step 2: Has obstruction been excluded?

- Complete anuria
- Palpable bladder
- Exclude post renal causes in all patient by renal ultrasound

Step 3: Does evidence of renal parenchymal disease exist?

- History and examination (systemic features)
- Urine dipstick and microscopy for sediments
  RBC cast – glomerulonephritis,
  WBC cast – pyelonephirtis,
  Eosinophils – interstial nephritis
- Renal tubular epithelial cells, tubular casts, coarsely pigmented granular castes – Acute tubular necrosis.

Step 4: Is this pre-renal? What is the patient's volume status?

- Pulse, JVP/CVP, postural blood pressure, daily weights, fluid balance
- Disproportional increase in urea: creatinine ratio, Urinary sodium concentration (unless on diuretics)
- Fluid challenge: Infuse 20ml/kg of normal saline in ½ -1 hour along with IV Frusemide 2-5 mg/Kg

	Pre-renal	*Established Renal*
Urinary sodium	<10mEq/L	>20mEq/L
Urinary osmolality	>500 mOsm U osm50mOsm/Kg more than plasma osmolality	<350 Urine osmolality equal to or less than plasma osmolality
Urine /Plasma urea	>8	<3
Urine /Plasma osmolality	>1.5	<1.1
Urine /Plasma creatinine	>40	<20
RFI(U Na/P Cr x U Cr.)	<1	>1
FeNa (U.Na/P.Na x P.Cr/U.Cr) x 100 plasma creatinine	<1	>1
Ratio of urine creatinine to	>14:1	<14:1
Specific gravity	> 1.020	1.012–1.018

Pre renal: Improvement in the urine output

Esatblished renal failure: Oiguria persists

Step 5: Has major vascular occlusion excluded?

- Renal asymmetry
- Loin pain
- Macroscopic haematuria
- Complete anuria

LABORATORY EVALUATION

Initial laboratory evaluation, including a full urinalysis with microscopy and culture, serum chemistries, blood urea nitrogen, creatinine, and complete blood count, will help establish current renal function and determine the presence of hematuria, proteinuria, and possible infection or anemia. Life threatening complications, electrolyte imbalance acidosis needs to be identified immediately and treated. Additional tests may be indicated for etiological diagnosis, such as serum complement levels, antinuclear antibodies, streptococcal serology, blood and stool cultures, and toxic screens. Renal imaging is important for the size of the kidneys and ruling out the obstructive causes.

THERAPY

The main stay of the therapy involves careful monitoring of blood pressure, volume status, and serum chemistries for potentially life threatening acidosis, and electrolyte imbalances.Dietary sodium restriction and possible diuretic therapy may be sufficient to control mild edema and blood pressure elevations during the acute phase of glomerulonephritis.

Conservative management includes judicious fluid therapy, control of hypertension (if present), and adjustment of drug doses to the level of renal function. The use of "renal-dose" dopamine and diuretics to improve urine output has not been shown to be beneficial in the long-term outcome of ARF

MANAGEMENT PRINCIPLES IN ACUTE RENAL FAILURE

- Identify and correct pre-renal and post-renal factors
- Optimise cardiac output and renal blood flow
- Review drugs: stop nephrotoxic agents; adjust doses and monitor concentrations where appropriate
- Accurately monitor fluid balance and daily body weight
- Identify and treat acute complications (hyperkalaemia, acidosis, pulmonary oedema)
- Optimise nutritional support: adequate calories, minimal nitrogenous waste production, and potassium restriction
- Identify and aggressively treat infection; minimising welling lines; remove bladder catheter if anuric
- Identify and treat bleeding tendency: prophylaxis with proton pump inhibitor or H2 antagonist, transfuse if required,
- Initiate dialysis before uraemic complications emerge

Fluid Management

Fluid management of the patient with ARF entails fluid resuscitation to improve perfusion and stabilize blood pressure in the patient with intravascular volume contraction and hypotension. Once renal failure is established management involves providing insensible fluid volume (300-400ml/m2) and replacement of urine output and other ongoing fluid losses. The type of fluid administered should be guided by composition of fluid losses. As a practical approach, the majority of the fluid is given as low sodium, potassium free, calori rich fluid (Dextose10%). The urinary loss and other loss are replaced by N/2 normal saline with 1meq/L of potassium.

SUMMARY OF THE FLUID MANAGEMENT

- **Insensible loss** (300-400 ml/m^2) + **sensible loss** (stool + vomitus/RTA + urine)
- Fluid order should be reviewed every 6 hr.
- Continuous CVP monitoring.
- K^+ free, Na^+ free, calorie rich usually 10% dextrose
- Urinary and RTA replacement is by N/2 with 5% Dextrose

Hyperkalemia

Hyperkalemia may develop as a potentially life-threatening complication of ARF, resulting in neuromuscular conduction abnormalities, ventricular dysrhythmias, and cardiac arrest. This is because of decreased excretion by the kidneys, also contributed by catabolic states, rhabdomyolysis, hemolysis, or extensive tissue injury and metabolic acidosis. Interventions for evolving hyperkalemia include the use of loop diuretics in patients who still have urine output, correction of acidosis, and avoidance of exogenous potassium administration both enterally as well as intravenously. Potassium sparing drugs should be used with extreme caution.

Once potassium levels have risen above 5.5 to 6.0 mEq/L, therapeutic maneuvers such as insulin and glucose infusions, additional bicarbonate administration,and beta-agonists serve as temporizing measures by redistributing potassium to the intracellular compartment. Calcium chloride/gluconate may help stabilize the myocardium but has no effect on potassium levels. Removal of potassium can be accomplished with sodium polystyrene sulfonate (SPS), an ion exchange resin. SPS may only be used in patients without gastrointestinal tract injury or compromise, because gut ischemia and perforation may develop. Hypernatremia,

Table 3: Summarizing the treatment modalities for hyperkalemia

Drug	*Dose*	*Onset and duration of action*
Ca-gluconate (10%)	1 ml/ Kg IV,	Immediate,30-60 min.
Dextrose(25%)- Insulin drip Dextrose	0.5- 1 gm/Kg + 1 U/gm IV, 1-2 Hr	15-30 min,3-6 Hrs.
Bicarbonate	1-2 mEq/Kg, IV	20 min,1- 4 Hrs
Salbutamol nebulization	0.15 mg/Kg, q 30 min	15-30 min
Ion exchanger (Kayexalate)	1 gm/Kg in 70% sorbitol	15-30 min,
Dialysis		Immediate

worsening hypertension, and congestive heart failure are other potential complicationsof SPS use, as potassium ions are removed in exchange for sodium.Dialysis provides the only other therapeutic modality for potassium removal.

Hypertension

The development of hypertension in ARF may be multifactorial, with contributions from fluid overload, high renin and catecholamine levels, and systemic inflammation or vasculitis; it may also be centrally mediated. Choice of antihypertensive agents depends on the underlying disease processes and the mechanism of action of each drug. While one lowers blood pressure into a safe range, one should avoid exacerbating renal injury and comorbid conditions. For example, angiotensin-converting enzyme inhibitors specifically target high-renin hypertension but may worsen kidney ischemia by affecting renal hemodynamics. Often, vasodilatory agents are the first-line drugs in hypertensive emergencies, but careful consideration should precede their use if central nervous system bleeding is present. Hypertension that is primarily due to fluid overload may respond partially to vasodilatory agents, but effective fluid removal remains the appropriate therapy.

Hyponatremia

Hyponatremia is usually a result of exesssive amount of hypotonic fluid to oligric-anuric patients.Correction may be accomplished by fluid restriction. If serum sodium levels acutely fall below 120mEq/L there is an increased risk of cerebral edema. 3% sodium chloride is used to elevated sodium to 125 mEq/L.The risk of using hyper tonic saline include volume expansion, hypertension and congestive coadiac failure.

Sodium Replacement = 0.6 x body weight x (125- serum sodium)

Hypocalcemia

Hypocalcemia is treated by lowering the phosphorous levels. A phosphate binding calcium carbonate antacid is given orally. Calcium supplements 0.5-1mMol/kg/day are given orally. Intravenous calcium should be avoided unless tetany develops.

Metabolic Acidosis

Acidosis occurs due to inadequate excretion of hydrogen ion and ammonia. Serum bicarbonate levels below 8mEq/l may increase

myocardial irritability and hence requires therapy. Partial correction of acidosis is done using the formula given below.
mEq NaHCO3 required= 0.3* weight(kg)* (12- serum bicarbonate[mEq/L])

Nutrition

Catabolism is to be avoided by supplementing bycalories which are initially are obtained from fats and carbohydrates and proteins are restricted to <1gram /kg/day. Restriction of sodium, potassium and fluid is also important.

RENAL REPLACEMENT THERAPY

Indications for Dialysis

Immediate indications for dialysis are

- Severe hyperkalemia;
- Unrelenting metabolic acidosis (usually in a situation where fluid overload prevents sodium bicarbonate administration);
- Fluid overload with or without severe hypertension or congestive heart failure
- Symptoms of uremia, usually manifested in children by CNS depression.

Methods of Dialysis

Any of the major dialysis modalities such as peritoneal dialysis, intermittent hemodialysis, and continuous modalities such as continuous venovenous hemofiltration (CVVH), continuous venovenous hemodialysis (CVVHD), or continuous venovenous hemodiafiltration (CVVHDF) may be used. Peritoneal dialysis is generally preferred in children because of the ease of performance and patient tolerance. Although peritoneal dialysis is technically less efficient than hemodialysis, hemodynamic stability and metabolic control can be better sustained because this technique can be applied on a relatively continuous basis. Hemodialysis should be considered (1) if rapid removal of toxins is desired, (2) if the size of the patient makes hemodialysis less technically cumbersome and hemodynamically well tolerated, or (3) if impediments to efficient peritoneal dialysis are present (eg, ileus). An important limitation of HD is the need for a good vascular access, anti coagulation and that the patient should be hemodynamically stable. CVVH and CVVHD can be used in children with hypotension and continuous dialysis are now being increasingly used in ICU setting.

OUTCOME

The outcome of children and infants with ARF is extremely varied owing to the diverse and multifactorial nature of ARF itself. The degree of persistent proteinuria, elevated serum creatinine and a tendency toward obesity (body mass index > 85%) correlate with deterioration in renal function and acted as prominent risk factors for the progression to chronic renal insufficiency. Surprisingly, the length of initial hospital stay, level of peak elevation of serum creatinine, loss of renal mass, and presence of nephrocalcinosis are noted to be unreliable prognostic indicators of disease progression.

CONCLUSIONS

With early recognition of signs and symptoms of renal injury, institution of better renal replacement therapies the immediate outcome of this medical emergency is improving in children and adults. However long term studies for development of end stage renal disease in future needs to be evaluated.

FURTHER READING

1. Benfield MR, Bunchman TE: Management of acute renal failure. In Pediatric Nephrology, 5th ed. Edited by Avner ED, Harmon WE, Niaudet P. Philadelphia: Lippincott Williams & Wilkins; 2004:1253–1266.
2. Andreoli SP: Acute renal failure in the newborn. Semin Perinatol 2004, 28:112–123.
3. Bellomo R, Ronco C, Kellum JA, Mehta RL, Palevsky P (2004) Acute renal failure – definition, outcome measures,animal models, fluid therapy and information technology needs: 2nd Int Consensus Conf Acute Dialysis QualityInitiative (ADQI) Group. Crit Care 8:R204–R212. http://www.adqi.net/
4. Maxvold NJ, Bunchman TE: Renal failure and renal replacement therapy. Crit Care Clin 2003, 19:563–575.
5. Strazdins V, Watson AR, Harvey B: Renal replacement therapy for acute renal failure in children: European guidelines. Pediatr Nephrol 2004, 19:199–207.

Wayne C. Rutledge, Jr.

44 Acute Scrotum

The diagnosis of acute scrotum presents a difficult clinical challenge to the Emergency Physician. Most commonly, acute scrotal pain is related to torsion of the testicular appendage, epididymitis, and testicular torsion (torsion of the spermatic cord). Testicular torsion is the least common of the three but remains the first diagnosis to consider and must be ruled out. These must be quickly evaluated to distinguish a surgical emergency from a condition that could be treated medically. This chapter will explore the various etiologies causing acute painful scrotum by describing the pathogenesis, clinical presentation, and therapy for each of these conditions.

TESTICULAR TORSION

Torsion of the testes or spermatic cord occurs in about 1 of 4000 males, with a peak incidence at age 13 but can present at any age.[1] It accounts for 30% of acute scrotal symptoms in those aged <10 years, but accounts for about 90% in post-pubertal boys. The left side is more commonly affected and exercise, trauma and cold weather may be risk factors.[2] Delay in diagnosis and treatment can result in a loss of spermatogenesis or necrotic, gangrenous testes. Prompt evaluation is necessary if the testicle is to be spared. There are two types of torsion, intravaginal and extravaginal. Intravaginal torsion occurs more commonly and most frequently in young adolescents. Intravaginal torsion is thought to be the result from the absence of posterior attachments between the tunica vaginalis and testis that normally stabilize the gonad within the scrotum.[3] This is considered the bell clapper deformity which is typically bilateral and predisposes to testicular torsion. The twisting of the spermatic cord within the tunica vaginalis causes venous compression and subsequent edema of the testicle and cord with ultimate ischemia of the testicle caused by arterial occlusion.[4] Extravaginal torsion (torsion of the entire spermatic cord and testis, outside the tunica vaginalis) occurs almost exclusively in neonates and may occur before birth. Its etiology may be the lack of adhesions between the scrotum and the testicular membranes. It usually presents as a small, hard, nontender mass replacing the testis in a discolored hemiscrotum[3].

Testicular torsion typically presents with acute onset of severe scrotal pain with associated nausea or vomiting usually of less than 12 hours duration.[5] However, lower abdominal or inguinal pain may be the presenting complaint so it's important to examine the scrotum in patients with abdominal complaints as well. A typical presentation, particularly in children, is for the patient to awaken with scrotal pain in the middle of the night or in the morning. Many boys report a previous episode of pain which could indicate an intermittent torsion.[6] However, one study reported only 8 percent of the patients with torsion had a history of pain in the past.[7]

On physical examination, the scrotum may be edematous with associated erythema and the affected testis usually is severely tender, swollen, and slightly elevated because of shortening of the cord from twisting with a horizontal lie. The cremasteric reflex (elevation of the testis in response to stroking of the upper inner thigh) is absent in nearly all cases of torsion, but it also may be absent in boys without torsion, particularly if they are younger than 3 months.[8]

The diagnosis of testicular torsion can be made clinically as previously described, however, if the certainty of the diagnosis is in question and the performance of imaging studies will not significantly delay treatment then a color Doppler ultrasound or nuclear scan of the scrotum should be done to assess testicular blood flow. Demonstration of decreased testicular perfusion with either of these scans is consistent with testicular torsion. Color Doppler ultrasound and scintigraphy show similar sensitivity for the diagnosis of testicular torsion. A small number of false-negative cases can occur with either modality. The two studies may provide complementary information in indeterminate cases.[9, 10] However, if torsion is strongly suspected then prompt surgical exploration and detorsion are mandatory, as irreversible changes in the testis may occur within 4 hours. If treatment is not provided promptly, orchiectomy may be required for a necrotic gonad. Because the abnormality (absence of posterior testicular attachment) often is bilateral, a contralateral scrotal orchiopexy should be performed whenever an intravaginal torsion is diagnosed.[3]

TORSION OF THE TESTICULAR APPENDAGES

Torsion of the testicular appendage may be the most common cause of acute scrotal pain overall. The appendix testis and appendix epididymis are remnants of the Müllerian and Wolffian ducts, respectively. Hormonal stimulation in adolescence increases their mass, making them more likely to twist on their vascular pedicle[6]. Torsion of theses embryonic remnants in the scrotum account for 60% of cases of the acute scrotum in childhood. Torsion more commonly affects the appendix testis and peak incidence occurs between 10 and 12 years of age.[2]

Patients will usually present with sudden onset of scrotal pain as seen in testicular torsion or they can have a gradual onset as well. However, pain will be less severe usually without associated systemic symptoms such as vomiting.[11] At an early stage, it may be possible to detect a tender nodule at the upper pole of the testis or epididymis or even visualize the infarcted appendage through the skin ('blue dot sign'). The cremasteric reflex should be present and the testis should be mobile[6].

The diagnosis of torsion of the appendix testis or appendix epididymis can be made clinically, as described above. Doppler ultrasound may be helpful in cases where testicular torsion cannot otherwise be excluded. Doppler ultrasound will show a normal blood flow to the testis with occasional increased blood flow if there is inflammation.[11] The diagnosis of torsion of the appendages is difficult, and emergency surgical consultation is advisable.

The treatment of a torsed appendix testis or appendix epididymis is supportive, with analgesics (preferably NSAIDS), bed rest, and scrotal support to help alleviate swelling. The pain should resolve in 5 to 10 days. Surgery to remove the testicular appendix is reserved for patients who have persistent pain while the contralateral hemiscrotum need not be explored.[1, 2, 3, 2, 6].

EPIDIDYMITIS

Epididymitis is a nonspecific term describing inflammation of the epididymis. It is most often caused by infection but can be caused by trauma or may be reactive. In sexually active males, chlamydia is most common microbial agent, followed by N. gonorrhea, E. coli, and viruses[7]. Epididymitis occurs more frequently among late adolescents, but also occurs in younger boys who deny sexual activity[7, 12]. Prepubertal boys with bacterial epididymitis often have structural or functional genitourinary (GU) ab-normalities. Risk factors include a history of urinary tract infection, recent urethral endoscopy or manipulation, indwelling Foley catheter, neurogenic bladder, dysfunctional voiding, or a history of GU surgery. The likely pathogens in these patients are coliform bacteria[11]. Epididymitis in young boys and adolescents also may occur after infection (i.e. Mycoplasma pneumoniae, enteroviruses, and adenoviruses).[13]

Epididymitis usually presents with a slow onset of scrotal pain but occasionally will present with a more sudden onset. Other presenting symptoms include fever, urethral discharge, dysuria and other lower urinary tract symptoms[6]. Physical exam may reveal a tender swollen epididymis, however, the entire hemiscrotum can be inflamed, erythematous, and swollen. In contrast to patients with testicular torsion, patients with epididymitis usually have a normal cremasteric reflex (if they have one under normal conditions)[4, 7].

The diagnosis of epididymitis can be made clinically as described above. However, if the diagnosis is uncertain, Doppler ultra-sonography or nuclear scan may be helpful, revealing increased blood flow to the affected epididymis[14]. Additionally, this helps rule scrotal abscess as well. Laboratory data such as leukocytosis, pyuria, and bacteriuria suggest a diagnosis of epididymitis.

Once testicular torsion has been ruled out a urine culture should be obtained. In addition, the CDC recommends a gram stained smear and culture of urethral exudates or intraurethral swab specimen, or nucleic acid amplification tests for N. gonorrhea and C. trachomatis, urine culture and first void urine for leukocytes, and syphilis and HIV testing. The CDC recommends, for first line treatment when the most likely cause is chlamydia or gonorrhea, it should be ceftriaxone (250 mg IM in one dose) plus doxycycline (100 mg PO twice a day for 10 days)[15, 16]. For acute epididymitis most likely caused by enteric organisms or with negative gonococcal culture or nucleic acid amplification test, ofloxacin (300 mg PO twice a day for 10 days) or levofloxacin (500 mg PO once daily for 10 days) may be used[16].

INGUINAL HERNIA

Although most inguinal hernias present as a bulge in the groin area they can also extent and present as a painless scrotal mass or swelling. Incarceration or strangulation of an inguinal hernia can present as an acutely painful, red, and swollen scrotum which requires prompt evaluation and treatment.

Most infantile hernias occur within the first year of life with the diagnosis usually made in the first month. The overall incidence is reported as from 1.0 to 4.4 percent. Prematurity and low birth weight may raise the incidence to as high as 17 percent. The condition occurs in boys from six to nine times as frequently as it does in girls.[17]

Inguinal hernias occur because the processus vaginalis remains open after birth, allowing abdominal contents to traverse the passage. The processus develops as a result of testicular migration from the abdomen to the scrotum. By the seventh month, the testis has usually completed its descent, and the processus or peritoneal investment begins to obliterate. Patency persists in 80 percent to 90 percent of newborns and decreases to 10 percent to 20 percent in the adult. Many of the adults with patent processes are not clinically evident and persist undetected.[17]

Like a communicating hydrocele an inguinal hernia may get larger with crying, bowel movements or coughing. With a hernia a mass should be palpated from the internal inguinal ring extending down through the inguinal canal to the scrotum[7]. This should help differentiate a hernia from a hydrocele. An incarcerated hernia should be suspected if there is severe scrotal pain, bilious vomiting and abdominal distention. Emergent surgical exploration is indicated if nonoperative reduction fails. Sedation and elevation of the lower extremities with manipulation of the bulge may reduce the hernia, allowing elective repair after the edema resolves[17].

HYDROCELE

A hydrocele is an accumulation of fluid that passes through the patent processus into the tunica vaginalis[17]. It presents as a painless swelling to the scrotum that will transill-uminate easily. It is usually confined to the scrotum which can help differentiate it from and inguinal hernia. If there is any pain to the testis or if the overlying scrotal skin is erythematous or edematous then testicular torsion, torsion of the testicular appendage, or epididymitis should be considered. If the testis is normal then a simple hydrocele can be diagnosed. For a persistent hydrocele the patient can be referred for surgery as an outpatient.

HENOCH-SCHÖNLEIN PURPURA

Henoch-Schönlien purpura is a type of vasculitic syndrome that can include the skin, joints, gastrointestinal and genitourinary system. In up to one third of patients, pain, erythema, and swelling of the scrotum, and spermatic cord may occur.[18] A history of rash on the buttocks and lower limbs may precede this illness which would aid in diagnosis[7].

IDIOPATHIC SCROTAL EDEMA

Idiopathic scrotal edema is typically seen in asymptomatic boys aged 4-7 years who present with marked swelling and erythema to scrotum which can extend into the perineum and abdominal wall.[2] Palpation of the scrotal swelling usually reveals normal nontender testes and epididymis. Diagnostic workup is usually not indicated as a good history and physical exam can help distin-guish from more serious conditions.

Management is supportive and reassurance, but antibiotics and antihistamines (of no proven benefit) have been used. The edema resolves in 1-2 days and recurrence is unusual[18].

TESTICULAR TRAUMA

Although most testicular injuries are caused by minor contusions, testicular rupture or testicular torsion secondary to the trauma must always be considered. With testicular rupture, pain is usually severe and the scrotal sac appears full, ecchymotic and tender. The testical may feel enlarged and irregular. Ultrasound is usually helpful in this case, and if a testicular rupture is suspected then urgent urologic consultation is necessary. Minor contusions of the scrotum may be treated with ice packs, scrotal support and analgesia[7].

CONCLUSION

Acute scrotal pain in the child or adolescent male is a common event, but should always be suspected as an emergent condition. Of most importance is the prompt diagnosis of testicular torsion of the spermatic cord to avoid permanent ischemic damage to the testicle. Patients with signs and symptoms that are suspicious for testicular torsion or strangulated inguinal hernia should undergo immediate surgical exploration. With a thorough history, physical examination, and imaging if warranted, an accurate diagnosis can usually be made.

REFERENCES

1. Knight PJ, Vassy LE. The diagnosis and treatment of the acute scrotum in children and adolescents. Ann Surg 1984 ; 200 : 664-73.
2. O'Brien Mike, Chandran Harish: The Acute Scrotum in Childhood. Surgery: Paediatric; 2005, 22 :10, 255-57.
3. Roth David R., Gonzales Edmond T. Title: Oski's Pediatrics, 4th Edition, Disorders of Renal Development and Anomalies of the Collecting System, Bladder, Penis and Scrotum. Chapter 320 pgs 1831-1833, Editors: McMillan, Julia A.; Feigin, Ralph D.; DeAngelis, Catherine; Jones M. Douglas, Copyright © 2006 Lippincott Williams & Wilkins.
4. Kass EJ, Lundak B. The acute scrotum. Pediatr Clin North Am 1997; 44 : 1251.
5. Karmazyn B, Steinberg R, Kornreich L, *et al.* Clinical and sonographic criteria of acute scrotum in children: retrospective study of 172 boys. Pediatr Radiol 2005; 35: 302.
6. Shipstone David. Pain and swelling of the scrotum, epididymitis and torsion. Surgery: Renal and Urology. Copywrite 2004 Elsevier Ltd., volume 24, issue 5, pages 160-62.
7. Kadish HA, Bolte RG. A retrospective review of pediatric patients with epididy-mitis, testicular torsion and torsion of testicular appendages. Pediatrics 1998; 102: 73.
8. Rabinowitz R: The importance of the cremasteric reflex in acute scrotal swelling in children. J Urol 132 : 89, 1984.
9. Blask Anna R. Nussbaum, *et al.* Color Doppler sonography and scintigraphy of the testis: A prospective, comparative analysis in children with acute scrotal pain. PEDIATRIC EMERGENCY CARE. Vol. 18, No. 2, 67-71. 2002.
10. Dennis F. Bentley, Daniel J. Ricchiuti, Phillip F. Nasrallah and Daniel R. McMahon. Spermatic Cord Torsion with Preserved Testis Perfusion: Initial Anatomical Observations. The Journal of Urology. Vol. 172, 2373 – 2376, December 2004.
11. Stephen W. Burgher, The Difficult Diagno-sis, ACUTE SCROTAL PAIN. Emer-gency Medicine Clinics of North America - Volume 16, Issue 4, 781-809, 1998.
12. Pillai SB, Besner GE. Pediatric testicular problems. Pediatric Clinics of North Ame-rica 1998; 45:813.
13. Somekh E, Gorenstein A, Serour F. Acute epididymitis in boys: Evidence of a post-infectious etiology. J Urol 2004; 171:391.
14. Johannes Schalamon, Herwig Ainoedhofer, Juergen Schleef, George Singer, Emir Q. Haxhija, Michael E. Hollwarth J. Manage-ment of acute scrotum in children—the impact of Doppler ultrasound. J Pediatr Surg 2006; 41:1377.

15. Workowski KA, Berman SM. Sexually transmitted diseases treatment guidelines, 2006. MMWR Recomm Rep 2006; 55:1.
16. Updated recommended treatment regimens for gonococcal infections associated condi-tions — United States, April 2007. (www.cdc.gov/std/treatment/2006/Gon Update April 2007.pdf). Accessed on April 18, 2007.
17. J. Stephen Archer, Phillip C. Jones, Synopsis of Pediatric Emergency Medicine, Acute Scrotum, Chapter 26.
18. John M. Gatti *et al.* Current Management of the Acute Scrotum, Seminars in Pediatric Surgery, 2007 16, 58-63; 2007.

In the previous edition this chapter was written by J. Stephen Archer, MD, FAGS Clinical Assistant Professor Urology—OUHSC University of Oklahoma Health Sciences Center Oklahoma City, Oklahoma

and

Philip L. Jones, MD Chief Resident Department of Urology University of Oklahoma College of Medicine Oklahoma City, Oklahoma

Jerry Ray Baskerville and Arun Bansal

45 Diabetic Ketoacidosis

Diabetic ketoacidosis (DKA) is a true metabolic emergency that emergency physicians as well as primary care physicians must be continually aware of as a sentinel reason for a patient's presentation with variable and often complex medical symptomatology. DKA is defined by hyperglycemia (>200 mg/dL), ketonemia (>3 mmol/L) and acidosis (<pH 7.30) with the severity classification as in Table 1.[1]

Table 1: Severity classification of DKA

Severity Classification of DKA	
Mild	pH < 7.30; HCO_3- < 15
Moderate	pH < 7.20; HCO_3- < 10
Severe	pH < 7.10; HCO_3- < 5

General malaise, weight loss, abdominal pain, infection, vision changes, alteration in mood and mentation, and even extremity numbness may be presenting symptoms of this serious disorder. It is not unusual for even experienced physicians to be surprised at the unusual presentations of this metabolic emergency. Once the clinical diagnosis is considered the definitive diagnosis is straightforward. However, the failure to consider the clinical diagnosis can have devastating effects if DKA is missed and treatment delayed.

BACKGROUND

The world incidence of diabetes mellitus is expected to double by 2030. The worldwide prevalence of diabetes for all age groups was estimated to be 2.8% in 2000 and is predicted to reach 4.4% by 2030. It is predicted that the total number of people with diabetes will rise to 366 million in 2030, up from 171 million in 2000.[2]

In the United States there are 20.8 million people with diabetes mellitus or 7% of the US population. An estimated 14.6 million have been diagnosed and 6.2 million unaware that they have the disease.[3] Insulin deficiency is the primary etiologic factor in the development of DKA. The non-diagnosed Type 1 diabetic is at high risk of presenting to the emergency department in DKA. Upto two thirds of DKA presentations and 65 percent of DKA admissions in the USA and developed countries are due to previously undiagnosed Type 1 patients with this life threatening disorder.[4] Fifteen percent to 70% of all newly diagnosed infants and children who have DM present with DKA.[5] Because the diagnosis of DM with DKA is not suspected in the young child, the duration of symptoms may be longer, leading to more severe dehydration and acidosis and the possibility of obtundation progressing to coma.[6] In a carefully analyzed cohort of pediatric patients who had new-onset DM with DKA, 23.3% of the children presented with DKA. Thirty-six percent of children under 5 years of age presented with DKA as the initial diagnosis, compared with 16% of adolescents older than 14 years of age.[7] Mortality is significant with between 0.15 and 0.31 percent of patients dying from each DKA presentation.[8] The major reason for death is cerebral edema which occurs in 0.5-2 percent of DKA pediatric cases and has a 40-90% mortality rate and is able to produce sequelae in 10-25% of survivals.[9-13] In diagnosed Type 1 patients DKA occurs at a rate of 1-10% per patient annually.[14] Type 1 diabetes is one of the most frequent metabolic diseases of children and has a variable incidence in different ethnic groups with upto 35/100,000 per year in Finland and Sardinia, Italy to a low of 3/100,000 in Asians.[15] Genetic and environ-mental factors are etiologic in the penetrance of this autoimmune disorder. The HLA-DQ locus on chromosome 6 appears to be the single best genomic predictor of disease susceptibility. Coxsackie virus B (CVB) and other viral agents can directly or through autoimmune stimulation destroy beta pancreatic cells.[16]

PATHOPHYSIOLOGY

Interestingly, DKA is best described as the patient being in a profound starvation state in the presence of plenty. The bodies' cells are surrounded by substrate in the form of glucose, free fatty acids and amino acids without the ability to utilize them as insulin is relatively deficient. This concept is critical to the understanding of the vicious catabolic cycle of DKA induced acidosis, hyperglycemia, dehydration and electrolyte deficiency.

With insulin insufficiency, the passage of glucose into cells is impaired, and the mobilization of free fatty acids from adipose tissue rapidly follows because of counter regulatory hormones. This process is enhanced by the lipolytic and glycogenolytic actions of glucagon, norepinephrine, corticosteroids, and growth hormone. Glucagon enhances both ketosis and hepatic gluconeogenesis. The primary ketone bodies β-hydroxybutyric acid (βHB) and acetoacetic acid (AcAc) results in metabolic acidosis. Intracellular potassium exchanges for the serum hydrogen ions and passes out into the plasma. The serum potassium may be elevated even in the presence of total body potassium deficiency due to this acidosis related shift.

Osmotic diuresis results when glucose concentration exceeds the resorptive capacity of the renal tubule approximately 180 mg/dL. Phosphate resorption in the proximal tubule is inhibited by glucose accounting for phosphate losses.

Cerebral Edema

When the brain is exposed to a hypertonic insult it protects itself from excess fluid loss through the production of particles from cellular metabolism termed idiogenic osmoles; taurine, glycine, glutamine, sorbitol and inositol are some of these osmotically active substances. An increase in these idiogenic osmoles has been detected in brain cells as early as 4 hours after an acute hypertonic challenge.[17] The rapid treatment of acidosis and hyperglycemia promotes the development of acute cerebral edema. It is for this reason that the blitz to normalization should be avoided in children at all costs. The gradual and studied approach is difficult for emergency physicians who are trained to respond with immediacy; however it is essential in children to have patience awaiting acid base, electrolyte, and especially glucose normalization. In adults the rapid tonic shifts do not appear to cause cerebral edema and protocol driven rapid treatment regimens have been effective in reducing ICU and hospital length of stay.[18] There remains to be differing opinions on the role of rapid correction of DKA in the development of childhood cerebral edema.[19] This debate is unlikely to be resolved definitively in the near future due to the rarity of the condition and the many confounding variables in each individual case.

EMERGENCY PRESENTATION

Constitutional

Insulin deficiency in new onset Type 1 diabetes does not occur instantly. The clinical effects of insulin deficiency are most often subacute with a tipping process such as infection, dehydration or stress being the provocative event. This event and initial diagnosis is often preceded by a two to three weeks period of polydipsia, progressive dehydration, weight loss and malaise. In known insulin dependent diabetics' insulin maladministration, stress, infection and/or end organ dysfunction can precipitate DKA. In severe diabetic ketoacidosis, there is associated dehydration manifested by sunken eyes, dry mouth, and decreased tissue turgor and poor capillary refill. The vital signs show tachycardia, tachypnea, hypotension and narrow pulse pressure. Fever may be present as evidence of concurrent infection.

CNS

On initial presentation the patients' mentation may range from normal to comatose. The emergency management of altered mental status must be structured and guideline based to avoid errors in management. It is very possible that there may be two or more causes of mental status changes in a given patient. The AEIOU TIPS mnemonic (Alcohol, Epilepsy, Insulin related, Opiate, Uremia, Trauma, Infection, Poison, Sepsis) is helpful in the algorhythmic management of this multifactorial sign. The bedside testing of glucose is primary in making a timely diagnosis.

The patients' mental status can worsen within the next 24 hours of management as this is the most common time for cerebral edema to present. The signs of cerebral edema include failure to feed, somnolence, vomiting and in older children mood changes and confusion. Parents and significant others are often the first to notice subtle changes and physicians are well advised to heed any concerns of these individuals.

Risk factors that predispose children to cerebral edema include an early drop in plasma osmolality, aggressive fluid balancing and precipitous serum glucose reduction. Other factors include an extended history of poor metabolic control, acidosis with a pH less than 7.2, an initial corrected sodium value in the hypernatremic range, and a rapid decrease in serum sodium during treatment.

Cardio vascular

Myocardial dysfunction and cardiac arrest is related to intracellular potassium status. A total body depletion of potassium occurs during prolonged acidosis, and at the time of presentation in DKA, cardiac stores of potassium are often dangerously low. It is important that the clinician manage the EKG abnormalities as needed. In the case of a normal EKG and high potassium no effort should be made to reduce serum potassium by using bicarbonate or kayexelate. Treat the EKG and/or arrhythmia and not the laboratory test. The serum potassium will normalize on correction of the systemic acidosis with fluid therapy and insulin alone. Correction of the acidosis results in restoration of the intracellular deficit and rapid depletion of plasma potassium, which requires replacement to offset arrhythmias and the danger of cardiac arrest.

Respiratory

Hyperventilation with the characteristic rapid, deep breathing of Kussmaul respirations is a feature of profound acidosis. This sign can be easily missed in early DKA unless the physician decodes vital signs that are accurately taken. It is critical to all emergency patient care that accurate vital signs are recorded and acted on. The sweet odor of acetone may frequently be detected on the child's breath. The DKA patient may present with the primary complaint of numb extremities and be misdiagnosed with idiopathic hyperventilation syndrome.

Gastrointestinal

Abdominal pain with associated anorexia, nausea and vomiting is a frequent presenting complaint in the emergency department. The DKA patient may be misdiagnosed with gastroenteritis and managed with anti-nauseants and antispasmodics with damaging and possibly deadly results. The marked dysmotility in the diabetic patient is a contraindication to any medication with anticholinergic effects as this may worsen ileus and gastroparesis. Treatment for nausea is best managed by gastrointestinal rest. In the event that an antinauseant is needed a medication that improves intestinal transit and gastroparesis is advisable. Prokinetic agents such as metoclopramide (Reglan) are recommended. The usage of erythromycin has been shown to induce premature phase 3 activity via stimulation of motilin receptors and may be considered in some cases of refractory gastroparesis.[20]

Urogenital

Polyuria with frequency and monilial infection is not uncommon in DKA patients. Balanitis and vulvitis may be the presenting primary diagnosis. Cystitis and pyelonephritis can be the precipitating event in the development of DKA.

Other

An attempt should be made to identify the circumstances that tipped the patient into ketoacidosis (Table 2).

Table 2: Contributing factors to DKA in Type 1 diabetics on insulin

Insulin maltreatment: • Patient abstaining from treatment • Laxity of control • Non-compliance • Misunderstanding of the management routine
Inadequate health care resources
Psychosocial stress and depression
Alcoholism and/or drug abuse
Infection or a secondary illness
Trauma with inability to medicate

It should be stated that dietary indulgence does not precipitate DKA. One simply cannot eat oneself into DKA without insulin insufficiency.

Diagnostic Testing

The most important diagnostic testing that the physician can utilize is the clinical evaluation. This evaluation is primary in the assignment of pretest probability of precipitating etiology and treatment urgency. Vital signs with an accurate weight are very valuable especially if a recent accurate recorded weight is available. The utilization of a flow chart to assess progress or decline is good medical practice and should be used by physicians and nurses that manage these patients. The following tests will assist in the management of these patients the test and rationale is specified in Table 3.

TREATMENT

Goals

The goals of therapy in patients who have DKA[23] include: (1) improvement of circulatory volume and tissue perfusion, (2) gradual reduction of serum glucose and plasma osmolarity, (3) correction of electrolyte imbalance and steady resolution of ketosis, and (4) identification and prompt treatment of comorbid precipitating causes.

Supportive

Supportive therapy is critical to the management of the DKA patient with the ABC's of resuscitation competently followed. It is important to understand that this illness occurred in a subacute fashion and that the

Table 3: Diagnostic test in management of a child with diabetic ketoacidosis

Test	*Rationale*
CBC	Hematocrit is a rough measure of fluid contraction. The WBC is expected to be moderately elevated in DKA but if > 15,000 or shift to left consider infection.
Glucose and electrolytes	Glucose, Na, K, Anion Gap are all essential to patient management.
Phosphate	*Serum level must be ordered in DKA patients.* Total body phosphate is often decreased in DKA despite a normal serum phosphate level.
Serum osmolality	$2(Na^+)$ (mEq/L) + glucose (mg/dL)/18 + BUN (mg/dL)/2.8. Patients with DKA who are in a coma typically have osmolalities >330 mOsm/kg H_2O. **Seek other etiology if sOsm < 330.*
Calcium	Treatment of hypophosphatemia may induce hypocalcemia.
Venous pH	The management of the DKA patient does not require arterial blood gases unless the patient is in respiratory failure or is hemodynamically unstable. Venous blood gases are equivalent in pH management.[21]
Serum acetone	*The value is immaterial in the diagnosis or treatment of DKA.* The presence or absence of acetone is best evaluated by urinalysis. Urine ketones are 97% sensitive for DKA.[22]
Glycosylated Hb	Useful in differentiating chronic hyperglycemia of uncontrolled diabets from acute metabolic decompensation, in a previously well-controlled patient who has diabetes.
Urinalysis	Urine Specific Gravity, Glucose, Ketonuria, Urinary Infection, Proteinuria.
EKG	Hyperkalemia, Hypocalcemia, Arrhythmia.
Chest X-ray	Pneumonia, ARDS, CHF.

speed of correction of glucose, fluid, electrolyte and substrate be measured and purposeful. The sometimes irrepressible need of the less experienced physician to correct the hyperglycemia, acidosis, fluid deficits and electrolyte abnormalities is counterproductive at best and harmful at worst. The fastidious calculation of fluid and electrolyte deficits is marred by the inexact nature of the formulae. These formulae are not well validated and should be considered estimations only. The temptation is that once the deficits are calculated that they MUST be corrected as soon as possible. This is not the considered physiology based approach that physicians should have. *The most important aspect of management should be the continuous monitoring of the physiology of the patient with titration of treatment to effect.*

Fluids and Electrolytes

In the unstable patient volume expansion is primary with 15-20 ml/kg of normal saline being given immediately intravenously. The administration of insulin without fluid replacement in such patients with hypotension may aggravate hypotension. Furthermore, the use of hydrating fluid in the first hour of therapy before insulin has multiple advantages in that it (1) provides a chance to obtain serum potassium value before insulin administration, (2) prevents possible deterioration of hypotensive patients with the use of insulin without adequate hydration, and (3) is well-known that insulin effectiveness is lessened in hyperosmolar state.[24] The goal should be to correct the fluid and electrolyte deficit over no less than 48 hours. The normal body homeostatic mechanisms should be assisted but not overridden with oral fluid and electrolytes being administered as soon as acidosis correction allows. A good indicator is when the patient requests or tolerates oral intake. The intravenous fluids should contain normal saline until urine output is adequate for weight (0.5-1 ml/kg/hr) then based on the corrected serum sodium ½ normal saline with D5W should be substituted. All DKA patients have low body stores of potassium and magnesium and should have these salts administered by oral or I.V. route as soon as possible. In the hyperkalemic patient the addition of potassium to the intravenous mixture should take place as soon as renal function is deemed adequate. Patients without serum hyperkalemia can have potassium added as soon as bolus therapy is complete. Magnesium can also be added as soon as the initial bolus therapy is complete.

Insulin

The goal of treatment of DKA is correction of acidosis. The glucose level should not be looked at as a marker of therapeutic effectiveness. Insulin is used to enable the cellular metabolism of glucose, fatty acids, amino acids and ketoacids. It is interesting and axiomatic to understand that to clear these substrates that glucose will need to be given along with insulin. If the serum glucose level is lowered below 300 mg/dL without ongoing glucose administration hypoglycemia may occur without improvement of acidosis or closure of the anion gap.

Insulin should be initiated continuously by intravenous administration in the unstable patient. Insulin should not be given to patients unless the serum potassium value is greater than 3.3mEq/L. The need for an initial insulin loading dose is unnecessary.[25] Regular insulin at a continuous dose of 0.1 U/kg/hr should achieve adequate serum levels (50-200 mU/mL) within 60 minutes. The dose of insulin should remain at 0.1 U/kg/hr until resolution of ketoacidosis (pH > 7.30, bicarbonate >15 mmol/L, closure of the anion gap and especially no ketonuria). To prevent an excessive fall in blood glucose concentration and hypoglycemia, dextrose should be added to the intravenous fluid when the plasma glucose has fallen to approximately 300 mg/dL. Serum glucose must be maintained above 200 mg/dL until acidosis is cleared and catabolism is arrested. The urine ketone test is an accurate indicator of ketone production. If the serum glucose cannot be maintained > 200 despite a 12.5% dextrose administration at maintenance fluid rates then the insulin dosage must be reduced at a rate of 0.02 U/kg/hr per hour until stabilized. The half life of insulin is 5 minutes therefore intermittent stoppage of the insulin drip is discouraged. If an insulin drip is not possible then subcutaneous (SC) insulin can be considered. Hourly subcutaneous dosing of regular or short acting insulin has proven safe and effective in adults with DKA but as yet is unproven in children.[26] There are instances of insulin resistance where the acidosis does not show adequate clearance. In those cases the insulin administration, concentration and admixture should be closely checked. If administration is vetted then insulin may need to be increased by a factor of two to three above normal dosage.

The insulin types in the USA are listed in Table 4.

The continuous insulin drip should be maintained until the arrest of catabolism and the correction of acidosis. The patient should be able to sustain fluid and caloric requirements by oral intake before initiation of subcutaneous insulin. Agus suggests the starting dose of subcutaneous insulin can be based on a total daily dose (TDD) of insulin of 0.75 U/kg/d in prepubertal children and 1 U/kg/d in older patients.[27] Two thirds of the TDD is given before breakfast (one third as rapid-acting insulin and two thirds as intermediate-acting insulin; in young children, one fourth is given as rapid-acting insulin and three fourths are given as intermediate-acting insulin). One third of the remainder of the TDD is given before dinner as rapid-acting insulin, and two thirds of the remainder of the TDD is given as intermediate-acting insulin at bedtime shown in Table 5.

Potassium

Potassium is best replenished by oral replacement in the DKA patient with a functioning gastrointestinal tract. Intravenous potassium administration is potentially dangerous with errors of calculation or mixture potentially life-threatening. A total body potassium deficit exists in DKA patients even with normal or high serum concentrations. Potassium should be infused shortly after the I.V. insulin infusion is started because of the immediate action of insulin and fluid therapy on the intracellular passage of potassium. Initial fluid bolus therapy with normal saline should occur prior to the infusion of potassium. The administration of potassium to a poorly perfused patient with low urine output can induce dangerous hyperkalemia and cardiac arrhythmias.

Intravenous potassium at a concentration of 30 to 40 mEq per liter of I.V. solution should be administered once urine output is established and hyperkalemia > 5.5 mEq/L is excluded. Central line venous access and cardiac monitoring is required if > 40 mEq/L is necessary or a rate of administration is > 20 mEq/Hour. Acidosis increases potassium serum levels by a factor of 1 mEq/L for every

Table 4: Types of insulin that are commericially available

Insulin brand (Type)	*Onset*	*Peak*	*Duration (Hours)*	*Role in blood glucose management*
Rapid-Acting				
Humalog (lispro)	15-30 min.	30-90 min	3-5	Rapid-acting insulin covers insulin needs for meals eaten at the same time as the injection. This type of insulin is used with longer-acting insulin.
Novolog (aspart)	10-20 min.	40-50 min.	3-5	
Apidra (glulisine)	20-30 min.	30-90 min.	1-2½	
Short-Acting				
Regular (R) (humulin, novolin)	30 min. - 1 hour	2-5 hours	5-8	Short-acting insulin covers insulin needs for meals eaten within 30-60 minutes.
Velosulin (for use in the insulin pump)	30 min.- 1 hour	2-3 hours	2-3	
Intermediate-Acting				
NPH (N)	1-2 hours	4-12 hours	18-24	Intermediate-acting insulin covers insulin needs for about half the day or overnight. This type of insulin is often combined with rapid- or short-acting insulin.
Lente (L)	1-2½ hours	3-10 hours	18-24	
Long-Acting				
Ultralente (U)	30 min.- 3 hours	10-20 hours	20-36	Long-acting insulin covers insulin needs for about 1 full day. This type of insulin is often combined, when needed, with rapid- or short-acting insulin.
Lantus	1-1½ hour	No peak time; insulin is delivered at a steady level	20-24	
Levemir (detemir)	1-2 hours	6-8 hours	Upto 24	
Pre-Mixed*				
Humulin 70/30	30 min.	2-4 hours	14-24	These products are generally taken twice a day before mealtime.
Novolin 70/30	30 min.	2-12 hours	Upto 24	
Novolog 70/30	10-20 min.	1-4 hours	Upto 24	
Humulin 50/50	30 min.	2-5 hours	18-24	
Humalog 75/25	15 min.	30 min.- 2½ hours	16-20	

* Premixed insulins are a combination of specific proportions of intermediate-acting and short-acting insulin in one bottle or insulin pen (the numbers following the brand name indicate the percentage of each type of insulin).

Table 5: Starting dose of insulin after recovery from DKA

		Breakfast TDD						***Breakfast*** TDD			
Units/Kg/ Day	*Weight*	*Insulin*	*Regular*	*Intermediate*	***Total***	*Units/Kg/ Day*	*Weight*	*Insulin*	*Regular*	*Intermediate*	***Total***
1.00	10	10	3	4	**7**	0.75	10	8	1	4	**5**
1.00	15	15	3	7	**10**	0.75	15	11	2	6	**8**
1.00	20	20	4	9	**13**	0.75	20	15	3	8	**11**
1.00	25	25	6	11	**17**	0.75	25	19	3	9	**12**
1.00	30	30	7	13	**20**	0.75	30	23	4	11	**15**
1.00	35	35	8	16	**24**	0.75	35	26	4	13	**17**
1.00	40	40	9	18	**27**	0.75	40	30	5	15	**20**
1.00	45	45	10	20	**30**	0.75	45	34	6	17	**23**
1.00	50	50	11	22	**33**	0.75	50	38	6	19	**25**
1.00	55	55	12	24	**36**	0.75	55	41	7	21	**28**
1.00	60	60	13	27	**40**	0.75	60	45	8	23	**31**
1.00	65	65	14	29	**43**	0.75	65	49	8	24	**32**
1.00	70	70	16	31	**47**	0.75	70	53	9	26	**35**

		Noon Meal TDD					***Noon Meal*** TDD		
Units/Kg/Day	*Weight*	*Insulin*	*Available*	***Regular***	*Units/Kg/Day*	*Weight*	*Insulin*	*Available*	***Regular***
1.00	10	10	3	**1**	0.75	10	8	3	**1**
1.00	15	15	5	**2**	0.75	15	11	4	**1**
1.00	20	20	7	**2**	0.75	20	15	5	**2**
1.00	25	25	8	**3**	0.75	25	19	6	**2**
1.00	30	30	10	**3**	0.75	30	23	8	**3**
1.00	35	35	12	**4**	0.75	35	26	9	**3**
1.00	40	40	13	**4**	0.75	40	30	10	**3**
1.00	45	45	15	**5**	0.75	45	34	11	**4**
1.00	50	50	17	**6**	0.75	50	38	13	**4**
1.00	55	55	18	**6**	0.75	55	41	14	**5**
1.00	60	60	20	**7**	0.75	60	45	15	**5**
1.00	65	65	22	**7**	0.75	65	49	16	**5**
1.00	70	70	23	**8**	0.75	70	53	18	**6**

	Bedtime TDD				***Bedtime*** TDD		
Units/Kg/Day	*Weight*	*Insulin*	***Intermediate***	*Units/Kg/Day*	*Weight*	*Insulin*	***Intermediate***
1.00	10	10	**2**	0.75	10	8	**2**
1.00	15	15	**3**	0.75	15	11	**3**
1.00	20	20	**4**	0.75	20	15	**3**
1.00	25	25	**6**	0.75	25	19	**4**
1.00	30	30	**7**	0.75	30	23	**5**
1.00	35	35	**8**	0.75	35	26	**6**
1.00	40	40	**9**	0.75	40	30	**7**
1.00	45	45	**10**	0.75	45	34	**8**
1.00	50	50	**11**	0.75	50	38	**8**
1.00	55	55	**12**	0.75	55	41	**9**
1.00	60	60	**13**	0.75	60	45	**10**
1.00	65	65	**14**	0.75	65	49	**11**
1.00	70	70	**16**	0.75	70	53	**12**

0.1 change of pH < 7.4. With PICU monitoring > 60 mEq/L of potassium may be used. This concentration (60 mEq/L) may be used if the initial K < 3.5 mEq/L. Consider delaying insulin infusion until potassium is > 3 mEq/L.

Potassium chloride is the initial parenteral replacement salt with potassium phosphate used if a serum phosphate deficit is present and oral phosphate administration is not possible.

When in doubt about serum potassium, immediate information may be obtained from an electrocardiogram (EKG). If hypokalemia is present, prolongation of the QT interval with wide, low amplitude T waves may be seen.

Phosphate

Signs of hypophosphatemia include weakness, paresthesias, confusion, stupor, seizures, coma, hemolysis, platelet dysfunction, metabolic acidosis, rhabdomyolysis, respiratory compromise and/or CHF. Importantly the serum phosphate may not be a part of the electrolyte or metabolic panel in your institution and may require a separate order. If the serum phosphate is PO_4 < 1 mg/dL immediate phosphate replacement is required. Replacement of the phosphate deficit improves oxygen delivery to tissues by replacing red blood cell 2,3-diphosphoglycerate (2,3-DPG) so that impaired brain and myocardial oxygenation is avoided. Determination of initial ionized calcium is also advisable since excessive phosphate may precipitate with calcium and decrease the serum calcium level. Table 6 presents oral and parenteral options for treatment.

Bicarbonate

The only indication for bicarbonate is in the management of acute cardiac arrhythmia from hyperkalemia. The calculation of deficit should be expeditiously forgotten in DKA. There is no evidence that bicarbonate improves

Table 6: Oral and parenteral preparations for correction of phosphate deficit

Preparation oral	Phosphate mmol	Na+ mEq	K+ mEq
Neutra-Phos® (capsule/pkt)	8	7.1	7.1
Neutra-Phos K® (capsule/pkt)	8	0	14.25
Skim milk per 8 oz (1 cup)	8	3	5
K-Phos ® Neutral (tablet)	8	13	1.1
Preparation Intravenous	**Phosphate mmol/ml**	**Na+ mEq/ml**	**K+ mEq/ml**
I.V. preparations include sodium phosphate (Na_2HPO_4 and NAH_2PO_4) or potassium phosphate (K_2HPO_4 and KH_2PO_4). Pediatric Dose: 0.25-0.5 mmol/kg IV over 4-6 h; repeat if symptomatic hypophosphatemia persists			
Potassium Phosphate (ml) *3 mmol = 93 mg phosphorus (MW = 31)*	3	0	4.4

Phosphate equivalence: 22 mEq = 15 mmol = 465 mg (Conversion conventional to SI 0.0323).
Maintenance dosing
Children: 0.5-1.5 mmol/kg/24 hours Intravenous or 2-3 mmol/kg/24 hours orally.

outcomes and considerable evidence of associated risks to its usage. Cerebral edema, paradoxical CSF acidosis, hypokalemia, salt load excess, ARDS and hemoglobin – oxygen association curve shift are all directly associated with bicarbonate administration. A summary of management is outlined in Table 7.

Recovery

Oral intake of fluids and solids should be encouraged, but never forced. As the patient recovers oral correction of fluid balance, electrolytes and nutrition is the fastest road to homeostasis. Ketoacidosis causes anorexia. Acidosis will require correction before the patient will want to eat or drink. Hypotonic oral fluids should be avoided in large volumes because of the risk of cerebral edema. Nursing care should include accurate intake and output. Urine specific gravity and ketone assessment is helpful in fluid management.

In order to determine an approximate insulin dose requirement, most children will need a short period of in-hospital adjustment during which blood sugars are monitored under conditions that simulate the home environment with respect to diet and activity. Dietary counseling and compliance are essential to proficient patient care. It is of little value to enforce a strict hospital diet when on going home the patient will return to a free feeding routine. The initial period after diagnosis is an important phase of therapy that involves education and encouragement of both parents and child. At this time factors such as age, level of education, maturity, and acceptance of diabetes should be taken into consideration.

Table 7: Outline of emergency management of DKA

Fluids	• Use 5 - 7% dehydration in moderate DKA and 10% in severe DKA. • Fluid bolus of 15 – 20 ml/kg in 1st hr with isotonic saline. • Subsequent fluid is N/2 saline. • Rate of infusion is calculated to rehydrate evenly over 48 hours. • Add 5% dextrose once the blood sugar is 250 - 300 mg/dL. • If the blood glucose concentration declines below 150 mg/dL, the dextrose content may need to be increased to 10% or even 12.5%.
Potassium	• May present with high, normal, or low serum potassium values. • All affected patients have total body potassium depletion. • Unless the patient exhibits hyperkalemia or anuria, potassium should be added to the intravenous fluids at the beginning of the second hour of therapy. • Otherwise, potassium is added as soon as urine output is stablished or the hyperkalemia abates.
Insulin	• Low-dose insulin infusion of regular insulin at 0.1 units/kg/h. • Continue insulin infusion until resolution of DKA (pH>7.30, bicarbonate > 18 mEq/L). • The resolution of academia invariably takes longer than normalization of blood glucose concentrations.
Phosphate	• There is no evidence that replacement has clinical benefit. • Severe hypophosphatemia should be treated. • Potassium phosphate salts may be used as an alternative to or combined with potassium chloride/acetate.
Bicarbonate	• Treatment with bicarbonate confers no clinical benefit. • Bicarbonate therapy may cause paradoxical CNS acidosis.

DISPOSITION

DKA patients most often require admission to the hospital for the complex management decisions necessary to good outcomes. There are those patients and families that refuse admission, are turned away from care by the health care establishment for financial reasons, or are unable to spend time in the hospital for other reasons. Unfortunately these patients will most often return back to the emergency department in a deteriorated condition. In minors the assistance of child protective services for non-compliant patients and families is essential. Emancipated patients are especially difficult to assure compliance in, however all available resources should still be used to prevent worsening of the condition. The patient should always be given an open door for care to the ED as needed as it is unlikely that they will be able to access care otherwise unless they have adequate financial resources. Discharge instructions should be explicit and as detailed as possible with significant others and family used as agents to assist compliance.

Follow Up

In known Type 1 diabetics successful prevention of DKA and associated complications depend on effective communication between the patient, family, and health care team. The team should consist of a physician, diabetes nurse educator, and dietitian. Additional availability of social workers and psychologists may be necessary. Following discharge, good personal contact should be insured so that decisions on dose, diet and activity changes can be altered as needed between clinic visits. A strong support system is essential to the management of these patients.

REFERENCES

1. Dunger DB, Sperling MA, Acerini CL, *et al.* European Society for Paediatric Endocrinology/Lawson Wilkins Pediatric Endocrine Society consensus statement on diabetic ketoacidosis in children and adolescents. Pediatrics 2004; 113: e 133– 40.
2. Global prevalence of diabetes: Estimates for the year 2000 and projections for 2030. Sarah Wild, Gojka Roglic, Anders Green, Richard Sicree, Hilary King. *Diabetes Care*, May 2004 v27 i5, p1047(7).
3. American Diabetes Association: http://www.diabetes.org/about-diabetes.jsp.
4. Levy-Marchal C, Papoz L, de Beaufort C, *et al.* Clinical and laboratory features of Type 1 diabetic children at the time of diagnosis. Diabet Med 1992;9:279–84.
5. Wolfsdorf J, Glaser N, Sperling MA. Diabetic ketoacidosis in infants, children and adolescents. A consensus statement from the American Diabetes Association. Diabetes Care 2006; 29: 1150–9.
6. Orlowski JP, Cramer CL, Fiallos MR. Diabetic Ketoacidosis in the Pediatric ICU. Pediatr Clin N Am 2008; 55: 577-587.
7. Rewers A, Klingensmith G, Davis C, *et al.* Diabetic ketoacidosis at onset of diabetes: The SEARCH for diabetes in youth study (abstract). Diabetes 2005; 54 (suppl 1): A63.
8. Curtis JR, To T, Muirhead S, *et al.* Recent trends in hospitalization for diabetic ketoacidosis in Ontario children. Diabetes Care 2002;25:1591–6.
9. Edge JA, Hawkins MM, Winter DL, *et al.* The risk and outcome of cerebral oedema developing during diabetic ketoacidosis. Arch Dis Child 2001; 85:16–22.
10. Lawrence SE, Cummings EA, Gaboury I, Daneman D. Population-based study of incidence and risk factors for cerebral edema in pediatric diabetic ketoacidosis. J Pediatr 2005; 146: 688-92.
11. Glaser NS, Wootton-Gorges SL, Marcin JP, Buonocore MH, Dicarlo J, Neely EK, *et al.* Mechanism of cerebral edema in children with diabetic ketoacidosis. J Pediatr 2004; 45: 164-71.

12. Glaser N, Barnett P, McCaslin I, Nelson D, Trainor J, Louie J, *et al.* Risk factors for cerebral edema in children with diabetic ketoacidosis. The Pediatric Emergency Medicine Collaborative Research Committee of the American Academy of Pediatrics. N Engl J Med. 2001; 344: 264-9.
13. Piva JP, Czepielewski M, Garcia PC, Machado D. Current perspectives for treating children with diabetic ketoacidosis. J Pediatr (Rio J) 2007; 83: S 119-27.
14. Smith CP, Firth D, Bennett S, et al. Ketoacidosis occurring in newly diagnosed and established diabetic children. Acta Paediatr 1998;87:537–41.
15. Dorman JS, Bunker CH. HLA-DQ locus of the human leukocyte antigen complex and type 1 diabetes mellitus: A Huge review; Epidemiologic Reviews 2000;22:218-227.
16. von Herrath MG, Holz A, Homann D, *et al.* Role of viruses in type I diaktes. Semin Immunol 1998;10:87-100.
17. Regulation of Cell Volume; Fluid Physiology by Kerry Brandis - http://www.anaesthesia MCQ.com.
18. Bull, SV, *et al.* Mandatory protocol for treating adult patients with diabetic ketoacidosis decreases intensive care unit and hospital lengths of stay: Results of a non-randomized trial; Crit Care Med 35(1):41, January 2007.
19. Brown TB, Cerebral oedema in childhood diabetic ketoacidosis: Is treatment a factor? Emerg Med J 21:141, March 2004.
20. Frazee LA, Mauro LS. Erythromycin in the treatment of diabetic gastroparesis. Am J Ther 1994;1:287-95.
21. Kelly A.M, The case for venous rather than arterial blood gases in diabetic ketoacidosis; Emerg Med Australasia 18(1):64, February 2006.
22. Hendey GW, Urine ketone dip test as a screen for ketonemia in diabetic ketoacidosis and ketosis in the emergency department; *et al.* Ann Emerg Med 29(6):735, June 1997.
23. Kitabchi AE, Nyenwe EA. Hyperglycemic
24. crises in diabetes mellitus: Diabetic ketoacidosis and hyperglycemic hyperosmolar state. Endocrinol Metab Clin N Am 2006; 35: 725-751.
25. Lindsay R, Bolte RG. The use of an insulin bolus in low-dose insulin infusion for pediatric diabetic ketoacidosis. Pediatr Emerg Care 1989;5:77– 9.
26. Umpierrez GE, Latif K, Stoever J, *et al.* Efficacy of subcutaneous insulin lispro versus continuous intravenous regular insulin for the treatment of patients with diabetic ketoacidosis. Am J Med 2004;117:291– 6.
27. Michael SD Agus, MDa,b, Joseph I. Wolfsdorf, MB, BCh, Diabetic Ketoacidosis in Children; Pediatr Clin N Am 2005; 52: 1147–1163.

In the previous edition this chapter was written by Pierce R. Blackest, MD
Assistant Professor of Pediatrics Children's Hospital of Oklahoma
University of Oklahoma Health Sciences Center Oklahoma City, Oklahoma
and
Adolfo D. Garnica, MD Associate Professor of Pediatrics, Children's Hospital of Oklahoma
University of Oklahoma Health Sciences, Center Oklahoma City, Oklahoma
and
David B. Domek, MD, Assistant Professor of Pediatrics, Children's Hospital of Oklahoma
University of Oklahoma Health Sciences Center Oklahoma City, Oklahoma

Joseph M. Koza and Radheshyam Miryala

46 Acute Adrenal Insufficiency/Crisis

The two emergencies that relate to the adrenal gland are adrenal insufficiency and adrenal crisis. These emergencies occur due to structural or functional lesions of the adrenal cortex, the anterior pituitary gland, or the hypothalamus which lead to decrease in levels of hormones produced by the adrenal gland. This inability of the adrenal gland to meet the physiologic requirements of the body, leads to the clinical manifestations of adrenal insufficiency and adrenal crisis. Adrenal insufficiency can present as a chronic, insidious disorder, or as an acute, life-threatening emergency. In the acute manifestation, patients usually present with hypotension and hypoglycemia. Due to effective public health measures, infant screening, and the decreased prevalence of tuberculosis in the developed world, adrenal crises has become a less frequently faced medical emergency in the United States. Although it is a rare occurrence, the skilled clinician should be able to recognize and treat this disorder as it carries a high morbidity and mortality.

PHYSIOLOGY

The adrenals are tiny glands located on top of the kidney, and are composed of the adrenal cortex and the adrenal medulla. The adrenal cortex produce three groups of biologically active steroid hormones known as the glucocorticoids, the mineralo-corticoids, and the adrenal sex hormones[1,2,3,4,5,6]. The adrenal medulla produces catecholamines which are regulated by the autonomic nervous system. The two most physiologically important hormones produced by the adrenal cortex are cortisol and aldosterone, and these are regulated by the hypothalamic-pituitary-adrenal axis and the rennin angiotensin system respectively. Cortisol and the other glucocorticoids regulate a variety of important functions including energy metabolism, mineral homeostasis, immune function, and other cellular functions. Their overall action is catabolic, promoting protein and lipid breakdown. They also increase gluconeogenesis, thereby also being antagonistic to insulin. In low doses, cortisol stimulates glomerular filtration and decreases water resorption, thus increasing urine flow. During times of stress and at high concentrations, cortisol promotes sodium and water retention like a mineralcorticoid, increases angiotensinogen levels, increases vascular reactivity to vasoconstrictors, helps with the conversion of norepinepherine to epinephrine, and decreases production of nitrous oxide and vasodilatory kinins and prostaglandins. The central nervous system releases corticotrophin releasing hormone during periods of stress. This then increases the release of adrenocorticotropin (ACTH) which in turn acts upon the adrenal cortex, increasing the release of cortisol. The increased circulating cortisol inhibits the release of ACTH[1,2,3,5,7]. The mineralocorticoid, aldosterone, acts primarily on the kidneys. There, it stimulates increased sodium reabsorption and secretion of potassium and hydrogen ions[6].

PATHOPHYSIOLOGY

Adrenal insufficiency can be characterized by being either primary or secondary and either congenital or acquired[6,7,8,9,10]. Primary occurs because of improper gland development, gland responsiveness, or steroid biosynthesis. In developed countries, primary insufficiency is uncommon[11], with autoimmune adrenalitis being the most frequent cause. Here, the individuals commonly have antibodies against the adrenal tissue[12,13,14,15]. Other causes are Addison's, tuberculosis [formerly the most common reason][2,3,6,16], HIV, adrenoleukodystrophy, congenital adrenal hypoplasia, and various syndromes (i.e. triple A). It may also be associated with other endocrinopathies[17]. The signs and symptoms of adrenal insufficiency usually do not appear until after 90% of the cortex becomes nonfunctional.

Congenital adrenal hyperplasia (CAH) refers to histological alterations in adrenocortical tissue that occur as a consequence of chronically elevated circulating ACTH levels[2,3]. CAH comprises a group of inborn errors of adrenocortical hormone biosynthesis resulting from specific deficiencies in the activity of one of the enzymes involved in cortisol synthesis, with 21-hydroxylase deficiency being the most common[6]. Each enzyme deficiency produces specific, recognizable alterations in concentrations of serum adrenal steroid hormones and their precursors. The primary presentation is salt wasting in infants.

There are also a number of rare, genetically determined disorders that affect either adrenocorticosteroid production or function. Congenital aplasia or hypoplasia of the adrenals and the adrenoleukodystrophies present with features of cortisol and aldosterone deficiency[18, 19]. ACTH unresponsiveness and familial glucocorticoid deficiency demonstrate findings of cortisol deficiency[20, 21], while the inborn errors of aldosterone synthesis and pseudohypoaldosteronism present with symptoms of salt wasting[22, 23, 24].

Secondary adrenal insufficiency is caused by disruption of the hypothalamic-pituitary-adrenal axis. Glucocorticoid withdrawal or omission in patients with chronic doses is the leading cause of both secondary and overall adrenal insufficiency. Children who have received chronic suppression may take 12 – 16 months afterwards for their hypothalamic-pituitary-adrenal axis to recover[25]. As little as a two-week course may suppress cortisol production[6, 7]. It may also arise secondarily from hypopituitarism and steroid producing tumors.

Acute adrenal insufficiency may cause a crisis due to sepsis or surgical stress. Adrenal hemorrhage secondarily from septicemia induced Waterhouse-Friderichsen or anti-coagulation complications are examples[26]. Relative insufficiency in the septic or critically ill child also may be observed[27, 28, 29]. Steroid withdrawal, however, is the most common cause. Patients receiving high dose steroids for acute lymphoblastic anemia and flutica-sone for asthma are examples[30, 31, 32, 33].

Acute adrenal insufficiency accompanying overwhelming infection has been well documented[34]. The dominant features include fever, rash, and meningitis. Over-whelming meningococcemia, cutaneous purpura, and bilateral adrenal hemorrhage progress rapidly to shock, coma, and death[34, 35]. Unlike adults, children are more likely to have absolute adrenal insufficiency defined by a basal cortisol <18 μg/dL and a peak adrenocorticotropic hormane (ACTH)-stimulated cortisol concentration <18 μg/dL[36]. Nonsurvivors have exceedingly high ACTH/cortisol ratios within the first 8 hrs of meningococcal shock[37]. Aldosterone levels are also markedly depressed in meningococcemia.[38] Patients at risk of inadequate cortisol/aldosterone production in the setting of shock include children with purpura fulminans and Waterhouse-Friderichsen syndrome, children who previously received steroid therapies for chronic illness, and children with pituitary or adrenal abnormalities. Approximately 50 percent of patients develop petechiae or purpura, usually on the chest, upper arms, and axillae; a petechial rash extends rapidly and coalesces, forming large ecchymoses; a maculopapular rash may also be present even in the absence of petechiae. In the fulminant form, meningitis may be absent, but signs of cardiovascular collapse and septic shock may progress rapidly and lead to death within a few hours. Children with overwhelming septicemia and bilateral adrenal hemorrhage are incapable of normal stress cortisol release; circulatory collapse has been attributed to impaired adrenocortical function, but the serum cortisol is appropriately elevated in many patients[34]. Although the syndrome has been associated most commonly with overwhelming meningococcemia, similar crises have been observed less frequently with overwhelming pneumococcal, streptococcal, and diphtheritic infections.

SIGNS AND SYMPTOMS

Diagnosing a patient with adrenal crisis can be difficult primarily due to its nonspecific presentation. A detailed history and physical with a high index of suspicion is necessary. A history of steroid use, pituitary failure, or results of newborn screenings can be an asset. The trigger (i.e. infection, trauma) must also be determined.

Patients will present with vague complaints. Fatigue, anorexia, nausea, vomiting, loss of appetite, weight loss, abdominal pain, polyuria, diarrhea, and poor feeding in infants are common complaints[2, 3, 6, 16, 26]. These have often been occurring for the past one to two weeks. Other symptoms may include intermittent fever, headache, dehydration, developmental delay, and poor school performance. Less frequently, psychological disturbances (depression) or seizures may be the presenting symptoms[33]. In primary adrenal insufficiency, salt craving is common. Secondary insufficiency is usually associated with other pituitary hormone insufficiencies, such as hypothyroidism.

The physical exam will help in diagnosing those with primary adrenal insufficiency. Primary insufficiency may have increased skin pigmentation in areas of no sun exposure, while secondary insufficiency does not. Females may exhibit ambiguous genitalia. Orthostatic hypotension may also be demonstrated[2,3,6,16,26]. Otherwise, the physical findings are nonspecific.

Acute adrenal insufficiency will often present as severe dehydration, hypotension, hypoglycemia, or altered mental status. In infants, the presentation may mimic overwhelming sepsis or intracranial hemorrhage or other causes of circulatory collapse[34, 35]. At times, suspicion may not begin until a patient's hypotension remains refractory to fluids and pressers[39].

INVESTIGATIONS

After initial stabilization and treatment, ancillary testing can be performed[6, 26]. Blood work should be sent including complete blood count, electrolytes, blood urea nitrogen, creatinine, cortisol level, serum calcium, and thyroid studies. Hypoglycemia can be observed in both primary and secondary adrenal insufficiency. In primary insufficiency, hyperkalemia and hyponatremia are common due to the lack of aldosterone. However, hyponatremia may be seen in secondary adrenal insufficiency secondary to water retention from non-antagonized vasopressin. Diagnosis for primary insufficiency is backed by low cortisol and high ACTH levels while both will be low in secondary insufficiency. Thyroid functions tests will help to identify other co-existing endocrine deficiencies, which can mask the adrenal insufficiency[17].

A computed tomography of the abdomen may show adrenal hemorrhage, calcification, or metastasis[26]. These findings will help pinpoint the underlying cause.

TREATMENT

Initial treatment should focus on the resuscitation of the individual patient. Basic airway, breathing and circulation issues must be resolved foremost. Intravascular volume replacement should be aggressively performed with dextrose 5 normal saline (20 ml/kg bolus). If hypoglycemia is present correct with dextrose 25. After restoring the intravascular volume and glucose, any electrolyte abnormalities can be corrected.[6,15,26,31] Treatment of the underlying precipitating event also needs to be addressed.

The acute adrenal crisis is treated with hydrocortisone due to its equal glucocorticoid and mineralcorticoid activity.[6,11,26]. Dosage is recommended at 50-75 mg/m^2 intravenously, and then 50-75 mg/m^2 intravenously daily divided into four doses. Typical doses are 10 mg for infants, 25 mg for toddlers, 50 mg for older children and 100 mg for teens. If no intravenous access is available, it may be administered either intramuscularly or rectally. Cortisone at 1 mg/kg may be used, but not intravenously. Methylprednisolone (10-15 mg/m^2) and dexamethasone (1.5-2 mg/m^2, 0.2 mg/kg) may be utilized but these have little mineralocorticoid activity. Dexamethasone, however, will not interfere with further in-patient diagnostic ACTH stimulation testing. After stabilization and if not vomiting, fludrocortisones should be administered orally at 0.1–0.2 mg daily.

If hypothyroidism is detected, thyroxine should not be administered until after appropriate steroid replacement. Thyroxine can worsen the crisis, most likely due to its effect on enhanced cortisol clearance. If an underlying adrenal insufficiency is unknown, correction of the hypothyroidism may precipitate a crisis[17].

CONCLUSIONS

Acute adrenal insufficiency remains a life-threatening childhood condition. A high index of suspicion should be maintained when treating the critically ill child; especially since the presentation is often nonspecific[36]. It is helpful if the patient has a known history of steroid use, but insufficiency may also be seen in the formally healthy child who is now septic or under severe physiologic stress. High risk factors such as long-term glucocorticoid therapy, the presence of a mental disorder, and untreated hypogonadism have also been identified by Bykazue Omori *et al.*[40] In those patients with inadequately treated chronic adrenal insufficiency, crises may be precipitated by infection, trauma, excessive fatigue, or drugs such as morphine, etomidate[26], alcohol[26], thyroid hormone[17], or insulin[6]. Aggressive management is required and patients need to be admitted, often to the intensive care unit. Avoidance of a crisis will benefit the patient most and emphasis on patient education is essential.

REFERENCES

1. Simpson ER, Waterman MR. Steroid hormone biosynthesis in the adrenal cortex and its regulation by adrenocorticotropin. In DeGroot LJ, ed. *Endocrinology*. Philadelphia: Saunders, 1989.
2. Job JC, Chaussain JL. The adrenals. In Job JC, Pierson M, eds. *Pediatric Endocrinology*. New York: Wiley, 1981.
3. New MI, del Balza P, Crawford C, *et al.* The adrenal cortex. In Kaplan SA, ed. *Clinical Pediatric Endocrinology*. Philadelphia: Saunders, 1990.
4. Kenny FM, Richards C, Taylor FH. Reference standards for cortisol production and 17-hydroxycorticosteroid excretion during growth: Variation in the pattern of excretion of radio labeled cortisol metabolites. *Metabolism* 1970;19:280-90.
5. Stewart PM. The adrenal cortex. In: Larsen PR, Kronenberg HM, Melmed S, Polonsky KS, eds. Williams *Textbook of Endocrinology*. 10th ed. Philadelphia: Saunders 2003:491-551.
6. Shulman DI, Palmert MR, Kemp SF. Adrenal insufficiency: Still a cause of morbidity and death in childhood. *Pediatrics* 2007;119:484-494.
7. Root AW, Shulman DI. Clinical adrenal disorders. In: Pescovitz OH, Eugster EA, eds. *Pediatric Endocrinology, Mechanisms, Manifestations and Management*. Philadelphia: Lippincott, Williams and Wilkins 2004 : 568-600.
8. Ten S, New M, MacLaren N. Clinical review 130: Addison's disease 2001. *J Clin Endocrinol Metab* 2001; 86 : 2909-2922.
9. Perry R, Kecha O, Paquette J, *et al.* Primary adrenal insufficiency in children: Twenty years experience at the Sainte-Justine Hospital, Montreal. *J Clin Endocrinol Metab* 2001 ; 86: 2958-2965.
10. Kwon K, Tsai V. Metabolic emergencies. *Emerg Med Clin North Am*. 2007; 25 (4) 1041-60.
11. Arlt W, Allollo B. Adrenal insufficiency. *Lancet* 2003;361:1881-1893.
12. Nerup J. Addison's disease-clinical studies: A report of 108 cases. *Acta Endocrinol* 1974; 76: 127-41.
13. Ketchum CH, Riley WJ, McLaren NK. Adrenal dysfunction in asymptomatic patients with adrenocortical autoantibodies. *J Clin Endocrinol Metab* 1984 ; 58 : 1166-70.
14. Betterle C, Zanette F, Zanchette R. *et al.* Complement-fixing adrenal autoantibodies as a marker for predicting onset of idiopathic Addison's disease. *Lancet* 1983; 1 : 1238-41.
15. Simm PJ, McDonnell CM, Zacharin MR. Primary adrenal insufficiency in childhood and adolescence: Advances in diagnosis and manage-ment. *J Paediatr Child Health* 2004; 40 (11) : 596-599.
16. Bethune JE. The diagnosis and treatment of adrenal insufficiency. In DeGroot LJ, ed. *Endocrinology*. Philadelphia: Saunders, 1989.
17. Shaikh MG, Lewis P, Kirk JM. Thyroxine unmasks Addison's disease. *Acta Paediatr* 2004;93(12):1663-1665.
18. Peterson KE, Bille T, Jacobsen BB. Ivensen T. X-linked congenital adrenal hypoplasia: Study of five generations of Greenlandic family. *Acta Pediatr Scand* 1982;71:947-51.
19. Benke PJ, Reyes PF, Parker JC. New form of adrenoleukodystrophy. *Hum Genet* 1981 ; 58 : 204-8.
20. Franks RC, Nance WE. Hereditary adrenocortical unresponsiveness to ACTH. *Pediatrics* 1970; 45 : 43.

21. Allgrove J, Clayden GS, Grant DB, Macaulay JC. *et al.* Familial glucocorticoid deficiency with achalasia of the cardia and deficient tear production. *Lancet* 1978; 1 : 1284-6.
22. Visser HK, Cost WS. A new hereditary defect in biosynthesis of aldosterone. *Acta Endocrinol* 1964; 47:589-612.
23. Veldhius JD, Kulin HE, Santen RJ. Inborn error in the terminal step of aldosterone biosynthesis: Corticosterone methyloxidase type II deficiency in a North American pedigree. *Engl J Med* 1980; 303 : 117-121.
24. Roy C. Familial pseudohypoaldosteronism. *Arch Fr Pediatr* 1977; 34 : 37-54.
25. Chamberlain P, Meyer WJ. Management of pituitary-adrenal suppression secondary to corticosteroid therapy. *Pediatrics* 1981 ; 67 : 245.
26. Klauer K. Adrenal insufficiency and adrenal crisis. Available at www.emedicine.com/EMERG/topic16.htm. January 30,2007.
27. Menon K, Clarson C. Adrenal function in pediatric critical illness. *Pediatr Crit Care Med* 2002;3(2):112-116.
28. Hahner S, Allolio B. *Expert Opin Pharmacother* 2005; 6 (14) : 2407-2417.
29. Langer M, Modi BP, Agus M. Adrenal insufficiency in the critically ill neonate and child. *Curr Opin Pediatr* 2006; 18(4) : 448-453.
30. Felner EI, Thompson MT, *et al.* Time course of recovery of adrenal function in children treated for leukemia. *J Pediatr* 2000; 137 : 21-24.
31. Todd GR, Acerini CL, Buck JJ, *et al.* Acute adrenal crisis in asthmatics treated with high-dose fluticasone propionate. *Eur Respir J* 2002; 19(6): 1207-9.
32. Rix M, Birkeback NH, Rosthoi S, *et al.* Clinical impact of corticosteroid-induced adrenal suppression during treatment for acute lymphoblastic leukemia in children: A prospective observational study using the low-dose adrenocorticotropin test. *J Pediatr* 2005; 147(5) : 645-650.
33. Donaldson MD, Morrison, C, less C, *et al.* Fatal and near-fatal encephalopathy with hyponatremia in two siblings with fluticasone-induced adrenal suppression. Acta *Paediatr* 2007; 96(5): 769-772.
34. Hodes HL, Moloshok RE, Markowitz M. Fulminating meningococcemia treated with cortisone: Use of blood eosinophil count as a guide to prognosis and treatment. *Pediatrics* 1952; 10: 138-49.
35. Black J, Williams DI. Natural history of adrenal hemorrhage in the newborn. Arch Dis Child 1973; 48: 183-90.
36. Brierley J, Carcillo JA, Choong K, Cornell T, DeCaen A, Deymann A, *et al.* Clinical practice parameters for hemodynamic support of pediatric and neonatal septic shock: 2007 update from the American College of Critical Care Medicine. Crit Care Med 2009; 37:666-688.
37. Sakr Y, Reinhart K, Vincent JL, *et al.*: Does dopamine administration in shock influence outcome? Results of the Sepsis Occurrence in Acutely Ill Patients study Crit Care Med 2006; 34:589-597.
38. Lichtarowicz-Krynska EJ, Cole TJ, Camacho-Hubner C, *et al.*: Circulating aldosterone levels are unexpectedly low in children with acute meningococcal disease. J ClinEndocrinol Metab 2004; 89: 1410-1414.
39. Kwok MY, Scanlon MC, Slyper AH. Atypical presentation from acute adrenal insufficiency in an adolescent male. Pediatr Emerg Care 2005; 21:380-383.
40. Omori K, Nomura K, Shimizu S, Omori N, Takano K. Risk factors for adrenal crisis in patients with adrenal insufficiency. Endocrine J. 203; 50: 745-752.

In the previous edition this chapter was written Adolfo D. Garnica, MD Associate Professor of Pediatrics Children's Hospital of Oklahoma University of Oklahoma Health Sciences Center Oklahoma City, Oklahoma

and

Pierce R. Blackest, MD Assistant Professor of Pediatrics Children's Hospital of Oklahoma University of Oklahoma Health SciencesCenter Oklahoma City, Oklahoma

Suresh Gupta

47 Bleeding Child

Children are often brought to emergency room with bleeding emergencies. For discussion and approach point, we can categorize these children into three groups. The first group is children with underlying bleeding disorder. The second group is those with traumatic bleed and the third is those with underlying local problem of the part from where they are bleeding. Irrespective of the site and cause of bleeding, the emergency room management begins with assessment and stabilization of airway, breathing and circulation. Once the hemodynamic stability is achieved, simultaneous efforts should be made to control the ongoing bleeding and treat the underlying etiology.

BLEEDING DISORDERS

The bleeding disorders may be congenital and hereditary or acquired in later life (Table-1). Children with known bleeding disorders may present to the emergency department

Table 1: Common Causes of Bleeding Diathesis in Children

CONGENITAL		
Platelet Disorders	Thrombocytopenia	Secondary to bone marrow disease or defective megakaryocyte maturation
	Platelet dysfunction	Bernard-Soulier syndrome, Glanzmann thrombasthenia, storage pool diseases
Clotting Factor Deficiency	Factor VIII def. (Hemophilia A)	X-linked disorder with reduced factor VIII activity. It is characterized by prolonged aPTT and normal PT
	Factor IX def. (Hemophilia B)	X-linked disorder with low factor IX activity. It is characterized by prolonged aPTT
Combined	Von Willebrand (vW) disease	It is characterized by decreased quantity of functional vW Factor. Factor vW binds platelets to subendothelial surfaces and carries and stabilizes factor VIII.

Contd.

Contd.

ACQUIRED	
Vitamin K Deficiency:	Factors II, VII, IX, X, protein C, and protein S are vitamin K dependent. Early vitamin K deficiency may present with isolated prolonged PT because factor VII has the shortest half-life. Fibrinogen levels are normal.
Disseminated Intravascular Coagulation (DIC):	It is an acquired coagulopathy due to sepsis, hypoxia, or trauma. It is characterized by prolonged PT and aPTT, decreased fibrinogen and platelets, increased fibrin degradation products, and elevated D-dimers.
Liver Diseases:	There is deficiency of liver dependant factors like V, VII, IX, X, XI, XII, XIII, prothrombin, plasminogen, fibrinogen, protein C and S, and ATIII.
Hemolytic-Uremic Syndrome (HUS) and Thrombotic Thrombocytopenic Purpura (TTP):	HUS is characterized by the triad of microangiopathic hemolytic anemia, uremia, and thrombocytopenia. HUS does not typically include coagulation abnormalities of DIC. TTP is characterized by the triad of HUS in addition to fever and CNS changes. TTP is more common in older adolescents and adults. HUS or TTP is often triggered by bacterial enteritis, especially caused by *Escherichia coli* O157:H7.

due to a fresh bleeding episode or it may be the first time a child with an undiagnosed bleeding diathesis is coming to emergency room. The management and investigation of a child with bleeding disorder depends on the suspected etiology. There is a long list of bleeding disorders but only common ones will be discussed here. A platelet count, prothrombin time and aPTT may give valuable diagnostic clues (Figure 1).

Emergency Room Management of a Child With Hemophilia

Bleeds in hemophilics should be treated with factor replacement therapy at the earliest and one should not wait for the appearance of physical signs. Even young children can usually tell when a joint hemorrhage starts. Treatment at this early stage will lead to more rapid recovery with fewer requirements of factor concentrates. If in doubt, its always better to treat. Veins of these patients are lifeline and must be treated with care. For control of pain one should use acetaminophen with or without narcotic analogues and avoid non-steroidal anti-inflammatory drugs (NSAIDs) and intramuscular injections.

Hemophilia A (F-VIII Deficiency)

- *Factor VIII concentrates:* Each F-VIII unit per kilogram of body weight will raise the plasma F-VIII level approximately 2%. The half-life is approximately 8–12 hours. Dose of F-VIII = 0.5 X Patient Wt X Factor levels desired (Tables 2, 3).
- *Cryoprecipitate/fresh frozen plasma:* It should be used only if factor concentrates are not available. Each bag of cryoprecipitate (30-40 ml) contains 60-100 units of F-VIII. Fresh frozen plasma (FPP) may also be used if factor concentrates are not available. One ml of FFP has one unit of F-VIII.
- *Desmopressin (DDAVP):* DDAVP is useful in the treatment of persons with mild hemophilia who have a 5% or greater F-VIII level.

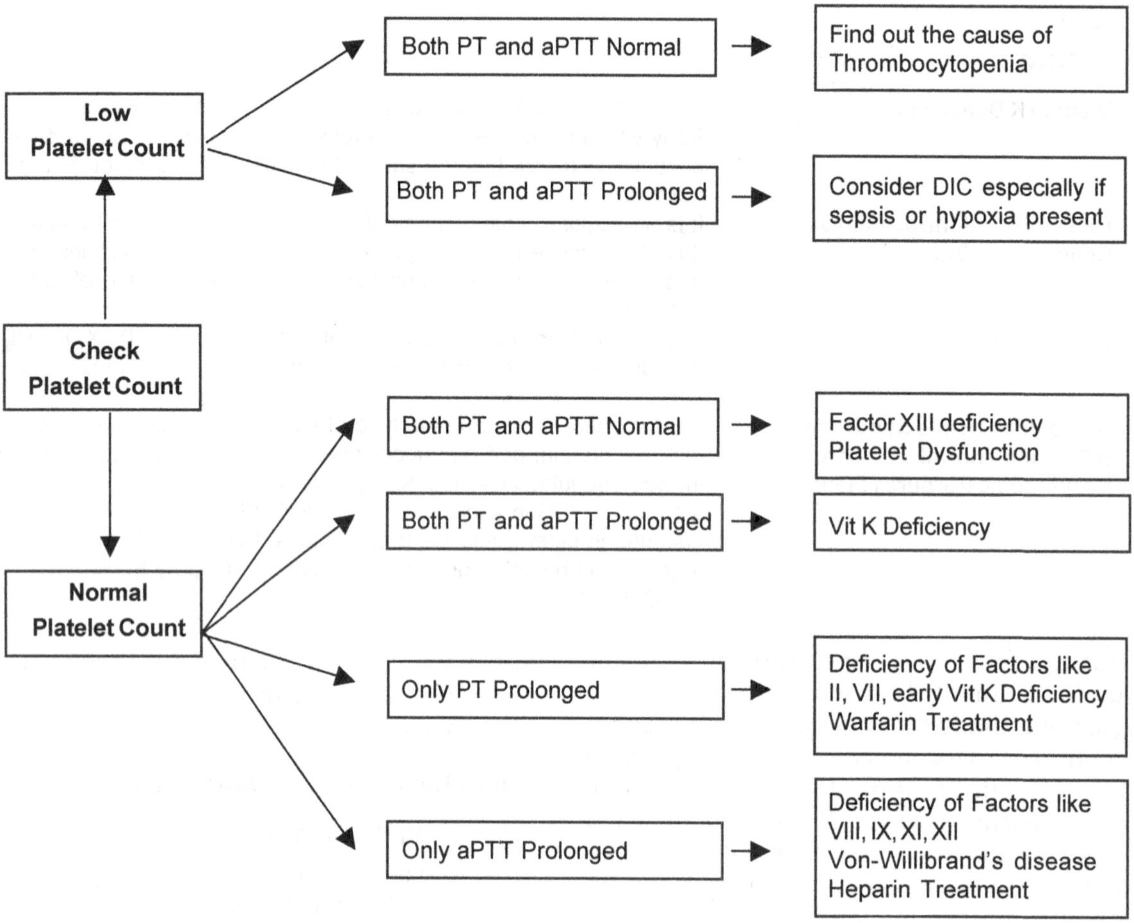

Fig. 1: Approach to a Child with bleeding diathesis in Emergency Room

Hemophilia B (F-IX Deficiency)

- ***Factor IX concentrates:*** F-IX concentrates fall into two classes: Pure coagulation F-IX products, and Prothrombin complex concentrates (PCCs). Purified F-IX products are preferable as these are largely free of the risks of thrombosis or DIC, which may occur with large doses of intermediate purity PCCs. Each F-IX unit per kilogram of body weight infused intravenously will raise the plasma FIX level approximately 1%. The half-life is about 18-24 hours. To calculate dosage, multiply the patient's weight in kilograms by the factor level desired.
- ***Fresh frozen plasma (FFP):*** FFP should only be used if F-IX concentrates are unavailable. The acceptable starting dose is 15-20 ml/kg but its unlikely to achieve F-IX levels above 25%. (Tables 2, 3)

Hemophilia: Practical tips

- Factor concentrates are expensive. In developing countries, factor availability is severely restricted and often unavailable, as it is dependent on finances of the family. Physicians frequently have to manage with FFP or cryoprecipitate. Local haemostatic measures including Tranexamic acid can aid in limiting mucosal bleeding. Dexamethasone is valuable in controlling raised intracranial pressure in CNS bleeds. Hydration and steroids complement factor replacement in managing hematuria.

– If there is recurrent bleeding from a single site in a patient with hemophilia despite adequate factor replacement, surgical etiology of bleeding should be considered, e.g. a torn vessel that requires suturing.

Table 2: Recommended plasma factor levels and duration of administration in hemophilic patients*

	Hemophilia A		*Hemophilia B*	
Type of hemorrage	**Desired Level**	**Duration (days)**	**Desired Level**	**Duration (days)**
Joint	40%-60%	1-2, may be longer if response is inadequate	40%-60%	1-2, may be longer if response is inadequate
Muscle	40%--60%	2-3, sometimes longer if response inadequate	40%-60%	2-3, sometimes longer if response inadequate
Iliopsoas				
• initial	80%-100%	1-2	60%-80%	1-2
• maintenance	30%-60%	3-5, sometimes longer as secondary prophylaxis during physiotherapy	30%-60%	3-5, sometimes longer as secoundary prophylaxis during physiotherapy
CNS/ head				
• initial	80%-100%	1-7	60%-80%	1-7
• maintenance	30%	8-21	30%	8-21
Throat and neck				
• initial	80%-100%	1-7	60%-80%	1-7
• maintenance	50%	8-14	30%	8-14
Gastrointestinal				
• initial	80%-100%	1-6	60%-80%	1-6
• maintenance	50%	7-14	30%	7-14
Renal	50%	3-5	40%	3-5
Deep laceration	50%	5-7	40%	5-7

Table 3: If significant resource constraint the desired levels may be kept in following ranges

Site of Bleeding	*Initial*	*Maintenance*
Joint/Muscles except iliopsoas	10-20%	10-20%
Iliopsoas	20-40%	10-20%
CNS/Head	50-80%	30-50%
Throat/Neck/GIT	30-50%	10-20%
Renal/Deep Laceration	20-40%	20-40%

Immune thrombocytopenic purpura (ITP)

Typical clinical picture of ITP is of acute skin and mucosal bleeding in an otherwise well child. Anemia is absent or proportionate to the bleeds. Absence of hepatosplenomegaly, lymphadeno-pathy, bone pains and fever are the clues that aid in distinguishing from acute leukemia. Children with platelet counts below 20,000/μL or those with significant bleeds are generally treated with specific drug therapy. Options include IVIg, anti-D immunoglobulin (in Rh +ve patients) or steroids. Choice depends on severity of bleeding, finances and individual centers pre-ference. A bone marrow examination is preferred prior to administrating steroids to avoid masking acute leukemia. Platelet transfusions are superfluous, as transfused platelets are rapidly destroyed by circulating antibodies. Platelet transfusions are rarely indicated as adjunct in managing life threatening bleeds (e.g. NS bleeds), while awaiting response to specific therapy.

Treatment of Other Bleeding Disorders

Vitamin K should be given to patients with liver disease with clotting abnormalities and hemorrhagic disease of newborn and childhood. Treatment of DIC includes identifying and treating underlying disorder. Replacement of depleted coagulation factors with FFP may be necessary in severe cases, especially when bleeding is present. FFP in the dose of 10–15 mL/kg will raise levels of clotting factors by 20%. Fibrinogen if depleted can be given as cryoprecipitate. Platelet transfusions may also be necessary.

Use of Blood Components in a Bleeding Child

1. **Packed RBC (PRBC) transfusion:** The decision to transfuse RBCs should be made with consideration of clinical symptoms and signs, the degree of cardiorespiratory compromise. Typed and cross-matched blood product is always preferred when possible. O-negative (or O-positive) blood may be used if transfusion cannot be delayed. O-negative is preferred for females of child-bearing age to reduce the risk for Rh sensitization.
2. **Platelets:** Indicated to treat severe or symptomatic thrombocytopenia. Hemorrhagic complications are rare with platelet counts above 20,000/μL. Many people consider the platelets count < 10,000/μL as transfusion trigger even in the absence of serious bleeding complications. A platelet count >50,000/μL is advisable for minor procedures and level >100,000/μL is advisable for major surgery. One unit/m^2 of platelets concentrate raises the platelet count by 10,000 to 15,000/μL. For infants and children, 10 mL/kg of platelets concentrates will increase the platelet count by approximately 50,000/μL.

3. **FFP:** Contains all clotting factors except platelets. It is used in patients with severe clotting factor deficiencies with active bleeding or to reverse effects of warfarin. It also replaces anticoagulant factors like antithrombin III, protein C, and protein S. FFP is useful in treatment of DIC, vitamin K deficiency with active bleeding, or thrombotic thrombocytopenic purpura (TTP). The usual dose is 10 to 15 mL/kg and repeat doses may be given as needed. In acquired TTP, plasma exchange is the treatment of choice.
4. **Cryoprecipitate:** Enriched for factor VIII (5–10 U/mL), vWF, and fibrinogen. It is useful for children with factor VIII or vWF deficiency when concentrates or recombinant products are not available.

TRAUMATIC BLEED

Trauma is a worldwide problem, with severe and wide ranging consequences for individuals and society as a whole. Injury to the central nervous system (particularly head injury) is the leading cause of death accounting for 40–50% of fatalities. Hemorrhage is the other major reason accounting 30–40% of deaths and significant morbidity. Most severe bleeding occurs during the acute phase of injury, typically as a result of the injuries sustained. There are many factors that place injured patients at increased risk for severe bleeding in which traditional hemostatic methods may prove inadequate. Hemorrhage is an important dilemma in the care of trauma victim. For management and understanding point of view, the traumatic hemorrhage can be put in three overlapping categories.

Surgical Bleeding

Surgical bleeding is not a well defined term, but it can be described broadly as including those injuries that can only be addressed through direct operative visualization and controlled with suture, packing, pressure, or application of a hemostatic agent. These traumatic hemorrhages need urgent surgery for control. More than 80% of trauma deaths that occur in the operating room are the result of these hemorrhages. These surgical bleedings account for about 50% of hypotensive patients. If surgical bleeding is not controlled in this manner, it is likely to be fatal. Given the large proportion of operative deaths secondary to hemorrhage, early intervention to control bleeding is paramount.

Nonsurgical Bleeding

Not all bleeding can or should be controlled surgically. Non-surgical bleeds are those in which operative intervention has limited or no ability to control hemorrhage, and in which attempts at surgical control have the potential to exacerbate traumatic hemorrhage and lead to severe bleeding and coagulopathy. Trauma care is constantly evolving, and the trend is toward nonoperative management of hemorrhage that was previously considered 'surgical' in nature. Coagulopathic bleeding can be addressed only by restoring normal hemostatic physiology. Surgical intervention in a patient with traumatic coagulopathy has disastrous consequences like further blood loss, physiologic derangement, and possibly death. Conservative, nonoperative management of splenic and hepatic parenchymal bleeding without operation is well described and studied, and is becoming standard practice for all but the most severe injuries. Keeping patients with these problems out of the operating room probably reduces morbidity and improves outcomes.

Acquired Coagulopathy of Trauma

The acquired coagulopathy of trauma is an important clinical entity that is undergoing intensive study. The phenomenon is responsible for the majority of postoperative traumatic hemorrhagic fatalities. The development of traumatic coagulopathy is associated with massive transfusion and resuscitation, increased injury severity, and the presence of hemorrhagic shock. Lethal triad of hemodilution, hypothermia, and acidosis has sequential and additive effects on the coagulation cascade producing 'bloody vicious cycle'. Unless interventions are done to break this cycle, it can rapidly lead to the demise of the injured patient from coagulopathic exsanguinations.

Other Factors: The underlying medical condition and some of the medications can contribute to excessive bleeding in trauma victim.

Management of Traumatic Hemorrhage: (Figure-2)

In a patient with traumatic hemorrhage, the three overlapping management phases of care are resuscitative, operative, and critical care phases. The diagnosis and control of bleeding should be a high priority especially if the patient is in hemorrhagic shock. Early attempts at hemorrhage control include direct control of visible sources of severe bleeding with direct pressure, pressure dressings, or tourniquets; stabilization of long bone and pelvic fractures; and keeping the patient warm. Table 4 presents a summary of these measures to enhance hemostasis during various phases of care.

Early Prehospital Interventions

Prehospital care practices and interventions are widely variable among different parts of the world, depending on resources and policies. In general, the prehospital trauma care focuses on management of airway, breathing and circulation along with control of bleeding. The basic principles of control of external hemorrhage in prehospital settings are followings:

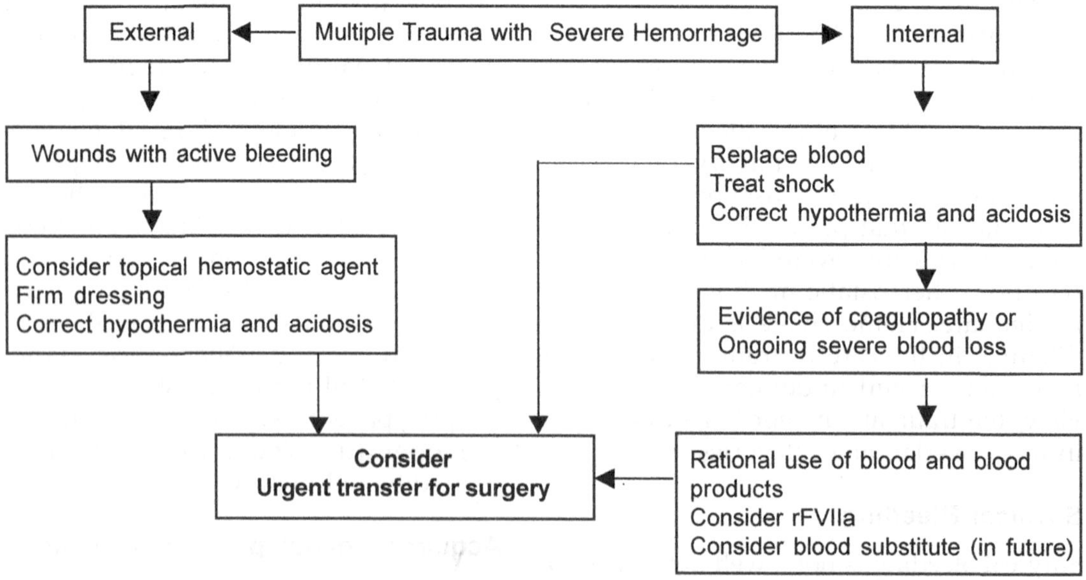

Fig. 2: Proposed algorithm for the application of new haemostatic products in trauma patients in the military setting

Table 4: Interventions to improve hemostasis in trauma care

Management Phase	*Treatment Strategies*
Early Prehospital Phase	• Control overt hemorrhage – Direct pressure – Pressure dressing – Tourniquet • Diagnose and treat occult hemorrhage – Stabilization of pelvis and long bone fractures • Keep patient warm
Resuscitative Phase	• Warm intravenous fluids • Avoid overaggressive fluid resuscitation prior to surgical control of hemorrhage • Appropriate transfusion of blood and blood products
Operative Phase	• Surgical control of life-threatening hemorrhage • Damage control surgery for critically ill patients • Appropriate transfusion of blood and blood products
Critical Care Phase	• Effective resuscitation – End-point should be adequate tissue perfusion • Physiologic support to prevent coagulopathy

Elevation: Keeping the wound above the level of the heart will decrease the pressure at the point of injury, and will reduce the bleeding. This mainly applies to limbs which are not fractured.

Direct pressure: Placing pressure on the wound will constrict the blood vessels manually, helping to stop any blood flow. Ideally a barrier, such as sterile, low-adherent gauze should be used between the pressure and the wound, to reduce the chances of infection.

Pressure points: If direct pressure and elevation are not possible or ineffective, and there is a risk of exsanguinations, one may use pressure points to constrict the major artery which feeds the point of the bleed. This is usually performed at a place where a pulse can be found, such as in the femoral artery. With pressure points, there is significant risk of necrosis below the constriction. So pressure time should not exceed more than 10 minutes.

Emergency tourniquet: A tourniquet is always considered to be the *last resort* as it can lead to eventual loss of the limb below application. Some argue that tourniquets should never be used in the pre-hospital setting, not even for amputations.

Haemostatic Agents

Haemostatic dressings aim to stop bleeding at the entrance or exit point of the injury. These agents induce coagulation at different points within the coagulation system.

QuikClot: It consists of zeolite volcanic mineral granules and has the potential to stop even high-volume bleeding from open wounds. When poured into a wound, these absorb the water content of blood through microscopic holes in the granules. This concentrates the clotting factors and blood cells resulting in a stable clot that can be removed by irrigation and suction. QuikClot dressings are being used by the US Marine Corps in Afghanistan and Iraq.

American Red Cross haemostatic dressing: It contains microfibrillar collagen, thrombin, oxidised cellulose and poly-*N*-acetyl-glucosamine. Allergic reaction is a potential problem. This product is not commercially available.

Rapid Deployment Hemostat (RDH) bandage: It consists of fully acetylated poly-*N*-acetyl glucosamine (p-GlcNAc) applied to a gauze bandage. It is still being evaluated for clinical application.

Chitosan bandage: It is a biodegradable carbohydrate found in prawns and lobster shells and many other animals. This dressing is currently being trialled by the US Army.

Resuscitative Phase

The resuscitative phase in the care of the hemorrhaging patient begins with Prehospital Trauma Life Support and Advanced Trauma Life Support (ATLS). Intravenous fluids are administered during this phase, which can continue through the subsequent operative phase. Fluid resuscitation in hemorrhagic shock should never overshadow the importance to curtail bleeding and prevent coagulopathy. It has been realized that excessive fluid resuscitation may be detrimental to hemostasis. According to the current ATLS guidelines each milliliter of lost blood should be replaced by three times the amount of isotonic crystalloid, while giving careful attention to the physiologic response of the patient.

The transfusion of blood and blood products is a cornerstone of resuscitation for trauma victim. Packed RBCs should be administered if a patient does not respond or responds only transiently to the initial 2 boluses of crystalloid infusion. Fresh frozen plasma, cryoprecipitate, and platelet concentrate are used to treat coagulopathy and prevent the bloody vicious cycle.

Operative Phase

The operative phase follows the initial resuscitative phase, but fluid resuscitation often continues while the patient is in the operating room. Most severe hemorrhages require surgical intervention, and approximately 50% of patients in hemorrhagic shock are moved to the operating room from the emergency department. Efforts to control bleeding and repair damaged tissue are made. But in the critically ill patients, an abbreviated 'damage control' procedure is done to tackle only life-threatening injuries and shift the patient to ICU immediately for continued resuscitation and restoration of physiology.

Critical Care Phase

The critical care phase is the continuation of resuscitation phase or operative phase. Restoring physiology involves attempts to interrupt the bloody vicious cycle through rewarming, effective resuscitation, and correction of acidosis. The aim of all these measures is to ensure adequate tissue perfusion and oxygenation. The oxygen delivery to tissues is better assessed by mixed venous oxygen saturation, base deficit and lactate, end-tidal carbon dioxide rather than standard hemodynamic parameters such as blood pressure and heart rate. The most devastating complications which can occur during this phase are infections, primarily sepsis, and multi-organ failure.

Newer Modalities for Control of Traumatic Hemorrhage

Timely surgical control of hemorrhage saves lives and remains a fundamental component of trauma care. Recombinant activated factor VII (rVIIa) is a hemostatic agent useful in uncontrolled bleeding. The rVIIa has great potential to improve the survivability and outcome from uncontrolled hemorrhage. Advanced hemostatic dressings and rFVIIa do not replace the need for surgical control of hemorrhage. But it may helpful to prevent life-threatening exsanguination hemorrhage and stabilize the patient until surgical care is undertaken. The rVIIa is also suitable in desperate cases of severe bleeding due to general ooze where surgical control is not the answer or fails to respond to appropriate surgical measures and blood component therapy.

NON-TRAUMATIC LOCAL BLEEDINGS

Gastrointestinal bleed, epistaxis, and vaginal bleed are the three local bleedings which are usually not due to major trauma. In most of these children a local cause is responsible for bleeding rather than underlying coagulopathy.

A. Gastrointestinal Bleeding

Gastrointestinal (GI) tract bleeding emergencies include hematemesis, hematochezia and melena. The initial evaluation and management of a child with GI bleed in emergency room proceeds as follows:

- The first priority is assessment of airway, breathing, and circulation with hemodynamic stability.
- Perform physical examination to look for the evidence of bleeding. Verify bleeding with rectal examination and/or testing of stool or emesis for occult blood. Consider gastric lavage to differentiate upper from lower GI bleeding and to assess for ongoing bleeding (Table 5).
- Obtain baseline laboratory tests and one can consider the following laboratory studies depending on clinical suspicion: Complete blood count (CBC), prothrombin time/partial thromboplastin time (PT/PTT), blood type and cross-match, reticulocyte count, blood smear, blood

Table 5: Differential Diagnosis of GI Bleeding in Children

Age	*Upper GI Bleeding*	*Lower GI Bleeding*
Newborn (0–30 days)	Swallowed maternal blood	Necrotizing enterocolitis Malrotation with midgut volvulus Hirschsprung disease
Infant (1m –1 year)	Esophagitis Peptic ulcer disease	Allergic proctocolitis Intussusception Meckel's diverticulum Lymphonodular hyperplasia Intestinal duplication
Preschool (1–5 years)	Esophagitis Peptic ulcer disease Esophageal varices Epistaxis	Juvenile polyps Lymphonodular hyperplasia Meckel's diverticulum Hemolytic-uremic syndrome Henoch-Schönlein purpura
School age and adolescent	Esophageal varices Peptic ulcer disease Epistaxis	Inflammatory bowel disease Juvenile polyps Hemorrhoids Anal fissure
All age group	Gastritis	Infectious colitis

urea nitrogen/creatinine, electrolytes, and a panel to assess for disseminated intravascular coagulation.

- Begin initial fluid resuscitation with normal saline or lactated Ringer's solution. Consider transfusion if there is continued bleeding, symptomatic anemia, and/or a hematocrit level <20%. Initiate intravenous acid suppression therapy, preferably with a proton pump inhibitor (PPI).
- Provide specific therapy based on assessment and site of bleeding.

Management:

- ***Immediate:*** Patients with significant bleeding should be placed on nothing by mouth (NPO) status. Begin rehydration and consider nasogastric decompression along with serial abdominal examinations. The need of evaluation by pediatric surgeon or gastroenterologist depends on the suspected etiology.
- ***Known esophageal varices and severe bleeding:*** Octreotide infusion, starting with 1mcg/kg IV bolus followed by a continuous infusion of 1 mcg/kg/hour, increasing every eight hours if there is no reduction in the bleeding up to 4-5 mcg/kg/hour as a continuous infusion. When there is no active bleeding after 24 hours the dose could be halved every 12 hours. Side effects of octreotide include nausea, abdominal cramps, diarrhoea, bradycardia and hyperglycemia which usually resolve spontaneously. As a last resort, a Sengstaken tube can be used but this has significant complications including aspiration and oesophageal rupture. When possible one can consider emergency esophageal band ligation or sclerotherapy for obliterating oesophageal varices.
- ***Peptic disease such as gastritis or oesophagitis:*** H_2 antagonists such as Ranitidine (2-4mg/kg/dose, maximum 150 mg/dose, twice a day) or proton pump inhibitors such as Omeprazole (0.7-1.4mg/kg/dose, max 40mg, once every day) are indicated in selected cases. Sucralfate (250 mg q.i.d. for children < 2 years old, 0.5-1g q.i.d. for children over 2 years) as a barrier agent is used for peptic ulcers and after sclerotherapy. Liquid antacids are a useful adjunct for breakthrough symptoms in older children. These should be given after meals and two hours apart from other medicines.
- ***Definitive Treatment:*** Surgical or laproscopic exploration may be warranted depending on the suspected etiology like in case of Meckel's diverticulum.

EPISTAXIS

The nose has a rich vascular supply, making it vulnerable to episodes of bleeding, either spontaneously or as a result of localized trauma. Mostly it is mild and self-limited following nose picking or a recent upper respiratory infection, but at times it can be profuse and life threatening. Various causes of epistaxis in children, are listed in Table 6.

Approximately 90% episodes of epistaxis arise from a venous vascular plexus on the anterior nasal septum, known as Kiesselbach's plexus. Anterior bleeds tend to be slow with persistent oozing as it is mostly from capillary or venous sources. Posterior bleeds originate from the sphenopalatine artery in the posterior nasal cavity and nasopharynx and tend to bleed more profusely.

Management

Most cases of mild epistaxis require minimal intervention.

- Mild epistaxis without active bleeding should focus on prevention of recurrence by limiting local trauma and applying nasal hydration with saline mist or ointments and increasing ambient humidity with a cool mist vaporizer.

Table 6: Etiology of Epistaxis

Common	Less Common
• Nose Picking	• Systemic causes: Hepatic disease, leukemia, Idiopathic thrombocytopenic purpura.
• Upper Respiratory Tract Infection	• Coagulopathies: – Congenital – Acquired
• Facial Trauma • Foreign body • Sinusitis	• Local causes: cocaine or heroin sniffing

- If minor bleeding recurs, the patient (or parent) may be instructed to pinch the nostrils together for 5 to 10 minutes nonstop and keep the head elevated but not hyperextended.
- A gauze-piece soaked with decongestant like epinephrine (1:1000), or phenylephrine may be placed in the affected nostril.

Major epistaxis needs a proper assessment and stabilization.

- Emergency room evaluation involves the assessment of the airway, breathing, and circulation (ABC). A posterior bleed is more likely than an anterior bleed to cause airway compromise or blood aspiration and may rarely require intubation to protect the airway. Hemodynamic stability must be ensured quickly.
- Once cardiopulmonary stability is established, nasal examination with a good light source and a handheld nasal speculum should be done. The nasal cavity should be cleared of clots to visualize the nasal mucosa and sources of bleeding. If a active source of bleeding is identified, thermal cautery or cautery with silver nitrate sticks may be helpful. One must be careful while cauterizing so as to prevent damage and perforation of the nasal septum.
- Unresponsive anterior bleeding may require anterior nasal packing with petroleum jelly gauze strips or a commercial packing that expands when it becomes wet to tamponade the bleeding vessel.
- The failure to identify an anterior source of bleeding is a possible indication of posterior bleeding. Posterior epistaxis is less amenable to cautery and often requires posterior nasal packing or epistaxis balloons. These patients should be managed in conjunction with an ENT specialist. Children with a posterior nasal packing should be given antibiotics to prevent staphylococcal and streptococcal related sinusitis or toxic shock syndrome.

VAGINAL BLEEDING

Vaginal bleeding in the prepubescent child is concerning both to parents and to care providers. It is infrequently encountered by primary care providers and may be referred to the emergency department for evaluation. Vaginal bleeding as symptom is less common than vaginal discharge. The etiology is mostly benign but it requires a thorough evaluation. Potential etiologies include foreign bodies, accidental trauma, urologic conditions, endocrine disorders, bleeding disorders, dermatologic conditions, and vaginal tumors. Sexual abuse is also a consideration in children with genital complaints.

Foreign Bodies: Vaginal foreign bodies account for approximately 4% of gynecologic problems in children. Vaginal bleeding or blood-tinged vaginal discharge is much more common than vaginal discharges alone. It occurs almost up to 100% of girls with vaginal foreign bodies. The recommended evaluation is direct visualization via pelvic examination under anesthesia and/or vaginoscopy. These modalities are typically both diagnostic and therapeutic as these allow for the removal of the foreign body.

Urologic Conditions: Urethral prolapse often presents as apparent vaginal bleeding. The characteristic appearance is a doughnut-shaped, edematous mass distinctly surrounding the urethra. Nonoperative management includes sitz baths, topical estrogen creams, and topical or oral antibiotics if infection is suspected. Operative resection is indicated if voiding is compromised or if conservative management fails.

Physiologic Vaginal Bleeding in the Newborn: It is due to the decline of circulating levels of maternal estrogens. Bleeding is typically mild and occurs most often during the first week of life. This condition is self-limited and resolves without intervention.

Precocious Puberty: Vaginal bleeding may be the presenting symptom of precocious puberty which may be a true precocious puberty or precocious pseudopuberty. Physical examination findings of additional secondary sexual characteristics should raise clinical suspicion for precocious puberty in children presenting with vaginal bleeding. Further evaluation is warranted. Exposure to estrogencontaining preparations should be discontinued.

Bleeding Disorders: Although vaginal bleeding may be the initial presentation of bleeding disorders in the postpubescent female but in prepubescent children, bleeding disorders rarely present with isolated vaginal bleeding.

Dermatologic Conditions: A variety of dermatologic conditions of vulva may present with apparent vaginal bleeding. These include lichen sclerosus, seborrheic dermatitis, atopic dermatitis, and psoriasis.

Vaginal Trauma: Trauma to the female perineum is relatively common, with the highest incidence in the 4- to 12-year-old age group. Frequent mechanisms of injury include straddle injuries, accidental penetration, abduction injuries, injuries associated with pelvic fractures, and sexual abuse. Accidental penetrating injuries are the result of falling onto a sharp or pointed object or self-manipulation with foreign objects. They occur most often in the 2- to 4-year age group. Presenting symptoms include pain, hematuria, vaginal discharge, vaginal bleeding, rectal pain, or rectal bleeding. Sexual abuse must be considered in all children presenting with genital trauma.

FURTHER READING

1. Pearl R: The approach to common abdominal diagnoses in infants and children. Part II. Pediatr Clin North Am 1998; 45:1287–1326.
2. Molleston J. Variceal bleeding in children. J Pediatr Gastroenterol Nutr 2003; 37; 538-545.
3. Johns Hopkins: The Harriet Lane Handbook, Editors W. Custer and Rachel E. Rau, 18th ed. Mosby, an Imprint of Elsevier, 2008.
4. Streiff MB, Kickler TS: The Johns Hopkins Hospital Hemostatic Testing and Antithrombotic Therapy Manual, 3rd ed. Baltimore, 2007.
5. Monagle P, et al: Antithrombotic therapy in children: Seventh ACCP Consensus Conference on antithrombotic and thrombolytic therapy. *Chest* 2004; 126:645S-687S.
6. Guidelines for the Management of Hemophilia published by the World Federation of Hemophilia 2005 at www.wfh.org.
7. Morgen Bernius, and Donna Perlin: Pediatric ear, nose, and throat emergencies. Pediatr Clin N Am 53 (2006) 195– 214.
8. David S Kauvar and Charles E Wade: The epidemiology and modern management of traumatic hemorrhage: US and international perspectives, *Critical Care* 2005, 9(Suppl 5):S1-S9.
9. Bridgette Guthrie: Vaginal bleeding in the prepubescent child, Clinical Pediatric Emergency Medicine -2009; 10 (1); 14-19.

48 Anemia in the Emergency Room

Deepak Bansal

It is relatively common for Paediatricians to face children with severe anemia in day-to-day practice. Goal of this chapter is to briefly describe approach to a child with severe anemia and to outline emergency management. Red cell transfusion practices in the pediatric intensive care unit are briefly discussed as well. Transfusion needs of neonates are not addressed here. Clinical disturbances are uncommon until the hemoglobin drops below 7-8 g/dL. Symptoms of anemia are particularly uncommon when moderately severe anemia develops slowly. Symptoms of severe anemia include weakness, tachypnoea, shortness of breath on exertion, tachycardia, cardiac dilatation, and congestive heart failure.

INITIAL APPROACH AND EVALUATION

Although the causes of anemia in childhood are plentiful, a rational presumption can frequently be made on preliminary assessment. A good history, physical examination and a reliable hemogram is all it takes to arrive at a probable diagnosis. Normal levels of haemoglobin and Mean corpuscular volume (MCV) are tabulated in Table 1. Attempt for initial diagnosis, based on findings of organomegaly and bleeds/thrombocytopenia is an easy and realistic approach, and illustrated in Figure 1.

Table 1: Normal haemoglobin and MCV during childhood

Age	*Hemoglobin (g/dL)*		*MCV (fL)*
	Mean	**Range**	**Lowest**
Cord blood	16.8	13.7 – 20.1	110
2 wk	16.5	13.0 – 20.0	
3 mon	12.0	9.5 – 14.5	
6 mon – 6 yr	12.0	10.5 - 14.0	70 - 74
7 – 12 yr	13.0	11.0 – 16.0	76 - 80

Complete Blood Count: Electronic Vs. Manual

It is advisable to obtain a hemogram (Hb, WBC, DLC and platelet count) from a lab equipped with an electronic cell counter. A hemogram from an electronic cell counter is more informative, reliable and value for money, than a manual count. In author's experience, a manual blood count from less well equipped labs is typically unreliable and often misleading. MCV is a measure of red

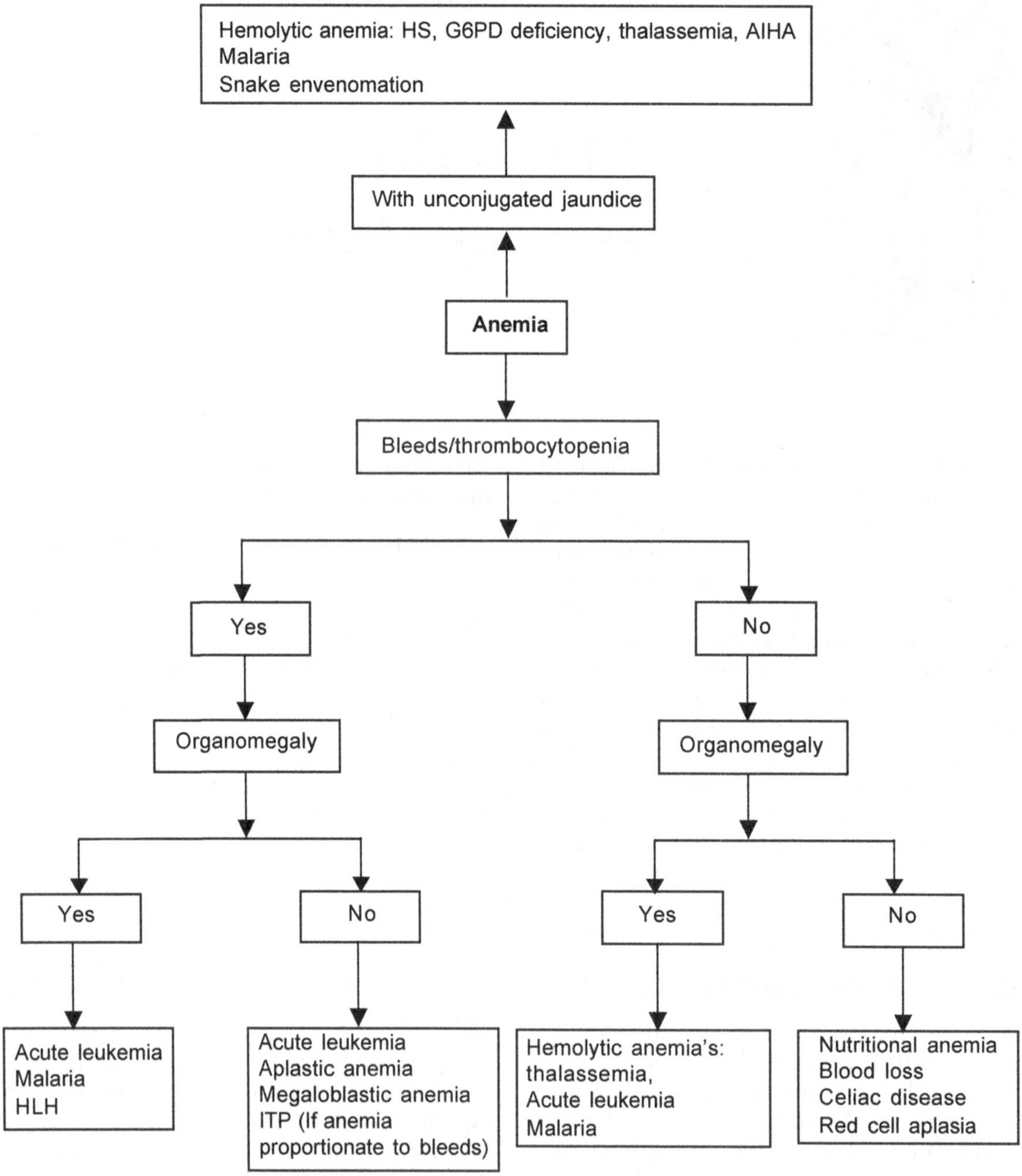

HLH: hemophagocytic lymphohistiocytosis, AIHA: Autoimmune haemolytic anemia, HS: Hereditary spherocytosis

Fig. 1: Flowchart for differential diagnosis of common causes of anemia in the emergency room

cell size. It is readily available from an electronic cell counter report and often aids in diagnosis (Table 2). However, as iron deficiency anemia is wide spread in our country, a low MCV may be confounding.

Table 2: Common causes of anemia, based on MCV

A. **Low MCV**
   i. Iron deficiency
   ii. Thalassemia
B. **Normal MCV**
   i. Mixed nutritional deficiency (e.g. Iron with folate deficiency)
   ii. Acute blood loss
   iii. Chronic renal failure
   iv. Hereditary spherocytosis
C. **Raised MCV**
   i. Vitamin B12 or folate deficiency
   ii. Newborns, prematurity
   iii. Aplastic anemia

Tips During Initial Evaluation

Erratic history of fever is often a mystifying factor for differential diagnosis of anemia. Undocumented fever ('warm forehead') is often described by parents of children with chronic haemolytic anemia (e.g. thalassemia). It plausibly could be due to hyperdynamic circulation secondary to long standing anemia. Documentation of temperature by a thermometer is obligatory to authenticate history of fever.

If haemolytic anemia is suspected, it is a good practice to draw a pre-transfusion blood sample for appropriate investigations (e.g. Hemoglobin electrophoresis). If feasible, obtain additional blood samples (EDTA, as well as plain vial), prior to blood transfusion. The samples may be exploited later for diagnostic studies. If the patient needs to be referred to a tertiary centre following the transfusion, transporting the blood samples along, may be valuable. A blood transfusion does not alter bone marrow picture.

An indirect clue to the diagnosis of autoimmune haemolytic anemia is the information from the blood bank about the cross match being repeatedly incompatible. In such cases, blood in which the RBCs give the least positive in vitro reaction by Coombs technique should be chosen and transfused under the cover of steroids.

WHEN TO TRANSFUSE BLOOD?

Initial evaluation should include assessment for the need and urgency for a blood transfusion. In general, no specific cut-off level of haemoglobin is recommended below which a red cell transfusion is indicated. Hemodynamic instability, aetiology and duration of anemia, ongoing blood loss, etc, are the factors that aid in decision making for a blood transfusion. Tolerance of the body for degree of anemia is higher when anemia develops over a period of time, e.g. thalassemia, as compared to acute blood loss, e.g. trauma. Transfusion of blood for nutritional anemia, in the absence of signs and symptoms of congestive cardiac failure should be avoided. In the large majority, oral hematinics suffice. It may be possible to hold a red cell transfusion in children with nutritional anemia, even with very low hemoglobin levels of upto 3 – 5 g/dL, if there is no hemodynamic instability and close monitoring can be ensured. A rapid haematological response can be confidently predicted in typical iron deficiency; blood transfusion is indicated only when the anemia is very severe or when superimposed infection may interfere with the response. Tachycardia alone should not be an indication for transfusion. On the other hand, threshold for transfusion should be much higher, if there is rapid drop in haemoglobin and ongoing blood loss. E.g. a child with hematemasis from portal varices should be transfused early to ensure a reserve.

Acute Hemorrhage

The most important measure in acute hemorrhage is first, to control the hemorrhage and to restore tissue with crystalloid and/or colloid solution. If the estimated blood loss is > 25% of the circulating blood volume, (i.e., > 17 ml/Kg) and the patient's condition remains unstable, red cell transfusion is indicated.

Perioperative Period

Transfusions may be given more stringently to children because normal haemoglobin levels are lower in healthy children than in adults and, except in defined circumstances, children do not have the underlying cardiorespiratory and vascular diseases that develop with aging in adults. Thus, children are better able to compensate for RBC loss. In the perioperative period, it is often unnecessary for most children to maintain Hb of 8 g/dL or greater, a level frequently desired for adults.

Choice and Volume of Red Cell Product

The RBC product of choice for children and adolescents is the standard suspension of RBCs separated from whole blood by centrifugation and resuspended in an anticoagulant/preservative storage solution at a hematocrit value of about 60%. The usual dose is 10-15 ml/Kg, transfused over 2-3 hours. If the anemia has developed slowly, over a period of time (e.g. iron deficiency anemia), it is not necessary to attempt rapid correction of severe anemia by transfusion; the procedure may be dangerous because of associated hypervolemia and cardiac dilatation. Packed red cells should be administered slowly in an amount sufficient to raise the haemoglobin to a safe level. In general, severely anemic children with haemoglobin values less than 4 g/dL should be given only 2-3 ml/Kg of packed cells at any one time. Furosemide (Lasix) may also be administered as a diuretic in children with long standing severe anemia. Needless to say, use of diuretic is contraindicated if the cause of anemia is rapid blood loss.

Duration of Transfusion

A RBC transfusion should not take longer than 4 hours because of the risk of bacterial proliferation in the blood component at room temperature. If the patient cannot tolerate an infusion rate necessary to complete the transfusion within 4 hours, a partial unit should be administered. If this is indicated, the hospital transfusion service should be contacted to arrange for a 'split' unit, one half of which can be retained in the transfusion service refrigerator until infusion of the first half unit is complete.

When to Request for 'Fresh' Blood?

The traditional use of 'fresh' RBCs has largely been abandoned, though requests are not uncommon, largely in ignorance. Time is required for the mandatory screening of infections. It is a good practice to restrict donor exposure in neonates by using a single unit of red cell to obtain aliquots for transfusing each infant, regardless of the duration of RBC storage. Risk of hyperkalemia for regular transfusions is often overestimated. Use of relatively fresh red cell product (< 7 days) does however apply to large-volume (> 25 ml/Kg) transfusions that are infused rapidly, in which greater doses of potassium may be harmful.

How to Request Blood in Urgent Situations?

Clinical assessment of the urgency for RBC transfusion will determine whether the patient receives unmatched emergency group O RBCs, group-specific RBCs, or a fully crossmatched RBC unit. In all cases, a pre-transfusion sample of appropriately identified and labelled blood should be obtained and sent to the blood bank for typing and initiation of compatibility testing. Risks of ABO transfusions errors are potentially high, particularly in urgent clinical situations involving multiple-trauma patients. Particular care and attention must accompany patient identification procedures in this setting. Group O, Rh-negative, unmatched RBCs can be used in children if the patient's blood group is unknown and transfusion is urgently required. Type-specific unmatched blood can usually be provided within 10 minutes; however, completion of an antibody screen and crossmatch often takes 30-60 minutes. Transfusing physicians should familiarize themselves with the policies and procedures of the hospital blood bank in providing blood for emergency use.

Exchange Transfusion Beyond the Neonatal Period

An exchange transfusion is sometimes indicated beyond the neonatal period. Indications include severe anemia with hyperleukocytosis in a patient with acute leukemia or chronic myeloid leukemia. Hyperleukocytosis is defined as a peripheral WBC count exceeding 100,0000 per µL. Clinically significant hyperleukocytosis occurs with WBC count of greater than 200,0000 per µL in acute myeloid leukemia, and greater than 300,0000 per µL in acute lymphoid leukemia and chronic myeloid leukemia. A regular red cell transfusion can be detrimental in such a situation as it can either worsen hyperviscosity or precipitate congestive cardiac failure. Leukaphereses is another option. Limitations with leukapheresis include need for anticoagulation, difficulty with access in small children and limited availability.

When to Request for Irradiated Blood Products?

Availability of irradiator in blood banks of tertiary hospitals is increasing. Gamma irradiation of blood products is done to prevent transfusion associated graft versus host disease. It is a life threatening condition with high mortality. Irradiated blood products are indicated in immunocompromised patients (e.g. leukemia on chemotherapy, bone marrow transplant, etc) and for directed donations (e.g., parents to children).

ANEMIA IN THE CRITICALLY SICK

The most important consequence related to anemia is a reduction of oxygen delivery. Blood transfusions are administered to increase oxygen carrying capacity and oxygen consumption. The risks and benefits of RBC transfusion should be weighed prior to any transfusion. There are a number of risks associated with transfusions, including transmission of infectious diseases and transfusion reactions. RBC transfusion may have proinflammatory activities which could be detrimental in primed patients with a systemic inflammatory response syndrome or in sepsis, two frequent problems in PICU. RBC transfusion may also be immunosuppressive. The latter two statements may seem contradictory. It is however a frequent occurrence to observe simultaneously, in the same critically ill patients, an immunosuppression and a systemic inflammatory state.

The optimal hemoglobin threshold for red cell transfusions in critically ill children is unknown. In acutely ill children with severe pulmonary disease requiring assisted ventilation, it is common practice to maintain the hemoglobin level close to the normal range. Up to 50% of children who are hospitalized in an intensive care unit (ICU) receive red-cell transfusions, yet children whose condition is stable may tolerate the decreased oxygen delivery associated with a moderate degree of anemia. On the other hand, children in the ICU could benefit from transfusions because of enhanced oxygen delivery. A study titled 'TRIPICU study' was conducted in 19 tertiary-care pediatric ICUs in four countries. 637 stable, critically ill children, with hemoglobin concentrations below 9.5 g/dL were enrolled. 320 patients were randomly assigned to an Hb threshold of 7 g/dL for red-cell transfusion (restrictive-strategy group) and 317 patients to a threshold of 9.5 g/dL (liberal-strategy group). Patients in the restrictive-strategy group received 44% fewer transfusions. Multiple-organ dysfunction syndrome (the primary outcome) developed in 12% in both the groups. There were 14 deaths in each group. No significant differences were found in two groups. Authors concluded that in stable, critically ill children, a hemoglobin threshold of 7 g/dL for red-cell transfusion can decrease transfusion requirements without increasing adverse outcomes. This recommendation, however, is not applicable to premature infants, or children with severe hypoxemia, hemodynamic instability, active blood loss, or cyanotic heart disease. One also has to note that leukocyte-reduced red-cell units were transfused in the study– a resource with limited availability in our country. Transfusions containing leukocytes might result in organ dysfunction through stimulation of the inflammatory cascade by the transfused leukocytes.

With an aim to understand anemia, blood loss, and red cell transfusions in the PICU, a prospective, multicenter, observational study was conducted involving 977 children in 30 PICUs in North America. 49% of children received transfusions. After adjusting for age and illness severity, compared with nontransfused children, children who underwent transfusion had significantly longer days of mechanical ventilation and PICU stay, and had increased mortality, nosocomial infections and cardiorespiratory dysfunction. Authors concluded that transfusions in the PICU were associated with worse outcomes. They suggested introducing measures to minimize blood loss from blood draws and to set clear transfusion thresholds.

Children with Cyanotic Heart Disease

Children with cyanotic heart disease deserve special consideration in relation to tolerable levels of anemia. Most textbooks recommend that a higher hemoglobin concentration should be maintained in children with uncorrected cyanotic congenital cardiopathy. It is suggested that in critically ill children with uncorrected cyanotic congenital cardiopathy, red cell transfusion should be administered if hemoglobin concentration falls below 10.0 or 11.0 g/dL. All thresholds are based upon expert opinion, given that there are no randomized clinical trials and very limited clinical physiological and observational studies in this very distinct pediatric population.

FURTHER READING

1. Oski FA, Brugnara C, Nathan DG. A diagnostic approach to the anemic patient. *In:* Nathan DG, Orkin SH, Ginsburg D, Look AT (eds). Nathan and Oski's Hematology of Infancy and Childhood. 6th edn. Philadelphia: WB Saunders Company; 2003, p. 409 -418.
2. Glader B. The Anemias. In: Behrman RE, Kliegman RM, Jenson HB, eds. Nelson textbook of Pediatrics. 17th ed. Philadelphia: Saunders; 2004:1604-1606.
3. Clarke G, Blajchman M. Clinical guide to transfusion. 4th edn. Toronto; Canadian blood services, July 2006. (http://www.transfusionmedicine.ca/)
4. Rheingold SR, Lange BJ. Oncologic emergencies. *In:* Pizzo PA, Poplack DG (eds). Principles and practice of Pediatric Oncology. 5th edn. Philadelphia: Lippincott Williams & Wilkins; 2006, p. 1202 - 1230.

5. Lacroix J, Hébert PC, Hutchison JS, et al; TRIPICU Investigators; Canadian Critical Care Trials Group; Pediatric Acute Lung Injury and Sepsis Investigators Network. Transfusion strategies for patients in pediatric intensive care units. N Engl J Med. 2007; 356:1609-19.
6. Desmet L, Lacroix J. Transfusion in pediatrics. Crit Care Clin. 2004; 20:299-311.

Jerry Ray Baskerville MD FACEP

49 Sickle Cell Disease

Sickle cell disease is an inherited blood disorder that affects between 50,000 and 75,000 people in the United States. Two million Americans carry the trait gene. Patients with Sickle Cell Diseases (SCDs) come to the emergency medicine environment frequently and with variable presentations. It is unusual for an emergency physician who treats patients of African heritage on a frequent basis to not see many hundreds of patients with variable presentations of SCDs in their career. The multitude of variable and yet common presentations demand the physician to have a standardized approach to facilitate the expeditious treatment of these complex patients without committing errors of management. Unfortunately there is great variability of management of SCD patients by physicians including those working in academic emergency departments.[1] It is very common for emergency medicine caregivers to have a high degree of knowledge about given patients that commonly present for pain medication. These patients are especially challenging as they can become so familiar that they may give the physician a false sense of security. It is very important that every presentation of every SCD patient be professionally evaluated to rule out the bad before settling for the common.

BACKGROUND

Sickle cell diseases are perhaps the most common human hereditary disorders worldwide. These disorders are found in people of African, Mediterranean, Indian and Middle Eastern heritage. In the United States, they are most commonly observed in African Americans and Hispanics from the Caribbean, Central America, and parts of South America. Approximately 250,000 babies worldwide and 2,000 in the USA are born with sickle cell disease annually. The incidence of sickle cell trait is 8% in African Americans.[2] SCD is a generic term that encompasses a group of symptomatic disorders having in common the predominance of hemoglobin S. The type of hemoglobin produced is determined by the two globin genes located on chromosome 11 and the four globin genes located on chromosome 16. Individuals who are homozygous for sickle globin gene have the most common form of SCD; this abnormal gene causes valine replacement of glutamic acid at the sixth position from the N-terminal end of the â chain. The other relatively common SCDs are sickle cell hemoglobin C disease (Sickle β gene and a hemoglobin C β gene), sickle cell beta thalassemia (Sickle β gene and a β thalassemia gene). Sickle cell anemia is an autosomal recessive disease with the homozygous progeny of two recessive parents being the unfortunate patient with SCD. Sickle cell trait is not a disease but rather a carrier state and should rarely be used to explain any illness of individuals carrying the trait; the exceptions to this rule are trait patients exposed to hypoxemia or severe physiologic stress. Although there is tremendous variability and overlap between disease groups with respect to clinical severity and manifestation, the genotypic distinction between SS and other SCD is important for several reasons. Individuals with Hb SC disease and sickle cell beta thalassemia are less likely to be symptomatic early in life so that these disorders may remain undiagnosed until adolescence or adult life, have higher steady state hemoglobin levels that are important considerations in the detection of anemic crises, retain splenomegaly well into the late adolescence and adulthood and thus are at risk for splenic sequestration crises. They also are more prone to certain complications such as acute and chronic eye complications and sickling related hematuria, and rarely have sickled red cells on a routine blood smear.

Patients with SCD frequently suffer from acute painful vaso-occlusive crises (VOC) and therefore become high consumers of emergency medical care. Complacency may lead to a tendency to label all medical illnesses of these patients as sickle cell crises. While crises tend to be self-limited and may require only conservative supportive treatment, SCD patients are at high risk for many serious and multi-system problems causing similar signs and symptoms that may require more aggressive and specific care. These patients therefore present a complex challenge for the emergency physician who must be constantly vigilant to rule out potentially life-threatening disease.

The diagnosis of SCD is made by Sickledex© screening followed by hemoglobin electrophoreses to define trait verses disease. When available, parents and siblings should be evaluated. Clinical and laboratory correlation is important in the diagnosis of SCD.

PATHOPHYSIOLOGY

There are three cardinal pathophysiologic features of SCD, chronic hemolytic anemia, vaso-occlusion resulting in ischemic tissue injury, and end organ and immunologic compromise. The hemolytic anemia is caused primarily by the abnormal properties of Hb S, which causes the red cells to undergo repeated cycles of sickling and unsickling. This eventually leads to irreversibly sickled red cells, which, being rigid and fragile, undergo mechanical lysis in the circulation. The hemolysis is predominantly intravascular. Hemosiderinuria and depletion of serum haptoglobin therefore are consistent laboratory findings in addition to the elevated indirect bilirubin and lactate dehydrogenase. The severity of hemolysis and related abnormalities are directly proportional to the intensity of sickling. Since sickling in general is less intense in Hb SC disease and sickle cell beta thalassemia, the anemia and laboratory features of hemolysis are less prominent in these disorders than they are in Hb SS. Chronic hemolysis is responsible for the increased incidence of cholelithiasis

from hemosiderin and of gout caused by hyperuricemia.

Vaso-occlusive episodes (VOE) have multi-factorial causes. On the molecular level the affected hemoglobin chain causes an interlocking of the affected chain with adjacent hemoglobin in a deoxygenated and acidotic state. This causes tactoid formation; these are interconnected parallel rods that grow to form a p-crystalline gel and then a crystal. This causes a deformed and non-malleable red blood cell (RBC) that obstructs capillaries and propagates deoxygenation of tissue in a vicious cycle of hypoxemia and acidosis.

In the past, pathophysiology of vaso-occlusive tissue injury was dominated by an emphasis on the sickling phenomenon. It is now recognized widely that SCDs are exceedingly complex and that attempts to explain the vascular occlusion on the basis of a single feature are artificial.[3] Available information supports an important contributory role for vascular endothelial cells, plasma proteins, granulocytes, lymphokines, and co-existing genetic factors in the genesis of vaso-occlusive episodes both acute and chronic. The organs at greatest risk are those with venous sinuses where the blood flow is slow and oxygen tension and pH are low (spleen, kidney, bone marrow) or those with a limited terminal arterial blood supply (eye, head of the femur, brain). Symptoms of vaso-occlusion may be acute (Pain crises, stroke and acute chest syndrome) or chronic (Aseptic necrosis of femoral head, splenic fibrosis and retinopathy).

EMERGENCY PRESENTATION

Common acute illnesses of SCD children relevant to the emergency physician are infection, painful events, acute splenic sequestration, other anemic crises, acute chest syndrome, cerebro vascular event and priapism. It is important to remember that one syndrome does not reduce the likelihood of another. Clinical manifestations of Hb SS begin to appear by 6 months of age in about 6 percent of the children with mortality peaking at age 1 to 3 years. Infection is the primary cause of death in this young age group. By 8 years of age 96% of Hb SS children manifest sickle cell-specific symptoms. SCD is no longer only a disease of children with 85% of these patients surviving beyond age 18.[4] The median age of death among SCD patients is 42 years for males and 48 years for females.

Infection

Children with SCD are very susceptible to bacterial infections. This is a consequence of impaired splenic function (With 14% and 94% of children functionally asplenic at 6 months and 5 years respectively), defective complement pathways, and serum opsonizing activities. Infections are a major cause of morbidity and mortality in the first few years of life. Indeed a life-threatening infection may be the first clinical manifestation of SCD in a child not detected during the newborn period. The organisms most frequently involved include S. pneumoniae, H. influenzae, E. coli, S. aureus, and S. typhi. Blood, lungs, bone, meninges and urinary tract are the areas most often involved.

Pulmonary infections account for the majority of the cases. S. pneumoniae and H. influenzae are the organisms most often involved but mycoplasma and chlamydia infections also occur commonly. Although prophylaxis with pneumococcal vaccine and oral penicillin have greatly reduced the frequency of pneumococcal infections, one must recognize that suboptimal antibody response against certain strains of pneumococci in some children and poor compliance to penicillin prophylaxis may leave such children at risk of pneumococcal sepsis.

Osteomyelitis is to be considered in all patients with one or more localized areas of bone pain and high fever. It is most often caused by salmonella infection although staphylococcal infection can also occur. Osteomyelitis is often multifocal and may be confused with aseptic necrosis. The unique predisposition of SCD patients to salmonella osteomyelitis probably represents the ability of this organism to survive in the necrotic bone. The reservoir for salmonella is often the gallbladder. Urinary tract infections are most often caused by E. coli and are frequently complicated by septicemia.

The general guidelines for evaluation and treatment are given in Table 1. The emphasis should be on prompt and aggressive evaluation and institution of empiric antibiotic therapy. A few hours delay can make a significant difference for the patient.

It is important to hospitalize all febrile SCD patients, especially those under five years of age and with a documented temperature over 101° F. If meningitis is ruled out or not suspected, treatment with appropriate antibiotic to cover S. pneumoniae and H. influenzae is still indicated. *Treatment should be given even for minimal clinical indications if pneumococcal sepsis is suspected.*

If antibiotic therapy is considered it must be initiated in the emergency department as the delay that can occur on the inpatient service can be life threatening. In some institutions, febrile children over the age of 5 years are not routinely hospitalized; such an approach should require close consultation with the consulting or primary hematologist and very specific and timely follow up within 24 hours or less is required. The social situation of the family should be strongly considered.

Infections in SCD patients can be reduced by immunization and prophylactic penicillin and morbidity reduced by educating parents to seek prompt medical care for their febrile child.

Pain

Pain is the most common reason that SCD patients present to the emergency department. Patients and their family rightfully expect their pain to be managed effectively and efficiently. Pain is believed to be caused by ischemia resulting from the obstruction

Table 1: Management of the febrile child with SCD

Physical examination (Evaluate each aspect)	*Laboratory studies (Consider)*
Oxygenation	Pulse Oxymetry
Hydration (Clinical Evaluation)	Vital Signs / Urine Specific Gravity
Sepsis	CBC & Reticulocyte Count / Blood Cultures
CNS Infection	Lumbar Puncture
Pulmonary Infection	Chest X-ray / Mycoplasma / Chlamydia titer
Hepato-Biliary Infection / Obstruction	Lipase / Amylase / LFT
Renal Infection / Obstruction	Urinalysis / Culture
Bone Infection	Bone X-ray / CT with directed aspiration
Colitis	Stool guaiac, leukocytes and reducing substance with Stool Culture if Diarrhea
Skin and Soft Tissue	Cultures as needed

of blood flow produced by sickled erythrocytes. The associated mediators proximate to the process accentuate the pain response. The frequency and severity of painful events are extremely varied. It is difficult for the caregivers to gauge the degree of pain that the patient is experiencing. Musculoskeletal pain is the most common complaint. Dactylitis, or hand-foot syndrome, is the first manifestation of vaso-occlusive crises in many infants. The pain can be symmetrical, asymmetrical, or migratory, and it may or may not be associated with swelling, low grade fever, redness, or warmth. Abdominal pain is the second most common SCD pain syndrome.

The possibility that the pain is precipitated by a concurrent medical condition such as infection should always be considered. It is extremely important to exclude non-sickle causes of pain such as cholecystitis, peptic ulcer, perforated viscous, urinary tract infection, intra-abdominal infection, osteomyelitis, or septic arthritis before labeling the patient as having a vaso-occlusive crises. Pneumonia in children can often present with abdominal pain.

Diagnostic evaluation of the painful events is dictated by site of pain and other associated manifestations and aimed primarily at ruling out non-sickle causes of pain. If fever higher than 101°F or if marked leukocytosis is present, an aggressive search for infection should be made. If chest symptoms are present acute chest syndrome (ACS) must be ruled out. Direct aspiration of a joint or bone lesion may be indicated in cases of suspected septic arthritis or osteomyelitis. Electrolytes and venous blood gas should be obtained in all severely ill patients. Computed tomographic (CT) scan or an ultrasound of the abdomen is often helpful in detecting medical or surgical causes of abdominal pain.

Management of pain crises has three essential elements; identification and treatment of precipitating or associated events, hydration and prompt relief of pain with analgesics. Dehydration occurs frequently in these patients because of decreased fluid intake, increased insensible water loss and limited ability of the kidney to concentrate urine. Intravenous (IV) hydration is indicated in most cases and is mandatory for clinically dehydrated patients. The choice of fluid is dictated by the patient's hydration status and electrolyte values. For uncomplicated pain crises, 5 percent dextrose with 0.45 percent normal saline is recommended as initial fluid. Children should receive 150 ml/kg/day with close monitoring to avoid precipitating congestive heart failure.

Analgesics are used with the goal of providing prompt pain relief. This is often not achieved because of inadequate understanding of the clinical pharmacology of

Table 2: Clues to non SCD disease pain

Fever> 101° F with lethargy	Localized bone pain with high fever
Severe abdominal pain with rebound and guarding	Headache with vomiting
Isolated extremity weakness or loss of function	Acute pulmonary symptoms
Significant dehydration	Marked leukocytosis > 20,000
Acute joint swelling	Pain unrelieved by conservative measures

analgesics, excessive concern about narcotic addiction, or misguided use of placebos. Despite the frequent need for analgesics, narcotic addiction is remarkably uncommon in this patient population.

The choice of therapy is based on severity of pain and potency, mode of action, and side effects of the drugs. Medication should be administered on a fixed schedule with dosing intervals not exceeding the duration of the desired effect. Potent narcotics should be used with the usual precautions and monitoring to avoid respiratory depression.

The goal of emergency management is to assess the clinical problem, exclude nonsickle illnesses, to undertake a brief trial of therapy, and to decide whether to hospitalize the patient. Certain high-risk patients, such as those with abdominal pain, high fever, lethargy, or neurologic deficit, should be promptly investigated, treated and admitted.

If the patient with severe pain remains comfortable for 2-3 hours after a parenteral narcotic, an oral narcotic may be administered and discharge may be contemplated. If moderate or severe pain returns, the parenteral narcotic dose should be repeated. If significant pain persists, the patient has failed out patient management and should be admitted to the hospital. If pain is under control, the patient can be discharged on an adequate dose of effective oral narcotic rescue medication. It is important to be perceptive and responsive to the wishes of the patient and family regarding hospitalization.

Acute Splenic and Hepatic Sequestration Crises

Splenic sequestration is a medical emergency demanding prompt, aggressive and focused therapy. The mortality rate of splenic sequestration is 10% with 29.9% of SCD patients experiencing at least one episode.[5] Sequestration crises usually occur in the 3 months to 6 years age group whose spleens have not yet undergone multiple infarctions and fibrosis. In Hb SS, sequestration occurs after five months of age and is unusual after age two. In those with other sickle cell diseases whose spleens remain enlarged, this complication can continue to occur later in life. Infection is often the precipitating cause.

These catastrophic events are clinically identified by abdominal pain with sudden massive enlargement of the spleen, anemia, weakness, pallor, dyspnea and fever. The resultant severe anemia and hypovolemia occur as a result of splenic third spacing of blood volume. This is the most acutely dangerous crises in the life of a young child with Hb SS. Infants can die within hours of the first sign of this disturbance.

Diagnostic Testing

- Ultrasonography.
- CBC shows profound anemia and thrombocytemia.
- Reticulocyte count elevation.
- LDH and LFT elevations.

Minor episodes characterized by modest increases in spleen size associated with a two to three gm decrease in hemoglobin level are very common. Although these resolve spontaneously, they predict for later severe episodes. Their recognition, therefore, is important in educating parents to look for pallor, to palpate for spleen size changes, and to seek prompt medical attention if either abnormality develops. Recognition of such episodes is facilitated by accurate documentation of steady state spleen size in every child with SCD.

Treatment

- Expeditious correction of hypovolemia, hypoxemia and anemia.
- Transfusion with 5-10 ml/kg of packed red blood cells (PRBC) within the first hour of presentation.[6]
- Evaluation for evidence of infection and other vaso-occlusive events and / or infection

If shock or hypotension can be reversed, there is rapid regression of splenomegaly and remobilization of trapped red cells. As a result, a rapid rise in hemoglobin can occur in a short time. Parents should be cautioned about the recurrent nature of this complication and educated in the recognition of the complication.

Aplastic and Megaloblastic Crises

Transient red blood cell aplastic crises patients can present with any combination of dyspnea, weakness, fatigue, CVA, splenic sequestration and CHF. These patients are found to be much more anemic than usual with very few < 0.5% reticulocytes. In aplastic crises, the bone marrow shows a selective suppression of erythropoiesis. Viral illness, particularly human parvovirus B_{19} (HPV) can cause aplastic crisis. HPV causes erythema infectiosum (fifth disease) which is highly contagious and usually occurs prior to age 15 years. HPV is spread by respiratory droplets or blood exposure with an incubation period of 14 to 21 days and is generally mild and self limited.[7] In the SCD patient however aplastic crises and severe anemia may last 12 to 14 days and require repeat transfusion. As of January 2008 there is no vaccine for HPV in the USA. The diagnosis is made by clinical evaluation, CBC and reticulocyte count. Treatment is supportive with transfusion therapy as needed to prevent worsening anemia or treat other SCD crises. These cases resolve spontaneously in 5 to 10 days. Oxygen administration for prolonged continuous periods of 5 days or more can markedly decrease erythropoietin levels.[8] Oxygen should be used intermittently as needed to maintain pAO_2 levels at 70 mm Hg.

Megaloblastic crises are rare in SCD and are characterized by megaloblastic erythropoiesis. The optimization of therapy with Vitamin B_{12}, folic acid and Vitamin B_6 is important in SCD patients due to the increased utilization by their disease process.[9] Folate deficiency is most often implicated in this syndrome that is most often precipitated by the stress of other SCD crises. Treatment is symptomatic with transfusion with folate and B_{12} replacement.

Acute Chest Syndrome (ACS)

The acute chest syndrome in sickle cell disease is defined as a new infiltrate on chest imaging associated with clinical symptomatology such as chest pain, respiratory distress, fever, cough, sputum production, tachypnea, dyspnea, or new-onset hypoxia.[10] ACS is most common in the 2 to 4 years age group and gradually declines in incidence with age. In young children infectious etiology either viral or bacterial is most frequent however with age and into adulthood pulmonary infarction is most common. Streptococcus pneumoniae is decreasing in incidence with mycoplasma and viral infections especially rhinovirus now most common in younger children and with age chlamydia becomes predominant.[11] Human Parvovirus B_{19} can cause very severe ACS and is second only to rhinovirus in viral agents responsible for this syndrome. No causative organism is identified in 55% of patients.

ACS can develop as an isolated event or occur in the course of vaso-occlusive crises. It often progresses rapidly from mild respiratory symptoms to respiratory failure with mechanical ventilation required in up to 13% of patients. The oxygen-hemoglobin saturation curve is shifted to the right in SCD and thus hypoxemia has a very profound effect on tissue oxygenation. The infiltrates are often multi-lobar and are very slow to resolve taking 10-12 days to improve.

The diagnosis of ACS is largely clinical however there are certain tests that may be employed to assist in the management of the patient.

Diagnostic Testing

- Complete blood count (CBC).
- Reticulocyte count.
- Blood gases (Venous or Arterial).
- Chest X-ray (May not show changes for 2-3 days).
- Chest multi-detector computerized tomography (MDCT) for pulmonary embolism.
- Serology for mycoplasma and chlamydia.
- Cultures of blood, and pleural fluid if present (Sputum cultures are rarely of value).

Severe hypoxia with pAO_2 below 60 indicates severe and potentially life threatening ACS. Ventilation perfusion lung scans are generally not helpful in the etiologic diagnosis or in therapeutic decisions.

The treatment and management should be expeditious. All patients with acute chest syndrome (ACS) should be stabilized promptly in the emergency department and hospitalized. Intensive Care Unit (ICU) admission may be required for observation and intensive supportive treatment. Pulmonary hypertension which has a prevalence of 32% should be considered in all ACS patients as it increases mortality and may require inhaled nitric oxide and transfusion therapy.[12]

Treatment Considerations

- Oxygen administration is required to raise the pAO_2 to 70 mm Hg.
- Empiric therapy for infection should be started promptly.
- Hydration by IV or oral methods.
- Analgesia administration.
- Incentive spirometry and pulmonary therapy with bronchodilators.
- Bronchoscopy to diagnose and treat plastic bronchitis[13]
- Exchange transfusion may be indicated in refractory patients.

It should be emphasized that supportive care should be the major therapeutic focus in ACS.

Neurologic Events

Strokes occur in 10% of SCD patients before age 20. In patients with Hb SS, CVA from infarction or hemorrhage, and transient ischemic attacks (TIAs) are the most common presentations. SCD patients also have an increased risk of cerebral aneurysm and intracranial hemorrhage over the general population. It is highly recommended that transcranial Doppler studies be performed to risk stratify patients for possible transfusion therapy.[14] In high risk patients CVA can be reduced by 90% with transfusion therapy aimed at reducing HbS to <30%.

Clinical signs are often obvious but may be difficult to distinguish from a limp caused by pain in young, nonverbal children. Hemiparesis is most common followed by aphasia, dysphasia, seizures, or monoparesis. Associated headache is common. Occasionally the patient may present in a complete or nearly comatose state. In about a quarter of the patients, the stroke may occur concurrently with other sickle cell complications such as pain crises, anemic crises, and acute chest syndrome.

Diagnosis is made on clinical grounds, but imaging procedures are necessary to distinguish between hemorrhage and infarction and to delineate the physical and functional location of the stroke. Most useful initial study is a CT without contrast or magnetic resonance imaging (MRI). CT may be normal at the onset of infarction, but it is helpful in ruling out bleeding, abscess, tumor, or other space occupying lesions. Lumbar puncture is indicated when infection or subarachnoid hemorrhage is suspected but must be undertaken only if CT or MRI shows no evidence of increased intracranial pressure.

Visipaque™ (iodixanol) at all iodine concentrations is the only iso-osmolar contrast medium available for intravascular use and should be the only contrast used in SCD patients. It can be used with caution in SCD considering the risk benefit of investigation. There is the potential of vaso-occlusive disease (VOD) and SCD pain crises aggravation. It is important that hydration and hematocrit be optimized prior to the administration. Angiographic MDCT and MRI are much safer and less invasive than arteriography.

For the patient with acute stroke, rapid evaluation, treatment and close monitoring are essential. Neurologic and possibly neurosurgical consultation is encouraged.

Partial exchange transfusion to reduce the Hb S level to less than 30% will help prevent progression of acute stroke and must be undertaken as soon as possible. Simple transfusion is not recommended if the Hb will be or is > 11gm. The outlook for intracranial hemorrhage is poor, but should be managed similarly.

Priapism

This disorder can occur in 30-80% of male patients with SCD.[15] Recurrent or severe, priapism is a predictor of other end organ damage and increased mortality. Pain control, hydration, urologic consultation and possible transfusion are required.

Diagnostic Testing

The testing armamentarium has improved over the last several years with the emergency medicine utilization of emergency medicine directed ultrasonography(EMDUS). Emergency physicians now utilize EMDUS for many aspects of SCD care including diagnostic testing and procedure facilitation. The other common emergency medicine tests necessary to manage SCD and their utilization are displayed (Table 3).

Treatment

Standardized treatment for SCD pain crises has been shown to decrease ED visits and hospitalizations.[16] The American Pain Society (APS) recommends initial analgesic administration within 15-20 minutes for patients presenting to the ED with acute sickle cell pain. APS recommends use of the IV route or the subcutaneous route if venous access is not available and initial use of morphine (0.1-0.15 mg/kg, or 5-10 mg if weight is above 50 kg) or hydromorphone (0.015-0.02 mg/kg). A recent multi-center study has shown that the median time to pain medication admini-stration is 90 minutes with only 55% receiving analgesia by IV or SC route.[17] It should be mentioned that the IM route is

Table 3: Emergency medicine testing utility

Test	*Utilization*
CBC	The Hb, Hct, WBC count, granulocyte count with shift, platelet count are all important to know in all SCD patient that present to the ED.
Reticulocyte Count	Essential in all SCD presentations.
Pulse Oxymetry	Essential to rule out systemic hypoxemia. Pulse Ox of 95% = pAO_2 of 74.9 mm / Hg therefore if < 90 patient must be placed on oxygen after ABG. Maintain pAO_2 = 70.
Urinalysis	Microscopic testing important for infection and blood but Specific Gravity > 1.015 means dehydration and + Ketones means catabolism.
Electrolyte Panel	BUN and Creatinine are both critical to know. Other electrolytes can be surprising.
Hepatic Panel	Especially important in hepatic and splenic sequestration.
Cranial MDCT	All CVA, altered mental status (AMS), headache and seizure patients.
Abdominal MDCT	If guarding and fever is especially cogent.
Abdominal Ultrasound	Splenic sequestration. Usually EMDUS (Emergency Medicine Directed Ultrasonography) is adequate.
MRI	In the event of acute spinal cord syndromes the differential includes not only vasoocclusion but also spinal abscess and hematoma.

unreliable due to poor muscle mass in these patients. A major issue is venous access in the SCD patient. Lines are often difficult and central access is often necessary. The utilization of ultrasound guided peripheral access has been shown to improve the likelihood of success when performed by either physicians or nurses.[18] In the event of delay in venous access patients should receive SC analgesia within 20 minutes of presentation. *In the real world of emergency medicine this means that SC analgesia should be used in virtually all SCDs pain crises patients.*

Supportive Care

Supportive care is the most important aspect of the management of the SCD patient with the clinician managing oxygenation, fluid balance, physiologic dysfunction and emotional needs. These aspects of care are covered in other chapters of this synopsis.

Pain Medication

Pain crises are responsible for up to 97% of hospital admissions for SCD. The application of a quality pathway has been shown to reduce hospitalizations by 40% and length of stay by 50%.[19]

Meperidine: The meperidine controversy continues to remain however renal failure and history of seizure are well recognized contraindications to meperidine. Seizure prevalence ranges from 1-12% in SCD patients receiving meperidine.[20] The half life of meperidine is 3 hours however the toxic metabolite normeperidine has a half life of 18 hours. Normeperidine can cause anxiety, tremors, myoclonus, and generalized seizures. These adverse effects occur almost exclusively in the setting of massive doses repeated every 1-2 hours for several days. Pediatric hospitalized SCD patients rarely have seizures. Nadvi found a rate of only

1:1700 hospitalizations.[21] It is important to recognize that patients prefer meperidine over morphine for acute painful syndromes.[22] It is very evident when treating SCD patients that those that have had prior success with meperidine are loath and often hostile at even the thought of a change of analgesic. This is a no win position for the treating physician. There is no evidence that meperidine is more addictive than morphine thus the mistaken thought that physicians should protect patients from meperidine for this reason is misguided. Meperidine inhibits the re-uptake of serotonin and can precipitate the serotonin syndrome in patients taking monoamine oxidase inhibitors, serotonin-reuptake inhibitors, cocaine, tramadol, amphetamines, dextromethorphan, and lithium. In the commonplace world of selective serotonin reuptake inhibitor (SSRI) drug usage the administration of meperidine is just an interaction away from a disaster.

Morphine: This is the heir apparent to meperidine however morphine also has significant disadvantages; it has metabolites that produce neuroexcitatory effects similar to those seen with meperidine and has been reported to cause acute non-cardiogenic pulmonary edema. Morphine is associated with a high incidence of marked dysphoria which can be very distressing to the patient, family and physician alike. Acute chest syndrome is the most common cause of death in SCD patients and morphine has been associated with an increased risk of this syndrome.[23]

Hydromorphone (Dilaudid): Administered by protocol has been successful in reducing SCD pain crises patient admissions from 38% to 20% and may be considered a valid player in the analgesic competition.[24]

Ketorolac (Toradol): and other NSAIDS: There is no convincing evidence to suggest ketorolac or other NSAIDS are more effective than narcotics in the treatment of acute painful SCD. There is potential for significant renal side effects due to inhibition of vasodilatory prostaglandins. Since SCD patients are at risk of renal compromise from their primary disease there is little evidence to support their usage.[25]

Narcotic addiction and tolerance are sometimes considered synonymous. This thought however is simplistic and not in the patients best interest. Addiction is persistent dysfunctional opioid use with adverse consequences, loss of control, or preoccupation, despite adequate analgesia.[26] Tolerance and physiologic dependence are intrinsic to chronic narcotic usage and should not be confused with addiction.[27] The dose response curve for opioids also has up to ten fold variability between patients. Physicians who treat chronic pain patients must become comfortable with titrating medication to effect by monitoring the behavioral and physiologic parameters available. The adequate narcotic dosage in these patients is 'Enough'. A case report by Eugenio describes a patient with malignancy requiring morphine infusion that was increased to a rate of 35 mg/hr with additional bolus doses of 15 mg intravenously every 15 minutes as needed.[28] This is not to suggest a cavalier approach to pain management with excessive dosages of narcotics but as a request to treat the patient and not the pharmacist.

Transfusion Therapy

The administration of blood by either simple transfusion or exchange transfusion is life saving in many SCD patients. Its routine for blood banks in the USA to screen all blood for transfusion to SCD patients with a sickle screening test such as Sickledex©.

Accepted indications for transfusion are:[29]

- Acute ischemic cerebrovascular accident (CVA).
- Acute chest syndrome.
- Primary and secondary ischemic CVA prevention.
- Retinal artery occlusion.
- Acute and recurrent Splenic and Hepatic sequestration.
- Aplastic crises.
- Acute hemorrhage.

Less well accepted indications are: preoperative transfusion, priapism, progressive renal failure, pulmonary hypertension, pregnancy with anemia and unusually frequent or severe pain crises.

New Treatments

Hydroxyurea is not used in the emergency management of SCD however emergency physicians may see patients on this medication. It is an oncologic schedule D drug that can cause severe pregnancy defects. Seizures, myelosuppression, anemia and secondary leukemia are adverse reactions to this powerful drug. Hematologists may use this drug for secondary prevention of CVA in patients who can no longer tolerate blood transfusion therapy as it increases HbF.[30]

Omega-3 fatty acids may reduce SCD pain crises by up to 50% however definitive trials have yet to be done.[31]

Nitric oxide has been successful in treating ACS[32] and VOC[33]. Further study is needed before FDA approval and routine usage. Nitric oxide is a potent vasodilator and is best given by inhalation therapy.

DISPOSITION

Prophylaxis

It is important to assess the immunization status and effectiveness of follow up of SCD children. All routine childhood immunizations as well as pneumococcal, meningococcal, and influenza vaccines are critical to good outcome. Penicillin prophylaxis until age 5 is also essential.[34]

Rescue Medication and Follow-up

Patients who go home after emergency treatment for pain crises without adequate rescue analgesic medication will return to the emergency department. Effective patient directed narcotic administration is essential to the care of the SCD patient. It is critical to not only assure adequate follow-up but also pain control for these patients. The administration of prescription narcotics should be based on the experience and comfort level of the physician. Certainly the illicit usage of prescription pain medication makes certain drugs highly prized and the realities of economics may press the SCD patient and their family to engage in profit making behavior. The United States Drug Enforcement Agency believes that illegal trafficking in prescription drugs is a 25 billion dollar per year industry.[35] Certainly the patients' primary care physician is in the best position to monitor this behavior. The emergency physician should always notify the PCP of the patients visit to the emergency department and the medication administered. All SCD patients must have adequate PCP care or patient directed narcotic administration should be limited.

Acknowledgement: I would like to thank Dilip L. Solanki for allowing pertinent content of the previous version of this chapter to be utilized in this publication.

REFERENCES

1. Silbergleit, R., et al,: Management of sickle cell pain crises in the emergency department at teaching hospitals. J Emerg Med 17(4):625, July-August 1999.

2. Wright SW, *et al.*, Screening for sickle cell trait in the emergency department, J Gen Intern Med 9:421, August 1994.
3. Ataga KI, Orringer EP. Hypercoagulability in sickle cell disease: A curious paradox. Am J Med 2003;115:721-8.
4. Orah S. Platt, Donald J. Brambilla, Mortality In Sickle Cell Disease — Life Expectancy and Risk Factors for Early Death; NEJM, Vol. 330:1639-1644, June 9, 1995.
5. Emond AM, Collis R, Darvill D, *et al.* Acute splenic sequestration in homozygous sickle cell disease: Natural history and management. J Pediatr 1985;107(2):201-6.
6. Rosse WF, Telen MJ, Ware RE. Transfusion support for patients with sickle cell disease. Bethesda (MD): AABB Press; 1998.
7. Jessica T. Servey *et al.* Clinical Presentations of Parvovirus B_{19} Infection; Am Fam Physician 2007;75:373-6, 377.
8. Embury SH, Garcia JF, Mohandas N, Pennathur-Das R, Clark MR. Effects of oxygen inhalation on endogenous erythropoietin kinetics, erythropoiesis, and properties of blood cells in sickle-cell anemia. N Engl J Med 1984;311:291-295.
9. Fey P.L. van der Dijs,1 M. Rebecca Fokkema; Optimization of Folic Acid, Vitamin B_{12}, and Vitamin B_6 Supplements in Pediatric Patients with Sickle Cell Disease. American Journal of Hematology 69:239-246 (2002).
10. Vichinsky EP, Neumayr LD, Earles AN, *et al*, National Acute Chest Syndrome Study Group. Causes and outcomes of the acute chest syndrome in sickle cell disease. N Engl J Med 2000;342:1855–65.
11. Tsolia MN, Psarras S, Bossios A, *et al.* Etiology of community-acquired pneumonia in hospitalized school-age children: Evidence for high prevalence of viral infections. Clin Infect Dis 2004;39:681–6.
12. Gladwin MT, Sachdev V, Jison ML, *et al.* Pulmonary hypertension as a risk factor for death in patients with sickle cell disease. N Engl J Med 2004;350(9):886–95.
13. Moser C, Nussbaum E, Cooper DM. Plastic bronchitis and the role of bronchoscopy in the acute chest syndrome of sickle cell disease. Chest 2001;120:608–13.
14. Adams RJ, McKie VC, Hsu L, *et al.* Prevention of a first stroke by transfusions in children with sickle cell anemia and abnormal results on transcranial Doppler ultrasonography. N Engl J Med 1998; 339 (1) : 5–11.
15. Mantadakis E, Cavender JD, Rogers ZR, *et al.* Prevalence of priapism in children and adolescents with sickle cell anemia. J Pediatr Hematol Oncol 1999;21(6):518–22.
16. Givens, M., *et al.*,: Impact of an emergency department pain management protocol on the pattern of visits by patients with sickle cell disease. J Emerg Med 32(3):239, April 2007.
17. Tanabe, P., *et al.*,: Emergency department management of acute pain episodes in sickle cell disease. Acad Emerg Med 14(5):419, May 2007.
18. Brannam, L., et al,: Emergency nurses' utilization of ultrasound guidance for placement of peripheral intravenous lines in difficult-access patients, Acad Emerg Med 11(12):1361, December 2004.
19. Montanez, A., et al,: First steps in quality improvement a pilot program for the management of acute sickle cell pain, J. Clin Outcomes Man 9(1):19, January 2002
20. Nadvi S, Sarnaik S, Ravindranath Y. Association of seizures with meperidine in sickle cell disease. In: *Book of abstracts, 0th Meeting of the National Sickle Cell Disease Program*. Boston, MA, March 18-21, 1995, p 210.
21. Nadvi SZ, Sarnaik S, Ravindranath Y. Low frequency of meperidine associated seizures in sickle cell disease. *Clin Pediatr* 1999;38: 459-462.
22. Richardson P, Steingart R. Meperidine and ketorolac in the treatment of painful sickle cell crises. *Ann Emerg Med* 1993;22: 1639-1640.
23. Kopecky EA, Jacobson S, Joshi P, *et al.* Systemic exposure to morphine and the risk of acute chest syndrome. *Clin Pharmacol Ther* 2004; 75:140-146.
24. Kathryn M. Perlman, MS, RN (BC), CEN, Suzanne, Myers-Phariss, BS, RN, CEN, and Jeremy C. Rhodes, BS, RN, A Shift From Demerol (Meperidine) to Dilaudid (Hydromorphone) Improves Pain Control and Decreases Admissions for Patients in Sickle Cell Crises; October 2004 30:5 Journal of emergency nursing 439.
25. Simckes AM, Chen SS, Osorio AV, *et al.* Ketorolac-induced irreversible renal failure in sickle cell disease: A case report. Pediatr Nephrol 1999;13(1): 63–7.
26. Compton P, Darakjian MA, Miotto K. Screening for addiction in patients with chronic pain and 'problematic' substance use: Evaluation of a pilot assessment tool. J Pain Symptom Manage 1998;16(6):355–63.

27. Sees KL, Clark HW. Opioid use in the treatment of chronic pain: Assessment of addiction. J Pain Symptom Manage 1993;8(5):257–64.
28. Eugenio; Profound Morphine Tolerance Following High-Dose Methadone Therapy, Journal of Pain & Palliative Care Pharmacotherapy, Vol. 18(4) 2004.
29. Sam O. Wanko, MDa, Marilyn J. Telen, MD; Transfusion Management in Sickle Cell Disease, Hematol Oncol Clin N Am 19 (2005) 803–826.
30. Ware RE, Zimmerman SA, Sylvestre PB, Mortier NA, Davis JS, Treem WR, *et al.* Prevention of secondary stroke and resolution of transfusional iron overload in children with sickle cell anemia using hydroxyurea and phlebotomy. J Pediatr 2004;145:346-52.
31. Tomer A, Kasey S, Connor WE, *et al.* Reduction of pain episodes and thrombotic activity in sickle cell disease by dietary n-3 fatty acids. Thromb Haemost 2001;85:966–74.
32. Sullivan KJ, Goodwin SR, Evangelist J, *et al*: Nitric oxide successfully used to treat acute chest syndrome of sickle cell disease in a young adolescent. *Crit Care Med* 1999; 27:2563–2568
33. Weiner DL, Hibberd PL, Betit P, *et al.*: Preliminary assessment of inhaled nitric oxide for acute vaso-occlusive crisis in pediatric patients with sickle cell disease. *JAMA* 2003; 289:1136–1142.
34. Satyen R. Mehta,.*et al.*: Opportunities to Improve Outcomes in Sickle Cell Disease. American Family Physician, July 15, 2006
35. Conlan, MF, "States starting to target prescription drugs sold on the streets", *Drug Topics* (Aug 1990).

In the previous edition this chapter was written by Dilip L. Solanki, MD Professor of Medicine Director of Clinical Oncology/Oklahoma Medical Center Hematology Oncology Section University of Oklahoma Health Sciences Center Oklahoma City, Oklahoma

Rayne H. Rouce and Frederick S. Huang

50 Oncological Emergencies

Although childhood cancer is fairly uncommon, it is the second leading cause of death in children between the ages of 5 and 14 and the third leading cause of death in children between the ages of 1 and 4. It is the most frequent cause of disease-associated death in children between the ages of 1 and 15 in the developed world. Infections continue to remain leading cause of childhood mortality in developing countries; however children with cancers constitute a significant burden in developing countries as well, due to large population base. Cancer can affect virtually every organ system and cause life-threatening emergencies. Therefore, it is vitally important for emergency physicians to be able to promptly and appropriately recognize and manage these complications.

This chapter is divided into 2 sections. The first section is devoted to emergencies that may present at the time of diagnosis, and the second one is reserved for emergencies that may occur as a consequence of treatment. With all of these emergencies, initial stabilization and management by the emergency physician is critical, but timely consultation with a pediatric oncologist is equally important.

EMERGENCIES AT DIAGNOSIS

Cardiopulmonary Emergencies

Superior Vena Cava Syndrome and Superior Mediastinal Syndrome

Superior vena cava syndrome (SVCS) is caused by the extrinsic compression of this blood vessel by a tumor or group of involved lymph nodes. The signs and symptoms include cough, dyspnea, orthopnea, stridor, and dysphagia. Clot formation and reduced venous return can lead to edema, plethora, and cyanosis of the face and upper extremities. Venous stasis and carbon dioxide retention can result in altered mental status and seizures. SVCS is rare in children, but when it occurs, it is usually in patients with a mediastinal mass, especially lymphoma. Acute leukemias, germ cell tumors, neuroblastoma, and soft tissue sarcomas are other mediastinal masses that can cause SVCS. These masses often lead to concurrent compression of the trachea and respiratory distress, which is known as superior mediastinal syndrome (SMS). SVCS and SMS can occur together or separately.

After the patient's airway is stabilized, a chest radiograph should be obtained immediately in order to assess for the presence of a mediastinal mass. If the patient is sufficiently stable, computed tomography of the thorax should also be performed in order to delineate the extent of the mass more clearly. Because the supine position may prompt or exacerbate respiratory distress, the prone position may be necessary during the study. Conscious sedation and drugs that decrease the respiratory drive should be avoided because the ensuing relaxation may make the patient's airway difficult or impossible to secure. An urgent diagnostic procedure e.g. fine needle aspiration cytology or needle biopsy of the mass under local anaesthesia is often necessary.

In cases of SVCS and SMS, emergency treatment, typically with chemotherapy but occasionally with radiotherapy, is indicated in order to shrink the mediastinal mass and relieve the blood vessel compression or airway compromise. Symptomatic improvement can be expected within days but may be seen within hours.

Pleural Effusion

Pleural effusions must be considered in the differential diagnosis of the child with respiratory distress. Malignancies can cause a pleural effusion by direct or indirect effect. Direct mechanisms include injury or inflammation and usually yield exudates. Indirect mechanisms include congestive heart failure or nephrosis and typically create transudates.

Intervention is not required for small pleural effusions in clinically stable patients, but measures must be taken for large or symptomatic pleural effusions, especially those that have developed rapidly. If a thoracentesis is performed, the fluid should be sent for cytological analysis because a preliminary or even definitive identification of the malignancy may be possible. Most patients will experience immediate improvement following a thoracentesis and will not require additional treatment, such as the placement of a chest tube or introduction of a sclerosing agent.

Gastrointestinal Emergencies

Gastrointestinal Obstruction

Tumors that arise in the abdomen or pelvis can cause an obstruction of the small or large intestine. They include lymphomas, soft tissue sarcomas, hepatoblastoma, neuroblastoma, and Wilms tumor. Burkitt lymphoma must be considered in the differential diagnosis of the child with a mass in the right lower abdomen that is causing signs and symptoms of obstruction, intussusception, perforation, or even appendicitis. Computed tomography of the abdomen and pelvis can confirm the presence of a tumor and define its extent.

The standard approach to the evaluation and management of gastrointestinal obstruction should be employed.

Hematological Emergencies

Children with a new malignancy may have one or more hematological abnormalities at initial presentation. Malignancies that affect the bone marrow can originate there, as in leukemia, or metastasize there, as in neuroblastoma.

Anemia

Without active bleeding, anemia usually develops gradually, and children are typically asymptomatic until their hemoglobin falls below 8 mg/dl. At this level, they may have fatigue, irritability, pallor, or tachycardia.

A packed red blood cell (PRBC) transfusion should be reserved for patients who are significantly symptomatic or hemodynamically compromised. In addition to being appropriately typed and crossmatched, the blood should ideally be irradiated and leukofiltered. A volume of 15 ml/kg should be administered over a period of 4 hours. Patients with a hemoglobin less than 5mg/dl or evidence of congestive heart failure should receive half of the calculated volume over 4 hours and the other half over another 4 hours. A diuretic, such as furosemide, may be given between the 2 aliquots in order to avoid pulmonary edema.

Thrombocytopenia

Many children are largely asymptomatic until their platelet count drops below 20,000/µL. At this point, they may develop petechiae, bruises, epistaxes, or gingival bleeding. The risk of spontaneous and life-threatening bleeding, such as an intracranial hemorrhage, increases when the platelet count is less than 10,000/ml.

The decision to administer a platelet transfusion should be based on the degree of thrombocytopenia, the presence or absence of active bleeding, the presence or absence of a coexisting coagulopathy, and the need for an invasive procedure. Like PRBC, platelets should ideally be irradiated and leukofiltered. The calculated volume should be administered over a period of 1 hour. One unit of random donor platelets for every 10 kg of body weight should raise the platelet count by 40,000-50,000/µL within 1 hour after the transfusion. A rough estimation is 2 units of random donor platelets for infants, 4 units of random donor platelets for children, and 6 units of random donor platelets for adolescents, with the caveat that the calculated volume does not exceed 10 ml/kg.

If possible, procedures that may cause bleeding, such as intramuscular injections, and medications that alter platelet function, such as nonsteroidal antiinflammatory drugs, should be avoided.

Neutropenia

Neutropenia is defined as an absolute neutrophil count (ANC) less than 1,500/µL. Mild neutropenia is an ANC between 1,000/µL and 1,500µL, moderate neutropenia is an ANC between 500/µL and 1,000/µL, and severe neutropenia is an ANC less than 500/µL.

Treatments for neutropenia, such as filgrastim and granulocyte transfusions, often involve special considerations, and their use should generally be left to the discretion of the pediatric oncologist.

The evaluation and management of neutropenia in the context of fevers are discussed in the section entitled *Febrile Neutropenia* under "Emergencies During Treatment."

Hyperleukocytosis

Hyperleukocytosis is defined as a white blood cell (WBC) count more than 100,000/mm^3. It is present in 5-22% of children with acute leukemia at the time of diagnosis and is more common in those with the myeloid type. Hyperleukocytosis leads to the occlusion of critical blood vessels by abnormally large numbers of white blood cells. The brain, lungs, and kidneys are most frequently affected, but any organ can be involved. Because the main cause of early death for patients with hyperleukocytosis is intracranial hemorrhage, neurological manifestations, such as headache, visual changes, altered mental status, papilledema, and even stroke, deserve special attention.

The infusion of intravenous fluids is a rapid way to dilute the concentration of the white blood cells and decrease the viscosity of the blood. The composition of the fluids and rate of infusion should also be appropriate for tumor lysis syndrome, which is discussed in the section entitled *Tumor Lysis Syndrome* under "Emergencies At Diagnosis." Leukapheresis should be arranged and initiated as quickly as possible, especially if the WBC count is greater than 200,000/mm^3. Ultimately, intravenous fluids and leukapheresis are only temporizing measures, so emergency chemotherapy should be started as soon as possible. A child with acute leukemia may present with severe anemia along with hyperleukocytosis; a scenario more likely to be encountered in developing countries, where patients tend to present late. A blood transfusion is unsafe in such a situation, as it may worsen hyperviscosity. Leukapheresis may not be readily available universally. An exchange transfusion may be restored to in such emergent setting. Platelet transfusions are indicated for patients with a platelet count less than 20,000/µL because they can decrease the risk of an intracranial hemorrhage, but PRBC transfusions should be avoided because they may increase the viscosity of the blood.

Disseminated Intravascular Coagulation

Disseminated intravascular coagulation (DIC) is associated with many cancers, especially acute leukemia and particularly acute promyelocytic leukemia. Up to 13% of children with acute leukemia will have DIC at the time of diagnosis. If actue promyelocytic leukemia is suspected from peripheral smear findings, initiation of all-trans retinoic acid (ATRA) along with plasma and platelet support is imperative to arrest ongoing DIC.

The standard approach to the evaluation and management of DIC should be employed.

Metabolic Emergencies

Diabetes Insipidus

Craniopharyngioma, pineal tumors, germ cell tumors, and Langerhans cell histiocytosis can perturb the function of the hypothalamus and cause diabetes insipidus. Magnetic resonance imaging of the brain can confirm the presence of a tumor and define its extent.

The standard approach to the evaluation and management of diabetes insipidus should be employed.

Neurological Emergencies

Children with a new tumor of the central nervous system may present with one or more of the following complications: increased intracranial pressure, focal neurological deficits, and spinal cord compression. Magnetic resonance imaging of the brain and spine can confirm the presence of a tumor and define its extent.

Increased Intracranial Pressure

Headache, vomiting, and lethargy form the classical triad of signs and symptoms for increased intracranial pressure, but other manifestations in children include poor academic performance, developmental delay, personality changes, irritability, fatigue, and anorexia. The physical examination may reveal papilledema and oculomotor cranial nerve deficits.

The standard approach to the evaluation and management of increased intracranial pressure should be employed.

Focal Neurological Deficits

Cerebellar dysfunction, cranial nerve palsies, and a partial Horner's syndrome suggest an infratentorial tumor, which is more common in pediatric patients. Headache, seizures, and upper motor neuron abnormalities suggest a supratentorial tumor.

Spinal Cord Compression

Primary and metastatic tumors of the central nervous system, as well as neuroblastoma, lymphomas, and soft tissues sarcomas, can cause spinal cord compression.

Spinal cord compression often presents with back pain. The differential diagnosis of the child with back pain is extensive, but a malignancy must be considered when it is associated with a neurological deficit, such as weakness of the extremities or abnormalities of the reflexes. Magnetic resonance imaging of the spine should be obtained in a timely fashion in order to avoid the possibility of irreversible damage to the spinal cord. Dexamethasone at a dose of 1-2 mg/kg IV may be indicated even before the study is ordered, especially if the history or physical examination is suggestive. It is certainly recommended if the study is confirmatory.

Radiotherapy is generally the treatment of choice for rapid decompression of the spine. Chemotherapy is an option if the tumor is sensitive. Surgery is a consideration if the spine is unstable.

EMERGENCIES DURING TREATMENT

Gastrointestinal Emergencies

Mucositis

Mucositis is a common side effect of many chemotherapeutic agents and radiotherapy. The lesions usually involve the oropharynx, but may affect other parts of the gastrointestinal tract, such as the esophagus and rectum. They are typically ulcerative and almost always painful. They often cause significant discomfort with swallowing, which can lead to decreased oral intake and dehydration. They may also become infected with herpes simplex virus or *Candida*.

The treatment is supportive in nature. Topical or oral analgesia may be appropriate if the lesions are few in number and limited to the mouth, but systemic analgesia is usually required. Any dehydration should be corrected with intravenous fluids, and any infection should be treated with an appropriate antimicrobial drug.

Typhlitis

Typhlitis is a necrotizing inflammation of the cecum and colon that may represent a more severe and extensive form of mucositis. It usually presents with fever, abdominal pain and distention, and watery or bloody diarrhea. Factors that are associated with the development of typhlitis include intensive chemotherapy, neutropenia and thrombocytopenia, and recent antibiotic treatment. Organisms that have been isolated with typhlitis include *Pseudomonas*, *Escherichia coli*, *Staphylococcus aureus*, *Clostridium difficile*, *Cryptosporidium*, *Candida*, and *Aspergillus*.

Computed tomography of the abdomen will reveal bowel wall thickening, and may even demonstrate pneumatosis intestinalis or frank perforation. The treatment is supportive in nature and includes bowel rest, nasogastric suction, and broad-spectrum antibiotics that cover gram-negative bacteria, gram-positive bacteria, and *Clostridium difficile*. Surgery is reserved for perforation, hemorrhage, or failure to improve with medical management.

Genitourinary Emergencies

Hemorrhagic Cystitis

Hemorrhagic cystitis is a complication of chemotherapeutic agents like cyclophosphamide and ifosfamide. It is characterized by gross hematuria with or without clots, dysuria, urgency, and frequency. It usually manifests while the chemotherapeutic agent is being administered but occasionally presents several days after the infusions have been completed.

Radiological studies are not typically necessary, but ultrasonography will reveal an edematous and hemorrhagic bladder. An infusion of intravenous fluids should be started. If clots are present, then the placement of a Foley catheter for continuous irrigation of the bladder may be necessary. If the patient also has thrombocytopenia, then a platelet transfusion should be considered.

Hematological Emergencies

Children receiving chemotherapy or radiotherapy frequently develop anemia, thrombocytopenia, neutropenia, or some combination of these hematological complications.

The evaluation and management of anemia are discussed in the section *Anemia* under "Emergencies At Diagnosis."

The evaluation and management of thrombocytopenia are discussed in the section *Thrombocytopenia* under "Emergencies At Diagnosis."

The evaluation and management of neutropenia in the context of fevers are discussed in the section entitled *Febrile Neutropenia* under "Emergencies During Treatment."

Infectious Emergencies

Children receiving treatment for cancer are often profoundly immunosuppressed and particularly prone to serious and occasionally life-threatening infections. Many patients have an indwelling venous catheter for the purposes of access and treatment, and this device poses additional infectious risks for them.

Febrile Neutropenia

Febrile neutropenia is one of the most common reasons for a pediatric oncology patient to seek an evaluation at an emergency facility. A timely and careful assessment is critical because fever may be the first and only manifestation of a significant infection in a patient with neutropenia.

The risk of a serious bacterial or fungal infection is inversely proportional to the ANC, and it is greatest when the ANC is less than 500/µL.

For neutropenic patients, a fever is defined as an oral temperature greater than or equal to 38.4°C. An oral temperature greater than or equal to 38°C for more than 1 hour or 2 oral temperatures greater than or equal to 38°C within 12 hours are also considered significant. A rectal temperature is not necessary, and should be avoided because of the possibility of mucosal injury and bacterial translocation.

A detailed history and meticulous physical examination should be performed. Special attention should be paid to the skin, nail beds, sites of indwelling venous catheters, sites of recent procedures, sinuses, oropharynx, gingiva, lungs, abdomen, perineum, and rectum because the skin, mucosa, and lungs are the most frequent sites of infection.

A complete blood count, aerobic and anaerobic blood cultures from each lumen of all indwelling venous catheters, and a urine culture should be obtained for all patients with febrile neutropenia. Cultures of the sputum, stool, and spinal fluid should be ordered for patients with a specific indication based on the history and physical examination. A chest radiograph may be informative for patients with respiratory findings.

An infectious organism is identified in approximately 40% of patients with febrile neutropenia. In the remainder, clear evidence of a specific infection is never established. The most commonly isolated gram-positive organisms are coagulase-negative *Staphylococcus, Streptococcus viridans*, and *Staphylococcus aureus*, while *Escherichia coli, Klebsiella, Pseudomonas, Acinetobacter*, and *Enterobacter* account for the majority of the gram-negative organisms. *Candida* and *Aspergillus* are identified occasionally, but are more likely to be the culprit after a prolonged period of neutropenia or a prolonged course of antibiotics.

Empiric administration of broad-spectrum antibiotics within 2 hours of arrival is the foundation of the treatment of febrile neutropenia. The antibiotic combination should not only cover the aforementioned bacteria, but it should also be consistent with the local antibiotic resistance profiles. Some centers use a 3-drug regimen that consists of an aminoglycoside, antipseudomonal penicillin, and fourth-generation cephalosporin or carbapenem. Some institutions studies employ a 1-drug strategy that features a third-generation or fourth-generation cephalosporin or carbapenem. The antibiotics may be adjusted in the event that an infectious organism is identified.

Catheter Infection

A catheter infection must be considered when a child with cancer presents with fevers with or without neutropenia. Erythema, warmth, tenderness, and drainage may or may not be observed.

Blood cultures from each lumen of all indwelling venous catheters and a peripheral vein should be obtained. Gram-positive cocci are associated with infections of the exit site, but gram-negative bacilli are associated with infections of the catheter track. Exit site infections can usually be managed with care of the skin and appropriate antibiotics. Catheter track infections typically require removal of the catheter and appropriate antibiotics.

Perirectal Cellulitis

Perirectal cellulitis is a common complication for neutropenic cancer patients, particularly when their ANC is less than 100/µL. Mucositis due to chemotherapy or radiotherapy is a predisposing factor. Constipation due to vincristine can lead to anal fissures, which is another risk factor. Anorectal pain with defecation and brawny edema may be the only indications that a perirectal cellulitis is present. The causative organisms are usually members of the fecal flora, which includes a mixture of anaerobes, *Pseudomonas*, *Escherichia coli*, and *Staphylococcus*.

Sitz baths and appropriate antibiotics are usually sufficient, but an incision and drainage may be necessary if an abscess has formed.

Pneumonia

The usual organisms, as well as some opportunistic ones, can infect the lungs of an immunocompromised child and cause a pneumonia. Opportunistic pneumonias may involve *Mycobacterium tuberculosis*, *Nocardia*, and *Legionella*.

An evaluation should include a rapid assay for respiratory syncytial virus, rapid assay for influenza virus, nasopharyngeal aspirate culture for viruses, sputum culture, chest radiograph, and pulse oximetry. Computed tomography of the chest and bronchoalveolar lavage may be indicated if better delineation of a pulmonary abnormality is needed.

If the chest radiograph demonstrates focal pulmonary infiltrates, then an infection with a spectrum of the usual and opportunistic bacteria, viruses, and fungi must be considered. Bacterial organisms are more common with shorter periods of neutropenia, while viral and fungal organisms are more likely with longer periods of neutropenia. Treatment should include a combination of antimicrobial drugs that cover these pathogens.

If the chest radiograph reveals diffuse pulmonary infiltrates, then an infection with the opportunistic pathogen *Pneumocystis jirovecii* must also be entertained, even if the patient has been receiving appropriate prophylaxis. These patients often have fevers, a nonproductive cough, tachypnea, and hypoxemia. Treatment should include trimethoprim-sulfamethoxazole and a corticosteroid.

Viral Infection

Cancer patients and healthy children are vulnerable to the same viruses, but varicella-zoster virus (VZV) and herpes simplex virus (HSV) in immunocompromised hosts deserve special mention.

VZV infections are usually limited to the skin, but the virus can disseminate and cause serious complications, such as a pneumonitis or encephalitis. Patients who are exposed to

VZV should receive intravenous immune globulin at a dose of 500 mg/kg within 72 hours and complete a 7-day course of acyclovir. Depending on the ANC of the patient and severity of the infection, the acyclovir may be given orally or intravenously.

HSV infections typically involve the oropharynx or skin and generally respond to acyclovir. Depending on the ANC of the patient and severity of the infection, the acyclovir may be given orally or intravenously.

Metabolic Emergencies

Tumor Lysis Syndrome

Tumor lysis syndrome (TLS) is a metabolic derangement that is caused by the massive release of contents from numerous malignant cells that have died. It is more likely to occur with cancers that have a large cellular burden or high proliferative index, such as leukemias and lymphomas. Although TLS can be present before the start of treatment, it usually becomes evident 12-72 hours after the initiation of chemotherapy. The release of potassium and phosphorus into the circulation leads to hyperkalemia and hyperphosphatemia. The hyperphosphatemia, in turn, can cause a secondary hypocalcemia. The release of DNA and its metabolism into uric acid leads to hyperuricemia. The precipitation of the uric acid in the acidic environment of the kidneys can result in an obstructive uropathy and renal failure.

The cornerstone of the management of TLS is copious hydration with intravenous fluids consisting of dextrose, 0.225% saline, and sodium bicarbonate at a rate of 125-250 ml/m^2/hr. The goal is a urine output greater than 100 ml/m^2/hr, urine specific gravity less than 1.010, and urine pH between 7 and 7.5. The alkalization of the urine and its high flow through the kidneys is designed to minimize the precipitation of the uric acid. Allopurinol, which inhibits xanthine oxidase and blocks the formation of new uric acid, can be given at a dose of 100 mg/m^2 PO BID-TID. Rasburicase, which converts uric acid to allantoin and reduces the amount of existing uric acid, can be administered at a dose of 0.15 mg/kg IV qD. The allopurinol and rasburicase should be discontinued when the hyperuricemia is no longer a concern. Rasburicase is expensive and unlikely to be readily available in developing countries. Corner stone of management is maintaining hyper-hydration along with rapid diuresis. Attendant anemia should be managed with blood transfusion to check pulmonary oedema in face of hydration.

The standard approach to the evaluation and management of hyperkalemia, hyperphosphatemia, and hypocalcemia should be employed.

Syndrome of Inappropriate Antidiuretic Hormone Secretion

The syndrome of inappropriate antidiuretic hormone secretion (SIADH) can be a manifestation of a central nervous system tumor but is more commonly a complication of chemotherapeutic agents like vincristine, vinblastine, cyclophosphamide, ifosfamide, cisplatin, and melphalan.

The standard approach to the evaluation and management of SIADH should be employed.

Neurological Emergencies

Altered Mental Status and Encephalopathy

Altered mental status and encephalopathy are complications of chemotherapeutic agents like corticosteroids, cytarabine, methotrexate, ifosfamide, and cisplatin. They may also be manifestations of an infection or hemorrhage due to treatment toxicities or signs of a recurrent tumor due to treatment failure.

The standard approach to the evaluation and management of altered mental status and encephalopathy should be employed.

Cerebrovascular Accident

A cerebrovascular accident is a complication of chemotherapeutic agents like L-asparaginase and intrathecal chemotherapy with cranial radiotherapy. It may also be due to thrombosis, hemorrhage, hyperleukocytosis, or recurrent tumor.

The standard approach to the evaluation and management of a cerebrovascular accident should be employed.

FURTHER READING

1. Adler AL, Casper C, Boeckh M, et al. An out-break of varicella with likely breakthrough disease in a population of pediatric cancer patients. *Infect Control Hosp Epidemiol*. 2008; 29:866-870.
2. Albano EA, Pizzo PA. Infectious complications in childhood acute leukemias. *Pediatr Clin North Am*. 1988;35:873-901.
3. Allegretta GJ, Weisman SJ, Altman AJ. Oncologic emergencies I: metabolic and space-occupying consequences of cancer and cancer treatment. *Pediatr Clin North Am*. 1985;32:601-611.
4. Allegretta GJ, Weisman SJ, Altman AJ. Oncologic emergencies II: hematologic and infectious complications of cancer and cancer treatment. *Pediatr Clin North Am*. 1985;32:613-624.
5. Auletta, JJ, O'Riordan MA, Nieder ML. Infections in children with cancer: a continued need for the comprehensive physical examination. *J Pediatr Hematol Oncol*. 1999;21:501-508.
6. Basu SK, Fernandez ID, Fisher SG, et al. Length of stay and mortality associated with febrile neutropenia among children with cancer. *J Clin Oncol*. 2005;23:7958-7966.
7. Ben Abraham R, Toren A, Ono N, et al. Predictors of outcome in the pediatric intensive care units of children with malignancies. *J Pediatr Hematol Oncol*. 2002;24:23-26.
8. Haut C. Oncological emergencies in the pediatric intensive care unit. *AACN Clin Issues*. 2005;16:232-245.
9. Hobson MJ, Carney DE, Molik KA, et al. Appendicitis in childhood hematologic malignancies: analysis and comparison with typhlitis. *J Pediatr Surg*. 2005;40:214-219; discussion 219-220.
10. Hughes WT, Armstrong D, Bodey GP, et al. 2002 guidelines for the use of antimicrobial agents in neutropenic patients with cancer. *Clin Infect Dis*. 2002;34:730-751.
11. Jaffe D, Fleisher G, Grosflam J. Detection of cancer in the pediatric emergency department. *Pediatr Emerg Care*. 1985;1:11-15.
12. Kuga T, Inoue T, Taniguchi S, et al. Management of respiratory distress in children and adolescents with cancer. *Med Pediatr Oncol*. 1999;33:577-579.
13. Loblaw DA, Laperriere, NJ. Emergency treatment of malignant extradural spinal cord compression: an evidence-based guideline. *J Clin Oncol*. 1998;16:1613-1624.
14. McCarville MB, Adelman CS, Li C, et al. Typhlitis in childhood cancer. *Cancer*. 2005;104:380-387.
15. Pizzo PA; Management of fever in patients with cancer and treatment-induced neutropenia. *N Engl J Med*. 1993;328:1323-1332.
16. Porcu P, Cripe LD, Ng E, et al. Hyperleukocytic leukemias and leukostasis: a review of pathophysiology, clinical presentation and management. *Leuk Lymphoma*. 2000;39:1-18.
17. Rheingold SR, Lange BJ. Oncologic emergencies. In: Pizzo PA, Poplack DG, eds. *Principles and Practice of Pediatric Oncology*. 5th ed. Philadelphia, PA: Lippincott Williams & Wilkins;2005:1202-1230.
18. Sloas MM, Flynn PM, Kaste SC, et al. Typhlitis in children with cancer: a 30-year experience. *Clin Infect Dis*. 1993;17:484-490.
19. Stokes DN. The tumour lysis syndrome: intensive care aspects of paediatric oncology. *Anaesthesia*. 1989;44:133-136.
20. Wiegering VA, Kellenberger CJ, Bodmer N, et al. Conservative management of acute appendicitis in children with hematologic malignancies during chemotherapy-induced neutropenia. *J Pediatr Hematol Oncol*. 2008;30:464-467.

In the previous edition this chapter was written byNirmal Bhaya, MD Assistant Professor of Pediatrics Wayne State University School of Medicine Director: Pediatric Emergency Medicine Fellowshir Children's Hospital of Michigan Detroit, Michigan

Roger Barkin

51 The Febrile Child Under Two Years of Age

Infectious diseases represent a large percentage of encounters in the emergency department. Although many of these are self-limited and require support and recognition to institute appropriate therapy on an ambulatory basis, several of them do require immediate intervention to minimize morbidity and mortality. Children present unique challenges in that their clinical presentation varies by age as do the disease processes and the etiologic agents.

The febrile child, particularly the child under two years of age, presents unique challenges to the clinician. Over 10 percent of visits in this age group are for acute fevers. It is difficult to determine the etiology in the young child because of problems of obtaining a specific history and defining physical findings.

Children are generally considered febrile when their rectal temperatures are 38.0°C (100.4°F) or higher. Oral temperatures greater than 37.6°C (99.7°F) are considered to be elevated. Although this figure is controversial, 37.3°C is defined as a febrile axillary value.

The *site* for temperature measurement must reflect proximity to major arteries, absence of inflammation, degree of precision required, safety, and insulation from external factors (drinking, and so forth). *Rectal* temperatures provide much more precision but obviously run the risk of rectal perforation and emotional trauma. Axillary temperatures are not practical in children under four years of age but are appropriate in thermostable environments or when absolute precision is not mandatory. Temperatures are not totally reliable in mildly febrile children (38-38.5 °C). The oral or sublingual site is useful in cooperative older children who do not have rapid respiratory rates. The tympanic membrane has been used with great accuracy and reproducibility, using new technology that is increasingly available, particularly in children over 6 months of age.

As temperatures rise above 40°C, the risk of meningitis increases. However, fevers higher than 42°C (107.6°F) usually are not infectious in origin (for example, central nervous system [CNS] involvement or heat stroke).

CLINICAL PRESENTATION

Historically parents usually report nonspecific observations related to behavior and associated signs and symptoms rather than those that permit an early focus on the involved system. It is particularly important, however, to define these alterations in behavior, activity, and eating habits and to determine if respiratory, gastrointestinal (GI), musculoskeletal, and dermatologic findings have developed. Urinary tract and CNS symptoms are reflected in changes in behavior, such as irritability and lethargy. Exposures to children with similar complaints are important to note as are recent events such as diphtheria and tetanus toxoids and pertussis vaccine (DTP) immunizations.

Early antipyretic therapy is imperative in facilitating observation. Many children who initially are irritable and disinterested in their environment will improve markedly with aggressive antipyretic management. Acetaminophen (15 mglkgldose *per os* [PO] or per rectum [PR]) should be considered to all children with temperatures higher than 38.5°C (101.3°F) on arrival in the clinic or emergency department to ensure optimal observation by reducing temperature and permitting a more accurate assessment of the child. Children with temperatures higher than *39,SO* C (103°F) should also be sponged with tepid water. The response to antipyretics does not predict the prevalence of bacteremia.

The physical examination to assess responsiveness must be done systematically, focusing on careful observation of the child at play and encouraging the youngster to follow lights, bright objects, or a parent. Components of this overall assessment that are useful and reassuring include that the child

Looks and focuses on the clinician and spontaneously explores the room
Spontaneously makes sounds or talks in a playful manner.
Plays and reaches for objects.
Smiles and interacts with the parent or the practitioner.
Quiets easily when helped by parents.

While the child is distracted with play objects, obvious physical abnormalities such as limitation of limb movement, rashes, and points of tenderness or pain should be defined. The chest, heart, and abdomen require a gentle hand and patience. Tachypnea disproportionate to fever must be carefully evaluated, usually by means of a chest X-ray. Once these areas have been assessed, a full examination of the ears, throat, neck, and so forth is required.

In most children, the initial evaluation will define the cause of fever, and appropriate therapy can be initiated at the time of assessment. Historically, in patients under 24 months of age who have an acute onset of temperatures of 40°C (104°F) or over, the common causes identifiable are otitis media, pneumonia, recognizable viral syndromes (exanthem/enanthem, meningitis/encephalitis, gastroenteritis, croup), and recognizable bacterial diseases (bacteremia, cellulitis, meningitis, urinary tract infection).

Routine laboratory considerations must be individualized to reflect the findings of the physical examination and history. This may include a complete blood count (CBC), urinanalysis and urine culture, blood culture, lumber puncture and radiologic studies. A C-reative protein measurement is increasingly used. Procalcitonin lavel may prove useful and are being studied.

SPECIFIC CLINICAL CIRCUMSTANCES

Infants under 12 Months of Age

Infants usually require a more extensive evaluation because the history is rarely more specific than the triad of fever, irritability and poor feeding. The physical examination may fail to reveal specific focal findings despite the presence of systemic infection.

Infants **under 4 weeks of age with fever** are often difficult to evaluate clinically and generally require admission for parenteral antibiotics and monitoring until cultures prove negative. Prospective studies have demonstrated that clinical judgment alone is not useful in these young infants. There are no clear factors that are sensitive or specific to be relied upon in decision making. *No single laboratory or historical factor should be used to exclude underlying bacterial infection.*

Ill appearing febrile infants between 4 and 12 weeks of age require hospitalization for parenteral antibiotics and monitoring after a full sepsis workup.

Well appearing infants in this age group may be followed closely as outpatients if they have normal evaluations including a negative past history, nontoxic appearance, no focal infections, good follow-up and compliance, along with a normal CBC, urinalysis and no WBC's in the stool if diarrhea is present. This group is often treated with a single injection of ceftriaxone after a sepsis evaluation and rechecked within 24 hours, if not earlier.

Immunocompromised Children

Children with a history of recurrent serious bacterial infections should be evaluated for immunodeficiency. Children undergoing cancer chemotherapy or with a history of asplenia (congenital, traumatic, and so forth) are obviously at risk. Those with sickle cell disease have a 400-fold increased risk of pneumococcal septicemia if they are under five years of age and a 4-fold risk of H. *influenzae* septicemia if they are under nine years of age.

Such children require an aggressive and anticipatory approach to potential infections. A blood culture, ancillary tests, and early initiation of antibiotics is warranted.

Occult Bacteremia

Bacteremia occurs in association with a host of clinical entities including meningitis, arthritis, epiglottitis, cellulitis, pneumonia, and kidney infections. Additionally children may have bacteremia in the absence of an obvious source for fever. The most common pathogen in this later group is *Streptococcus pneumoniae.* Less common organisms are *H. influenzea* type B, *Neisseria meningitides,* and Salmonella. The incidence of *S pneumoniae* has markedly decreased with the widespread use of vaccines as it has with *H. Influenzae* earlier. In fact, the entire incidence of occult bacteremia has been reduced with active immunizations in recent years.

Historically, the high risk group has been defined as children 24 months and younger, those with a fever of 39.4 C (102.9F) or higher, a white count over 15,000 mm^3 and a sedimentation rate of 30 mm/hr or greater. This group of children without a specific focus are often started on amoxicillin or ceftriaxone.

MANAGEMENT

The management of the febrile child must reflect specific conditions that are diagnosed and those that must be considered in the differential diagnosis. Often the history and the physical examination may be useful. Laboratory studies may be confirmatory but often must await final culture results. In those patients in whom signs and symptoms are nonspecific, laboratory data is incomplete, and toxicity is present, anticipatory management is often warranted.

1. Early antipyretic therapy will facilitate assessment. Previous antipyretic therapy requires a lower temperature threshold for initating laboratory evaluation.
2. Underlying cardiac, pulmonary, neurologic, and immunodeficient (sickle cell, neoplasm, steroids, and so on) diseases require early evaluation and treatment, regardless of age and the height of fever.
3. Meningitis must be considered in any febrile child who has a seizure. Children 12 months of age and younger should generally have a spinal tap. A temperature of 41.1 °C or higher is associated with a

higher incidence of meningitis in children under 2 years of age, although this risk has decreased with immunization.

4. Children with fever and petechiae may have a viral illness, Rocky Mountain spotted fever, or invasive bacterial disease. Rapid intervention is required. Children with fever and petechiae who have a normal lumbar puncture, WBC that is neither elevated nor decreased, normal absolute PMN and band count, and a temperature of less than 40 °C have a reduced risk of bacterial infection than those with all or some of these findings presents.
5. If the temperature has been present for less than 24 hours, if the child looks well on the basis of overall assessment and is over six months old, and if no helpful history is detected, close follow-up for 6 to 12 hours may substitute for laboratory evaluation at the time of the first encounter. If the temperature remains elevated above 39.4° C at the follow-up appointment, evaluation should generally proceed.
6. Children with a WBC greater than 15,000 mm^3, from whom blood cultures have been obtained, may be treated with antibiotics with the potential of reducing complications. Alternative regimens include amoxicillin 50 to 100 mg/kg/24 hrs, ampicillin 50 mg/kg/dose **IM** or **IV**, or ceftriaxone 150 mg/kg/24 hrs IM or IV.
7. Follow-up is essential, usually in 6 to 12 hours, depending on clinical and logistic constraints if the child is discharged.
   a. If the cultures remain negative, antibiotics may be stopped after 48 hours unless there was a specific focus initially or unless one develops. Follow-up until resolution of the illness is necessary.
   b. If the culture is positive, thereby documenting bacteremia, reexamination of the patient should determine treatment.
      (1) A patient who has a totally normal examination should continue taking high-dose antibiotics as an outpatient if daily contact can be maintained or as an inpatient if compliance is questionable. A total 10-day course is necessary. Most patients who have been treated initially will be improved on follow-up, but this does not preclude the importance of continuing antibiotics.
      (2) Febrile or toxic patients or those who develop a focus should be admitted for **IV** antibiotics and further evaluation. A total course of 10 days is necessary, part of which may be done as an out patient depending on the patients response.

The febrile child under two years of age presents a unique challenge to the physician. The signs and symptoms are often nonspecific and the ancillary data is supportive of initial clinical impressions. Aggressive and anticipatory management is essential.

PARENTAL EDUCATION

Parental education is important in the management of the febrile infant. Obviously instructions are indicated in the management of the specific diagnosis entity, but additional information about fever control must be provided. This is of utmost importance in the initial assessment of the child and in addition may make the child more comfortable throughout the duration of the illness. Fever is a means of fighting infection, and the degree of fever does not always reflect the severity of illness.

1. Fever is a temperature over 100° F (37.8° C) orally or 100.4° F (38.0° C) rectally (Figure 1). If the fever is between 100° F and 101°F orally or rectally, the temperature should be taken again in one

hour. Temperatures may be temporarily elevated from excess clothing or too much exercise. Oral temperatures can be raised by recently eaten warm food. Teething does not cause marked elevations of temperature.

2. Take the rectal temperature.
   a. Shake the thermometer down to below 97°F (36 °C).
   b. Lubricate with Vaseline®, cold cream, or cold water.
   c. Gently insert the thermometer one-half inch into rectum. Often holding the child's stomach down on parent's lap is helpful.
   d. Leave in three minutes or until the silver line stops rising.
   e. Do not leave the child unattended. Hold the child still.
   f. Read by turning the sharp edge of the triangle toward you. Turn it slightly in each direction until you can see the end of the silver column.
   g. On the centigrade (Celsius) thermometer, each line is 0.1 °C; on the Fahrenheit thermometer, each line 0.2°F. In unusual circumstances, axiliary temperatures may be taken as a screen, holding the tip of thermometer under the dry armpit for four minutes. The elbow should be held against the chest. If the temperature is more than 99°F (37. 2°C), recheck it by taking a rectal temperature.
3. Fever medication should be used if the temperature is above 101.5° F (38.6°C), if the child is very uncomfortable, or if any fever is present at bedtime. If the child is acting normally, fever medicines may be delayed until the temperature is 102.2° F (39.0 °C).
   a. If the child is over three months of age, fever medicine should be given if the temperature is over 101.5° F (38.6° C). Acetaminophen (Tylenol or an equivalent) should be recommended every four to six hours.
   b. Do not recommend aspirin if the child has chickenpox or an influenza-like illness because of association between Reye's syndrome and aspirin.
4. The child should be dressed lightly, and fluids should be pushed.
5. The physician should be called if:
   a. The fever goes above 105°F (40.5 °C).
   b. The fever lasts beyond 48 to 72 hours.
   c. The child is under three months and has a rectal fever of over 38°C (100.4°F) or above.
   d. The child has a seizure (convulsion), abnormal movements of the face, arms, or legs; a stiff neck; purple spots; a fullness of the soft spot; looks sicker than expected; or develops difficulty brea-thing, burning on urination, decreased urination, abdominal pain; or marked change in behavior, consciousness, or activity.

FURTHER READING

1. Pusic MV . Clinical management of fever in children younger than three years of age. Pediatr Child Health 2007; 12(6): 469-72.
2. Sur DK, Bukont EL. Evaluating fever of unidentifiable source in young children. Am Fam Physician 2007; 75(12): 1805-11.
3. Antonyrajah B, Mukundan D. Fever without apparent source on clinical examination. Curr Opin Pediatr. 2008;20:96–102.
4. Ishimine P. Fever without source in children 0 to 36 months of age. Pediatr Clin North Am 2006;53:167–94.

Sunit Singhi

52 The Febrile Child Without Focus: Indian Perspective

The febrile child, particularly the child under two years of age, presents unique challenges to the clinician. Over 10 percent of visits in this age group are for acute fevers. It is difficult to determine the etiology in the young child because of problems of obtaining a specific history and of defining physical findings.

WHAT IS FEVER?

Fever is defined as a core (rectal) temperature of 38°C (100.4°F). Oral temperature of 37.6°C (99.7°F) and axillary temperature of 37.3°C (99°F) are equivalent. However, axillary temperatures are less accurate and should not be used as far as possible.

Hyperpyrexia is defined as a core temperature of 41°C or more. Fever is one of the commonest symptom in a sick child. It accounts for more than 50% of visits to our Pediatric emergency service.

Temperature Determination

The glass-mercury thermometer remains the gold standard for accuracy. Dis-advantages - relatively long dwell time (2 to 3 minutes), risk of cross-contamination and potential breakage. Electronic thermometers are as accurate as glass-mercury. They have the advantages of a shorter dwell time and disposable sheaths. The *site* for temperature measurement must reflect proximity to major arteries, absence of inflammation, degree of precision required, safety, and insulation from external factors (drinking, and so forth). *Rectal* temperatures provide much more precision but obviously run the risk of rectal perforation and emotional trauma. Axillary temperatures are not practical in children under four years of age but are appropriate in thermostable environments or when absolute precision is not mandatory. Temperatures are not totally reliable in mildly febrile children (38-38.5° C). The oral, or sublingual, site is useful in cooperative older children who do not have rapid respiratory rates. The tympanic membrane has been used with great accuracy and reproducibility, using new technology that is increasingly available.

FEVER IN NEONATE AND INFANTS < 3 MONTHS

In apparently healthy looking infants transient spikes in first week are not uncommon.

These are benign in nature and are often due to high environmental temperature.

- Pyrexial reaction to an infection is often absent in premature very low birth weight neonates.
- Temperature above 38.3°C is uncommon in first month. When present it indicates significantly higher risk of sepsis and serious bacterial infection such as meningitis, lower respiratory infections and otitis media and malaria.
- Fever is a frequent symptom of neonatal septicemia (in upto 1/3 patients). Other more suggestive physical signs are often present in such patients. Specificity of fever as evidence of infection is 50-90%.
- Febrile infants < 3 months have 21.5 times more risk of serious underlying bacterial infections.

FEVER IN CHILDREN 3 MONTHS TO 3 YEARS

- Most cases are due to benign viral upper respiratory infections, exanthematous illnesses, or viral fever.
- Bacterial infections with focus such as gastroenteritis and pneumonia, urinary tract infection account for about 25 % of all febrile illnesses.
- Malaria in endemic area is a common cause
- Bacterial infections and bacteremia without apparent focus on clinical examination occurs in a small number of patients.
- Teething is not a cause of fever at any age

Careful observation, history, physical examination and judicious use of screening laboratory tests are required to identify underlying serious illness (Table 1). Most of the febrile children have a variety of characteristic signs and symptoms indicative of a specific infectious or noninfectious disease. A specific diagnosis can therefore, be made in these children.

Table 1: Historical and physical examination helpful in assessment of acutely febrile child

History:

- Age: Infants < 3 months are more susceptible to severe infection and infections by unusual organizer because of immunologic immaturity.
- Fever: onset, degree, site of recording, duration
- Associated symptoms – localising, activity and responsiveness, abnormal cry and appetite, paradoxic irritability, playfulness, sleep.
- Concurrent febrile illness among family members, day care centre: suggests viral illness
- Local epidemiology and climate: useful in epidemic or endemic illness

Physical Examination: look for a focus

- Meningeal signs (tense fontanelle)
- Inspection of ear drum
- Eye signs
- Mouth, pharynx
- Lymph nodes
- All joints and limb movements
- Auscultation of lungs, heart
- Palpation of abdomen, examination of genitalia
- Observation of the interaction of the child with parents, facial expression, alertness, activity, breathing, cry, abnormal posture/position. Presence of these signs may help in deciding if the infant is toxic or sick
- If no signs re-examine after 24-48 hours.

WHAT IS FEVER WITHOUT FOCUS?

Many febrile children especially those under 36 months of age may have subtle and nonspecific signs of disease. The etiology of fever is not apparent in these children after a careful history and physical examination. Such patient's account of 4-5 % of total visits to our emergency. Both minor and life threatening infections are common in these patients. Infants with meningitis may present just with fever and irritability but no meningeal signs, Or an infant with urinary tract infection who is too young to complain of dysuria, may present with unexplained fever.

Life-threatening non-infectious illnesses especially heat- stroke and certain poisonings also present predominantly as fever and non-specific signs and symptoms. These account for a very small number of febrile illnesses. Common causes of fever without focus are shown in table-2.

Table 2: Common causes of fever without focus

A. Infectious causes
1. Viral fever and prodrome of viral exanthem
2. Malaria
3. Bacteremia / Septicemia
4. Urinary tract infection
5. Meningitis
6. Otitis media

B. Noninfectious causes
1. Heat stroke/ high environmental temperature
2. Malignancies - leukemia, lymphoma
3. Collagen vascular disease
4. Drug fever
5. Poisonings - Dhatura, atropine, phenothiazine
6. Miscellaneous - after immunisation, after seizure, internal bleeding.

In our Pediatric Emergency final diagnosis of 100 Febrile children who did not have an apparent focus on first clinical examination, after excluding malaria was nonbacterial illnesses - 62%, bacteremia - 19% urinary tract infections- 6%, meningitis - 8% and otitis media 5 %. Staph aureus was the commonest cause of bacteremia, accounting for two-third (13 out of 19 cases).

MANAGEMENT DECISIONS

In a febrile child with nonspecific symptoms and no evident focus thus, the major concern is rapid and early detection and treatment of serious bacterial infections.

Attention needs to be focused on the findings, which may help in deciding as to whether

(i) The fever is because of a viral or bacterial infection.

(ii) The child is seriously ill requiring hospitalization or has a self-limiting or mild illness, which can be treated on ambulatory basis.

Repeated clinical examination may help and disclose a localised bacterial infection after 12-48 hours, and a blood culture can give definitive answer in 48-72 hours in many. Nonetheless, highly febrile patients who do not show a positive blood culture may also develop subsequent bacterial infection or serious complications of viral disease requiring antibiotic therapy. In one study of 552 febrile children (temperature> 39°C, aged 3-36 months with a negative blood cultures) 11 % had bacterial infection on follow-up.

Children with a history of recurrent serious bacterial infections should be evaluated for immunodeficiency. Children undergoing cancer chemotherapy or with a history of asplenia (congenital, traumatic, and so forth) are obviously at risk. Those with sickle cell disease have a 400-fold increased risk of pneumococcal septicemia if they are under five years of age and a 4-fold risk of H. *influenzae* septicemia if they are under nine years of age.

Such children require an aggressive and anticipatory approach to potential infections. A blood culture, ancillary tests, and early initiation of antibiotics is warranted.

Occult Bacteremia

Although bacteremia occurs in association with a host of clinical entities, including meningitis, arthritis, epiglottitis, cellulitis, pneumonia, and kidney infections, about six percent of febrile patients without a defined focus have positive blood cultures. Occult bacteremia is a significant problem in children, the high risk group being defined as:

Age	:	5 24 months
Fever	:	39.4° C (102.9° F)
White blood cell count (WBC)	:	15,000 mm3 (differential does not increase prognostic value)

Erythrocyte sedimentation (ESR)	:	30 mm/hr (difficult to use because of the dissociation of time required to obtain a result)

It is essential to evaluate such children carefully to be certain that there is no underlying disease such a pneumonia or meningitis. There is no conclusive evidence that performing a lumbar puncture on a bacteremic child significantly increases the risk of subsequently developing meningitis.

Organisms that are frequently cultured include Streptococcus pneumonia and Haemophilus influenza. Staphylococcus aureus and Neisseria meningitides are less common pathogens. Children under two to three months of age may also have Escherichia coli and Listeria monocytogenes.

Children with occult bacteremia in whom a specific focus has been excluded are often started on antibiotics to produce an earlier clinical response and reduce potential complications.

What are the variables that may help in selecting those febrile children below 3 years of age who are 'at high risk' or 'low risk' of serious bacterial infection?

Is the Temperature Grade Helpful?

Mild elevation of temperature (37.8 - 38.3°C) are common, even in first few months and accounted for about 20% of infants visits in one study. Temperatures > 38.3°C are uncommon in first months but become frequent with each succeeding month. In infants < 3 months of age fever> 38.3°C was associated with a 21.5 times higher risk of serious underlying infection than infants> 3 months with a similar temperature.

Temperature 39°C and above have been linked with a higher risk of bacteremia and bacterial infections. Based on the published data of other authors, McLellan calculated the probability of a temperature > 39°C in children with proved bacteremia as > 90% and rated low grade fever as an excellent discriminator of absence of bacteremia.

The evidence that hyperpyrexia (temperature> 41°C) is associated with a higher risk of serious bacterial infection (SBI) is somewhat conflicting.

From the available data it may be said that in previously healthy children higher the fever greater the risk of serious illness at any age. The risk of bacteremia increases as the degree of fever increases. The limit of physiological temperature regulation is 41.1°C. Fever in this range or higher indicate not only bacteremia but also a possible presence of CNS infection or pneumonia. In children 2-36 months of age, a temperature between 39°C-41°C is associated with as much risk of SBI as any hyperpyrexia and should receive as much attention. Temperature < 39°C of short duration is more likely to be due to non-serious infections.

Clinical Assessment of 'Toxicity' or 'Sickness'

Experienced physicians often find an overall 'subjective' assessment of the severity of underlying illness useful in final decision-making. Most of this assessment is based on evaluation of behavioural and functional response of the child to the illness. In the last decade several studies have aimed at enlisting these signs for an objective assessment of febrile as well as afebrile sick children. The items identified as useful in the overall assessment of febrile children are listed in Table 3.

It may be said that mildly ill children have temperature less than 39°C and appear alert, playful and active. Children with temperature > 39°C and with abnormal functional and behavioural symptoms such as irritability, abnormal cry, poor feeding, lethargy,

Table 3: Six observation items and their Scales

Observation item	*1 Normal*	*3 Moderate Impairment*	*5 Severe Impairment*
Quality of cry	Strong with normal tone OR content and not crying	Whimpering OR sobbing	Weak OR Moaning OR High pitched
Reaction to parent stimulation	Cries briefly then stop OR content not crying	Cries off & on	Continual cry OR Hardly responds
State Variation	If awake-stays awake OR if asleep and stimulated-wakes up quickly	Eyes close briefly awake OR Awakes with prolonged stimulation	Falls to sleep OR will not rouse
Color	Pink	Pale extremities OR Acrocyanosis	Pale OR Cyanotic OR Mottled OR Ashen
Hydration	Skin normal, eyes normal and mucous membranes moist	Skin, eyes normal and mouth slightly dry	Skin doughy OR tented and dry mucous membranes and/or sunken eyes
Response (talk, Smile) to social overtures	Smile OR Alerts (< 2 mo)	Brief smile OR Alerts briefly (< 2 mo)	No anxious, dull expression less OR No alerting (<2 mo)

drowsiness, refusal to play, signs of poor peripheral perfusion (pallor, poor capillary refill) and rapid or irregular breathing are more likely to have severe illness. Lethargy may be inferred if the infants has poor or absent eye contact or fails to recognize parents or interact with the persons or object around. Scales formally quantifying this assessment are valuable but may not be completely predictive of severe illness. Studies in our own setting have found these signs useful and valid in very young febrile infants less than 2 months.

Response to Antipyretic and Severity of Infection

There is a common myth that if a child's fever does not come down in response to antipyretic therapy the child is more likely to have a serious infection. On the present evidence several studies clearly prove that temperature response to paracetamol is a poor discriminator between bacterial and viral infections, bacteremic and nonbacteremic illness and within different diagnostic categories.

LABORATORY TESTS AND 'SEPSIS SCREEN'

A vast array of laboratory and radiological tests may be helpful and requisitioned in a febrile child (Table 4). Some of these such as examination of blood film for malaria parasite, x-ray chest, bacterioscopy of freshly passed urine may give definite answer to the diagnosis and guide the therapeutic decision. Other tests such as blood counts, ESR, qualitative C-reactive protein (CRP) have been found helpful in identification of patients who have bacterial infections and bacteremia.

Table 4: Investigations useful in rapid identification of febrile child at increased risk of common serious illnesses

1. **Blood counts**
   i) Malaria parasite on smear exam
   ii) TLC > 15,000/mm^3, < 5000/mm^3
   iii) Absolute Neutrophil count > 10,000/mm^3
   iv) Unsegmented polymorphs > 500/mm^3 Unsegmented: Segmented Ratio 0.15 - 0.3
   v) Platelet Count – 100,000/mm3 ESR > 30 m/hr in children
2. **CRP Qualitative:** +ve, suggestive
3. **Urine Bacterioscopy:** > 2 bacteria / 16 small squares of Neubaur's chamber. 90% chance of UTI
4. **X-ray** chest not very useful in early stage of an acute fever of unknown origin. If pneumonia is suspected strongly – it is very likely to be present; often x-ray would not help more.

As shown in Table-4 WBC counts, absolute neutrophil counts and band cell counts in the specified ranges have been suggested as useful in screening for presence of sepsis. We found that WBC > 15,000 had a sensitivity of 25% and specificity of 100%. However, none of these tests individually or in different combination has been found to be sensitive enough. Moreover children with proven viremia may also have counts > 15000/ mm^3. It appears that absence of leukocytosis is an excellent discriminator of the absence of bacteremia in the febrile child but its presence is a poor indicator of bacteremia. Leukopenia (total WBC < 5000/mm^3) strongly suggests bacteremia. ESR > 30 mm in 1st hour, has been considered as the single best indicator of bactermia. At our centre we found mESR > 25 mm at 1st hour, had a specificity of 97% and a sensitivity of 63% to predict bacteremia in febrile children 3 months to 3 years.

Qualitative and quantitative C-reactive Protein (CRP) concentration also has been recommended as specific indicator of presence of bacteremia and bacterial infection.

Should blood cultures be obtained routinely in evaluation of febrile children, 3-24 months, temperature > 39°C, duration < 4 days, without evident focus? Not unnecessary! Hospitalisation and intravenous antibiotic treatment of relatively large number of children whose bacteremia would spontaneously resolve appears to out weight the benefit of preventing serious infectious sequelae in few children.

At present, identification of high risk group by means of blood, counts, and blood culture and expectant antibiotic treatment at first visit appears to be the most cost-effective and procedure effective method of clinical evaluation of febrile children at risk of bacteremia.

Combination of Clinical Observation and 'Sepsis-screen'

Noting the limited usefulness of clinical observation and sepsis screen individually in predicting serious bacterial infections (SBI) efforts have been made toward evolving a combination of clinical and lab criteria which may discriminate children at 'high risk' or 'low risk' of SBI. We define 'low risk group' as those having temperature < 39°C, non-toxic look, normal sepsis screen (WBC counts 5000-15000) and E5R < 10 mm.

TREATMENT DECISIONS

In every child with fever without focus one needs to decide the following:

1. Does child needs hospitalisation or can be treated at home?
2. Does the child require antibiotics?
3. Is there a need for antipyretic therapy?
4. What supportive therapy is needed

Does Child Need Hospitalisation?

Every child with undiagnosed fever does not require hospitalization and many can be managed at home. Only the following groups need hospitalization.

1. All toxic-sick children, irrespective of age
2. All these patients should receive full sepsis work-up (culture of blood, urine and CSF).
3. All newborn (< 28 days)
4. Infants: age 28-90-days if sepsis screen is +ve
5. Children: age 3 months to 3 years if fever> 39°C and sepsis screen +ve

Approach to a previously healthy child with fever without focus and who is not toxic looking should be as follows:

Antibiotics in Undiagnosed Fever

Do not give antibiotics for an undiagnosed fever' - Doctors have great difficulty in following this rule.

Use antibiotics in patients who need hospitalisation and are at high risk of bacterial infection after taking appropriate specimen for bacteriological studies. Discontinue if the results of sepsis -workup are negative.

Choice of Antibiotics: Inj. Ceftrixone/ Cefotaxime 50mg/kg in infants < 3 months. Oral amoxicillin/Augmentin (40-50 mg/kg) or cloxacillin (100 mg/kg) with amoxicillin should be used in older children.

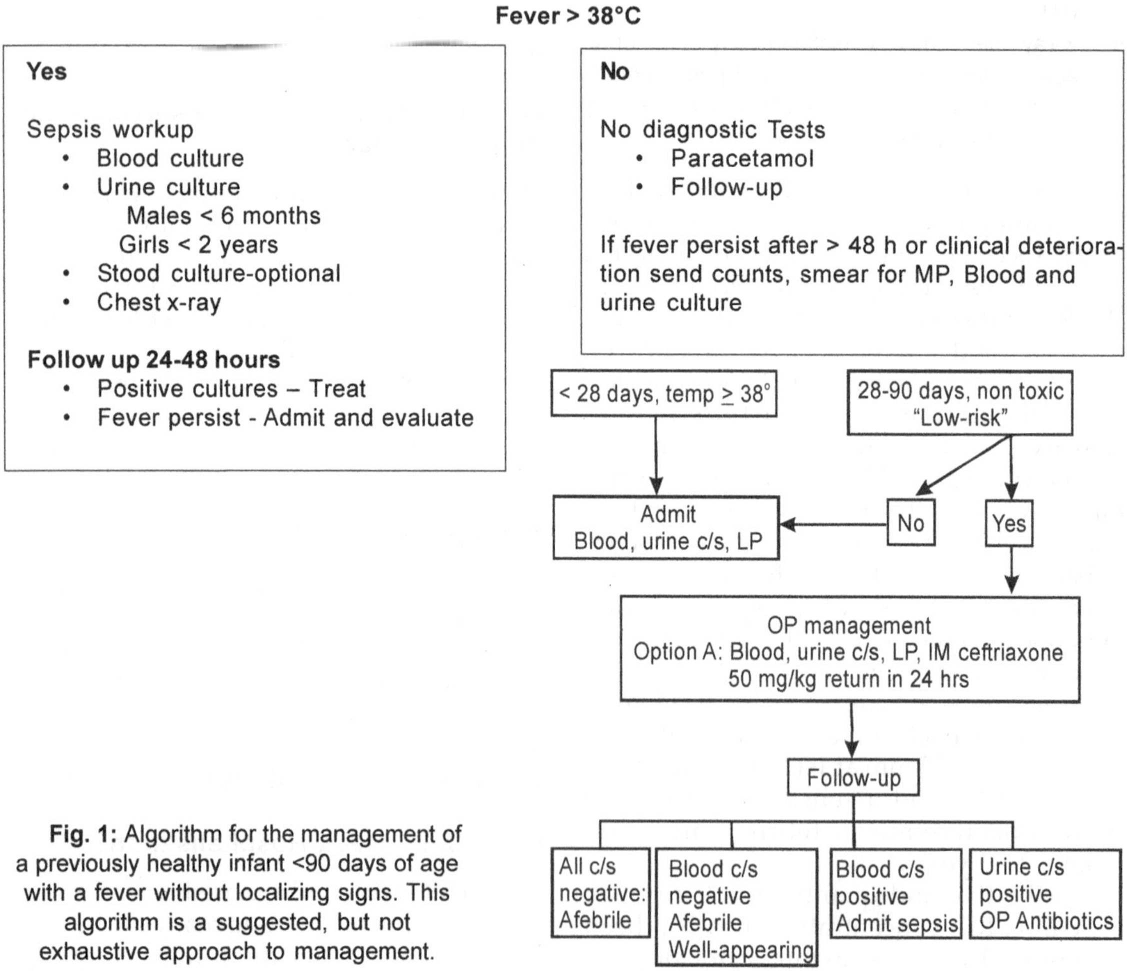

Fig. 1: Algorithm for the management of a previously healthy infant <90 days of age with a fever without localizing signs. This algorithm is a suggested, but not exhaustive approach to management.

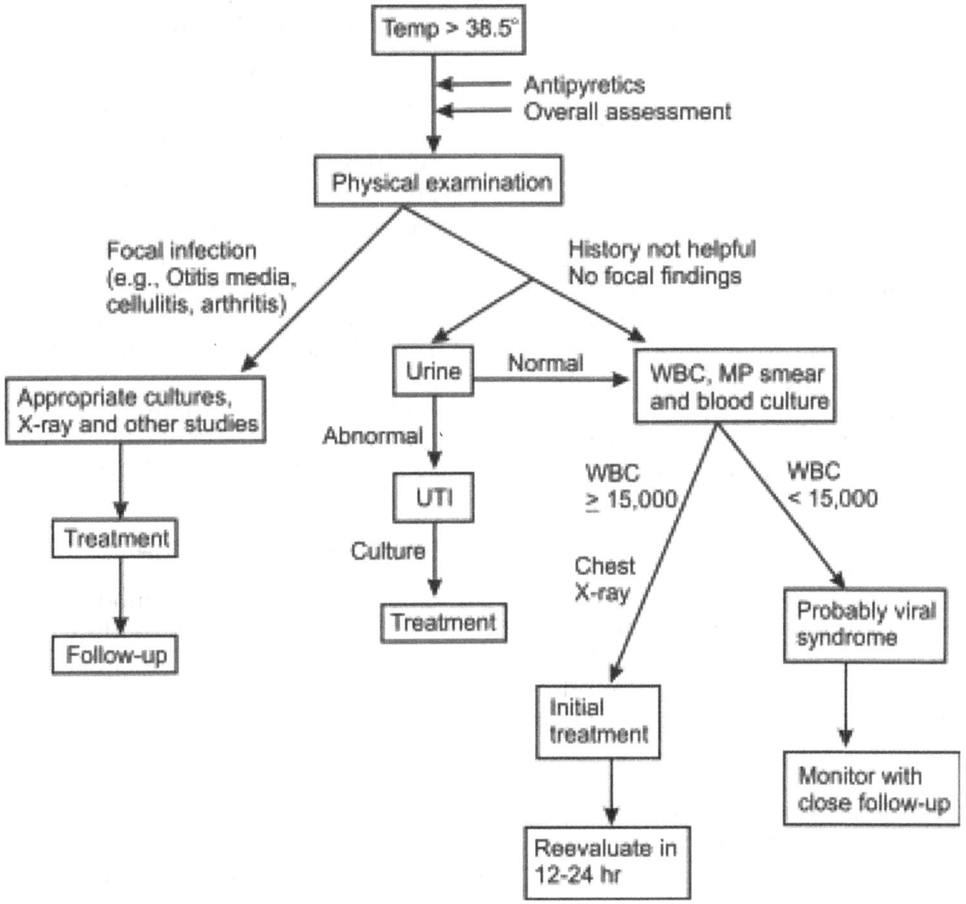

Fig. 2: Evaluation of the febrile child 3 months to 3 years of age. *Adapted from Barkin RM, Rosen P: Emergency pediatrics, ed 5, St Louis, 1999, Mosby.*

Disadvantages of Indiscriminate Antibiotic Use

i) mask physical signs of localization and delay the diagnosis
ii) vitiate subsequent bacteriological investigations
iii) increase chance of bacterial resistance
iv) occasionally, may be direct cause of fever, and other side effects

Antipyretic Therapy

Should temperature be lowered? Fever can cause irritability and convulsion; hyperpyrexia (> 41°C) may cause brain damage.

Early antipyretic therapy is imperative in facilitating observation. Many children who initially are irritable and disinterested in their environment will improve markedly with aggressive antipyretic management. Acetaminophen (15 mglkgldose per os [PO] or per rectum [PR]) should be administered to all children with temperatures higher than 38.5° C (101.3° F) on arrival in the clinic or emergency department to ensure optimal observation by reducing temperature and permitting a more accurate assessment of the child. Children with temperatures higher than 39.5^{O} C (103° F) should also be sponged with tepid water. The response to antipyretics does not predict the prevalence of bacteremia.

Antipyretics are Indicated in Following Group of Febrile Children

(i) If temperature > 39°C
(ii) If child is uncomfortable
(iii) If there is a known risk of febrile seizure

Choice of antipyretics: following drugs may be used

1. Paracetamol 10-15 mg/kg/6 hours
2. Ibuprofen 5 mg/kg/6 hours

Both are equally effective. The later has disadvantage of causing gastric irritation, but has advantage of better anti-inflammatory and analgesic activity. A combination may perhaps be more effective but also more toxic.

Cold sponging is necessary only if temperature is 40° or higher. The limit needs be lowered in children who have experienced a febrile seizure in past. It must cover whole body and use plain tap water. Antipyretic should be used an hour before cold sponging for maximum effect.

What Supportive Therapy

1. Sedation: Febrile children are very restless and may require sedation with Promethazine 1.0 mg/kg dose or Trichloryl 50 mg/kg/dose
2. Hydration - Febrile children have increased fluid requirement. Though there is no constant relationship between degree of fever and water loss, parents must be advised to give fluids liberally. There is no need, however to force fluids.
3. Diet - Anorexia is common. The best solution is to give food of child's liking and sweetened beverages. There is no need to force-feed.

DISPOSITION / FOLLOWUP

All children with mild to moderate febrile illness should be followed within 12 h, and 48 h. By that time about 50% are afebrile.

- In about 25 % focus may be identified - commonly otitis media.
- In about 25 % fever persists. Initiate diagnostic workup for infections/ noninfective causes in these.

PARENTAL EDUCATION: POINTS

The following should be highlighted while counselling the parents about fever:

1. Fever is a body temperature above 37.8°C (100°F) measured orally or 38°C when measured rectally.
2. Fever is not a disease by itself; it is due to some underlying illness.
3. Fever per se does not cause any harm unless the body temperature is 41°C. Generally the body keeps a check on the temperature and it seldom goes beyond 41°C.

4. Antipyretics are required only if the temperature exceeds 39°C (102°F) and/ or if the child is uncomfortable. If the child is comfortable and sleeping he need not be awakened for antipyretic medication.
5. Cold sponging is necessary only if the temperature is 40°C or higher. It must cover the whole body. Ordinary tap water at a temperature between 30°C - 37°C is good enough for the purpose, antipyretic one hour before cold sponging to derive the best effect from the sponging.
6. The limits for antipyretics and cold sponging need to be lowered for those children who have experienced a febrile seizure in the past.
7. A doctor must be consulted for fever if (i) the child is younger than 3 months; (ii) it persists for more than 2 days; (iii) the child appears sick or stop feeding; (iv) the temperature is > 39°C; and (v) the child has other symptoms.

CONCLUSIONS

In conclusion the following groups of febrile patients need careful diagnostic and therapeutic consideration:

1. All sick looking toxic children of any age
2. Fever> 39°C and sepsis screen positive
3. Young infants < 3 months. Among non-toxic appearing febrile infants upto 3 months, without a focus, clinical and laboratory evaluation can be used to define a population of low risk criteria. These are :
   i) Previously being healthy
   ii) Negative laboratory screen (WBC 5000 - 15000/mm^3, bands < 1500/mm^3 and normal urine-analysis)

   All these infants however, must have a complete sepsis evaluation and followed up.
4. If fever persists> 2 days

Sick Toxic looking infants and children have abnormal behaviour, (lethargy, poor activity, poor feeding, poor/continuous shrill cry, inconsolability), signs of poor peripheral perfusion (pallor, delayed capillary refill) or breathing abnormality (hyperventilation or irregular). All these infants/children should have full septic workup.

Further studies are needed to evaluate above criteria for assessment of illness severity in our population and to formulate criteria for hospitalization and empiric antibiotics therapy.

FURTHER READING

1. Singhi S, Kohli V, Ayyagiri A. Bacteremia and bacterial infections in highly febrile children without apparent focus. Indian Pediatr 1992 Oct; 29(10):1285–89.
2. Kohli V, Singhi S, Sharma P and Ganguly NK. Value of scrum C reactive protein concentration in febrile children without apparant focus. Anal Trop 1993; 13: 371-72.
3. Park JW. Fever without source in children. Recommendations for outpatient care in those up to 3. Postgrad Med 2000; 107(2); 259-62, 265-6.
4. Baraff LJ. Management of infants and young children with fever without source. Pediatr Ann 2008 Oct; 37(10):673-9.
5. Pusic MV . Clinical management of fever in children younger than three years of age. Pediatr Child Health 2007; 12(6): 469-72.
6. Sur DK, Bukont EL. Evaluating fever of unidentifiable source in young children. Am Fam Physician 2007; 75(12): 1805-11.
7. Antonyrajah B, Mukundan D. Fever without apparent source on clinical examination. Curr Opin Pediatr. 2008;**20**:96–102.
8. Ishimine P. Fever without source in children 0 to 36 months of age. Pediatr Clin North Am 2006;**53**:167–94
9. Newman TB, Bernzweig JA, Takayama JI, Finch SA, Wasserman RC, Pantell RH. Urine testing and urinary tract infections in febrile infants seen in office settings. Arch Pediatr Adolesc Med 2002;**156**:44–54.

M. Jayashree

53 Severe Malaria

Malaria is one of the leading cause of morbidity and mortality in developing countries. Nearly 2.48 million malaria cases are reported annually from South-East Asia especially India, Bangladesh, Nepal, Sri Lanka, Thailand and Indonesia. Plasmodium falciparum is the principal cause of severe disease with most deaths occurring in young children living in areas of intense transmission and that too due to cerebral malaria. In absolute terms, malaria kills 3000 children under age of 5 years every day.The rising incidence of malaria, especially P falciparum infections (50%), coupled with increasing resistance of P.falciparum to antimalarials has made severe malaria a serious illness in children. Severe malaria has a mortality of around 10-25% even in optimally treated cases and also carries the risk of neurologic morbidity in survivors.

DEFINITION

According to WHO guidelines a patient with P falciparum asexual parasitemia without any other obvious cause for symptoms, in the presence of one or more of the following clinical or laboratory feature qualifies for the diagnosis of severe malaria (Table 1, 2). These patients are at a higher risk for mortality and need immediate supportive care and parenteral antimalarials. Patients may not satisfy all the criteria for diagnosis nor is there any need to wait for laboratory confirmation to classify disease severity. Any evidence of organ dysfunction should be treated with utmost urgency as severe complicated malaria. The stringent criteria for definitions are mainly for ensuring uniformity for research purposes.

DIAGNOSIS

Peripheral Blood Film

Thick peripheral smears examined by a competent microscopist still remain the gold standard for diagnosis of malaria. Thick smears can detect 5-10 parasites/µl of blood provided at least 100 oil immersion fields are examined. Thin smears are needed for species identification. Conventional microscopy additionally helps in estimation of parasite density, detection of mature schizonts and malarial pigment in neutrophils, all of which are important prognostic indicators. Response to treatment can be assessed from serial blood films done every 6 hourly for the first 48 hours.

Table 1: Features of Severe Malaria.

(i) Cerebral malaria (Unrousable coma)
(ii) Severe normocytic anemia (Hb<5g/dL.)
(iii) Renal failure (Serum creatinine >3mg/100mL)
(iv) Pulmonary edema
(v) Hypoglycemia (<40mg/100mL).
(vi) Circulatory collapse/Shock (Systolic blood pressure <50mmHg in children below 5 years).
(vii) Spontaneous bleeding/disseminated intravascular coagulopathy.
(viii) Repeated generalized convulsions.
(ix) Acidemia/Acidosis
(x) Macroscopic hemoglobinuria.

Other manifestations:

(i) Impaired consciousness but rousable
(ii) Prostration, extreme weakness (inability to stand or sit)
(iii) Hyperparasitemia (>5% RBC infected)
(iv) Jaundice (total serum bilirubin >3mg/dL)
(v) Hyperpyrexia (axillary temperature >39.5^{0}C)

Adapted from:WHO Severe falciparum malaria.Trans R Soc Trop Med Hyg 2000;94:S1-S90

Table 2: General Danger Signs of Malaria

Danger Signs of Malaria
(i) Not able to drink or breast feed.
(ii) Vomiting everything.
(iii) Recent history of convulsion
(iv) Lethargic or unconscious state
(v) Unable to sit or stand up

The parent/guardian should be instructed to bring the child to the doctor if the patient develops any of the danger signs during the follow up.

Adapted from:WHO Severe falciparum malaria.Trans R Soc Trop Med Hyg 2000;94:S1-S90

However a peripheral blood film may be negative in a patient with malaria, due to previous treatment, highly synchronous infection or sequestration of parasitized RBC's in the internal organs. Multiple smears at 6-12 hourly intervals or during a spike of fever may improve the diagnostic yield. In case of mixed infection one species suppresses the other, making diagnosis of the suppressed species difficult. Thus a patient with severe manifestations but only P vivax on the peripheral smear should be treated for P vivax and P.falciparum coinfection.

Newer Methods

Although it is cost effective conventional microscopy has limitations of being highly observer dependent and time consuming. This has led to the development and evaluation of several newer diagnostic modalities. Acridine orange stained thick blood smears and quantitative buffy coat (QBC) provide rapid diagnosis with sensitivities/specificities of 42-93%/52-93% and 89%/>95% respectively. Limitations include non-quantitation of parasitemia by QBC, poor sensitivity of AO staining, need for special microscope and unreliable species diagnosis by both these methods.

Rapid diagnostic tests based on detection of parasitic antigens i.e. HRP II antigen of P falciparum (Parasite F) and detection of parasite LDH (Optimal test) are now being increasingly used as they require little or no training. Though these tests have been shown to have good sensitivity and specificity the major limitations are their higher cost, inability to quantify parasitemia, and diagnose non-falciparum species. Also these tests can remain positive even after 30 days of infection/treatment. The new tests cannot replace conventional microscopy for malaria diagnosis but are useful in situations where reliable microscopy is not available. There is no role of malarial antibodies in the diagnosis of malaria in endemic areas.

Tests for Disease Severity Assessment

These include complete blood count (Hb, TLC, DLC, platelet count), coagulogram, blood glucose, serum electrolytes and BUN, blood gas with anion gap, plasma lactate, chest X ray for respiratory distress syndrome, liver function tests, plasma hemoglobin and urine hemoglobin. Blood cultures should be sent in all patients presenting with shock. Serial blood glucose assessments are very important. The WHO consensus statement recommends that a lumbar puncture should be done in a child presenting with acute febrile encephalopathy even if asexual parasitemia is demonstrated in the peripheral smear. This is important as in the African/Indian context where bacterial meningitis and malaria can co exist. P falciparum parasitemia is fairly common in endemic areas posing difficulty in establishing a cause effect relationship.

MANAGEMENT OF SEVERE MALARIA

Effective care of a child with malaria includes antimalarial chemotherapy, supportive management and treatment of complications that are present at admission or develop later during the course. Severe life threatening malaria is nearly always due to P falciparum .It should be treated as a medical emergency preferably in an intensive care set up. Untreated severe malaria has a mortality of almost 100% that can be reduced to 15-20% with timely treatment. In cases of strong clinical suspicion prompt antimalarials therapy should be started pending lab results.

Initial assessment and stabilization: As for any other sick child a rapid cardiopulmonary assessment should be done at the outset in all children presenting to the ER. The sequence of clinical assessment should include the early recognition of impending respiratory failure, detection of shock and neurological assessment.

Airway and breathing: Airway must be secured in patients with Glasgow Coma Score (GCS) <8, shock and respiratory failure. Oxygen therapy and respiratory support should be given to all who present with distress and/or shock. The presence of respiratory depression or irregular breathing should alert the clinician to presence of seizures, raised intracranial pressure and hypoglycemia. Tachypnoea and increased work of breathing are very common in severe malaria and have been shown to be associated with metabolic acidosis which may be secondary to hypovolemia.

Circulation: Compensated and decompensated hypovolemic shock have been associated with base deficits of >8 mmol/l and >15 mmol/l respectively in patients with severe malaria. Shock should be resuscitated with initial bolus of 20 ml/Kg normal saline or Ringer's lactate to restore adequate perfusion and urine output. In the absence of coma, fluid therapy of 20-40 ml/Kg has been shown to correct hemodynamic imbalances safely. However a more cautious approach is warranted in patients with coma as over hydration may lead to pulmonary edema and neurological deterioration. It is safer to intubate, electively ventilate and use CVP guided fluid therapy in children in whom shock persists despite 40 ml/Kg of fluids.

Disability: Coma: Rapid assessment of neurological status can be done using the Glasgow coma scale. Other infections of the CNS or intracranial hemorrhage should be considered in a child with neck stiffness or bulging fontanel. Hypoglycemia may precipitate coma and needs to be excluded. Initial management of all comatose patients includes maintenance of airway, support of breathing, correction of hypoglycemia and volume deficits.

Seizures, hyperpyrexia should be appropriately treated. Patients should be monitored for features of raised intracranial tension.

Antimalarial Chemotherapy

Given the current situation of widespread chloroquine resistance the only two drugs recommended for use in severe malaria through parenteral route are quinine and artemisinin derivatives. Since death due to severe malaria often occurs within hours of admission it is very essential to ensure quick therapeutic concentration of antimalarials drugs by parenteral route. The WHO recommendations for antimalarials chemotherapy in severe malaria are as shown in Table 3.

Quinine: Acts primarily on the mature trophozoite stage of parasite development. It has no action on the pre-erythrocytic or sexual stage of the parasite and does not prevent sequestration or formation of meronts.

Bolus dose is recommended for quick therapeutic levels and should be avoided in patients who have received quinine/ halofantrine/mefloquine in the past 24 hrs as this can augment the risk of cardiotoxicity.

In centers where facilities for controlled IV quinine administration are not available IM quinine with similar efficacy can be used except in patients with coagulopathy.

Presence of G6PD deficiency and history of quinine allergy are the only known contraindications to use of quinine. Thrombocytopenia, jaundice, renal failure, hypotension are not contraindications for quinine administration. Hemolysis and hemoglobinuria at presentation is also not a contrain- dication to quinine even if the patient's G6PD status is not known. However any hemolysis developing during quinine therapy may warrant shift to artemisinin group. Conscious patients may experience tinnitus, deafness, headache, nausea and visual disturbances termed as "cinchonism" that does not warrant dose reduction or drug withdrawl. Severe and persistent symptoms however affect the drug compliance necessitating substitution with oral artemisinin derivatives.

Serious side effects with parenteral quinine are rare if it is administered properly. Though quinine produces prolongation of the QTc interval significant conduction abnormalities or dysrhythmias are rare. Hence routine ECG monitoring during quinine infusion is not required unless there is evidence of preexisting heart disease. Quinine can cause hypoglycemia due to stimulation of β cells although not associated with hyperinsulinemia in children. Frequent blood glucose monitoring is therefore mandatory in all patients receiving quinine.

The parasite count may remain unchanged or paradoxically increase during the initial 18-24 hrs with quinine therapy. Complete

Table 3: Drug and dosage of antimalarials in complicated and severe malaria

Drug	*Dosages*
Quinine salt	20mg salt/kg (loading dose)diluted in 10mL of isotonic fluid/kg infusion over 4 hours. 12 hours later give maintenance dose of 10mg salt/kg over 2 hours. To be repeated every 8 hourly, calculated from beginning of previous infusion, until the patient can swallow, then quinine tablets, 10mg salt/kg 8 hourly to complete a 7 day course of treatment(including both parenteral and oral). Tetracycline or doxycycline or clindamycin is added to quinine as soon as the patient is able to swallow and should be continued for 7 days. If controlled IV infusion cannot be administered then quinine can be given in the same dose by IM route in the anterior thigh (not in buttock). The dose of quinine should be divided between two sites, half the dose in each anterior thigh. If possible IM quinine should be diluted in normal saline to a concentration of 60-100mg salt/ml. (Quinine is usually available as 300mg salt/ml.) Tetracycline or doxycycline should be added as above.
Artesunate	2.4mg/kg IV at 12 and 24 hours, then once a day for total 7 days. If the patient is able to swallow, then the daily dose can be given orally. Tetracycline or docycycline or clindamycin is added to artesunate as soon as the patient can swallow and should be continued for 7 days.
Artemether	3.2mg/kg (loading dose) IM, followed by 1.6mg/kg daily for 6 days. If the patient is able to swallow, then the daily dose can be given orally. Tetracycline or doxycycline or clindamycin is added to artemether as soon as the patient can swallow and should be continued for 7 days.

(i) Loading dose of quinine should be avoided if patient has received quinine, quinidine or mefloquine within the preceding 12 hours. Alternatively loading dose can be administered as 7mg salt/kg by IV infusion pump over 30 minutes followed immediately by 10mg salt/kg diluted in 10ml isotonic fluid/kg by IV infusion over 4 hours.

(ii) Quinine should not be given by bolus or push injection. Infusion rate should not exceed 5 mg salt/kg/ hour.

(iii) If there is no clinical improvement after 48 hours of parenteral therapy, the maintenance dose of quinine should be reduced by one third to one half i.e. 5-7 mg salt/kg.

(iv) Quinine should not be given subcutaneously as this may cause skin necrosis.

(v) Previous maintenance dose of parenteral artesunate of 1.2mg/kg has been modified by WHO to 2.4mg/kg.

(vi) Artesunate, 60mg per ampoule is dissolved in 0.6mL of 5% sodium bicarbonate diluted to 3-5mL with 5% dextrose and given immediately by IV bolus (push injection).

(vii) Artemether is dispensed in 1mL ampoule containing 80mg of artemether in peanut oil.

Adapted from World Health Organization. Management of severe malaria. A practical Hand Book,2nd Ed Geneva:WHO;2000

clearance of asexual parasitemia takes about 5-6 days but the gametocytes persist, as the drug is not gametocidal. However counts remaining unchanged after 24 hr of quinine therapy may indicate quinine resistance.

The purpose of adding a second drug with quinine is mainly to shorten the duration of oral quinine therapy, to improve cure rates and to prevent the emergence of quinine resistance. The choice of second drugs to be added when the patient is able to take oral medication are either SP (pyrimethamine and sulfadoxine) single dose of pyrimethamine 1.25 mg/kg, or tetracycline (children > 8 years) as 5 mg/kg 6 hourly for 7 days, doxycycline 2 mg/kg twice a day for 7 days or clindamycin 20-40 mg/kg divided in 3 daily doses for 5 days. Mefloquine is not recommended because of additive toxicity.

Artemisinin Derivatives

Artemisinin and its derivatives (artemether, artesunate) are the most rapidly acting of all antimalarials; exerting their effect on all forms of the parasite from ring forms to mature trophozoites. Studies have shown similar efficacy and side effects amongst the artemisinin derivatives. A minimum of 3 days of parenteral therapy is recommended before switching to oral therapy. The total duration of therapy should be for 5 days, as shorter durations are associated with recrudescence (50% recrudescence risk with three days therapy). Monotherapy with artemisinin should be avoided as it increases the risk of recrudescence and development of resistance and a second antimalarial like Mefloquine is commonly added. Additional gametocidal drug like primaquine is not required as artemisinins themselves have a gametocidal effect. Artemisinin derivatives have a good therapeutic and safety profile. Unlike quinine both the onset and complete clearance are faster with artemisinins. The parasite counts start declining in 5-6 hours after institution of therapy and asexual parasitemia disappearing within a mean time of 72 hours. Local reactions after intramuscular administration, cardiotoxicity, hemolysis and seizures are some of the side effects that have been rarely reported. It will be prudent not to combine artemisinins with other cardiotoxic drugs such as quinine/halofantrine. Moreover there is no evidence to suggest that combination therapy of artemisinins and quinine would be additive or synergistic in severe malaria.

Quinine Vs Artemisinin:

The rapidity of action, better safety profile, cost effectiveness and increasing availability of artemisinin derivatives are making them more popular resulting in a danger of indiscriminate use that may potentiate the development of drug resistance. Hence the question that needs to be addressed before liberalizing the use of these drugs is whether artemisinin is superior to quinine with respect to survival outcomes in severe P falciparum malaria in quinine sensitive areas. A Cochrane meta-analysis of 16-randomised trials comparing quinine with artemisinin derivatives in severe malaria in both adults and children found that both the drugs were similar in efficacy in areas where significant quinine resistance has not been documented. Though the parasite clearance time was significantly faster with artemisinin derivatives, the fever clearance time was similar with both drugs. For clinicians it means that artemisinin is as good as quinine with no added survival advantage. Hence its use should be restricted to documented quinine resistance (suboptimal parasite clearance) or where facilities for controlled IV administration of quinine are suboptimal. Moreover given the history of development of resistance to other antimalarial drugs artemisinins must be used judiciously avoiding incorrect dosages and monotherapy.

Exchange Transfusion

There is no clear-cut evidence about the utility of exchange transfusion in severe malaria. Theoretically exchange transfusion helps in removing parasites, harmful metabolites, toxins, cytokines, and parasitized non-deformable red cells and also restores normal red cell mass, platelets, clotting factors, albumin and other depleted substances. However electrolyte disturbances, cardiovascular complications, infections, requirements for large volumes of blood and inability of exchange to remove sequestered parasites are some of the issues against this procedure which is quite labour intensive especially in older children.

The WHO guidelines for indications for exchange transfusion in non-immune individuals are as mentioned in Table 4.The important prerequisites are availability of safe and compatible blood and technical support for a safe procedure. Post exchange transfusion, doses of antimalarials should be repeated. Erythrocytapheresis is preferable to manual exchange if resources permit.

Table 4: Indications for exchange transfusion

1. Parasitemia > 30% in the absence of clinical complications
2. Parasitemia > 10% in the presence of severe disease like cerebral malaria, acute renal failure, acute respiratory distress syndrome, jaundice and severe anemia
3. Parasitemia >10% and failure to respond to optimal chemotherapy after 12-24hours
4. Parasitemia > 10% and poor prognostic factors e.g. late stage parasites in peripheral blood

Supportive Therapy

Careful monitoring of vitals that include pulse rate, blood pressure, respiratory rate, core body temperature, pallor, level of consciousness at least 4 hourly is important to detection complications. Indwelling catheter should be in situ for urine output monitoring and to watch for hemoglobinuria. Strict intake and output should be maintained. In patients with hemodynamic instability preload can be assessed by central venous pressure monitoring. All comatose patients must have a Ryle's tube in situ.

Blood glucose in children with coma should be ideally monitored every hour; this may be relaxed to every 2 hours and every 4 hours if there is no episode of hypoglycemia. In others blood glucose can be monitored every 4-6 hourly. Blood glucose should be checked at every instance of clinical worsening in a child with malaria. Convulsions should be treated with IV or rectal benzodiazepines. Hyperpyrexia should be treated with paracetamol, and tepid sponging. Hemoglobin, electrolytes, and blood urea should be monitored on a regular basis. Parasite count should be monitored 6 hourly for the first 48 hours. A combination of a third generation cephalosporin and aminoglycoside to provide a broad spectrum cover is indicated in children with shock or in presence of localized signs suggesting bacterial infection.

MANAGEMENT OF COMPLICATIONS

Among the various complications of falciparum malaria the common and important ones in children are as follows:
(a) Cerebral malaria
(b) Severe anemia
(c) Respiratory distress (acidosis)
(d) Hypoglycemia

Cerebral Malaria

Children usually present with fever and refusal to eat or drink. The progression to coma or convulsion is seen rapidly within one or two days of onset of symptoms. Generalized seizures associated with nystagmus or salivation is usually seen. Focal seizures are uncommon. Other causes for encephalopathy (e.g., bacterial meningitis, hypoglycemia) need to be excluded. The general principles of management will be same as for any comatose child with early institution of antimalarial chemotherapy. Harmful adjuvant treatment like corticosteroids, adrenaline and phenobarbital are contraindicated.

Severe Anemia

Children with hyperparasitemia may develop severe anemia due to acute destruction of parasitized red cells. Packed red cell transfusion should be given cautiously when PCV is 12% or less, or hemoglobin in below 4g%. In patients with less severe anemia, transfusion is indicated in the presence of respiratory distress (acidosis), impaired consciousness or hyperparasitema (>20% of RBCs infected).

Lactic acidosis

Effortless tachypnoea without chest indrawing or any localizing chest signs suggest lactic acidosis. It usually accompanies cerebral malaria, anemia or dehydration. Metabolic acidosis resolves with correction of hypovolemia and treatment of anemia. There is no evidence to support the use of sodium bicarbonate. Careful monitoring of acid base status, serum electrolytes, blood glucose and renal functions is needed in all patients with hypovolemia and acidosis.

Hypoglycemia

It is common in children below 3 years and correlates with hyperparasitemia and disease severity. It can also occur in patients treated with quinine. Children usually manifest with convulsions or altered sensorium. Manifestations can closely mimic those of cerebral malaria and can be often overlooked if not looked for carefully. The importance of serial blood glucose monitoring hence cannot be overemphasized. If facilities to monitor blood glucose are not available then hypoglycemia should be assumed in symptomatic patients and treated with IV dextrose (25% dextrose 2 to 4 mL/kg by bolus) followed by slow infusion of 5% or 10% dextrose containing fluid to prevent recurrence.

Hyperpyrexia

High fever is common in children with malaria and may lead to convulsions and altered consciousness. Antipyretics (Paracetamol 15mg/kg) and tepid sponging should be used to control fever.

Circulatory Collapse

There should be a high index of suspicion for complicating gram-negative septicemia in patients presenting with shock especially in a developing country scenario. Broad-spectrum antibiotics should be started after sending blood cultures. Septic shock should be resuscitated with judicious use of fluids.

Spontaneous Bleeding and Coagulopathy (DIC)

This complication is usually seen is non-immune children and should be treated with Vitamin K, blood or blood products as required.

FURTHER READINGS

1. Palmer CJ JA, Bruckner DA, Barnett ED, Miller NS, Haseeb MA, Et.al. Multicenter study to evaluate the Optimal test for rapid diagnosis of malaria in US hospitals.J Clin Microbiol 2003; 41:5178-82.
2. English M, Waruiru C, Amukoye E, Murphy S, Crawley J, Mwangi I, Et al. Deep breathing in children with severe malaria: indicator of metabolic acidosis and poor outcome. Am Trop Med Hyg 1996; 55:521-4.
3. Maitland K, Levin M, English M; Mithwani S, Peshy N, Marsh K, et Al. Severe P falciparum malaria in Kenyan children: evidence for hypovolaemia. QJ Med 2003; 96:427-34.

4. Maitland K, Pamba A, English M, Peshu N, Marsh K, Newton CRJC, et al. Randomized trial of volume expansion with albumin or saline in children with severe malaria: preliminary evidence of albumin benefit. Clin Infect Dis 2005; 40:538-45.
5. World Health Organization. Incorrect approaches to treatment. Guidelines for the treatment of malaria. Geneva: World Health Orgaization; 2006.p. 26-27.
6. White NJ. Protozoan infections: Malaria. In: Cook GC, Zumla A, eds. Manson Tropical Diseases, 21st ed. London: Saunders; 2003. p. 1205-1295.
7. World Health Organization. Management of severe malaria. A practical Hand Book, 2nd ed. Geneva: WHO; 2000.
8. Makler MT, Palmar CJ, Ager AL. A review of practical techniques for diagnosis of malaria. Am Tropp Med Parasitol 1998; 92:419-433.
9. WHO. A rapid dipstick antigen capture assay for the diagnosis of falciparum malaria. Bull WHO 1996; 74:47-54.S.
10. Severe falciparum malaria. World Health Organization, Communicable Diseases Cluster. Trans R Soc Trop Med Hyg 2000; 94 (Suppl) 1 : S1-90.
11. Imbert P, Gerardin P, Rogier C, Ka AS, Jouvencel P, Brousse V et al. Severe falciparum malaria in children: a comparative study of 1990 and 2000 WHO criteria for clinical presentation, prognosis and intensive care in Dakar, Senegal. Trans R Soc Trop Med Hyg 2002; 96 : 278-281
12. Singh N, Valecha N, Nagpal AC, Mishra SS, Varma HS, Subbarao SK. The hospital- and field-based performances of the optimal test, for malaria diagnosis and treatment monitoring in central India. Ann Trop Med Parasitol 2003; 97: 5-13.
13. Avila PĖ, Kirchgatter K, Brunialti KC, Oliveira AM, Siciliano RF, Di Santi SM. Evaluation of a rapid dipstick test, Malar-Check, for the diagnosis of Plasmodium Falciparum malaria in Brazil. Rev Inst Med Trop Sao Paulo 2002; 44 : 293-296.
14. McIntosh HM, Olliaro P. Artemisinin derivatives for treating severe malaria (Cochrane Review). In The Cochrane Library, Issue 4, 2003. Chichester, UK: John Wiley and Sons Ltd.
15. Newton PN, Chierakul W, Ruangveerayuth R, Silamut K, Teerapong P, Krudsood S et al. A comparison of artesunate alone with combined artesunate and quinine in the parenteral treatment of acute falciparum malaria. Trans R Soc Trop Med Hyg 2001; 95 : 519-523.
16. Woodrow CJ, Haynes RK, Krishna S. Artemisins. Postgard Med J 2005;81:71-78.
17. .Maitland K, Nadel S, Pollard AJ, Williams TN, Newton RJC, Levin M. Management of severe malaria in children: proposed guidelines for the United Kingdom.BMJ;331:337-343.

Sunit Singhi

54 Dengue and Dengue Hemorrhagic Fever

Dengue is a mosquito-borne disease caused by one of the four serotypes of dengue viruses. It is characterized by fever and mild constitutional symptoms to hemorrhagic manifestations and shock, or dengue hemorrhagic fever/dengue shock syndrome (DHF/DSS). Dengue fever is classically a self-limiting, nonspecific febrile illness. DHF is a more serious clinical entity. It began to emerge among children in Southeast Asia during the 1950s and has since become major public health problems worldwide. The affected children need very careful monitoring. The fluid therapy is challenging and needs modification frequently. Respiratory distress due to extensive pleural effusions, myocardial dysfunction, extensive bleeding and multi-organ failure including acute respiratory distress syndrome, acute liver failure, and acute renal failure are other potentially life threatening complications that may need attention in PICU.

GLOBAL BURDEN

The global prevalence of dengue has grown dramatically in recent decades. The disease is now endemic in 112 countries in tropical and subtropical belt. WHO estimates that 40% of world's population is at risk. Every year about 50-100 million cases of Dengue infection, 500,000 cases of DHF and at least 12000 deaths occur worldwide; ninety percent of these deaths occur in children less than 15 years of age.[1,2] An estimated 500 000 cases of DHF require hospitalization each year, of whom a very large proportion are children. At least 2.5% of cases die. Without proper treatment, DHF case fatality rates can exceed 20%. With modern intensive supportive therapy, such rates can be reduced to less than 1%.

DENGUE VIRUSES

Dengue is caused by 40 to 50-mm single-stranded RNA viruses belonging to Flavivirus group. Four species have been described, called serotypes: DEN-1, DEN-2, DEN-3, and DEN-4. The viral genome encodes three structural proteins (capsid, C, membrane protein M, and envelope glycoprotein, E) and seven non-structural proteins (NS1, NS2a, NS2b, NS3, NS4a, NS4b, and NS5). The main biological properties of the viruses are located in the E protein.

DEN-2 was the predominant serotype in the 1980s and the early 1990s, in the recent years it has changed to the DEN-3 serotype. Infection with one dengue virus serotype results in specific immunity to that serotype only; theoretically individuals can be infected with all four serotypes.

Transmission

Dengue is transmitted by female Aedes mosquito. The mosquito gets infected from biting an infected person during acute febrile illness (viremic phase). After an extrinsic incubation period of 8-10 days, the infected mosquito transmits infection by biting and injecting infected salivary fluid into the wound of another person. Vertical transmission from mother to child has been reported.

Aedes aegypti is the most important epidemic vector; in some areas *A. albopictus* and *A. polynesiensis* may act as vectors. It is found between latitudes 30° north and 20° south and at over 2200 meters above sea level. *Aedes* rest indoors, mainly in living rooms and bedrooms, and in small collections of water such as flower vases or coconut shells. This maximizes man-vector contact and contributes to difficulty in controlling this vector. Improper disposal of garbage or inadequate wastewater drainage facilitates may be responsible for high mosquito densities in endemic areas. Significant increases in the mosquito larval populations are seen during the rainy season. This is why epidemics of dengue tend to coincide with the rainy season.[5]

PATHOGENESIS

After the bite of an infected mosquito, the average incubation period is 4 to 7 days (range 3-14 days). Patient may or may not experience symptoms during this period. This is followed by viremia, which is associated with sudden onset of fever and constitutional symptoms lasting for 5-6 days (range 2 to 12 days).

The dengue virus replicates within cells of the mononuclear phagocyte lineage (macrophages, monocytes, and B cells). Additionally, infection of mast cells, dendritic cells, and endothelial cells are known to occur.[3] The virus may infect peripheral blood leukocytes, liver, spleen, lymph node, bone marrow, thymus, heart, kidney, stomach, lung, and possibly brain, suggesting a blood-brain barrier passage.[4]

Following the febrile (viraemic) phase the patient may either recover or progress to the leakage phase, leading to DHF and/or dengue shock syndrome. Peak plasma viremia and circulating levels of the dengue virus nonstructural protein NS1 correlates with the severity of dengue infections.[5] The increased number of infected cells results in increased production of the cytokines including TNF-á and IFN- α, and other chemical mediators. The release of various cytokines and mediators cause increased vascular permeability, abnormal leakage of plasma, hypovolemia, shock, and hemostatic abnormalities. Endothelial cells also undergo apoptosis causing disruption of endothelial cell barrier, which contributes to syndrome of generalized vascular leakage.[6] (Figure. 1).

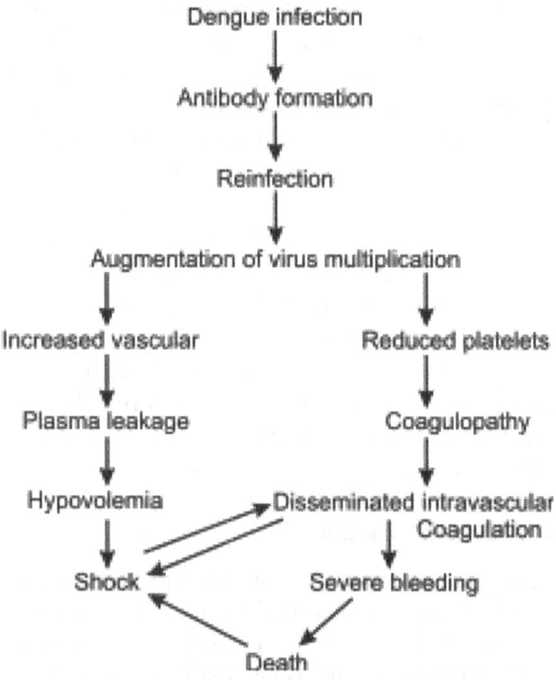

Fig. 1: Pathogenesis of Dengue

More severe infection occurs when a person is infected for a second time with a different serotype. How a second dengue infection causes a severe disease and why only some patients get severe disease remains unclear. It is suggested that residual antibodies produced during the first infection are unable to neutralize a second infection with another serotype, and the second infection under the influence of enhancing antibodies result in severe infection and disease. This phenomenon is referred to as antibody dependent enhancement.

Common gross pathologic findings in dengue infection include petechial hemorrhages and ecchymoses, serous pleural and peritoneal effusions, and pulmonary edema. Vasculitis of small vessels in visceral and soft tissues is found on microscopy as well as focal midzonal hepatic necrosis and subendocardial left ventricle and gastric mucosal hemorrhages.

CLINICAL FEATURES

Dengue virus infections may be asymptomatic or may have three main clinical manifestations.

1. Undifferentiated febrile illness (UF) or viral syndrome
2. Dengue Fever (DF)
3. Dengue Hemorrhagic Fever (DHF)
   - DHF without shock,
   - Dengue shock syndrome (DSS)

Dengue Fever

WHO defines dengue fever as an acute onset febrile illness of 2-7 days duration with two or more of the following: headache, retro-orbital pain, myalgia/arthralgia, rash (macular popular), and petechiae and positive tourniquet test. Hemorrhagic manifestation are uncommon.

Younger children tend to present with undifferentiated febrile illness, coryza, diarrhea, rash and seizure, and less commonly with vomiting, headache, and abdominal pain. Flushing, a characteristic feature is commonly observed on the face, neck, and chest. DF with bleeding complications such as epistaxis, gingival bleeding, gastrointestinal bleeding, and haematuria can be observed during some epidemics.

Dengue Haemorrhagic Fever (DHF)

DHF and DSS are severe manifestations of dengue infections. In Southeast Asia these are predominantly seen in children, whereas in the Americas, these are seen in all age groups. DHF usually follows secondary dengue infections, but may sometimes follow primary infections, especially in infants. These patients have a significantly higher viral load and a slower rate of clearance of viral load and virus-containing immune complexes than patients with dengue fever.

According to the current WHO guidelines, a case of DHF fulfills all of the following clinical criteria: acute onset fever, any hemorrhagic manifestation, thrombocytopenia <100,000 platelets/mm^3), and objective evidence of increased capillary permeability and plasma leakage manifested by one or more- 20% rise in hematocrit, > 20% drop in hematocrit following fluids, signs of plasma leakage (pleural-effusion, ascites, hypoalbuminemia or hypoproteinemia). When the only hemorrhagic manifestation is a positive tourniquet test, the case is categorized as DHF grade I, but a spontaneous hemorrhage, even if mild, indicates grade II illness. Grades III and IV DHF represent dengue shock syndrome (DSS). There are however, difficulties in using these definitions as these may underestimate disease severity. Modifications have been suggested to use higher cutoff for platelet counts <150,000/mm^3) and hematocrit for plasma leakage (either one hematocrit of 50% or over or hemoconcentration of 10% or over). Caution is needed as new case definition may affect estimation of dengue severity.

DHF usually begins with a sudden rise in temperature and other symptoms identical to those of dengue fever. The temperature remains so for 2 to 7 days. Hepatomegaly and splenomegaly is occasionally seen, especially in infants. Hemorrhagic tendency may manifest in many ways: positive tourniquet test; petechiae, ecchymoses or purpura; bleeding from mucosa. Easy bruising, and bleeding at venipuncture sites are common, while epistaxis and gingival bleeding are uncommon. Gastrointestinal bleeding, hemetemesis or malena, may occur in severe cases. Intracranial bleed is rare.

The bleeding may not correlate with the platelet counts and usually occur once the fever has settled. Mechanisms of bleeding are multiple: vasculopathy, thrombocytopathy and DIC. Thrombocytopathy consisting of thrombocytopenia and platelets dysfunction is caused by bone marrow suppression, immune injury, and infection of platelets by dengue virus.

In mild to moderate cases fever subsides with profuse sweating. Mild changes in pulse rate and blood pressure may be noticed with cold extremities and skin congestion. Patients recover spontaneously or after fluids and electrolyte therapy. **In severe cases** sudden deterioration may occur after few days with progression to DSS.

Dengue Shock Syndrome (DSS)

WHO define DSS as DHF plus signs of circulatory failure manifested by rapid and weak pulse, narrow pulse pressure ($\leq$20 mm Hg) or hypotension for age, prolonged capillary refill, cold and clammy skin and restlessness. Onset of shock is acute and occurs at time of defervescene, usually after 2-5 days of fever. The temperature is often subnormal, skin is cold and clammy, and pulse rapid and feeble.

Pleural effusion and ascites predict the development of DSS. Intense abdominal pain is a frequent complaint that appears shortly before the onset of shock. Consciousness is usually intact. The duration of the shock is short. It is at its worst during the first 48 hours and recovers rapidly after appropriate fluid replacement. Uncorrected shock will result in metabolic acidosis, severe bleeding from the gastrointestinal tract and other organs, and a poor prognosis. DIC and prolonged bleeding is more common in patients with shock, and causes fatality.

Convalescence in DHF is usually short and uneventful usually 2-5 days. Pleural effusions and ascites may be detected for a little longer. During the convalescent stage, bradycardia or arrhythmia may be noted. The return of appetite is a good indicator of recovery from shock. Many patients also complain of severe itching especially on the palms and soles, and may have recovery rash (confluent petechial rash with erythema and islands of pallor). The course of DHF/DSS is approximately 7 to 10 days.

Unusual Manifestations - Complications

Unusual manifestations of DHF/DSS include hepatitis, encephalitis and glomerulonephritis. Myocardial dysfunction has also been reported.

Central Nervous System Involvement

CNS involvement usually occurs as result of an encephalopathy. It manifests with irritability, lethargy, confusion and depression and sometimes convulsion, impaired consciousness/coma, and paresis. be due to metabolic acidosis, metabolic disturbances e.g. hypoglycemia and electrolyte imbalances (hyponatremia, hypocalcemia), cerebral anoxia, cerebral edema, intracranial hemorrhage, and vessel occlusion. Acute liver failure or Reye's syndrome and edema associated with leakage through the cerebral vasculature may contribute to encephalopathy.

True encephalitis may be seen rarely. Nuchal rigidity, mononeural palsies to encephalitis with seizures may be seen. Guillain-Barre syndrome, myelitis and acute flaccid paralysis caused by dengue myositis has been reported.

Acute Hepatic Failure

Acute liver failure because of hepatocellular damage caused directly by dengue virus or Reye's syndrome can occur. It presents with rapid change in the consciousness with rising, high level of liver enzyme. The case fatality rate is high. Rapid recovery in those who survive is more suggestive of Reye's syndrome than true viral hepatitis

Acute Renal Failure

Kidneys are rarely affected in DSS. Most reported cases are associated with late acute hepatic failure. Other risk factors for acute renal failure are use of nephrotoxic drugs, intravascular hemolysis e.g. G-6-PD deficiency, and abnormal hemoglobinopathy.

DIAGNOSIS AND DIFFERENTIAL DIAGNOSIS

During the early febrile phase dengue may mimic a spectrum of febrile illness including Infectious mononucleosis, chickengunya, cocksackie and other enteroviral infections, rubella, parvovirus B19 infections, rubella, measles, malaria, rickettsia and leptospirosis and bacterial sepsis. DHF can also mimic Kawasaki disease, meningococcemia and other viral hemorrhagic fevers. Acute onset of high fever for 1-2 days, flushed face without coryza or any other respiratory symptoms with a positive tourniquet test (inflate blood pressure cuff to a point midway between systolic and diastolic pressure for minutes; positive test: > 10 petechiae per 2.5 cm2) increases probability of DHF in an epidemic situation.

Two clinical observations plus one laboratory findings or at least a rising hematocrit are sufficient to establish a provisional diagnosis of DHF. These include thrombocytopenia (less than 100,000 cells/ mm^3) and hemoconcentration. Since patients are likely to present with symptoms suggestive of DHF, a drop in hemoglobin or hematocrit of more than 20% following volume replacement therapy can be taken as an indication of previous hemoconcentration.

LABORATORY DIAGNOSIS

For individual patient clinical diagnosis is adequate for starting treatment. A laboratory diagnosis of dengue infections can be accomplished by detecting either the virus, specific viral antigen/RNA or anti dengue antibodies in serum. Isolation of virus is most definitive way but it is not feasible and requires time, skills, expertise and equipments. The virus remains detectable during the febrile (viremic) period (on average 5 days after onset of symptoms).

Virus isolation by Cell Culture and Fluorescent Antibody Test is not needed for routine diagnosis but it is needed to determine serotype of the infecting virus for research and epidemiological studies.

Serological Tests That are Available are:

Haemagglutination inhibition test: Easy, simple and ideal for epidemiological studies. Haemagglutination inhibitor antibodies appear by day 5-6 of illness. A fourfold or greater rise in antibody titres is suggestive of a flavivirus infection (and not diagnostic of dengue infections). This test lacks specificity. However, a single antibody titre >1/2560 is accepted as indicator of secondary dengue infection if supported by a suggestive clinical history.

Complement fixation test: Difficult to perform. Not specific.

Neutralizing test: Most specific and sensitive but technically difficult and time consuming.

IgG ELISA: Can be used to differentiate primary and secondary dengue infection but it is non-specific and cross reacts with other flaviviruses. Does not give serotype diagnosis.

IgM ELISA test has sensitivity ranging from 83.9%–98.4% and a specificity of 100%.

RT-PCR is useful for early detection of dengue infection when antibodies are not yet detectable. It is less sensitive than viral isolation during early days of fever, but after 5 days of fever it is more sensitive than virus isolation, allows for rapid detection within in 24 hours and is able to detect virus up to 7-8 days of fever.

WHO defines a confirmed case as one who has positive viral identification and/or a serological test HI antibody 1:1,280 or positive IgM/ IgG ELISA test in convalescence serum is also diagnostic.

MANAGEMENT

WHO has issued a document focusing on the guidelines for treatment of Dengue fever and DHF/DSS. These guidelines are easy to follow and can be used in any hospital until the patient is admitted to an ICU. Indications for admission to hospital are shown in Table 1. The WHO guidelines are useful in that they offer an algorithmic approach to fluid resuscitation of DHF and DSS. However, the usefulness of these guidelines is limited beyond the immediate resuscitation because they do not address the treatment of complicated forms of the disease including fluid overload and multiple organ function failure, which could cause disability or death.

Table 1: High Risk DHF Patients and Indication for admission to hospital/ICU

High Risk Dengue Patients that need special attention

1. Infants under 1 year of age
2. Overweight / obese patients.
3. Massive bleeding
4. Change of consciousness, especially restless and irritable or coma
5. Have underlying diseases e.g. thalassemia, G-6-PD deficiency, heart disease.

Indication for admission

1. Excessive family concern or cannot be followed up.
2. Very weak, cannot eat or drink,
3. Spontaneous Bleeding
4. Platelet counts < 100,000 cells/ cu mm and/or rising Hct 10-20%
5. Clinical deterioration during defervescence.
6. Severe abdominal pain/ vomiting
7. Significant dehydration requiring intravenous fluids.

Admit Immediately if signs of shock. These signs are as follows:

1. Rapid pulse with no fever
2. Prolonged capillary refill time
3. Cold clammy skin, mottling
4. Narrow of pulse pressure ≤20 mmHg e.g. 100/80,
5. Hypotension
6. Oliguria, no urine for 4-6 hours.
7. Change of consciousness : drowsy to stupor, restless, irritable (encephalopathy)

Adapted from - Prevention and Control of Dengue and Dengue Haemorrhagic Fever. Comprehensive Guidelines. New Delhi, WHO, 1999)

The treatment of dengue fever in febrile phase is symptomatic. Fever is treated with paracetamol. Salicylates and other non-steroidal anti-inflammatory drugs must be avoided as these may predispose a child to mucosal bleeds. In an epidemic setting all patients with dengue fever need regular monitoring by a primary care physician for clinical features of fluid leak &/or shock along with hematocrit and platelet counts, if possible, for early detection of DHF and DSS. Any patient who develops cold extremities, restlessness, acute abdominal pain, decreased urine output, bleeding and hemoconcentration should be admitted in a hospital. Children with rising hemotocrit and thrombocytopenia without clinical symptoms should also be admitted

With adequate and appropriate fluid replacement, DSS is rapidly reversible. In an Indian study, of 858 patients with dengue fever/DHF admitted to the hospital, 109 cases with severe forms of disease required PICU admission, The commonest indication for PICU admission was persistent shock (39 patients) followed by requirement for positive pressure ventilation in 29 patients (10 of whom had Acute Respiratory Distress Syndrome [ARDS]) and neurological symptoms in 24 patients. All patients had thrombocytopenia.[7]

In the hospital, all children without hypotension (DHF grades I and II) should be given oxygen and fluids. Ringer's lactate is infused at the rate of 7 ml/kg over one hour. After one hour if hematocrit decreases and vital parameters improve, fluid infusion rate should be decreased to 5 ml/kg over next hour and to 3 ml/kg/hour for 24 – 48 hours. When the patient is stable as indicated by normal blood pressure, satisfactory oral intake and urine output, the child can be discharged. If at one hour the hematocrit is rising and vital parameters do not show improvement, fluid infusion rate is increased to 10 ml/kg over next hour. In case of no improvement fluid infusion rate is further increased to 15 ml/kg over the third hour. If no improvement is observed in vital parameters and hematocrit at the end of 3 hours, colloids or plasma (10 ml/kg) is administered. Once the hematocrit and vital parameters are stable the infusion rate is gradually reduced and discontinued over 24 – 48 hours.

Children with hypotension (DHF grades III and IV) also need oxygen and fluids. In a small randomized study of DSS patients complicated by respiratory failure, oxygen administration by nasal continuous airway pressure (NCPAP) was a better option than oxygen by face mask. NCPAP reduced the need for intubation and ventilation.[8] Initial resuscitation with Ringer's lactate is acceptable for children with moderately severe dengue shock syndrome.[9] Six percent hydroxyethyl starch may be preferred in children with severe shock. Ringer's lactate solution, 10-20 ml/kg is infused over one hour or given as bolus 20 ml/kg if blood pressure is unrecordable (DSS grade IV). The bolus may be repeated twice if there is no improvement. If there is no improvement in vital parameters and hematocrit is rising, colloids 10 ml/kg are rapidly infused. If the hematocrit is falling without improvement in vital parameters, blood is transfused, presuming that lack of improvement is due to occult blood loss. Once improvement starts the fluid infusion rate is gradually decreased.

Monitoring of children DHF/ DSS should include—

1. Vital signs every 15-30 minutes till stable, then 1-2 hourly
2. Hematocrit every 2 hr for 6 hr, then every 4 hr for till the patient is stable. Monitor 12 hourly during recovery.
3. Fluid balance sheet: type of fluid, amount, rate etc.
4. Accurate urine output
5. Serum electrolytes and blood gases every 12 hr.
6. DIC profile and liver function tests as and when indicated.
7. Weight every 12 hr.

In those at high risk of complicated DHF one should obtain Blood glucose, Blood electrolyte (Na, Ca, K, CO_2), Liver function test, Renal function test (BUN, Creatinine, uric acid), Blood gases, Coagulogram (PTT, PT, TT) and Blood grouping/cross matching

Patients who are unresponsive to fluids may have myocardial dysfunction and decreased left ventricular performance, which may be easily detected by echocardiography. They need vasoactive drugs (dopamine, epinephrine) infusion. In these patients also look for and correct massive plasma leakage, concealed internal bleeding –decrease in hct; give blood, hypoglycemia – blood sugar < 60 mg%, hyponatremia, hypocalcemia – electrolyte and metabolic acidosis.

Infusion of fresh frozen plasma and platelet concentrates may be beneficial in patients with disseminated intravascular coagulation or significant bleed. Platelets or blood should not be transfused based upon platelet count alone unless the platelet count is < 5000/mm^3. Low platelet count may not be predictive of bleeding.[10] In children with severe thrombocytopenia in absence of significant bleeding platelet infusion do not alter the outcome.[11] A good dictum to follow in patients with thrombocytopenia is ***"If the patient is not bleeding do not transfuse platelet".*** Treatment with methylprednisolone did not show any benefit in a double blind placebo controlled trial in patients with DSS.

Duration of IV fluid infusion is between 24-48 hours as plasma loss may continue for 24-48 hrs. It should be discontinued when the haematocrit level falls to approximately 40%, with stable vital signs. Good urine flow indicates sufficient circulating volume. Reabsorption of extravasated plasma occurs 48 hours after the termination of shock (manifested by a further drop in haematocrit after intravenous fluids has been stopped), and hypervolemia, pulmonary edema or heart failure may be caused if more fluid is given. *It is extremely important that a drop in haematocrit at this later stage is not interpreted as a sign of internal bleeding.* Strong pulse and blood pressure and adequate diuresis are good signs at this stage. The return of the patient's appetite is also a sign of recovery.

Patients may be discharged from hospital if following criteria are met:

- Absence of fever for at least 24 hours without the use of anti-fever therapy
- Minimum of three days after recovery from shock: stable pulse, blood pressure and breathing rate

Table 2: Complications and their treatment

1. Electrolyte imbalance
   - Hyponatremia
   - Hypocalcemia –10% Ca gluconate 1 ml/kg/dose, IV push slowly q 6 hrs.
2. Fluid Overload: Avoid the common causes of fluid overload, which are:
   - Early IV fluid therapy- from febrile phase
   - Excessive use of hypotonic solutions.
   - Non reduction in the rate of IV fluid after initial resuscitation.
   - Blood loss replaced by fluids in cases with concealed bleed.
   - Judicious fluid removal using colloids with controlled diuresis (frusemide 1mg/kg infusion over 4 hours) or dialysis.[12]
3. Large pleural effusions, ascites
   - Careful titration of intravenous fluids.
   - Large pleural effusions during the recovery phase after 48 hours - small doses of frusemide (0.25-0.5mg/kg 6 hourly for 1 to 2 doses). Avoid insertion of intercostal drains and tracheal intubation.
4. Disseminated Intravascular Coagulation:
   - Some seriously sick patients with bleeding and DIC have benefited from heparin therapy and cryoprecipitate (1 unit per 5 kg body weight) followed by platelets (4 units/m2 or 10-20 ml/kg) within one hour and fresh frozen plasma (FFP – 10-20 ml/kg). Frequent clinical assessment and regular coagulation profile (PT, aPTT, fibrinogen, platelet and FDP) are mandatory as indicated.

- No respiratory distress from pleural effusion and no ascites
- No evidence of external or internal bleeding
- Good urinary output and stable haematocrit
- Platelet count of > 100,000/mm^3

The treatment of complications are outlined in Table 2.

PROGNOSIS

Early recognition of illness, careful monitoring and appropriate fluid therapy alone has resulted in reduction in mortality to 1 %.[9] If shock is identified when pulse pressure starts getting narrow and intravenous fluids are administered, the outcome is excellent. If left untreated, the mortality in patients with DHF or DSS may be as high as 40 – 50%. Recovery is fast and most patients recover in 48 hours without any sequelae. The outcome may not be as good once patient develops cold extremities. The most death in DHF/DSS are caused by prolonged shock, massive bleeding, fluid overload and acute hepatic failure with encephalopathy. Severe refractory shock, DIC, ARDS, hepatic failure and neurological manifestations singly or in combination were the commonest causes of death in a recent series.[7] The case fatality rate is high with shortage of experienced medical teams.

PREVENTION AND CONTROL

At present no specific drug or vaccine is available against dengue virus. Vaccines is under development. A tetravalent live attenuated DEN vaccine trial has been done in Thailand and another one is licensed by GlaxoSmithKline. The control is primarily dependent on Personal protection (Protective clothing, insecticide treated mosquito nets and curtains and mats & coil), and Vector Control (by Biological control using larvivorus fishand Chemical control (1% temephos sand granules, space sprays – malathion, fenitrothion, pirimiphos only in major DHF epidemics).

CONCLUSIONS

The global prevalence of dengue has grown dramatically in recent decades. Dengue hemorrhagic fever/dengue shock syndrome (DHF/DSS) are the serious clinical forms. The fluid therapy is main stay of treatment but it is challenging and needs frequent modification based on careful monitoring. Data on DHF and DSS in infants is very limited. Better understanding of immuno-pathogenesis in this immunologically distinct group is needed. Clinical studies defining the role of myocardial dysfunction and inotropes and vasoactive support in fluid refractory DSS, and evaluation of specific immune globulins to treat thrombocytopenia are needed.

REFERENCES

1. WHO. Strengthening implementation of the global strategy for dengue fever and dengue haemorrhagic fever, prevention and control. Report of the informal consultation, 18–20 October 1999.Geneva: WHO, 1999.
2. WHO. Scientific working group on dengue. Meeting report, Geneva, Switzerland, 3–5 April 2000. Geneva: WHO, 2000.
3. King CA, Marshall JS, Alshurafa H, Anderson R. Release of vasoactive cytokines by antibody-enhanced dengue virus infection of a human mast cell/basophil line. J Virol 2000; 74:7146–50.
4. Hayes EB, Gubler DJ: Dengue and dengue hemorrhagic fever. Pediatr Infect Dis J 1992; 11:311-17.
5. Libraty DH, Young PR, Pickering D, Endy TP, Kalayanarooj S, Green S, et al. High circulating levels of the dengue virus nonstructural protein NS1 early in dengue illness correlate with the development of dengue hemorrhagic fever. J Infect Dis 2002;186:1165–8.
6. Lin CF, Lei HY, Shiau AL, Liu HS, Yeh TM, Chen SH, et al. Endothelial cells apoptosis induced by antibodies against dengue virus nonstructural protein I via production of nitric oxide. J Immunol 2002; 169:657-664.

7. Kamath SR, Ranjit S. Clinical features, complications and atypical manifestations of children with severe forms of dengue hemorrhagic fever in South India. Indian J Pediatr. 2006; 73:889-95.
8. Cam BV, Tuan DT, Fonsmark L, Poulsen A, Tien NM, Tuan HM, Heegaard ED. Randomized comparison of oxygen mask treatment Vs nasal continuous positive airway pressure in dengue shock syndrome with acute respiratory failure. J Trop Pediatr 2002; 6: 335-9.
9. Wills BA, Nguyen MD, Ha TL, Dong TH, Tran TN, Le TT, et al. Comparison of three fluid solutions for resuscitation in dengue shock syndrome. N Engl J Med. 2005; 353:877-89.
10. Lum LC, Goh AY, Chan PW, El-Amin AL, Lam SK. Risk factors for hemorrhage in severe dengue infections. J. Pediatr 2002; 5: 629-31..
11. Kabra SK, Jain Y, Madhulika, Tripathi P, Singhal T, Broor S, et al. Role of platelet transfusion in dengue hemorrhagic fever. Indian Pediatr 1998; 35: 452-454.
12. Ranjit S, Kissoon N, Jayakumar I. Aggressive management of dengue shock syndrome may decrease mortality rate: a suggested protocol. Pediatr Crit Care Med 2005; 6: 412-9.
13. Halstead SB, Lan NT, Myinet TT, Shwe TN, Nisalak A, Kalyanarooj S et al. Dengue Hemorrhagic Fever in Infants: Research Opportunities Ignored. Emerging Infectious Diseases 2002; 8: 1474-79.

Sunit Singhi

55 Exanthems and Rashes

Children are often brought to emergency department for acute onset rashes with or without fever. Some of these may be presentation of life threatening illnesses, while other may be trivial. Common causes of fever with rash in children are as follows:

Macular rash:	Measles, Rubella, Roseola infectiosum Infectious mononucleosis ECHO, Coxsackie infection. Drugs: Ampicillin; penicillin, Barbiturates, INH, Erythema infectiosum.
Vasicular	Vericella, Herpes simplex, Herpes zoster, Vaccinia
Purpuric	Meningococcal septicemia Henoch-Schönlein Thrombocytopenia
Urticarial	ECHO, Coxsackie, Allergy: drugs and food.
Multiple	Erythema multiformae.

MEASLES

Symptoms include fever malaise and cough. Physical examination findings include: conjunctivitis, coryza, on day 3: Koplik's spots on buccal mucosa and on day 5: erythematous macular rash that appears on face and neck, and spreads to trunk. The rash coalesces, turns coppery brown, and may desquamate. Acute complications that are seen commonly include laryngotracheitis (stridor), bronchitis or pneumonia (cough, tachypnea and respiratory distress) and otitis media. Myocarditis, pericarditis, and appendicitis are uncommon.

Diagnosis is best made by recognition of the characteristic rash. Measles can be distinguished from rubella by presence of the toxic appearance and high spiking fever.

Treatment: Measles runs a self-limited course. Treatment is supportive. Children with complications of measles should be admitted to the hospital. Other children may be discharged home with outpatient follow-up in 1 week (Table 1).

RUBELLA

Rubella occurs in epidemics every 6-9 years in unimmunized children or adolescents in whom immunity may have faded. Outbreaks have occurred in college students.

Symptoms may include prodrome of fever, malaise, cough and conjunctivitis. On

Table: 1 Differential diagnosis of erythematous maculopapular rash in children

Disease	*Causative organism*	*Main clinical features*
Chicken pox	Varicella zoster virus	Erythematous vesicles on face and trunk, progressing to crusted lesions
Drug rash	Variable	Generalized rash commonly associated with ampicillin use in infectious mononucleosis
Erythema infectiosum	Parvovirus B19	"Slapped cheek" rash followed by maculopapular rash on trunk and extremities. May look lacey
Herpangina	Cocksackievirus A4	Bright red macules on face, with vesicle formation, ulcerative lesions on palate and mouth
Infectious mononucleosis	Epstein-Barr virus	Pink maculopapular rash on trunk and limbs, petechial hemorrhages on palate, cervical lymphadenopathy
Kawasaki disease (mucocutaneous lymph node syndrome)	Agent unknown	High fever lasting 5 or more days, conjunctivitis, oral changes (strawberry tongue), extremity changes, rash
Measles	Paramyxovirus	High spiking fever, cough, conjunctivitis, coryza followed by rash on face and neck progressing downward
Rocky Mountain Spotted fever	Rickettsia rickettsii	Maculopapular to hemorrhagic lesions spreading from wrists and hands to trunk
Roseola	Herpes-6 virus	Young child with high fever; pink maculopapular rash appears on trunk after fever drops in 2-4 days
Rubella	Togavirus	Low-grade fever, cough, conjunctivitis, rash on face and neck
Scarlet fever	Streptococcus pyogenes	Generalized punctate erythema (gooseteeth or sandpaper texture) on trunk and limbs, circumoral pallor, strawberry tongue
Stevens-Johnson Syndrome (Erythema multiforme rash)	Sulfa drugs, penicillins, Cefaclor, phenytoin	
Toxic shock syndrome	Staphylococcus aureus	High fever, headache, vomiting and diarrhea, rash, hypotensive shock

physical examination, there is erythematous maculopapular rash appearing on the face and spreading downward, low-grade fever and tender posterior cervical lymphadenopathy. Complications may include encephalitis, thrombocytopenia, arthritis or arthralgias. No specific diagnostic tests are necessary. CBC may be done to look for leukopenia and thrombocytopenia. However, any adolescent or young woman with suspected or known pregnancy should have rubella confirmed by titer.

Treatment is supportive. Patients with suspected complications of rubella should be admitted to the hospital. All other patients can be discharged home with outpatient follow-up. Care should be taken that patient's contacts do not include unimmunized pregnant women.

ROSEOLA (EXANTHEM SUBITUM)

Roseola is caused by herpesvirus-6. It usually is seen in children younger than 2 years old. Symptoms may include rapid onset of high fever followed by rash and febrile seizure. Physical examination findings include generalized, nonpruritic erythematous macular rash that appears upon defervescence (usually on day 2-3). This rash is most prominent on buttocks, back, and trunk. The child appears otherwise well: no pharyngitis, conjunctivitis, or hepatomegaly.

Diagnosis is made by the characteristic appearance of the rash following defervescence. It sometimes is misdiagnosed as a drug rash when antibiotics are given to combat the fever-producing infection. No specific diagnostic tests are necessary. Treatment is supportive. Patients can be discharged home with outpatient follow-up.

KAWASAKI DISEASE (MUCOCUTANEOUS LYMPH NODE SYNDROME)

Kawasaki disease (KD) is an inflammatory syndrome that causes a systemic vasculitis of small and medium sized arteries with predilection for the coronary arteries. The etiology is unclear; however, a wide variety of infections are associated with development of KD in children. Primarily it affects young children; 80% of the patients are <5 years.

Diagnostic Criteria

Clinical diagnosis is based on presence of fever for at least 5 days and following criteria:

- Conjunctival injection/nonpurulent conjunctivitis (red eyes)
- Oral changes: red, cracked lips/oral erythema, prominent follicles of lip (strawberry tongue), diffuse redness of oral cavity
- Cervical lymphadenopathy (> 1.5 cm in diameter)
- Polymorphous rash
- Swelling/redness of hands and feet

Typical KD has fever for at least 5 days plus meets 4 of 5 criteria. Atypical KD does not fully meet KD criteria (i.e. fever +3 of 5 KD criteria), but has evidence of coronary artery lesions on echocardiogram. Incomplete KD does not fully meet KD criteria. No echocardiogram data are implicated in this term. Infants and children >9 years often do not meet all criteria. Abnominal pain and vomiting may occur secondary to biliary obstruction.

Sometimes KD may also present with:

1. Cardiac manifestations-hypotension, tachycardia, myocarditis, pericarditis, pericardial effusion, arrhythmia, valvulitis (<1%), mitral regurgitation.
2. CNS manifestations: headaches, aseptic meningitis, acute encephalitis.
3. LN: lymph node abscess/severe adenitis, generalized lymphadenopathy
4. Lungs: pneumonitis, pleuritis.
5. Abdominal symptoms: gallbladder hydrops, noninfectious hepatitis, mesenteric vasculitis, ischemic strictures, pseudo-obstruction.
6. In subacute phase, patient may have

irritability, arthritis, arthralgias, myocarditis and more prominent desquamation of hands and feet, before gradual resolution of symptoms.

Laboratory tests that may be useful include: elevated erythrocyte sedimentation rate (ESR), leukocytosis and thrombocytosis on CBC, elevated IgE level (this test is not needed in the ED) and blood and throat cultures to identify causative organisms. ECG should be obtained to look for arrhythmias (tachycardia, bradycardia, blocks, ST changes). Chest radiograph to look for cardiomegaly and infiltrates and echocardiogram to look for valvular abnormalities and cardiomyopathy.

Differential Diagnosis

- Group A Streptococcal Tonsillitis/scarlet fever, other bacterial infections.
- Viral infections: adenovirus, EBV, other drug reactions.
- Toxin-mediated diseases.
- Leukemia.
- Macrophage activation syndrome (MAS).
- Systemic juvenile idiopathic arthritis (JIA).

Treatment

Children presenting in the acute phase should be admitted to the hospital for IVIG 2gm/kg followed by Aspirin : 20-30mg/kg 3-4 times a day. IVIG reduces risk of coronary aneurysms. Children presenting in the subacute or convalescent phase should be evaluated for development of cardiac complications, but may be discharged home with outpatient follow-up biweekly.

ERYTHEMA INFECTIOSUM (FIFTH DISEASE)

Erythema infectiosum (fifth disease) is caused by parvovirus B19.

Clinical features may include characteristic "slapped cheek" rash that progresses to erythematous maculopapular rash on trunk and extremities, and appears lace-like after a few days, arthralgias or arthritis (most often in hands, wrists and knees) and lamphadenopathy. It may cause transient aplastic crisis (TAC) in patients with hereditary hemolytic anemias or immunodeficiency, including: sickle cell disease, hereditary spherocytosis, alpha-thalassemia, autoimmune hemolytic anemia, G6PD deficiency, acute lymphocytic anemia, congenital immunodeficiency and HIV infection.

No specific diagnostic tests are necessary, but diagnosis may be confirmed by IgM-antibody assay.

Treatment

Treatment is supportive. Patients who develop TAC may require blood transfusion. Most patients can be discharged home with outpatient follow-up.

FURTHER READING

1. Burns JC, Glode MP. Kawasaki syndrome. Lancet. 2004;364:533-544.
2. Newburger JW, Takahashi M, Gerber MA, *et al.* Diagnosis, treatment, and long-term management of Kawasaki disease: a statement for health professionals from the Committee on Rheumatic Fever, Endocarditis, and Kawasaki Disease, Council on Cardiovascular Disease in the Young, American Heart Association. Pediatrics. 2004;114:1708-1733.

56

Sunit Singhi and Pratibha Singhi

Psychiatric and Behavioural Emergencies

Psychiatric emergencies are acute behavioral disturbances related to severe mental or emotional instability or dysfunction that require medical intervention. These are potentially preventable or treatable conditions that threatens the patient's own bodily integrity (by suicide, self-mutilation, or drug ingestion), someone else's bodily integrity (by assault or homicide), the patient's own psychological and functional integrity (i.e., ability to perceive reality, feel appropriately, make judgment, remember) or the psychological and functional integrity of the family unit. Since most children and adolescents are basically dependent on their parents, it is they who perceive the situation as an emergency and seek help and not the children themselves. If the parents feel too anxious or angry or inadequate to help or control the child, they may declare the situation as emergency and need immediate help.

Suicide ideation or suicide attempts are the most common childhood psychiatric emergencies, with approximately 9% of adolescents and 1% of pre-adolescents reporting one or more suicide attempts.

PSYCHOPATHOLOGY

Children often present to the emergency department in acute behavioural crisis / emotional upset arising from situational, developmental, or sociocultural sources resulting in temporary inability to cope. Most emergencies occur within the family or the school setting and often give warning signals before becoming emergent. Problems like suicide, drug abuse, aggression and conduct disorder occur commonly in dysfunctional families. The child may have some basic problems like low intelligence, specific learning disability, attention deficit hyperactivity disorder, psychosis etc. Such children may be abused, neglected, punished and condemned for their failure and consequently they develop major emotional and behavioral difficulties. In certain situations, the child is simply a victim of the external adverse circumstances such as disaster, or catastrophic events such as death of a parent or parental divorce.

The clinical presentations may take various forms irrespective of the diagnosis e.g.

1. Fits or impaired consciousness
2. Abnormal behaviour
3. Suicidal behaviour
4. Aggression and violence
5. Paralysis, paresis, loss of bodily sensations

6. Refusal to eat and severe weight loss.
7. Hyperventilation
8. Acute anxiety and panic attack.
9. Acute severe pain
10. Non-accidental injuries and neglect.

These presenting symptoms do not necessarily correspond to a specific psychiatric diagnosis. Since, most of the symptoms listed above can also occur in physical illnesses, a thorough physical examination and necessary investigations must be undertaken to rule out any underlying organic causes.

Some of the psychiatric disorders that can present to emergency rooms are:

1. Severe depression and suicidal behaviour
2. Dissociative disorders
3. Anxiety and panic disorder
4. Conduct disorders
5. Post-traumatic stress disorder
6. Drug abuse
7. Psychotic disorders.

Psychiatric causes are considered only after excluding organic causes.

EVALUATION

The goals of evaluation in emergency department are as follows:

1. Determine if behavior has an organic etiology (medical cause, Table 1)
2. Assess psychiatric manifestations of presenting condition.
3. Assess family and social situation and support.

First of all, all children should receive acute medical evaluation, including assessment of the airway, breathing, circulation, vital signs, and CNS function, an assessment for possible toxic ingestions including all possible medications accessible to the child at home or elsewhere and identification of possible toxidromes. History of potential traumatic injury, and past medical history suggestive of an organic basis for the acute emergency should be obtained (Table 1 Organic causes of acute psychiatric emergencies).

Table 1: Organic causes of acute psychiatric emergencies

Trauma: Intracranial hemorrhage

Drug intoxication: Alcohol, barbiturates, cocaine, opiates, amphetamines, marijuana, phencyclidine, anticholingergic antihistamines, tricyclics, corticosteroids, neuroleptics.

CNS lesions/infections: Meningitis, encephalitis, brain tumor, intracranial hemorrhage, temporal lobe epilepsy

Cerebral hypoxia: CO poisoning, cardiopulmonary failure

Metabolic/endocrinologic: Hypoglycemia, hypocalcemia, diabetes mellitus, adrenal insufficiency, uremia, liver failure, porphyria.

Collagen vascular diseases: Lupus erythematosus.

Miscellaneous causes: Malaria, typhoid fever, Wilson's disease

Consider laboratory evaluation if organic etiology is suspected. This should include serum electrolytes, blood glucose, plasma osmolarity, blood gas, toxicologic screen, ECG, and cranial CT scan and urine HCG in all adolescent females.

In organic disease onset is acute, vitals are abnormal and memory, intellect and orientation are impaired. In psychiatric disorder onset is often gradual, vitals are normal and orientation, intellect and memory are intact, auditory hallucination may be present.

Once the child has been medically evaluated, and organic etiologies of the mental disturbance have been ruled out, the psychiatric assessment may proceed. It should preferably be done in a quiet, undisturbed place away from the noisy distraction of the main ED. First establish rapport to develop trust. Avoid confrontation and escalation of the crisis. Psychiatric emergency services should be sought for the risk assessment of the crisis event.

Clinical History in the assessment of psychiatric emergencies should include the following

1. Chief complaint and history of present illness with attention to time of onset, duration, predisposing and precipitating factors, perpetuators, and severity.
2. Mood symptoms: Depression: irritable or depressed mood, loss of interest/ pleasure, reactivity, feeling sad, change in appetite or weight, sleep disturbance, loss of energy and fatigue, social isolation and withdrawal, poor concentration and indecisiveness, worthlessness, and feeling of guilt, low self-esteem, or feeling hopeless.
3. Mania: agitation, mood elevation, pressured speech or grandiosity
4. Anxiety symptoms: Isolated or generalized worries, phobias, panic, obsessions, compulsions, dissociations, flashbacks, and avoidance.
5. Psychotic symptoms: delusions, hallucinations-visual or auditory, loosening of associations, changed affect (flat or inappropriate)
6. Psychiatric history: Past hospitalizations, outpatient treatment, diagnoses, medications.
7. Medical and development history
8. Personal history; level of adjustment, social relations, academic performance, areas of interest and special competences, behavioral functioning, impulsiveness, substance abuse, aggression, violence, body image, eating problems, sexual orientation, personal crises of any nature, circumstances leading to shame,
9. Family history of psychiatric disorders and medications, relationships
10. Homicidality Assessment: Past or present homicidal behaviors: homicidal thoughts, thoughts about death or hurting or killing, and for how long, or previous attempts or rehearsals.

Red flags signs: possession of plan and means, such as knives, poison and firearms

ABC's of the mental status examination in the emergency department includes:

1. *Appearance:* facial expression, dress/ grooming; abnormal movements; eye contact; activity level and age appropriateness

   Affect: Depressed, blunted, flat anxious, constricted, hostile, euphoric.
2. *Behavior* (attitude): cooperative, manipulative, guarded, suspicious, angry, violent, withdrawn.
3. *Cognition:* Thought content: delusions, suicidal or homicidal; paranoia, depression, obsessions, fears, phobias; insight concerns, belief of special powers; depersonalization; feelings of helplessness or hopelessness; guilt. Thought process: coherence, goal directedness or flight of ideas, level of consciousness orientation, attention, concentration, abstraction, short and long-term memory.

DIFFERENTIAL DIAGNOSIS

Psychosis

There is major disturbances in thinking, relating, and reality testing manifesting in form of unclear expression, difficulty with direct questions, suspicious, hostile, suicidal or parasuicidal behaviour, self sleep deprivation, self-malnutrition.

Conduct Disorder

Significant behavioral disruption, manifesting as aggressiveness, stealing, fire- setting, truancy, or other forms of delinquency. Patient is angry and resentful (but may improve when behaviors not tolerated)

Table 2: Features of Agitated or Withdrawn Child

The Agitated Child	The Withdrawn Child
Anxious, upset, unresponsive	Unresponsive, quiet, non-rapport
Pacing, loud, abusive, disoriented	Clinging, whining, crying
Tantrums, crying, violent	Sullen, apathetic
Distraught, sullen, angry Improve in ED with structure	Different from shyness

Post-traumatic Stress Disorder (PTSD)

PTSD manifests in form of recurrent nightmares or flashbacks, lack of involvement in usual friendships or activities and fluctuating behavior (e.g., excitement, fearfulness, irritability). The patient can be upset or guilty, and may refuse to discuss.

Adjustment Reaction

Characteristically there is deterioration of functioning from a previously higher level because of some precipitating event or situation. The patient can usually explain the problem. The usual precipitating events are either developmental triggers such as new school, peer pressure, emergence of secondary sexual characteristics during puberty, or acute trigger such as loss of a parent through death or divorce.

Depressive Syndromes

Depressive syndromes include four categories primary depressive disorders, depression as a response to a stressful event, depression caused by a medical condition, medication, and depression coexisting with other psychiatric or medical disorders. Treatment strategies are based upon this categorization.

Depression in response to a stressful event: Usually there is history of personal crises such as parental divorce or separation, loss of a parent through death, recent setback to personal abilities (e.g. poor academic performance), peer rejection or onset of significant physical illness.

Medical conditions associated with depression are as follows:-

Neurologic: Hydrocephalus, migraine, myasthenia gravis, seizure, tumor,

Endocrine: Adrenal insufficiency, diabetes mellitus hyper/hypothyroidism, menses related, post-partum

Metabolic: Hyper/hypocalcemia, hyponatremia, uremia, porphyria, Wilson's disease

Infectious/Inflammatory: HIV, influenza, EBV, Epstein Barr Virus infections, hepatitis, collagen vascular diseases.

Medications that may be associated with depression include neuropsychiatric drugs (antipsychotics, barbiturates, benzodiazepines, carbamazepine, phenytoin), antimicrobials (ampicillin, griseofulvin, metronidazole, trimethoprim), anti- inflammatory/ analgesics (corticosteroids, opiates), antihypertensives (Clonidine, propranolol), agents used for chemotherapy, ethanol, caffeine and oral contraceptives.

Suicidal Behaviour

Depression is the strongest co-morbidity to suicide attempt. Children under 14 have a lower risk than the older adolescent. Adolescent females make three times more suicide attempts than males. Presence of a conduct disorder, substance abuse, prior suicide attempt, family history of suicide attempt, and access to weapons are other risk factors for suicide attempt.

Clinical Assessment of depression and suicidal potential may be accomplished with help of a modified SAD PERSONS Scale, which was originally developed for adult patients.

	MNEUMONIC	CHARACTERISTIC
S	Sex	Male
A	Age	<19 or >45 years
D	Depression/ hopelessness	Admits to depression, poor concentration, appetite, or sleep
P	Prior attempts/psych care	Prior in –or out-patient care
E	ETOH/drug use	Addiction or frequent use
R	Rational thinking lost	Psychosis
S	Single/separated/ divorced	
O	Organized/serious	Life-threatening presentation, careful plan
N	No social supports	No family, friends, religious associations
S	Stated future intent	Determined to repeat, ambivalent

From: Hockberger RS. Rostein RJ: Assessment of suicide potential by non-psychiatrists using the SAD PERSONS Score. J Emerg Med 1988:6:99-107.

A score>6 suggests one to one observation and acute psychiatric evaluation, a score > 10 suggest psychiatric inpatient hospitalization.

Management issues in emergency department

First assess the potential medical causes of the child's depression, with specific attention to evaluation of toxic ingestions. Hospitalization in a pediatric unit for treatment of injury or medical consequences of poisoning may be needed. Maintain suicide precautions with one to one observation until the patient has been fully evaluated. Search for possible harmful objects.

Outpatient therapy is possible if the family environment is supportive and the child is willing to engage in a contract of safety. If there is evidence of active suicidal ideation with a thoughtout plan, inadequate or unstable family support, or severe psychiatric disturbance, the child should be hospitalized for intensive psychiatric care.

Fits or Impaired Consciousness

One of the common and most dramatic presentations in ED is in form of "fits", which is characterized by a variable combination of impaired consciousness, abnormal movements or behaviour. Usually these 'fits' are episodic, lasts for a few minutes to few hours, and are interspersed with periods of recovery. The abnormal movements or abnormal behaviour does not conform to any known pattern. Consciousness is usually preserved, or impaired but not totally lost. Sometimes children present in a trance like state and do not remember some of their behaviour. They may exhibit psychosis like phenomenon like visual and auditory hallucinations, feeling of being controlled by external forces. These are known as dissociative disorders, and are seen in children who have experienced acute or chronic stress or abuse of a severe degree. If the symptoms are severe and disruptive, hospitalization is necessary. A reassuring, non-threatening and protective environment, isolation, establishing communication with the child and encouraging him/her to express feelings is helpful. Drugs have no role except for anxiolysis in patients displaying high degree of anxiety.

Aggressive and Violent Behaviour

Aggressive and violent behaviour may be a reaction of the child to interpersonal difficulties with parents, peers or teachers or may be a manifestation of underlying psychotic disorder. These children have low frustration tolerance, poor impulse control, and underlying personality difficulties. The patient who also exhibits abnormal speech, irrelevant talk, delusions and hallucinations is obviously psychotic, whereas, a child who has gross disorientation to time, and place, memory impairment, gross incoherence of speech, confusion, and ill organized, innovated acts of violence is likely to have organic brain pathology. The first task in such an emergency is to assess the risk and safety of the child and parents, and staff.

Sudden appearance of abnormal behaviour in the form of psychomotor excitement, stupor, irrelevant speech, abnormal motor movements, inappropriate acts, amnesias may occur in a psychiatric disorder or emotional stress. After the neurological causes are excluded, the possible causes of sudden abnormal behaviour include acute onset of functional psychosis, (schizophrenia), affective disorder or acute and transient psychotic disorder. In these conditions psychotic symptoms such as delusions, hallucinations, gross psychomotor excitement, stupor etc often coexist.

Management

Sometimes abnormal behaviour can occur following acute emotional stress as in dissociative disorder or post-traumatic stress disorder. Such a child is handled with psychological support in the form of reassurance, encouragement to ventilate the thoughts and feelings and positive guidance. Medication may be given as necessary to counteract anxiety or depression with short acting benzodiazepines like alprazolam or imipramine. Psychotic behaviour is managed with anti-psychotic drugs like haloperidol, resperidone, chlorpromazine. Hospitalization is needed for patients who show continuous or recurrent abnormal behaviour.

Paralysis, Paresis, Loss of Bodily Sensations

Sudden development of weakness of limbs, loss of superficial sensations (pain, touch, temperature) or of special sensations like loss of vision, hearing, smell or taste. Aphonia, mutism, agraphia, paraesthesias etc. these can be easily distinguished from true neurological syndromes by a good history and clinical examination. Sudden development of these symptoms that do not follow the known pattern of nerve distribution, based on the anatomical and functional segments of the central nervous system; and generally occur following a stressful event. These are known as a dissociative disorders (earlier called as conversion disorders). These occur generally in children who have relatively lower level of intelligence and who come from lower socio-economic status families.

Management

It should be cautious and sensitive. Such a child should be isolated and interviewed alone. Reassurance and positive suggestion, encouragement can be used to make the symptoms disappear. Drugs have no role in this situation except for using as placebo. Main mode of treatment is psychotherapy.

Acute Anxiety and Panic

Acute anxiety manifests as acute palpitation, sweating, trembling, choking, dizziness, numbness, tingling, heperventilation, fainting or acute chest pain. Feeling of unreality or depersonalization, fear of dying, symptoms may build up gradually or may start suddenly. A panic attack is a descrete period of intense fear or discomfort which builds up to its peak intensity within less than 10 minutes and is accompanied by acute anxiety symptoms, a sense of impending doom, and a desire to escape. In children it can occur as a reaction to traumatic event, (separation from parent figure) or sexual abuse. Separation anxiety is commonly seen in young children who join the school first time. Examination shows no evidence of an underlying medical disorder.

MANAGEMENT

Child should be palced in a calm, and

comfortable non threatening environment and reassured to reduce the distress. Oral or parenteral use of a short acting anxiolytic may be required for quick relief. Hospitalization may be necessary when the parents are unable to handle the problem at home. In separation anxiety disorder and post traumatic stress disorder imipramine may be used as adjunct to psychotherapy.

Acute Pain

Presentation of acute pain in any part of the body internal or external associated with emotional upset is not uncommon. Somatic pain is usually well localized, psychogenic pain is often variable and shifting in nature and is modified by situational stress and distraction. A sudden, dramatic onset of pain in the absence of a known history of physical disorder, occurring in a stressful situation is likely to be psychogenic pain. Pain may be a somatizing response to stress or an affective concomitant of stress in dissociative disorder, anxiety, depression or histrionic behaviour.

Psychogenic pains are not relieved by anti-inflammatory analgesic drugs. These may be respond to narcotic analgesics or to tricyclic antidepressants. After acute intervention, main treatment involves psychotherapy and tricyclic antidepressants.

RESTRAINT OR SECLUSION IN THE EMERGENCY DEPARTMENT

Very rarely this may be required in select cases.

Indications for the use of physical restraint or seclusion in the emergency department

1. When attempts to provide verbal restraint have been unsuccessful.
2. To prevent imminent harm to the patient or other persons.
3. To prevent serious disruption of the treatment plan or significant damage to the physical environment.
4. To decrease the stimulation a patient receives.
5. When the patient is feeling out of control and requests it.

There should be close supervision (one to one) while the patient is in physical restraints, and restraints should be assessed at least every 30 minutes and documented. Remove restraints only with adequate staff present, and when the patient has regained control either on his/her own volition, or with the use of chemical restraint (Table 3).

Table-3: Drugs of choice to use for chemical restraint

Drug	*Dose*
Benzodiazepines	
Diazepam	0.1 mg/kg PO or IM/IV, q 30 min
Lorazepam	0.05 mg/kg PO or IM/IV
Neuroleptics*	
Haloperidol	0.05 mg/kg PO or IM/IV q 30 min
Chlorpromazine	0.05 mg/kg PO or IM/IV q 30 min
Antihistamines	
Diphenhydramine (Benadryl)	10 mg/kg PO or IM/IV

*Concomitant use of antihistamine with neuroleptics may decrease the likelihood of dystonia.

For substance-induced psychosis due to hallucinogens, benzodiazepines administered at 30-60 minute are more effective. For substance-induced psychosis due to stimulant intoxication (such as cocaine or amphetamine), haloperidol may be the optimal choice.

Marcella M. Donaruma-Kwoh

57 Child Physical Abuse and Neglect

BACKGROUND

Physicians and nurses are mandated reporters of suspected abuse and neglect across the nation. Medical personnel have the obligation to notify the appropriate state agency about their reasonable suspicion of abuse and/or neglect on a patient's behalf. It is not necessary for the health professional to investigate the circumstances or identify a guilty party in such cases, but it is vital to bring these patients to the attention of an investigative authority to ensure that the child is living in a safe environment.

It is so critically important to recognize and report suspected abuse because children who are abused tend to present repeatedly for medical care with injuries that often escalate in severity. In some cases, this trend progresses to the point where a child may come to medical attention as an abuse victim only after irreparable damage or even death has occurred. It is not necessary to become accusatory or confrontational when informing a caretaker of your actions notifying protective services. Rather, explain that state law mandates the reporting of certain medical findings for all young children, and the investigation usually can corroborate a history of accidental injury if that is the true cause of the injury or condition.

Because it is quite likely that medical records will be subpoenaed for juvenile, civil or criminal court action, documentation should be thorough, detailed, explicit, and legible. Photographs and drawings are often helpful.

Overview

This chapter will focus on inflicted injuries to children that are likely to present to an emergency department. Physical abuse may include beating, shaking, burning, poisoning, scalding, or other traumas. Neglect may accompany abusive injury or present in isolation.

It is crucial to maintain a high index of suspicion for inflicted injury and to remain aware of abuse as a potential diagnosis. This happens most easily when history given by a caretaker is inconsistent with physical findings. In particular, developmentally incompatible histories (e.g., a 1 month old rolling over and falling off a piece of furniture); unexplained or multiple trauma;

alleged self- or sibling-inflicted injuries; or excessive delay in seeking medical treatment should raise suspicions about abuse.

Cutaneous Injury

Bruises and welts are the most frequent evidence of physical abuse. They can reflect the shape of the object used to hit a child and may vary in color and distribution. Bruises that are highly suspicious for inflicted injury are those which present in a non-ambulatory infant, regardless of size, shape or location. Suspicious areas for inflicted bruises are those which are naturally protected, such as the neck, oropharynx, abdomen, or the genitals and inner thighs. Additionally, sites which are often the focus of corporal punishment, such as the buttocks and lower back, cheeks and earlobes may demonstrate bruising as an indication of excessive force applied to the child's body. Also concerning is bruising present in a bilateral distribution, or distributed both dorsally and ventrally. Most falls result in a bruise on a single surface of the body.

Dating bruises is not something that can be done reliably because of the many factors which affect the appearance of a bruise, so it is not advisable to try to assign an age to bruises of varying colors. Simple description of each bruise size, pattern (if any), color and location is sufficient.

Accidental bruises, certain skin disorders, and cultural practices may be mistaken for abuse. Accidental bruises usually occur over bony prominences. The most common sites in children are on the knees and shins. Bruises on the forehead of toddlers are not uncommon. Bruises over the soft parts of the body should raise suspicion.

Child abuse is frequently a cause of pediatric **burns.** Scald or immersion burns are the most common causes of thermal injury to children who have been abused. Such injuries characteristically present during the frustration of the toilet-training years, although any age group may be affected. Immersion burns leave a characteristic stocking or glove pattern that is observed as a well-demarcated border between injured skin and normal skin, without splash or drip marks. In addition, forced immersions can cause what is called a "doughnut-sparing" pattern, in which the buttocks maintain a central island of intact skin where they were pressed against the relatively cool floor of the tub and protected from the higher temperature of the water. These types of burns are also more characteristically uniform in their depth of dermal injury than accidental scalds.

Contact burns are the second most frequent cause of abusive burns. Usually they result from contact with a hot object, such as a curling iron, clothes iron, or radiator grate, and can reflect the shape of the object. Cigarette burns are a type of contact burn and are round, sharply defined lesions with a rolled border. Accidental cigarette burns differ from those that are deliberately inflicted by demonstrating an irregular border with a "trailing" edge due to the irregular distribution of the hot ember over the skin. Burns located in body regions that are usually clothed, protected, or inaccessible are especially suggestive of abuse.

Bite marks are typically semicircular rings of abrasions. Measure the distance between the impressions from the canine teeth; a good guideline is that an inter-canine distance of greater than 3 cm is more likely to be the result of an adult bite than one from a small child.

Skeletal Injury

A child who presents with multiple fractures at multiple sites or in various stages of healing should be presumed to be abused until it is proven otherwise (Figure 1). Osteogenesis imperfecta is, after all, a rare condition. Epiphyseal-metaphyseal injury, also called a 'classic metaphyseal lesion' (CML) or 'bucket handle fracture', is virtually diagnostic of physical abuse in an infant. An infant cannot generate enough force to fracture a bone at the epiphysis. There is some evidence that CMLs can be associated with the obstetric procedure of external version of a breech fetus. This may easily be confirmed by history.

Skull fractures should arouse suspicion of abuse when found in a child less than one year of age and probably less than two years of age. While a linear parietal skull fracture may result rarely from a short household fall, any bilateral or diastatic fractures should raise concerns for abuse, as should a developmentally incompatible or inconsistent mechanism of injury.

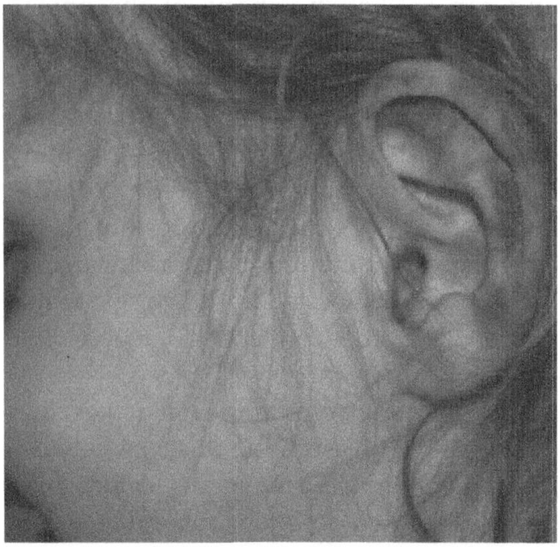

Fig. 1: Bruising in an infant. This is suspicious for abuse based on the age and limited developmental capabilities of the child

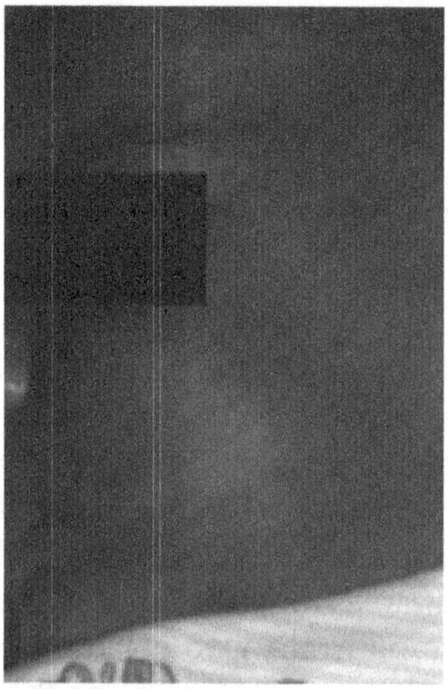

Fig. 2: Bruising over the pinna in toddler. This is both a suspicious location and an extensive bruise in a healthy child

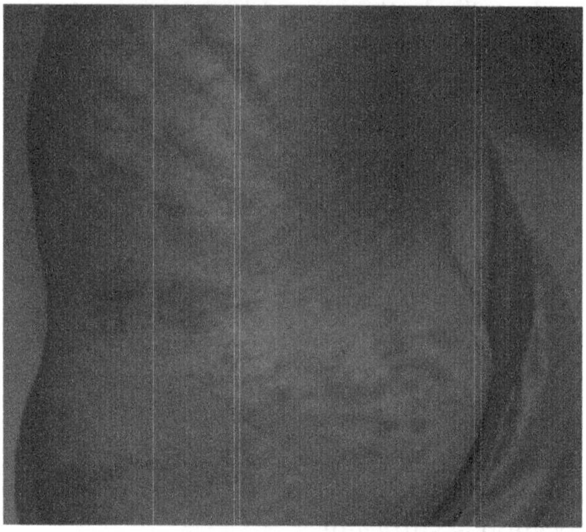

Fig. 3: Bruising over a soft area of the body that is typically protected

Rib fractures, particularly in the posterior chest, can indicate where the child was gripped during an abusive event and are often present in a succession of adjacent ribs. Like CMLs, rib fractures are highly suspicious for inflicted injury.

Figure 4 and 5 AP and lateral views of an angulated spiral femur fracture in an infant.

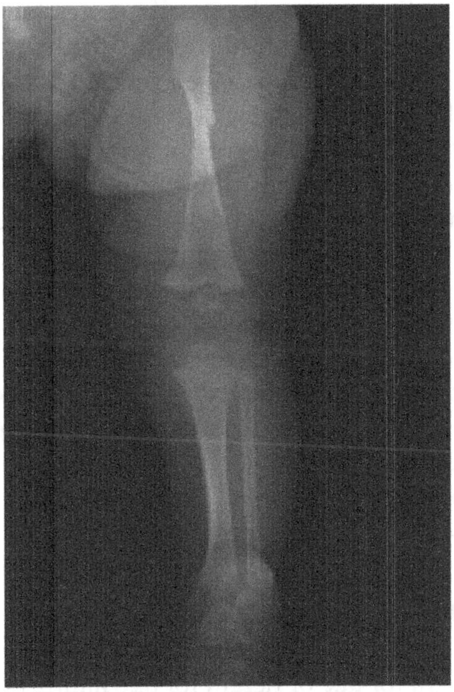

Figure 4

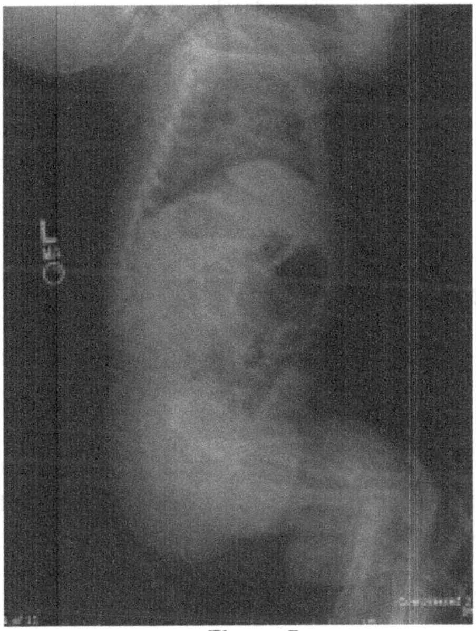

Figure 5

Inflicted Traumatic Brain Injury

Central nervous system (CNS) injury is the most common cause of death from child abuse.

Inflicted traumatic brain injury (ITBI) or abusive head trauma (AHT) is referred to as "shaken baby syndrome" in the lay press. Shaking an infant or young child is thought to produce a whiplash injury to the brain. As the infant is shaken, the head moves to and fro on the weak neck, with acceleration of the brain inside the skull, followed by sudden deceleration up against the inner edge of the skull at the end of each forward or backward motion. This may cause direct cortical injury and also can lead to rupture of bridging vessels which in turn results in subdural and/ or subarachnoid hemorrhage accumulation. Acceleration and deceleration of the brain within the skull also may cause diffuse axonal injury, which presents as loss of grey-white matter differentiation on CNS imaging with magnetic resonance imaging (MRI) or computed tomography (CT) scan.

These young children and infants may present with emesis, seizures, or an otherwise nonspecific depressed neurologic exam that is recognized only after a prolonged period of time has passed. There may be no bruises or signs of skull fracture to warn of CNS damage in a child who has suffered this type of injury.

An ophthalmologist may be able to describe retinal hemorrhages in upto 80% of cases of abusive head trauma. Commonly, retinal hemorrhages characteristic of AHT are distributed in multiple quadrants and multiple layers of the retina, and typically extend to the retinal periphery when viewed by indirect funduscopy. Retinal hemorrhages may be unilateral or bilateral.

The use of terminology such as 'shaken baby syndrome' or 'shake-and-slam syndrome' in the medical record should be avoided, because it implies that the physician knows the mechanism of injury. For clarity in documentation, it is preferable to describe the clinical picture of the infant or child.

Abdominal Injury

Abdominal injury is the second most common cause of death among battered children, after traumatic brain injury. Its incidence, while estimated as a relatively low 5% of hospitalized inflicted injury cases, also carries with it a 50% mortality rate. A perforated small intestine or pancreatic injury is the most common abusive intra-abdominal injury, and liver lacerations also occur frequently. Most injuries are caused by a blow which compresses the organ against the anterior spinal column, or causes an abrupt increase in intraluminal pressure and subsequent rupture. Unfortunately there are no visible bruises or marks on the abdomen in over half such cases. Therefore, a high index of suspicion is required in any abdominal crisis of undetermined etiology in a child. This is particularly important to remember in cases of inflicted traumatic brain injury, when it is often easy to attribute possible abdominal signs such as emesis to increased intracranial pressure, rather than the possible comorbid condition of an evolving acute abdomen.

NEGLECT

Children may also present to an emergency center with signs or symptoms of neglect. Common forms of neglect include:

1. Medical neglect, which is noncompliance with health care recommendations or non-adherence to a health care plan. This may also be manifested as a delay or failure in seeking health care.
2. Nutritional neglect is most often seen in patients who chronically suffer hunger, who demonstrate failure to thrive, or who have unmanaged morbid obesity.

Drug-exposed newborns or older children also fall into the category of neglect. Children who suffer injuries due to unsafe environments are victims of neglect as well: children with toxic ingestions, injuries related to poor firearms safety or injuries incurred due to failure to use car seats or seat belts all reflect inadequate protection from a potentially hazardous environment by their caretakers. Poor hygiene and inadequate clothing or housing can also contribute to medical problems.

Failure to Thrive

Failure to thrive (FTT) is simply growth that is less than expected. It is quantified as weight for age or height for age falling below the 5th percentile, the weight for height falling below the 10th percentile, or the weight for age falling down across two isopleths. Children's protein and energy needs are high due to their growth, and growth delay in the absence of an underlying medical condition should raise concerns about the adequacy of the child's diet.

EVALUATION

The evaluation of a suspected pediatric victim of inflicted injury varies based on the age of the child.

A **skeletal survey** should be performed on every child who is under the age of two. This is to assess for the presence of occult fractures. In children who are over the age of two, a skeletal survey may be indicated if there is localized tenderness on physical exam, or if they are developmentally delayed or non-ambulatory. A complete skeletal survey includes X-rays of the ribs (oblique views as well as AP and lateral view), shoulder girdle, hips, spine, long bones, bones of the hands and feet and skull. When arranging discharge, it is also helpful to order a follow-up skeletal survey to occur 2 weeks after the date of acute assessment. By doing so, it is possible to detect callus formation on subtle, non-displaced fractures that were undetectable at the time of initial presentation. The discovery of additional fractures often helps to support the diagnosis of inflicted injury and disproves a false history of accidental trauma.

CNS imaging with **Head CT** is indicated for every child who is under the age of one. This is done to evaluate for the presence of extra-axial bleeding and parenchymal injury. After the age of one, as the sensitivity of the neurological exam improves, a Head CT should be obtained for those children with a history or physical exam concerning for inflicted neurotrauma.

Laboratory evaluation may be tailored somewhat to the child's presentation, although in any case of suspected child abuse, **liver transaminases (AST/SGOT and ALT/SGPT)** as well as **amylase** and **lipase** measurements should be obtained in order to evaluate for possible occult abdominal injury. A urinalysis looking for microscopic hematuria can also be helpful in recognizing intra-abdominal injury, although this is a less useful test in the pediatric population than in adults.

When multiple fractures are present, a **complete blood cell count (CBC)** to screen for hematologic malignancy or disseminated infection, as well as serum **calcium**, **phosphorus**, and **alkaline phosphatase** concentrations to assess bone mineralization should be obtained. An elevation of alkaline phosphatase in the context of multiple fractures is to be expected. If rickets is suspected based on radiographic findings such as cupping and fraying of the epiphyses, demineralization, and cortical thinning, or due to certain aspects of the patient's history, such as unsupplemented breastfeeding or inadequate exposure to sunlight, then a serum 25-hydroxy-vitamin D concentration should be obtained.

In the presence of bruising or bleeding, a **prothrombin time (PT)** and **partial thromboplastin time (PTT)** are necessary to rule out major injury presenting after minor trauma. The interpretation of these studies in a severely brain-injured child can be challenging when the timeline for injury is not well-established; blood circulating through damaged brain distributes brain tissue factors which can lead to coagulation derangement. A **CBC** is also recommended to evaluate normal platelet morphology and number and again as screen for hematologic malignancy. In a child with extensive bruising and welts, a **creatinine phosphokinase (CPK)** level may also be helpful to determine the extent of injury and possible risk of comorbidity from renal complications.

In the evaluation of young infants, there are metabolic disorders which may mimic abusive head trauma. If urine and serum samples are obtained during the acute period of illness, then assessments for organic acidopathies and amino acidopathies may be performed. This determination should be made on a case by case basis.

CONCLUSIONS

A high index of suspicion on the part of the physician who must recognize and diagnose child abuse and participate with others to investigate and manage the case is vital.

FURTHER READING

1. Caffey J. The whiplash-shaken infant syndrome: Manual shaking by the extremities with whiplash-induced intracranial and intraocular bleedings, linked with residual permanent brain damage and mental retardation. Pediatrics 1974;54:396.
2. Coant PN, Kornberg AE, Brody AS, Edwards-Holmes K. Markers for occult liver injury in cases of physical abuse in children. Pediatrics 1992;89(2):274-8.
3. Dubowitz H, Giardino A, Gustavson E. Child neglect: Guidance for pediatricians. Pediatr Rev 2000;21(4):111-6; quiz 116.
4. Jenny C. Evaluating infants and young children with multiple fractures. Pediatrics 2006;118(3): 1299-303.
5. Kleinman PK. Diagnostic Imaging of Child Abuse. 2nd ed. Saint Louis: Mosby Inc.; 1998.
6. Reece R, Nicholson, Carol E., editor. Inflicted Childhood Neurotrauma. Bethesda: American Academy of Pediatrics; 2003.
7. Sugar NF, Taylor JA, Feldman KW. Bruises in infants and toddlers: Those who don't cruise rarely bruise. Puget Sound Pediatric Research Network. Arch Pediatr Adolesc Med 1999;153(4):399-403.
8. Swerdlin A, Berkowitz C, Craft N. Cutaneous signs of child abuse. J Am Acad Dermatol 2007;57(3):371-92.

In the previous edition this chapter was written by Gwendolyn Gibson, MD Assistant Professor of Pediatrics University of Oklahoma College of Medicine—Tulsa Tulsa, Oklahoma

and

Robert Block, MD Professor of Pediatrics Vice Chair—Department of Pediatrics University of Oklahoma, Tulsa Campus Tulsa, Oklahoma

Reena Isaac

58 Sexual Abuse

What was initially described a "hidden pediatric problem" in 1977 has become an increasingly unveiled entity in subsequent decades. Sexual abuse occurs when a child or adolescent is engaged in sexual activities that the child cannot comprehend, in which the child or adolescent is developmentally unprepared and unable to give informed consent, and/or when there is violation of the legal or social taboos of society. Sexual abuse includes a full spectrum of activities ranging from oral-genital, genital, or anal contact, and fondling by or to the child, to non-contact abuses, such as exhibitionism, voyeurism, or various forms of child exploitation such as pornography or prostitution. It is important to note that many forms of abuse may in fact occur simultaneously or evolve into the other forms.

As sexual abuse presents in many ways, and because the very nature of child sexual abuse results in its being cloaked in secrecy, a high level of suspicion may be required to identify and recognize the problem. The diagnosis of sexual abuse and the protection of the child and siblings from further harm depend on the physician's openness to consider abuse as a possibility. The primary responsibility of the physician is the protection of the child, and a healthy degree of suspicion of abuse to the child should prompt a report to law enforcement and / or child protective services so that further investigations can be conducted.

The time of the last incident is important information that should be obtained on initial presentation of a child to an emergency facility for alleged sexual abuse. If the incident occurred more than 72 hours prior to presentation, an appointment for evaluation can be scheduled in a more appropriate setting. If assault of a child has occurred less than 72 hours before the child's presentation, and/or the history reveals the likelihood of transfer of biological evidence from the perpetrator, forensic evidence collection is indicated. Some states and jurisdictions may have extended time allowances for forensic evidence collections, such as within 96 or even 120 hours of the last sexual contact. It is important to know such time recommendations of your community. However, recent studies of forensic collections of prepubertal children suggests that such guidelines do not suit this population, as no swabs taken from the children's bodies were positive for sperm/semen more than 9 hours after the alleged assault and the diminishing retrieval of such biological transfer evidence from the pediatric patient over time. The majority of forensic evidence was identified in these studies was identified either the child's clothing or from bed linens taken from the home by the police. Such results underscore the need for prompt collections of evidence in a timely manner. Clinical judgement and state statutes should assist in the physician's decisions in the collection of forensic evidence; however, it is always prudent to err on the side of caution. If there is physical evidence (e.g. clothing, bedding) that are not in police custody or present at the time of the child's medical evaluation, their retrieval and submission to authorities is important, as it found that there is greatest likelihood in retrieving forensic evidence from these items. If the child's contaminated clothing/linens are at home, have the parents place these items in a paper bag and the parents should bring this bag to the police themselves.

Prior to the physical examination, time should be taken to obtain a history from the child, preferably interviewing the child away from the parents. An extensive history is not required from a child who has previously disclosed, but enough information should be obtained to aid the physician in medical assessment and treatment. Disclosure of sexual abuse is a process. Commonly a child will initially give a history of minimal sexual contact, and may continue to disclose further in a continuum, disclosing more detailed information regarding the abuse in subsequent interviews. Other children may disclose fully on an initial interview. Consequently, thorough examinations need to be performed with any history of sexual abuse. In studies of legally confirmed cases of child sexual abuse, a majority of victims had no diagnostic physical findings, essentially normal physical examinations. An unbiased, neutral interview of the child, therefore, may be the most important part of the child's sexual abuse evaluation. Such an interview begins with open-ended, non-leading questions. A history of sexual abuse obtained in the course of medical diagnosis and treatment may be admissible in court as an exception to laws restricting hearsay testimony. If the child previously has given a full disclosure of sexual abuse to an experienced social worker or investigator, a physician's medical history can be curtailed to allow for determination of the tailoring of the medical evaluation, diagnosis, and management. The information should be carefully recorded, using the child's own words in quotation marks as often as possible. It is not unusual after an initial disclosure for a child to recant the history. This may be due to several reasons. The child may have received pressure from others to recant, may have become fearful from being removed from home and family, or may be overwhelmed by the consequences of the disclosure. In any case, the child's initial history should not be discounted. Document a concise history of the physical contact between the victim and the assailant. Document the presence and exchange of blood and secretions between the victim and the assailant. When closing the interview, tell the child that she or he did the right thing by telling about what happened. Assure the child that she or he did nothing wrong and is not in any trouble. This reassurance and validation may be the most important message the patient will hear during the entire evaluation.

The primary goal of the genital examination is to identify and treat trauma and other sequela of abuse and to provide physical evidence of sexual abuse. Prior to the examination, it is important to establish rapport and to comfort the child with a thorough explanation of what is about to happen in order to minimize the perceived unpleasantness of the situation and to alleviate fear. If the alleged sexual contact/abuse has occurred less than 72 hours, or there is bleeding or acute injury, the examination should be conducted immediately. Immediately assess for potential life-threatening physical trauma in addition to the sexual assault. The child's physical health and welfare takes precedence over any forensic investigation. Record the time elapsed from the assault. When the last alleged sexual contact/abuse has occurred less than 72 hours, protocols for child sexual assault victims should be followed to secure biological trace evidence such as epithelial cells, semen, saliva and blood. Maintenance of "chain of custody" is also paramount. When more than 72 hours has passed and no acute injuries are present, an emergency examination is usually not necessary. In these cases, if the parents and child agree, an evaluation may be scheduled at the earliest convenience in a more calm setting (i.e. clinic, outside of the emergency center).

To garner trust and comfort, begin with an unhurried, general physical examination, looking for evidence of related physical abuse (i.e. ligature marks, defensive wounds, bruises) or neglect. Discuss the anogenital examination before proceeding. Give an older child a choice about parental presence during this examination. It is prudent for the examiner to have a chaperone in the room during the examination.

When examining the anogenital area, position the child in a position that is comfortable for both child and examiner and that allows for the best visualization of anatomical structures. Respect the patient's modesty. Young female children are examined in the frog-leg position on the examination table. Young children may also be examined lying in their mother's or in a trusted caretaker's lap while the adult sits or lies on the examination table. A prepubertal girl's genital anatomy is diagrammed in Figure 1. Adolescent females may be examined in the lithotomy position. Confirmation of positive forensic findings of hymenal injuries secondary to trauma includes (1) examining the patient in a second position (i.e. knee-chest), or (2) the use of swabs or foley catheter to indicate interruption of tissue. The male genitals may be examined with the patient lying supine or standing. Signs of trauma should be carefully documented by detailed diagrams illustrating the findings or by photodocumentation. It is essential to have an adequate strong light source and magnification for a proper examination. A colposcope is ideal but not necessary. Colposcopy does not significantly increase the recognition of physical findings that are diagnostic of sexual abuse; however, it is an excellent tool for magnification of the anatomy and affords superb photo documentation of the examination. The latter's use allows for peer review on concerning or questionable examinations without having the child return for a repeat examination. In addition, it allows photodocumentation of forensically abnormal examinations and the subsequent chronicling of healing injuries. A speculum exam is not

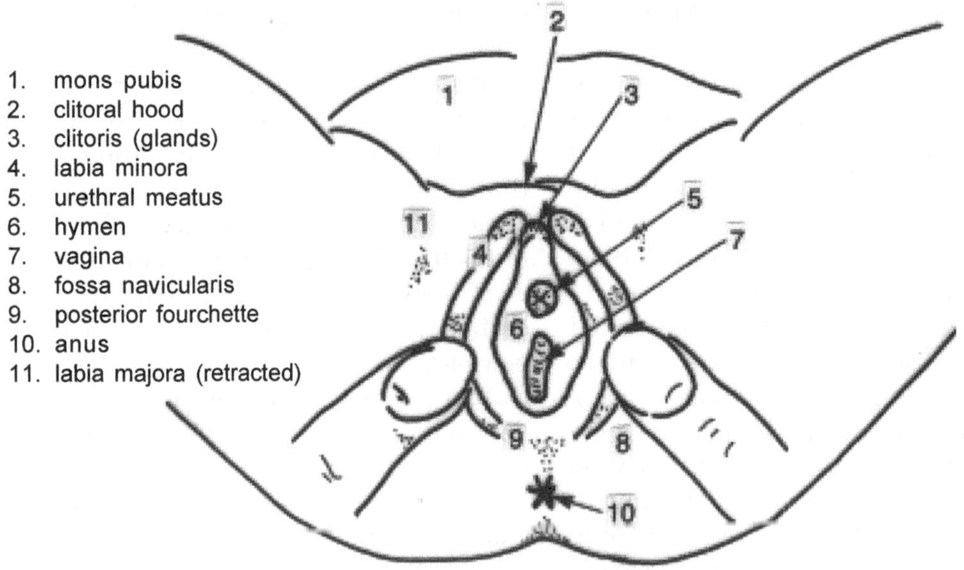

Fig. 1: Female child genital anatomy.

recommended for prepubertal children unless there is severe bleeding and intravaginal lacerations are of concern. In cases where one suspects severe vaginal lacerations, surgery or gynecology consultations should be contacted and the child should be examined under sedation. When the child is unable to cooperate and the examination must be performed because of the likelihood of trauma, infection, and/or the need to collect forensic samples, the use of sedation must be considered.

When the clinician is examining boys for possible sexual abuse, the oropharynx should be carefully examined for signs of trauma and/or infection. The penis should be inspected for signs of trauma, and the urethra carefully inspected for inflammation, bleeding or discharge. To examine the anus, the child may be placed in the lateral decubitus position or the supine, knee-chest position. Findings that are diagnostic of trauma and/or sexual contact include tears, abrasions, or scars of the anus; bleeding; discharge; or semen. Anal findings are very difficult to interpret, however, unless there is acute trauma. An acutely assaulted child or adolescent may demonstrate fresh lacerations, bruising, and hymenal tears with or without bleeding and discharge. Physical signs of chronic abuse may include missing or interrupted hymenal tissue, scarring; and discharge. The size of the hymenal opening is of negligible forensic value. It varies with age and the degree of relaxation of the child, the amount of labial traction used, and the shape of the hymen itself. Pregnancy and the identification of sperm found in specimens taken directly from the child's body are diagnostic of sexual contact. Ultimately, however, most often the physical examination will be normal, even with a clear history of penetration given by the child. Consequently a normal physical examination does not negate a history of sexual abuse. In contrast, a child may present with clear evidence of anogenital trauma without an adequate history. It is important to also note that abused child may initially deny abuse. A report to child protective services is necessary in these situations given the strong suspicions and indications.

Certain conditions may be mistaken for sexual abuse. Lichen sclerosis et atrophicus and labial adhesions are two. Nonabusive causes of vulvovaginitis may be a foreign body, a chemical irritation, or infections such as 13 hemolytic streptococci, salmonella, shigella, yersinia, and candida, or irritation. Diffuse erythema of the anogenital region is therefore a nonspecific finding. The differential diagnosis of genital trauma also includes accidental injury (i.e. straddle injury) and physical abuse. This distinction may be difficult and requires a careful history and possibly a multidisciplinary approach. Because many congenital malformations and infections or other causes of anogenital abnormalities may be confused with abuse, recognition and awareness of these other causes is important.

The extent to which a child victim of suspected sexual assault should be medically evaluated for the presence of sexually transmitted infections (STIs) should be determined on a case by case basis and based on the events of the assault, the child's age, the presence of symptoms, the prevalence of a STI in a community and any information available on the risk status of the perpetrator. The yield of positive cultures is very low in asymptomatic prepubertal children, especially those whose history indicates fondling only. The general rule that STIs beyond the neonatal period are evidence of sexual abuse has its exceptions. For example, rectal or genital chlamydial infections in young children might be the result of perinatally acquired infection, and has, in some cases, persisted for as long as 2-3 years. Genital warts have been diagnosed in children who have been sexually abused, but also in children who have no other evidence of sexual abuse. The possibility of sexual abuse should be strongly considered if no conclusive explanation for nonsexual transmission of a sexually transmitted infection can be identified. The Centers for Disease Control and Prevention and the AAP also provide recommendations on laboratory evaluation (Table of Suspicion/Diagnostic/Report MMWR).

When confronted with a child victim of an alleged sexual assault, the initial examination includes:

- Visual inspection of the genital, perianal, and oral areas for genital warts and ulcerative lesions.
- Cultures for *N. gonorrhoeae* specimens collected from the pharynx and anus in both boys and girls, the vagina in girls, and the urethra in boys. Again, culture of each is based on the circumstances as detailed by history. Cervical specimens are not recommended for prepubertal girls.
- Cultures for *C. trachomatis* from specimens collected from the anus in both boys and girls and from the vagina in girls. The likelihood of recovering chlamydia from the urethra of prepubertal boys is too low to justify the trauma of obtaining an intraurethral specimen. Pharyngeal specimens for *C. trachomatis* are not recommended for either sex because the yield is low, perinatally acquired infection may persist beyond infancy, and culture systems in some laboratories do not

distinguish between *C. trachomatis* and *C. pneumoniae*.

- In adolescents, nucleic acid amplification tests offer advantages of increased sensitivity if confirmation is available. If a nonculture is used, a positive test result should be confirmed using a second FDA-cleared nucleic acid amplification test that targets a different sequence from the initial test.
- Culture and/or wet mount of a vaginal swab for *T. vaginalis* infection.
- Collection of a serum sample to be used as a baseline for comparison with follow-up serologic tests. Sera should be tested immediately for antibodies to sexually transmitted agents. Agents for which suitable tests are available include *T. palladium* (Rapid Plasma Reagin (RPR), HIV, and HBV).

HIV infection has been reported in children whose only known risk factor was sexual abuse. Serologic testing for HIV infection should be considered for abused children. In circumstances in which transmission of syphilis, HIV, or hepatitis B is a concern but baseline tests are negative, an examination approximately 6 weeks, 3 months and 6 months after the last suspected sexual exposure is recommended to allow time for antibodies to infectious agents to develop.

When considering HIV Postexposure Prophylaxis (HIV PEP), in children that present within 72 hours of a sexual assault the following must be followed:

- Review HIV/AIDS local epidemiology and assess risk for HIV infection in the assailant.
- Evaluate circumstances of assault that might affect risk for HIV transmission.
- Consult with a specialist in treating HIV-infected children if PEP is considered.
- If the child appears to be at risk for HIV transmission from the assault, discuss PEP with the caregiver, including its toxicity and unknown efficacy.
- Perform HIV antibody test at original assessment, 6 weeks, 3 months, and 6 months.

The risk for a child's acquiring an STI as a result of sexual abuse has not been determined; however, it is believed to be low in most circumstances. Presumptive treatment for prepubescent children is not widely recommended because girls are at a lower risk for ascending infection than adolescent or adult women, and regular follow-up usually can be ensured. Patient or caregiver concerns may be an appropriate indication for presumptive treatment in some settings (provided that all specimens relevant to the investigation have already been collected). Adolescent victims should be offered STI prophylaxis for gonorrhoea, chlamydia, trichomonas, and bacterial vaginosis. (MMWR).

A follow-up medical visit approximately 2 weeks after the most recent sexual exposure should include a repeat physical examination and collection of additional specimens. To allow sufficient time for antibodies to develop, another follow-up visit approximately 12 weeks after the most recent sexual exposure may be necessary to collect sera (HIV, RPR, HBV).

Testing for pregnancy on the initial examination, discussion and offering of pregnancy prophylaxis, and a follow-up exam 2 weeks after the most recent sexual exposure that also includes a test for pregnancy should also be addressed in these cases.

When there is a concern for a possible drug-facilitated sexual assault (i.e. "I was at a party, I drank a Coke, and I don't remember anything after that"), necessary laboratory testing of specimens should be prompted when such history. "Date Rape" drugs (e.g. gamma hydroxybutyrate (GHB), GHB metabolites, rohypnol, ketamine) must be specifically ordered for the hospital lab, if such drugs are suspected. Blood and a refrigerated urine specimen sample should be included in the forensic evidence collection kit for processing by the crime lab. Positive results of these specimens are most likely when the child presents soon after an assault (less than 72 hours).

Physicians who see children who have been abused may be called as expert witnesses in court. Although court appearances are often seen by some doctors as time-consuming, frustrating experiences, failure to perform this role with the same professional abilities as are used in the medical environment can result in an unjust outcome for the patient. Physicians asked in court for opinions, explanations and conclusions, rather than merely a recitation of findings, will be qualified as experts. A pretrial conference with the appropriate attorney is helpful to both the doctor and the lawyer. Most courts will respect a cooperating physician's busy schedule and will place doctors on call for a targeted time.

REFERENCES

1. American Academy of Pediatrics, Committee on Child Abuse and Neglect and Kellogg, N. Clinical report: The evaluation of sexual abuse in children. *Pediatrics* (2005); 116(2): 506-512.
2. Adams JA. Approach to the Interpretation of Medical and Laboratory Findings in Suspected Child Sexual Abuse: A 2005 Revision. *The APSAC Advisor* 2005; 7-12.
3. Adams JA, Harper K, Knudson S, Revilla J. Examination findings in legally confirmed child sexual abuse: It's normal to be normal. *Pediatrics* 1994; 94: 310-317.
4. Bays J, Jenny C. Genital and anal conditions confused with child sexual abuse trauma. *Am J Dis Children* 1990; 144: 1319-22.
5. Centers for Disease Control and Prevention. Sexual Assault or Abuse of Children. MMWR 2006; 55 (RR-11): 83-86.
6. Christian CW, Lavelle JM, De John AR, Loiselle J, *et al.* Forensic evidence findings in prepubertal victims of sexual assault. *Pediatrics* 2001; 106: 100-104.
7. Heger A, Ticson L, Velasquez O, Bernier R. Children referred for possible sexual abuse: Medical findings in 2384 children. *Child Abuse & Neglect* 2002; 26: 645-659.
8. Kellogg ND, Menard SW, Santos A. Genital anatomy in pregnant adolescents: "Normal does not mean 'nothing happened'." *Pediatrics* 2004; 113:e67-e69.
9. Kellogg ND, Parra JM, Menard S. Children with anogenital symptoms and signs referred for sexual abuse evaluations. *Arch Pediatri Adolesc Med* 152:634-641.
10. Kempe CH. Sexual abuse, another hidden pediatric problem: The 1977 C. Anderson Aldrich Lecture. *Pediatrics* 1978; 62(3): 382-9.
11. McCann J, Miyamoto S, Boyle C, Rogers K. Healing of hymenal injuries in prepubertal and adolescent girls: A descriptive study. *Pediatrics* 2007; 199(5): e1094-e1106.

In the previous edition this chapter was written by Gwendolyn Gibson, MD Assistant Professor of Pediatrics University of Oklahoma College of Medicine—Tulsa Tulsa, Oklahoma

and

Robert Block, MD Professor of Pediatrics Vice Chair—Department of Pediatrics University of Oklahoma, Tulsa Campus Tulsa, Oklahoma

59 Approach to Poisoning in Children

Sunit Singhi

Poisoning is an important emergency encountered in children. Fortunately diagnosis is not usually a problem; most acute pediatric poisonings are witnessed or strongly suspected on presentation. Unsuspected poisoning may be very difficult to diagnose; physicians must keep intoxication in the differential diagnosis whenever a case is complex or confusing (Table 1), especially when life-threatening symptoms or multiple organ systems are involved.

Therapy should be rational and systematic but individualized; a "cookbook" approach is inappropriate. Assessment of severity is very important. Most poisonings are inconsequential, requiring only observation or minimal therapy, but some can

Table 1: Frequency of agents causing severe poisoning requiring hospitalization at PGIMER and other STATES.

POISON	*PGIMER 1970-79 (n=83)*	*PGIMER 1980-88 (n=217)*	*DELHI 1990-94 (n=213)*	*RAJASTHAN 1991-95 (n=1051)*	*TRIVANDRUM 1990-94 (n=933)*
Kerosene	42%	25%	54.9%	43.2%	30.9%
Barbiturate	12%	12%	-	-	-
Pnenothiazine	8%	6%	-	-	-
Organophosphates	7%	10%	2%	3.8%	9.2%
Opium	6%	4%	-	-	-
Corrosive	4%	6%	3%	4.3%	9.3%
Alum. Phosphate	0%	13%	-	1.6%	-
Iron	0%	5%	-	-	-
Atropine/dhatura	0%	2%	-	-	-
Others	0%	16%	15%	11.9%	13%
Drugs	-	-	23.4%	7.9%	29%
Plant toxin	-	-	1.8%	4.3%	7.8%
Food poisoning	-	-	-	17.6%	-
Animal bite	-	-	-	5.4%	-

be life threatening. In serious cases, supportive care takes precedence; if vital functions are sufficiently supported, most patients will recover. In other words, treat the patient, not the poison. Measures for decreasing absorption and/or increasing elimination of toxins are often helpful. Specific antidotes can be lifesaving when they are available. Reference sources (literature, consultant, poison information centers, and so forth) should be readily available and consulted routinely. Many poisons are encountered only rarely.

EPIDEMIOLOGY

Available literature indicates that poisonings constitute 0.33% to 7.6% of total hospital admissions in India. Accidental poisoning is commonest in young preschool children, 80-90% of reported cases being under the age of 5 years. Intentional poisoning is rare in this age group. Age related curiosity and exploratory behaviour puts this group at high risk for poisoning. Male gender, children from lower socio-economic status and psychologically stressed families are more prone to poisoning. In older children poisoning is generally intentional comprising about 10-15% of childhood poisoning. Agents commonly for poisoning in Indian children are shown in table 1.

Most acute pediatric intoxications occur in defined subgroups. These groups differ in clinical presentation and potential for morbidity and mortality.

The largest group consists of children under five years of age, usually presenting with accidental ingestions. Substances ingested are usually therapeutic drugs, common household substances, or environmental agents such as plants. Fortunately, large amounts of the toxic agent are rarely ingested unless it has a pleasant taste or the toddler is fed by an older child. Serious effects are usually limited to agents with high intrinsic toxicity. Child abuse should be suspected in atypical cases.

A second group consists of patients of any age with iatrogenic toxicity. Exposures are usually relatively benign except for a few highly toxic drugs (for example, theophylline, digitalis). It is important to keep in mind, however, that children often are treated with over-the-counter substances, home remedies, or folk medicines. Inquire about *all* treatment given, including over-the-counter and home remedies.

The last group consists of adolescents attempting suicide. Such intoxications are often difficult to manage. Large amounts of lethal substances may be ingested. History may be unavailable or unreliable. Patients may be uncooperative or actively resist therapy. Suicide gestures may prove lethal since the toxicity of readily available substances (for example, aspirin and acetaminophen) may not be appreciated. When dealing with suicide attempts, presume the worst.

MANAGEMENT

Poisoning is always a medical emergency and steps in initial stabilization should be similar to any other emergency. Management should proceed in the following order:

1. First aid and Emergency stabilization: Ensure airway-patency, breathing and circulation.
2. Clinical evaluation: Rapid identification of poison, if possible.
3. Removal and prevention of further absorption.
4. Use of antidote.
5. Enhancement of elimination.
6. Supportive therapy.

7. Symptomatic therapy.
8. Monitoring.

A general approach to a child with ingestion of an unknown substance is given in Figure. 1.

STABILIZATION PHASE

Emergency cardiorespiratory stabilisation and basic life support must precede any diagnostic steps in the poisoned child. Attention to standard ABC's of resuscitation must receive utmost priority at all times.

A. Airway and breathing: Failure to maintain a patent airway in a poisoned child may be due to increased secretions and CNS depression [e.g. organophosphates, opiates]. Respiratory failure may be due to respiratory centre depression [opiods] or failure to maintain reasonable gas exchange [tricyclic antidepressants].Airway maybe needed at times for prevention of aspira-tion. Airway patency measures include proper positioning, ensuring a patent oropharyngeal nasophary ngeal airway, suctioning whenever needed, endotracheal intubation, and if necessary tracheostomy. Early elective intubation is better because the poisoned patients are at a high risk for progression of respiratory failure. Rapid sequence intubation is the preferred method of intubation because it produces the highest success rate coupled with lowest complication rate. Some of the precautions that need to be kept in mind during RSI are adequate pre-oxygenation and

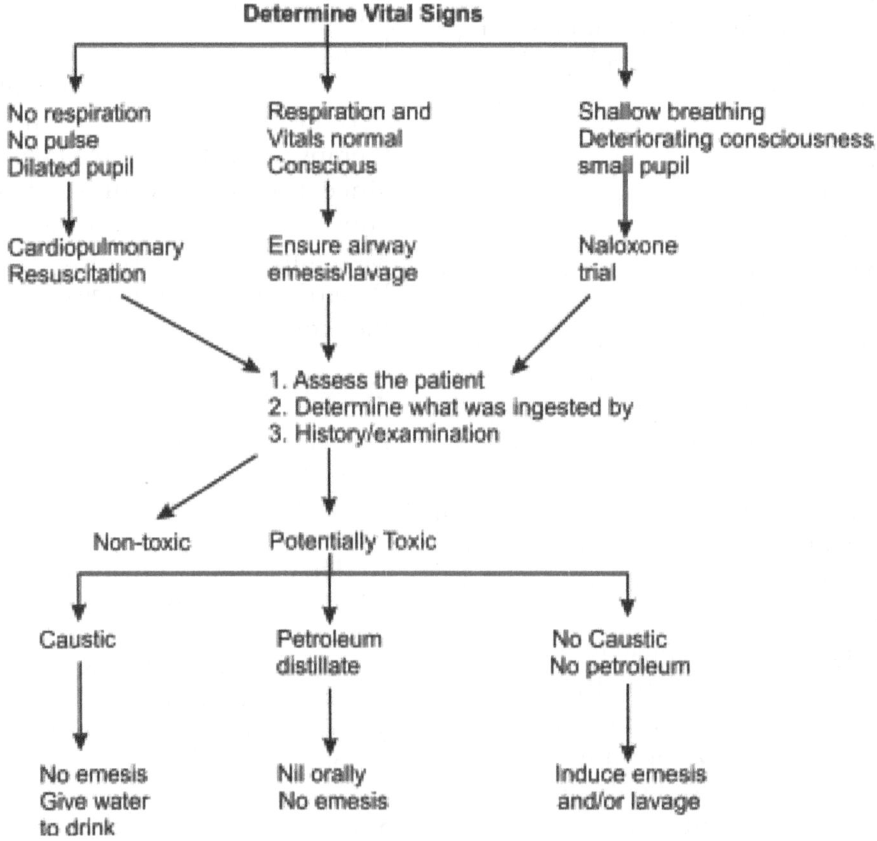

Fig. 1: General approach to a child with ingestion of an unknown substance

avoidance of hypercapnia, minimizing the risk of aspiration and choosing sedative drugs appropriate to the cardiovascular status of the child. Oxygen support and ventilatory support should be provided if there are signs of respiratory failure or shock.

B. Circulation: Shock secondary to critical poisoning results from decreased intravascular volume, decreased systemic vascular resistance, myocardial depression or combination of factors.

Initial treatment is always optimization of preload. Vasoactive agents are indicated for shocks that persist even after adequate volume loading.

Initial treatment for toxin-induced hypotension consists of fluids and Trendelenburg positioning. Should fluid therapy fail, vasopressors may be necessary, using appropriate monitoring devices to guide therapy. Many toxins (notably tricyclic antidepressants) deplete norepinephrine stores in autonomic ganglia and blood vessels; thus indirect-acting agents such as dopamine and phenylephrine may be less effective than usual. Norepinephrine is the preferred vasopressor for such patients. Hypo- and hyperthermia may produce hypotension and can best be corrected with physical measures. If hypotension cannot be reversed by the previously mentioned therapy, inotropic agents such as epinephrine, dobutamine, calcium (for calcium channel blocker toxicity), and/or glucagon (especially for beta-blocker and calcium channel blocker effects) should be considered. Digitalis should be avoided.

Control of cardiac dysrhythmias, usually seen in adolescents with suicidal ingestions and in children who have ingested cardioactive drugs, is important in preserving circulation. Hypoxia must be corrected first if possible; if dysryhthmias persist, pharmacologic intervention and correction of electrolyte or metabolic factors are required. Hemodynamically significant bradycardias are treated with atropine, or electrical pacing. Supraventricular tachydysrhythmias may be controlled with vagal maneuvers, adenosine, beta-blockers, alkalinization (for cyclic antidepressants), physostigmine (for severe anticholinergic toxicity. Digitalis, cholinergic agents, and vasopressors should be avoided. Ventricular dysrhythmias may be controlled with lidocaine, phenytoin (especially for cyclic antidepressant and digitalis-induced dysrhythmia), or alkalinization (cyclic antidepressants). Other drugs should be avoided. Correction of hypomagnesemia may be very helpful, and magnesium may be a useful agent for ventricular dysrhythmia (especially for *torsades de pointes,* often drug-induced). A significant dysrhythmia occurring in the setting of digitalis intoxication is an indication for digitalis Fab (Fragment antigen-binding) fragments.

Hypertension, which may be life threatening in certain intoxications (sympathomimetics, MAO inhibitor interactions) is best controlled by alpha- and betablockade. Pure beta agents are theoretically hazardous since unopposed alpha effects may occur. Nitroprusside may also be used, and calcium channel blockers are theoretically attractive but unproven in this setting.

Seizures are common serious manifestations of intoxications, and toxic causes should always be considered when evaluating a seizure. Treatment is similar to that of status epileptic us from other causes. Phenytoin may not have its usual effectiveness when used for toxin-induced seizures, notably theophylline, cyclic antidepressants, and salicylates. Benzodiazepines and barbiturates tend to retain their efficacy, but some toxic seizures may require general anesthesia. Alkali therapy should be given much more freely if the seizure was caused by cyclic antidepressants or salicylates; these agents penetrate the CNS (central nervous system) and myocardium much more readily in conditions of acidemia, increasing toxicity. Finally for refractory seizures, consider isoniazid-induced seizures, which may respond only to pyridoxine therapy.

DIAGNOSIS

History

If poisoning is definite or strongly suspected, the history (Table 2) can be focused to answer three questions: (1) What substance was involved? (2) How much was involved? (3) When did the exposure occur? Efforts should be made to obtain information from parents, siblings, or caretakers. The substance, in its original container, should be brought in for inspection. If it is not available, knowledge of its intended use may suggest its composition. Determining where the child was last seen and what medications or household or industrial products are in the home (particularly what substances or materials were used in the past 24 hours) may provide identification clues. When history is unavailable or inadequate, the clinician must presume a worst-case scenario.

Table 2 : Symptoms and signs helpful in diagnosis of poisoning

1. **CNS Signs**
   Delirium/hallucinations: Antihistamines, dhatura, atropine and related drugs, psychomimetics, bromides, salicylates, pesticides.
   Depression/coma: Barbiturates and other sedatives, hypnotics, tranquilliser, opiate group, organic solvents, carbon monoxide, cyanides.
   Convulsions: Organophosphates, organochlorines, phenol, amphetamine, atropine, kerosene, aminophylline, benzylebenzoate, salicylates, strychnine.
   Weakness or paralysis: Lead, arsenic, botulism, organic mercurials, tri-ortho cresyl phosphate, pesticides.
   Fasciculation's: Organophosphates
   Dilated pupil: Atropine group, Cocaine, Nicotine
   Small pupil: Opiate group, phenothiazines, Organophosphates
2. **Respiratory Signs:**
   Resp. difficulty: Organophosphate-insecticides, salicylates, botulism, carbon monoxide, cyanides, atropine.
   Cyanosis without respiratory distress: Methemoglobinemia
3. **Temperature abnormality**
   High fever: Salicylates, anticholinergic, atropine, organophosphates, nitrophenols, kerosene, paracetamol.
   Hypothermia: Opiates, barbiturates.
4. **CVS findings**
   Hypotension: b blockers, sedatives, hypnotics or narcotic
   Hypertension: Amphetamine or sympathomimetic overdose, sedative or narcotic withdrawal.
   Bradycardia: Digitalis, b-blockers, calcium channel antagonists, hypothermia
5. **Typical Odors:** Kerosene, Bitter Almond-Cyanides, Garlic- parathion, organophosphates, phosphorus, alcohol, paraldehyde, phenols and cresols, sulfides.

The important points in the history critical for assessment of patient with suspected poisoning are as follows:

(i) Age of the patient may suggest likelihood of accidental vs intentional poisoning.
(ii) History of available drugs/medications like aspirin, dapsone, iron etc.
(iii) History of chronic medical illnesses in the family members. This will give a clue to the classes of drugs available in the household. e.g.: dapsone for skin disorders; iron supplements during pregnancy and antidepressants for psychiatric illnesses.

(iv) Time of exposure, quantity of exposure
(v) Time of onset of symptoms with detailed symptomatology.
(vi) Complete circumstantial history elaborating on
- What the child was doing at the time of ingestion.
- Things /drugs/household products found at the scene.
- Approximate quantity ingested.
- Leftover of medications/drugs/household products.

Focused Physical Examination/ Toxidromes

The emergency physician should perform a rapid cardiopulmonary assessment to detect any abnormalities in the ABC's. Physical finding beyond those detected by the rapid cardiopulmonary assessment may have particular value and diagnostic significance. A constellation of characteristic clinical signs and symptoms of a specific poisoning or toxin is called a toxidrome. Some of the well known toxidromes are listed in Table 2. Many commonly ingested agents have low toxicity (Table 3).

Table 3: Common Ingestion of low toxicity

No treatment required	
Bar Soap	Lipstick
Dry Cells	Newspaper
Candles	Pencil
Chalk	Shampoo
Clay (modelling)	Shaving Cream and Lotions
Crayons	Shoe Polish
Dehumidifying packets	Striking surface of matches
Detergents	Sweetening agents
Hand lotion and creams	Thermometer
Ink	Toothpaste
Removal necessary only if large amounts ingested	
After-shave lotion	Body conditioners
Colognes	Deodarants
Fabric softners	Hair dyes
Hair Tonic	Marker Ink
Match Stick > 20	Oral Contraceptive
Perfumes	Toilet Water

Contd.

Reassessment at appropriate intervals is important; many toxins have a delayed onset of action. A period of observation is necessary for almost all toxic ingestions even if the initial examination is normal. For young children with seemingly benign ingestions, home observation is appropriate if the parents are reliable.

Diagnostic Studies

Routine toxicologic screens seldom add information to that already available from history and clinical findings. Laboratory evaluation may be helpful but has significant limitations. Simply detecting a drug on a "tox screen" does not mean that the substance detected is responsible for the patient's condition. Furthermore drug screening is not all inclusive; it is not possible to test for every potentially toxic substance. Laboratories vary in methods used and in technical expertise. Interpretation of results requires clinical correlation and judgement, and overreliance on drug screens should be avoided.

Appropriate use of the laboratory requires knowledge of specific tests to order, whether quantitative or qualitative results are needed, and what type of specimen (blood or urine) should be obtained. In general when the determination of the presence of a substance is the goal, urine screens are used since most substances have a much higher concentration in the urine than in the plasma. When determination of quantity is important, blood is preferred. Other specimens are of little value in the usual situation.

Serum concentrations of specific drugs like anticonvulsants, aspirin, paracetamol and digoxin may guide in the management wherever toxic ingestions of these drugs are suspected. Aspiration pneumonia and non - cardiogenic pulmonary edema can be diagnosed on a chest radiograph. Certain mediations such as iron, other heavy metals and enteric coated capsules might be seen on abdominal radiographs.

For serious poisoning general laboratory test are often needed. An arterial blood gas can give valuable information and help in differentiating a normal anion gap acidosis from a wide anion gap acidosis. Increased anion gap acidosis is suggestive of the presence of organically active acids, which can occur with toxin like salicylates, iron, isoniazid, methanol and cyanide. Serum osmolarity allows detection of an "osmolar gap" and rough calculation of the concentration of osmotically active substances (sugars and alcohols). This is especially helpful when ethylene glycol or methanol levels are unavailable.

Blood glucose, serum electrolytes, serum creatinine and liver function tests can assist in indirect evaluation of the end organ effects of the toxin. Electrocardiogram may be useful in detecting cardiac dysrhythmias (e.g. TCA poisonings).

Abnormal hemoglobins (methemoglobin, carboxyhemoglobin) may produce a "satiuration gap" (calculated arterial oxygen saturation minus the measured arterial saturation. Finally, hepatic and renal function tests estimate capacity to metabolize toxins and/or to determine whether the toxin has damaged these organs.

Radiographic evaluation may be helpful in poisonings. Abdominal X rays may reveal heavy metals; chest X-rays show hydrocarbon pneumonitis; contrast studies detect concretions due to salicylates.

POST STABILIZATION MANAGEMENT

Post stabilization management is based on the three general principles.

- Prevention or reduction of absorption.
- Enhancement of excretion.
- Administration of antidotes.

Prevention or Reduction of Absorption (Gastrointestinal decontamination).

Syrup of Ipecac

Induced emesis is no longer advocated for treatment of the acutely poisoned patient. It is most effective when given within 30min of ingestion of low risk substances and when the victims are alert and cooperative. Danger of aspiration coupled with lack of evidence with this drug has compelled paramedics to use it only if specifically directed. Induced emesis is contraindicated in hydrocarbons and acid-alkali poisonings.

Gastric Lavage

Gastric lavage is indicated in patients who arrive within 1 hour of ingestion and in those who have massive ingestions and for those substances that do not bind to charcoal. Most of the evidence suggests that lavage does not improve clinical outcome and may be associated with increased risk of aspiration and complications. Lavage should be performed with the largest bore tube available, with patient lying on his/her side and head lower than the body, using copious amounts of fluids (10-40 litres) to dissolve and remove as much of gastric contents as possible.

Lavage is contraindicated in obtunded patients, corrosive and hydrocarbon ingestions and in patients with unprotected airway. In massive ingestions with a suicidal intent a lavage if necessary should always be done only after proper airway protection has been achieved.

Activated Charcoal

The first line therapy for significant ingestion consists of a single dose of activated charcoal in water given either by mouth or by gastric tube. The dose is 1g/kg in children up to 1 year of age, 25 – 50 g in children 1-12 years of age and 25-100g in adolescents and adults. A heaped teaspoon of charcoal slurry in about a glassful of water is adequate. Once a 'charcoal' stool is seen, it can be assumed that absorption has ceased. Some authors suggest administration of a cathartic (Sorbitol 2ml/kg, or magnesium citrate 4 ml/kg or magnesium sulfate 250 mg/kg) mixed with charcoal to facilitate GI decontamination.

A patent and stable airway must be ensured before administering activated charcoal. It should be deferred in situations where the aspiration risk is high.(e.g. in hydrocarbon ingestions). In case of toxins that slow the GI motility, charcoal may lead to complications like regurgitation. It is contraindicated in patients with ileus, intestinal obstruction, and peritonitis and in corrosive ingestions. Charcoal is ineffective for alcohol, iron, lithium, petrochemical and essential oil ingestion.

Whole Bowel Irrigation

Whole bowel irrigation is done through rapid administration of polyethylene glycol electrolyte lavage solution given via a nasogastric tube. It is indicated for the ingestion of significant amounts of iron or sustained release preparations. The end point is a clear rectal effluent that takes several hours. It is contraindicated in patients with ileus, obstruction, perforation or GIT hemorrhage.

Gastrointestinal decontamination (e.g. syrup of ipecac, toxin absorption by activated charcoal or whole bowel irrigation) has not been shown to change outcome (mortality, morbidity or length of hospital stay).

Enhancing Excretion

Techniques of enhancing excretions are used in situation where prolonged exposure to high concentrations of toxin is likely to cause hemodynamic and respiratory compromise, intractable seizures or organ failure.

Repeated Doses of Activated Charcoal

Multidose charcoal is indicated with drugs that undergo enter enteric recirculation (eg barbiturates, theophylline, carbamazepine). This technique enhances the excretion of toxins by using the gastrointestinal epithelium as a dialysis membrane. There may be complications like bowel obstruction and perforation during the procedure. Careful monitoring of bowel sounds is very essential

Forced Diuresis

Urine flow can be increased through the administration of IV crystalloids in excess of maintenance rquirement thus enhancing elimination of toxins like salicylates and barbiturates. The risk of fluid overload is high with this method. Pulmonary edema, cerebral edema and renal failure are contraindications for this technique.

Urinary Alkalinisation

Urinary alkalinisation is used to enhance the excretion of weakly acidic drugs. Alkalinisation increases the proportion of ionized drug in the tubule preventing its reabsorption. The unionized form of the drug is filtered and reabsorbed. Toxins like salicylates, isoniazid and phenobarbitone may be eliminated by this method. For alkaline diuresis urine pH is maintained between 7.5-8.5 by giving sodium bicarbonate (1-2 ml/kg).Normal saline is given at a flow rate of 30 ml/kg/hr initially usually for 2 hours till diuresis is established and then followed by 5ml/kg/hr.

Decreasing urinary pH (acidification) conversely can be used to enhance the excretion of weakly alkaline drugs. For acid diuresis pH is maintained between 4-5 with ammonium chloride (75 mg/kg/day orally or 1-2% soln. IV).This is required for toxins like amphetamine, quinine etc. The dangers of acidosis, hyperammonemia and exacerbation of rhabdomyolysis outweigh the benefit of this method and hence should be avoided.

Dialysis

Dialysis is effective if the toxin is of low molecular weight (< 500 RMM i.e relative molecular mass), highly water soluble, has a small volume of distribution (<2L/kg)and poor protein binding. Examples of toxins that can be eliminated by dialysis are salicylates, methanol, ethylene glycol, theophylline and lithium. Dialysis is useful if toxin ingestion is associated with concomitant electrolyte or acid-base disturbances (Table 4).

Hemoperfusion

Hemoperfusion is effective if the toxin has low water solubility,high affinity for the adsorbent Fast rate of equilibrium from peripheral tissue to blood, Low affinity for plasma proteins Toxins which can be eliminated by this technique are carbamazepine, barbiturates and theophylline.

Hemofiltration

Is useful for removal of compounds with higher molecular weight (>500 – 40,000 RMM). It may be beneficial in iron, lithium, aminoglycoside and theophylline overdose.

Extracorporeal drug removal (ECDR) Is effective in removing very small particles (molecular weight 100-4000) if these are water or lipid soluble. The substance is removed from blood by adsorption in an extracorporeal circuit. Adsorbent may differ depending on the nature eg. charcoal for salicylate, amberlite for lipid soluble poisons such as digoxin, and barbiturates. It is not effective in alcohol poisoning, and does not correct acid-base disturbance.

Plasmapheresis

Plasmapheresis is effective in almost all commonly ingested intoxicants. It removes plasma bound drugs by centrifugation

SPECIFIC ANTIDOTES

It is a common error to search for a specific antidote to a poison. An Antidote is available for only about 5%-10% of all poisons. The common ones are given in Table 5.

While using antidotes in a child with unknown overdose one must weigh the benefits and risks of administering a specific antidote. The basic supportive management is hence very important in all toxin ingestions.

PATIENT DISPOSITION

The final decision in poison management is whether admission or transfer is required. Most toxins will manifest toxic effects within

Table 4: Poisonings where hemodialysis/perfusion may be of benefit

Hemodialysis	*Hemoperfusion through charcoal*
Salicylates	Salicylates
Phenobarbitol	Phenobarbitol
Barbitol	Barbitol
Methanol and ethanol	Short-and medium-acting barbiturates
Ethylene glycol	Trichlorethanol derivatives
Lithium	Trichlorethanol derivatives
Isopropanol	Disopyramide
Carbamazepine	Theophyllines

Table 5: Commonly available specific antidotes

Poison	*Antidote & dose*
Benzodiazepines	Flumazenil
Carbon monoxide	Pure oxygen
Cyanide	Sodium nitrite 3% soln, 0.2 ml/kg, IV,over 2 min followed by sodium thiosulphate (25% soln, 1 ml/kg, IV, over 10-20 minutes)
Nitrate and nitrites	If meth. hemoglobinemia, treat with methylene blue
Organophosphates	Atropine- 0.05 mg/kg, IV, every 10 min until signs of atropinism. PAM 25-50 mg/kg, IV, in older children, and 250 mg IV in infants over 5-10 minutes, 8 hourly upto 36 hours
Anticholinergics	Physostigmine (0.5mg, slow IV over 5 (atropine gp)min; repeated every 10 min till a maximum of 2 mg).
Narcotics (opium)	Naloxone - 0.1 mg/kg, I.V or, intratracheal, from morphine) birth upto 5 years or 20 kg of weight, at which time a minimum of 2 mg should be used.
Phenothiazine	Benadryl (Diphenhydramine) 1-2 mg/kg (promethazine)
Iron	Desferrioxamine 15 mg/kg/hr I.V in 100-200 ml 5% glucose soln (maximum 360 mg/kg, upto a total of 6 g.)
Paracetamol	N-acetylcysteine; Oral- intially 140 mg/kg, then 4 hourly, upto 72 hours. IV-150 mg/kg by infusion over 15 min followed by 50 mg/kg 4hourly for 72 hrs
β-blockers	Glucagon
Arsenic, mercury	Dimercaprol
Methanol,ethylene glycol	Ethanol
Lead	Sodium calcium edetate
Copper	Penicillamine
Warfarin	Vitamin K

a six-hour period of observation. Some, however, will not (for example, acetaminophen), and it is imperative that it be reasonably certain that delayed effects will not occur. Other factors to consider are the accuracy of the history, the possibility of recurring exposure (for example, CO), reliability of follow-up, and availability of diagnostic and therapeutic services (for example, dialysis). Most importantly, adolescents who have attempted suicide (even as a "gesture") are at great risk for further, perhaps more successful, attempts and should have psychiatric evaluation. When in doubt, one must err on the side of admission. Should home discharge be feasible, counsel parents in prevention and first aid when such instruction is appropriate.

CONCLUSIONS

Intoxications represent a frequent serious problem for the pediatric emergency physician. Diagnosis requires skill in obtaining historical and physical findings to confirm suspected poisonings and a high level of suspicion for unsuspected ones. Determining the actual and potential level of severity of poisoning is crucial for determining treatment and disposition. Therapy begins with good supportive care. Use of antidotes and measures to decrease absorption and increase excretion are common with additional methods such as hemodialysis being used in serious cases. New concepts and therapies are being rapidly developed. Traditional methods are increasingly being questioned, and many older therapies and concepts are being dismissed. The field is rapidly evolving, and clinicians must strive to remain cognizant of current developments. For optimum results, scientific knowledge must be combined with good clinical skills.

HYDROCARBONS (Kerosene, Petrol)

This is the most common accidental poisoning in children, usually in infants and toddlers. Significant toxicity does arise from the inhalation of vapours or pulmonary aspiration of the liquid. Large amounts (100 ml or more) must be swallowed to allow GI absorption to produce pulmonary lesion.

Pathology: In the lungs it causes chemical pneumonitis characterised by hyperemia, edema, inflammation, diffuse hemorrhages and cellular infiltration which lead to hypoxia. Liver damage, cardiomyopathy, renal toxicity and GI involvement may also occur. Temperature regulations is impaired because of direct effect on CNS.

Clinical Picture

Two major system affected by hydrocarbon ingestion are the respiratory and central nervous system. Respiratory symptoms resemble bronchopneumonia (cough, breathlessness, tachypnea and fever) and may appear as early as within 15 minutes and as late as 24 hours after kerosene ingestion. Hyperexpansion of chest is seen occasionally. In severe cases hemoptysis ensues. Cyanosis is accentuated and death may follow, usually within 24 hours. CNS involvement can cause lethargy, dizziness, headache, visual disturbances and may progress to seizures, hyperpyrexia, coma, respiratory paralysis and death. Symptoms usually subside between the second and fifth day.

Radiographic Findings

Radiographic findings consist of perihilar mottling, consolidation, areas of collapse or frank pulmonary edema. Pleural effusion may develop. Rarely cysts or pneumatoceles may form. The x-ray abnormality usually clears within 7-10 days but may rarely last for months.

Approach

Record vital signs and observe for 6-8 hours. If the child is asymptomatic it is unlikely that significant problems will occur. If significant symptoms appear, the patient should have a chest x-ray. It may identify pulmonary disease not appreciated by auscultation in upto 60% cases. Liver and renal functions tests, urine analysis and electrolytes should be evaluated.

Treatment

1. Prevention of aspiration is the main goal. Do not induce emesis.
2. Lavage with a cuffed endotracheal tube in situ has been advocated in comatose patients. If large amount (1-2 ml/kg) is ingested controlled gastric emptying must be done in an alert patient by a stomach tube.
3. Instillation of oils to slow gastric emptying and decrease intestinal absorption has not proved to have practical application.
4. Specific treatment is aimed at aggressive correction of hypoxia with humidified oxygen and CPAP.
5. Prophylactic antibiotics to prevent secondary bacterial infection may be used.
6. Value of corticosteroids to prevent chemical pneumonia is doubtful.
7. Proper supportive care especially to maintain fluid balance, and prevent hypoxia.

Pneumatocele, Pneumothorax, cardiomegaly or arrhythmia may occur occasionally. Recovery is usually complete. However, pulmonary fibrosis and bronchiectasis have been known on long term follow up.

ORGANOPHOSPHATE INSECTICIDES

Common agents Malathion, parathion (fatal dose 0.1 mg/kg)

Pathophysiology

This group causes cholinesterase inhibition with resultant accumulation of acetyl choline. Toxic effects therefore mimic muscuranic, nicotinic and CNS actions of parasympathetic stimulation.

Clinical Picture

Onset of symptoms is within 12 hours of exposure; usually following a household spraying. The common symptoms and signs are dizziness, headache, blurred vision, miosis, excessive lacrimation and salivation, nausea, vomiting, diarrhoea, epigastric pain, sense of constriction around chest, dyspnea, sweating, muscle twitching and fasciculations, convulsions, flaccidity and muscle weakness, loss of reflexes and coma. Fasciculations are less common in children than in adults. Bradycardia may occur in some pediatric patients.

Diagnosis

A high index of sucpicion is needed as the history of exposure may be denied. It may be confirmed by measuring red cell cholinestrase level, which is reduced to 20% of the normal values in clinically apparent poisoning (normal range 0.6-0.9 pH lH).

Assessment

Bradin and Van Eeden have suggested a clinical grading of the patient presenting within a few hours, which may help in planning the management and predicting the prognosis. Mild poisoning normal consciousness, mild secretions and few fasciculations) suggests eventless recovery. Severe poisoning (copious secretions, generalised fasciculations, and altered consciousness) indicates the likelihood of complications and the need for ventilatilon. Life threatening poisoning, generally associated with suicide attempts, is characterised by a pO_2<75 mmHg and abnormal chest X-ray. These patients need immediate ventilatory support.

Treatment

1. Establish **airway, suctioning, and oxygen**. This is most urgent as death occurs from respiratory failure. Establish an I.V line, monitor BP, do not rush fluids.
2. **Decontamination** of the skin, mucous membrane and gut (if skin is contaminated, clean with soapy water and change the clothings; gastric lavage and catharsis if poison has been ingested).
3. **Atropine IV 0.05 mg/kg every 10 minutes** until signs of atropinism appear; maintain it for **24 hours. The signs of atropinism are:** drying of all secretions and dilated pupils. As much as 10 times of usual dose of atropine may be required.
4. Pralidoxmine(PAM) in recommended doses (Table 3) given immediately in severe cases and repeated every 8-12 hrs. The drug is probably not useful after 36 hrs. of exposure.
5. Assisted ventilation may be required in upto 25% of patients.

BARBITURATES

Toxic dose: Ingestion of more than 6 mg/kg may be toxic.

Clinical Picture

CNS symptoms range from confusion and poor coordination to delirium and coma. Respiratory depression characterised by slow, deep and irregular respirations. Pupil are dilated (may be unequal). Respiratory acidosis is common and hypotension frequently occurs. Face is flushed and congested. Bullous skin lesions are seen in 10% cases. Hypothermia is common.

Diagnosis

Diagnosis is based on the very characteristic clinical picture of flaccid coma with reactive pupils, hypothermia and hypotension and Serum levels of barbiturate >10 mg/dl. Differential diagnosis includes other causes of coma and glutethimide poisoning (pupils are dilated and fixed).

Treatment

Death may occur from respiratory failure, therefore :

1. Keep airway clear, treat hypotension and maintain ventilation.
2. If the patient is awake-induce vomiting and give activated charcoal. Gastric lavage is useful in first 4-6 hours. In a comatose child do not undertake any of the above.
3. Forced alkaline diuresis, to aim at urine pH 7.5-8.5, and a urine flow > 2ml/kg/hour.
4. Mechanical ventilation and dialysis may sometimes be required. Analeptics are contraindicated.

OPIUM AND ITS DERIVATIVES

It is fccommonly seen in infants following its use for diarrhoea or sedation.

Fatal Dose

Oral > 0.3 gm, parenteral > 0.1 g.

Clinical Picture

Typically a 'sleepy' child with constricted pin-point pupils, and CNS and respiratory depression, which may progress to cyanosis, irregular breathing, depressed tendon reflexes, coma and aspiration pneumonia. Respiratory failure may occur.

Diagnosis

Diagnosis is evident from the history of ingestion and typical clinical picture.

Treatment

1. Specific antidote: Naloxone (see Table-II), 0.1.-0.2 mg I.V repeated

ever 30 min. Response is evident by an improved depth and rate of respiration. (Pupils-do not dilate).
2. Gastric lavage with saline is indicated, even after hours of ingestion.
3. Supportive therapy requires attention to oxygenation.

ATROPINE GROUP (BELLADONA ALKALOIDS)

Effects are due to parasympthetic blockade (anticholinergic effect)

Clinical Picture

Mild cases show dryness of the mouth, hyperpyrexia and widely dilated pupils. With higher doses tachycardia, flushing of face (red, hot, dry face), hyperpyrexia, mental disturbances (delirium, hallucinations and excitation) and Cardiac rhythm disturbances may occur.

Differential Diagnosis

Encephalitis, cerebral malaria, acute meningitis, intracranial bleed. Similar symptom complex is caused by over dose of antihistamines and tricyclic antidepressants.

Treatment

1. Gastric lavage, administration of charcoal and cathartics.
2. Administer antidote, (i) Neostigmine methyl sulfate 0.5 mg- 2.5 mg IM at frequent intervals. (ii) Physostigmine 0.5 mg slowly I.V / 1.M repeated every 5 min. till a maximum of 2 mg. Current thinking is that the antidote should be used only with severe cardiac disturbances.
3. If patient is excited and unmanageable phenobarbitone 100 mg, or diazepam 0.2-0.3 mg/kg/24 hours. in 6 hourly doses.
4. Supportive therapy requires attention to airways, oxygenation, prevention of aspiration, correction of fluid and electrolyte imbalance.

SALICYLATE POISONING

Toxic Dose

Acute dosage of salicylate necessary to produce serious intoxication is in the range of 200 mg/kg. Ingestion of less than 150 mg/kg are mild, and >300mg/kg serious. Fatal period varies from a few minutes to 10 hours.

Pathophysiology

Direct effect on respiratory center causes tachypnoea, CO2 elimination and resp. alkalosis.

Salicylates (i) alters proper functioning of Kreb's cycle and causes accumulation of lactate and other organic acids. (ii) cause uncoupling of oxidative phosphorylation.

Hypoglycemia/Hyperglycemia

Bleeding- as a result of local gastric irritation, alteration of platelet function and defective prothrombin synthesis.

Hypokalemia by direct effect on renal tubular excretion.

Signs and Symptoms

Clinical features are not diagnostic, but are fairly typical. Usual symptoms are nausea, vomiting, restlessness and confusion. Tachypnea is most frequent sign. Hyperpyrexia, tinnitus, hallucinations, convulsions, and coma may also occur. Bleeding from upper GIT and generalised respiratory depression, pulmonary edema, acute tubular necrosis and hepatotoxicity, bronchospasm is uncommon.

Diagnosis is usually made by history. A rapid bedside test may be done. Ferric chloride test (10% $FeCl_3$ soln.+ few drops to urine) will give a violet purple colour on urine. Quantification of serum salicylate level is of value in assessing the severity of the poisoning.

Differential Diagnosis

Encephalitis, diabetic ketoacidosis, lactic acidosis, bleeding disorders.

Treatment

1. Induce emesis/gastric lavage with saline or weak bicarbonate solution to remove unabsorbed poison.
2. Charcoal may be given.
3. Alkalinise the urine (i) sodium bicarbonate (1-2 mEq/kg over one hour) is preferable and has added advantage of counteracting systemic acidosis. Aim for a urine pH of >7.5. (ii) Acetazolamide (5mg/kg, 2 times/24 hr) has the advantage of rapidly and consistently producing an alkaline urine, after subcutaneous administration.
4. Fluid therapy- Prepare D5W 500 ml with sodium bicarbonate 25 ml. Start at 20-30 ml/kg/hour, after the urine flow is established maintain at 5ml/kg/hour. About 2000-5500 ml/m2/2 hr. may be required, with sodium 40-50 mEq/L/and potassium 40 mEq/L. This is needed to cover increased losses. A urine specific gravity of 1010 should be the goal. If diuresis is not established after 2-3 hours consider dialysis.
5. Hemodialysis or hemoperfuslon may be necessary in unresponsive acidosis renal failure and seizures.
6. Supportive: Vit. Kl, calcium gluconat, anticonvulsants.

Monitor temperature, respiratory rate, heart rate, B.P., urine pH and specific gravity, and acid-base values.

PARACETAMOL (ACETAMINOPHEN)

Paracetamol ingestion is most often seen in children under six years of age, but overdose may also be associated with suicide attempts in adolescents. Ingestions are potentially serious, especially in adolescents.

The drug is rapidly absorbed after ingestion. It is metabolized in the liver. When the glutathione stores are approximately 70% of normal, the highly reactive metabolite binds to hepatic macromolecules, and hepatic damage ensues.

Signs and Symptoms

The clinical course has been divided into four stages:

Stage 1 (first 24 hours after ingestion): Symptoms appear within on average of six hours after ingestion, with 60% of patients symptomatic by 14 hours. Young children may have vomiting, older children -nausea, vomiting, generalized malaise, and diaphoresis. Consciousness is not impaired unless other drugs have been taken. Liver enzymes and prothrombin times are normal.

Stage 2 (second 24 hours after ingestion): It is marked by a diminution of symptoms. Liver enzymes may becomes elevated. Biochemical evidence of liver damage become apparent. Transaminases greater than 1000 IU/L indicate severe hepatotoxicity.

Stage 3 (48 to 96 hours after the ingestion): In severe intoxication fulminant hepatic failure develop at 3-6 days with deepening jaundice, coma, hyperventilation, acidosis, hypoglycemia, cerebral edema, DIC and bleeding. Serum glutamic-oxalacetic transaminase (SGOT) levels may be as high as 20,000 or 30,000 IU/L. Death may occur either from hepatic failure or coagulopathy.

Stage 4: (7-8 days after ingestion) : The hepatic abnormalities are almost resolved in survivors. Persistently high liver enzyme abnormalities are seen in relatively few patients.

Diagnosis

It often is difficult to distinguish between toxic and nontoxic overdoses by history alone. Plasma acetaminophen levels should be determined in cases with potentially serious overdoses. Once the plasma level has been determined, plot it on the Matthews-Rumack nomogram to determine whether the level in relation to time is toxic. Alternatively, draw a line on semilogarithemic graph joining 200 ug/ml at 4 hours and 50 ug/ml at 12 hours after ingestion. With values above this line there is 60% chance of severe liver damage.

Treatment

If the drug level cannot be determined in an acceptable time, initiate treatment with N-acetylcysteine (NAC). Oral NAC is available as a 20% concentrate. It has a strong smell of sulfur that is generally unacceptable to patients. Dilute the concentrate by mixing one part with 3 parts of any carbonated beverage. Use a cup with a cap and hole for a straw to avoid the smell. Dose of NAC is shown in table-II. The advantage of IV NAC is in patient acceptance and in the patient with an altered state of consciousness.

An alternative drug is oral methionine 2.5g 4 hourly upto a total of 10 g . It is unreliable.

Supportive Treatment

(i) Maintain hydration and electrolyte balance
(ii) Glucose solution as and when needed to correct hypoglycemia
(iii) Vit K or fresh-frozen plasma for clotting abnormality.
(iv) Do not use diuretics or forced diuresis.
(v) Dialysis may be associated with increased mortality.

Monitoring

Follow liver function studies- prothrombin time, SGOT, SGPT and bilirubin for at least 4 days. If there is no abnormality with in 4 days, there is no need for further follow up. Also follow electrolytes, BUN, creatinine and blood glucose in case of serious poisoning.

Bilirubin >4 mg/dl or prothrombin time ratio > 2.2 are signs of hepatoxicity. Most patients (99%) will recover within a week.

IRON

Iron ingestion is common in children under five years of age. It can be fatal if proper management is not initiated. The *lethal oral dose* is between 200 and 500 mg/kg elemental iron. Gastrointestinal symptoms can be seen at doses of 15 to 30 mg/kg. Significant toxicity is uncommon at amounts less than 50 mg/kg. The toxic dose is not absolute, and fatal reactions have been reported with small amounts. All ingestions should thus be considered potentially dangerous.

Pathophysiology

Iron directly damages the gastrointestinal mucosa and can lead to massive fluid loss and hemorrhage. In addition vasodilation caused by ferritin and other compounds released from the metabolism of iron complexes in the liver, acidosis caused by the effects of iron on oxidative metabolism, and the coagulopathy and resultant bleeding contribute to circulatory failure. Iron is rapidly absorbed and causes direct damage to the liver parenchymal cells which can lead to massive hepatic necrosis and liver failure. The GI effects may contribute to systemic hypovolemia by the third spacing of fluid in the small bowel.

Signs and Symptoms

Clinical picture and course may have distinct phases:

1. *Gastrointestinal Stage* : The early symptoms include vomiting, rapid onset of

diarrhea, colicky abdominal pain and gastrointestinal hemorrhage.

2. *Relative Stability Stage:* Reports have suggested that there is a period of relative stability beginning three to four hours after ingestion and lasting as long as 48 hours. Subtle signs such as mild gastrointestinal bleeding, hyperventilation, and poor capillary refill may exist during this stage, but may go unrecognised.
3. *Shock Stage:* The third stage is characterized by circulatory failure and profound shock. Rarely, liver failure may occur.
4. *Gastric Scarring Stage:* This late manifestation which may occur two to six weeks after ingestion and is manifested by obstruction of the gastric outlet and portions of the small bowel.

Approach to Management (Fig. 2)

Assessment : The amount of iron ingested often is hard to quantify clinically. Serum iron levels, if obtained promptly, have been shown to correlate with the likelihood of developing symptoms. Iron levels below 350 mcg/dL, when drawn two to six hours after ingestion, predict an asymptomatic course. Levels greater than 500 mcg/dL suggest significant risk for phase III manifestations.

In absence of serum iron level early clinical assessment and several simple laboratory tests may be used to predict approximate iron levels. Vomiting, diarrhoea, serum glucose greater than 150 mg/dL, white blood cell count greater than 15,000/mm^3 and the finding of radio paque material on abdominal radiograph all show a high correlation with an elevated serum iron level greater than 300 mc/dL.

Patients with severe early symptoms (vomiting, diarrhoea, gastrointestinal bleeding, depressed sensorium, or circulatory failure) require urgent, intensive treatment in the emergency. Obtain a venous access and support blood pressure with normal saline or lactated Ringer's solution. Lavage should be started with as large a bore tube as possible.

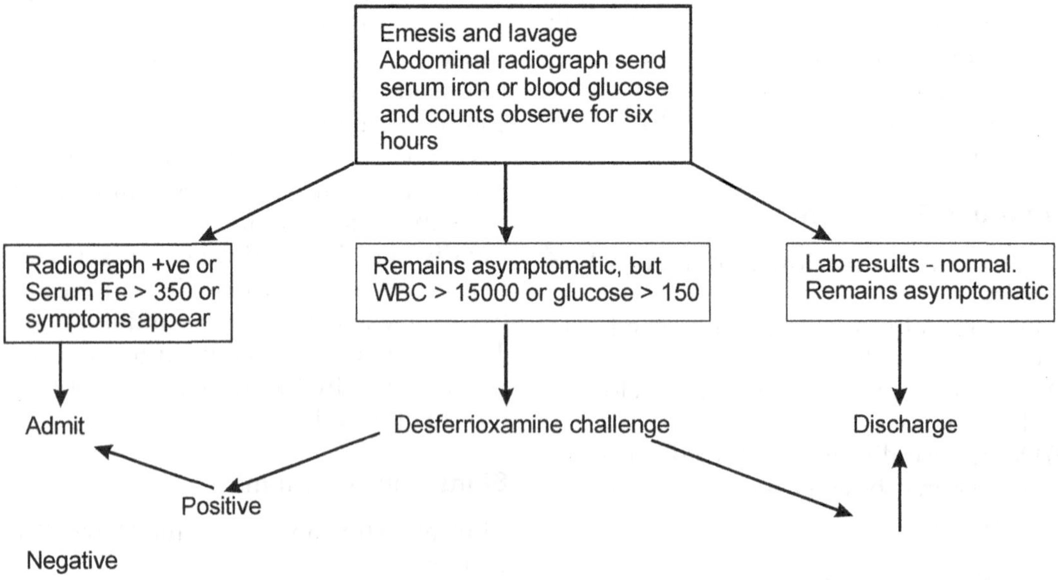

Fig. 2: Approach to a child with iron poisoning

In patients with mild symptoms (only mild vomiting and diarrhoea) emesis is induced, followed by lavage. In all symptomatic patients follow-up with a post lavage radiograph, and start specific chelation therapy as soon as possible. Blood should be drawn for complete blood cell count, blood glucose, electrolytes, BUN, liver function tests, serum iron, total iron binding capacity, and typing and cross matching.

In asymptomatic patient who has presumably ingested iron induce emesis. Obtain serum iron levels if possible, and a post-lavage abdominal radiograph. Observe the patient. When serum iron levels are not availlable on an emergency basis, a combination of the white blood cell count, and serum glucose and x-ray abdomen may be used as screening laboratory tests. Iron levels above 350 mc/dL (actual or from screening tests), the development of any symptoms, or a "positive" radiograph should lead to admission and management as described above for the mild to moderately ill patient.

Other patients should be observed for six hours in the emergency department. Those who have normal screening tests and remain asymptomatic may be discharged. Patients with abnormal screening laboratory tests should have an iron level sent for later reference, and be given a desferioxamine challenge (50 mg/kg intramuscularly up to a maximum of 1 g). The appearance of a pinkish to orange color to the urine indicates the presence of iron-desferioxamine complex. These patients need admission and further treatment as given below. Others who remain asyptomatic after six hours, and have a negative challenge, may be discharged.

Treatment

1. Ipecac-induced or saline induced emesis is the first step, followed by a thorough stomach wash.
2. *Gastric lavage:* Some authors recommend a 1 to 1.5% sodium bicarbonate solution or alkalinized desferioxamine, 2 g/L, in lavage fluid as well as giving a postlavage intragastric bolus of 10 g of this agent in 50 mL of water to minimize any direct mucosal injury due to residual particulate matter and in effecting the precipitation of residual iron salts to a less absorbable form. If the post-lavage abdominal radiograph shows significant amount of residual radiopaque material and the patient's condition allows, consideration should be given even to gastrostomy to effect the removal of iron. Early resort to whole bowel irrigation may be life saving in severe poisoining.
3. *Activated charcoal* is not effective in binding iron salts.
4. *Chelation therapy* with deferoxamine infusion enhances the excretion of iron. The maximum recommended dose is 15 mg/kg/hr (maximum daily dose, 360 mg/kg, up to 6g total). A higher infusion rate may itself be associated with hypotension. Patients with mild symptoms or those who are asymptomatic but have high serum iron or positive challenge test, should receive 20 to 40 mg/kg infused over 4 hours or 20 mg/kg I.M, 4-8 hourly. Chelation is continued until the urine color and serum iron level return to normal.

Supportive Treatment

Supportive treatment should include maintenance of proper fluid balance and correction of circulatory failure caused by hypovolemia, management of metabolic acidosis, hypo- or hypoglycemia or hyperglycemia, anemia and colloid loss due to gastrointestinal hemorrhage. Colloid transfusion should be considered.

Maintenance of an adequate urine output is essential to prevent renal failure and to promote excretion of the iron-deferoxamine complex. If renal failure supervenes, chelation may be continued with concurrent dialysis only. Iron-desferoxamine complex itself is toxic.

CORROSIVES

There are many households substances which contain toxic or caustic elements such as houdehold cleaners, detergents etc. Alkalis may produce significant, irreversible damage to eyes. Patient with significant ingestion may have vomiting, drooling, stridor, dyspnea, hemetemesis, fever and oral burns. Presence of two or more symptoms viz vomiting, drooling or stridor correlates well with oesophageal injury.

Treatment

Immediate dilution and irrigation with most readily available fluid. Emesis, lavage, charcoal and cathartics are contraindicated. Those with oral burns or definite history of ingestion must undergo an endoscopy within 12 hours from the time of injury. In presence of oral or oropharyngeal ulcers the risk of dangerous visceral burns is considerably increased. The current recommendation is that any patient with suspected ingestion of corrosive should undergo mandatory endoscopy within 24 hours from the time of injury. Antibiotics are indicated when GI perforation has occurred.Steroids have been shown to be efficacious in animal studies and uncontrolled human studies. They are recommended in cases where endoscopy cannot be performed or when there is definite circumferential burns on endoscopy.

ALUMINIUM PHOSPHIDE INGESTION

Aluminium phosphide (ALP) ingestion has became a chosen mode of suicide. There has been an explosion of reports of ALP poisoning predominantly from wheat growing regions of North and Central India, almost assuming epidemic proportions.

Clinical Features

The initial symptoms after ingestion are retrosernal burning, epigastric pain and recurrent profuse vomiting, followed by development of severe hypotension. Other common features are restlessness, tachypnoea, pulmonary crepitations, oliguria or anuria, jaundice, and impaired sensorium.

Later manifestations appear to be secondary to cardiovascular collapse. Profound hypotension is the hallmark of ALP ingestion. Global hypokinesia of left ventricle has been seen. Adult respiratory distress syndrome (ARDS) soon developed in severe cases.

Several ECG abnormalities have been described. These have been attributed to focal myocardial necrosis.

Both hypo and hypermagnesemia have been reported. In severe cases compromised adrenal function has been reported. However, all these changes appear to be secondary to cytotoxic effects of phosphine and the exact mechanism by which it acts is not clear.

Diagnosis

The diagnosis of ALP ingestion can be confirmed by detecting phosphine in exhaled air or in stomach aspirate. Strips impregnated with silver nitrate are good enough though dimethyl yellow cresol red and mercury (II) chloride or silver nitrate and mercury (II) chloride are more sensitive.The most specific and sensitive is gas chromatography.

Management

1. *Measures to decrease phosphine absorption* from the gastro- intestinal tract include :
   (i) Repeated gastric lavage with mild oxidizing agents (e.g., 1:10,000 potassium permanaganate) followed by sodium bicarbonate lavage.

(ii) Activated charcoal administered orally followed by a cathartic to increase phosphine excretion.
(iii) H2 receptor antagonist like intravenous rantidine and oral antacids can be used.
(iv) Liquid paraffin may be administered to increase the excretion of aluminium phosphide and phosphine from the gut.

2. *Adequate hydration* to maintain a satisfactory urinary output is recommended.
3. *Other supportive* measures include:
   (i) Oxygen.
   (ii) Treatment of shock with fluids, low dose dopamine, intravenous hydrocortisone.
   (iii) correction of acidosis with sodium bicarbonate.
   (iv) Assisted respiration may be required.
   (v) Hemodialysis is effective in cases with uremia.
   (vi) Magnesium sulphate has been tried with limited success.

Complications

Cardiogenic shock, renal failure, GI hemorrhage, hepatic failure are some of the well described complications. Death usually occurs due to acute cardiotoxicity within 24 hours. However, it may be delayed up to 4 days when adult respiratory distress syndrome supervenes. Other causes of death include metabolic derangements and hepatic failure.

Outcome

The reported mortality of all aluminium phosphide poisoning varies from 37% to 100%. The outcome depends on the number and freshness of ingested tablets and presence of shock and other poor prognostic factors like severe metabolic acidosis, hypoxia, electrolyte imbalance, arrhythmias, aspiration pneumonia and anemia.

FURTHER READING

1. Dutta AK. Seth A, Goyal PK, Aggarwal V, Mittal SK, Sharma R, et al. Poisoning in children: Indian scenario. Indian J Pediatr 1998; 65: 365-370.
2. Singh S, Singhi S, Sood NK, Kumar L, Walia BNS. Changing pattern of childhood poisoning (1970-1989). Experience of a large North Indian Hospital. Indian Pediatr 1995; 32: 331-336.
3. Singhi SC, Baranwal AK, M J. Acute iron poisoning: clinical picture, intensive care needs and outcome. Indian Pediatr. 2003 Dec;40(12): 1177-82.
4. Khadgawat R. Garg P, Bansal P, Arya A, Choudhary B. Accidental poisoning. Indian Pediatr 1994; 31: 1555-1557.
5. Singhal PK, Kumar H, Rastogi V, Saili A, Patwari AK, Mullick DN. Accidental poisoning. Indian Pediatr 1998; 25: 350-355.
6. Walton PJ, Fraser JJ Jr, Wilhelm GW. Gastrointestinal decontamination in the emergency department. Indian J Pediatr. 1997 Jul-Aug;64(4):451-5.
7. Tenenbein M. Recent advancements in pediatric toxicology. Pediatr Clin North Am. 1999 Dec;46(6):1179-88, vii.
8. Riordan M, Rylance G, Berry K. Poisoning in children 1: General management. Arch Dis Child. 2002 ;87(5):392-396.
9. Salgia AD, Kosnik SD. When acetaminophen use becomes toxic. Treating acute accidental and intentional overdose. Postgrad Med. 1999 Apr;105(4):81-4, 87, 90.
10. Bradberry SM, Vale JA. Poisons. Initial assessment and management. Clin Med. 2003 Mar-Apr;3(2):107-10.
11. Gupta S, Taneja V. Poisoned child: emergency room management. Indian J Pediatr. 2003 Mar;70 Suppl 1:S2-8.
12. Chugh SN. Aluminium phosphide poisoning: present status and management. J Assoc Physicians India. 1992 Jun;40(6):401-5.

Sunit Singhi

60 Snake Bite

Very few animal bites sustained by children elicit more emotional response and parenteral concern than do snakebites. From many parents' standpoint, almost every snake is poisonous and therefore life threatening. In reality, 70% of snakebites are non-venomous. Nonetheless, poisonous snakebites represent a true emergency to the physician requiring critical decisions in a timely manner.

INCIDENCE AND EPIDEMIOLOGY

Of the estimated 30,000 deaths per year from snake bite all over the world, an estimated 15,000-50,000 death occur in India, mainly in rural and semi rural areas, in a distinct seasonal pattern between April to October. Viper bites are commonest, followed by cobra and krait bites. In a recent study, about two-third of the victims were boys and 40% were in the age group of 11-15 years. Most bites occur during two periods—April to June and October to December. Time of bite may be any, however, krait bites generally occur at dusk and night. In India, 70% of the bites occur on the lower limbs. In contrast to this in USA, two-third of all pit viper bites tend to involve the hand and upper extremity.

SNAKES AND VENOM

Of more than 3000 species of snakes worldwide, only one-tenth are venomous. These belong to 4 major families: Elapidae (cobras, krait, mambas, coral snakes). Viperidae (true vipers), Hydrophidae (sea snakes) and Colubridae.

In India, 216 species are found, of which about 50 are poisonous. The important poisonous species are cobras, kraits, Russel's viper and saw-scaled viper. Important species of snakes found in India are shown in Table 1 and their characteristics in Table 2.

The poisonous snakes indigenous to the United States are members of the family Crotalidae (pit viper) or the family Elapidae. The rattlesnake (*crotalus* species), water moccasin (*Agkistrodon piscivorus*), and copperhead (*Agkistrodon contoris*) are pit vipers and are responsible for 95 percent to 99 percent of venomous snake bites. The coral snake is the only member of the Elapidae family in USA and along with imported exotic snakes, accounts for the remaining 1 percent to 5 percent of poisonous snakebites.

Table 1 : Important species of venomous snakes found in India.

A. Elapids	
I. Cobras :	i) Spectacled cobra (Naja naja) ii) Monocled kobra (Naja kaonthia) iii) King cobra (Ophiophagus hannah)
II. Kraits :	i) Common krait (Bugarus faciatus) ii) Banded krait (Bugarus faciatus)
B. Viperidae	i) Russell viper (Vipera russelli) ii) Saw scaled viper (Echis carinatus) iii) Bamboo pit viper, Himalayan pit viper, Levantine viper
C. Hydrophidae	Sea snakes (Enhydria schistose)

Table 2: Characteristics of individual snakes

	Elapids	*Vipers*	*Hydrophidage*
Head	oblong	triangular	Small sized
Head scales	large	small	
Pupils	round	vertical	
Fangs	Fixed and grooved	mobile and grooved	short and fixed
Habitat	kraits are nocturnal predators stay close to human habitation	stays far from human habitation	vicinity of coastline

Snake venoms are the most complex of all venoms. More than 90% of the dry weight is protein, comprising ~ 5-15 enzymes, 3-12 nonenzyme proteins and peptides, and nontoxic proteins, which exert toxic and lethal effects on various systems.

Phospholipase A_2 is the most widespread and extensively studied of all venom enzymes. It contributes to neurotoxicity, cardio-toxicity, hemolysis and increased vascular permeability of the venom.

The polypeptide neurotoxins are found almost exclusively in elapid and hydrophid venoms. Cobra venom contains postsynaptic (alpha) neurotoxins which bind to the acetylcholine receptors on the motor end plate and cause a neuromuscular block similar to d-tubocurarine. Krait and Sea snake venom produce pre-synaptic (beta) neuromuscular block by decreasing the acetylcholine output from the motor nerve endings.

Sea snake venom has a potent myotoxin that leads to muscle necrosis, myoglobinuria and hyperkalaemia.

The viper venom has both procoagulant and anticoagulant activity, and also contains a potent hemorrhagin which allows bleeding into various organs.

The **cardiotoxin** gives rise to irreversible depolarization of cell membrane resulting in cardiac asystole, circulatory and respiratory collapse.

The difference in toxicity and potential for lethality can be attributed to the variation in amounts of hyaluronidase, phospholipases, A,B,C,D proteases, L-amino acid oxidase, amino acid esters, thrombin-like enzymes, AT Pase, DNase, RNase, phosphodiesterase, and a host of other enzymes.

CLINICAL FEATURES

About 20-30% of all poisonous snake bites may not cause envenomation; 50% of elapid bites and 30% of viper bites are "dry bites", Clinical features and severity of envenoma-tion depends on size and species of snake, number and location of bites and quantity of venom injected, and age and health of victims (Table 3). The signs and symptoms following snake bite are therefore, quite variable and nonspecific.

Table 3 : Factors that increase the severity of envenomation

1. Small sized victims: children are more susceptible because of the effect of more venom per unit of body mass
2. Location of bite: bites on face, head and trunk
3. Penetration of a vessel: bites directly over a vessel
4. Size of snake: large
5. Angry and provoked bites
6. Previous bite by snake decreases the severity of the bite

Snake bite should be considered in any severe pain or swelling of a limb or in any unexplained illness that presents with bleeding or neurological signs.

Local Symptoms

Local symptoms predominate in case of viperine as well as cobra bites. Pain and swelling are most intense with viper bites and least with krait, so much so that the bite may go unnoticed till neurological signs appear. Envenomation by a coral snake causes minimal localized tissue reaction. Cobra bite result in severe radiating local pain. Viperine bite causes inflammatory swelling, bleeding, ecchymosis, and blister formation leading to necrosis of wound.

Nonspecific systemic symptoms include weakness, nausea, vomiting, sweating, perioral anesthesia, metallic taste in mouth, and muscle fasciculations. Early in krait bite, only these feature may be there. Excessive pain abdomen, explosive diarrhoea, and characteristic loss of taste and smell sensation may follow.

SYSTEMIC SYNDROMES

Hematological, cardiovascular, pulmonary and renal syndromes predominate in case of viperine bites, whereas neuroparalysis is the hall-mark of elapid envenomation, and musculoskeletal problems of hydrophid envenomaton.

Neuroparalytic syndrome is characteristic of cobra, krait and sea-snake bite. It may be heralded by weakness, paresthesia and numbness at bite, and sets in with involvement of muscle supplied by cranial nerves in form of ptosis, diplopia, ophthalmoplegia, palatal palsy, dysphagia, inability to speak, cough or swallow. This is followed by weakness of respiratory muscles-first the intercostals and the diaphragm, then the neck and trunk muscles and finally distal muscles. Respiratory arrest, coma and death may occur. Conciousness is usually preserved.

Hematological manifestations are characteristically seen in viperine bite, and may occur in form of consumptive coagulopathy, hemolysis, thrombocytopenia and serious bleeding from internal organs such as lungs and kidneys.

Cardiovascular: Early collapse, hypotension and shock may occur because of direct toxic effect of venom and vascular intimal damage. Myocardial depression, cardiogenic and or vasogenic shock, and systolic cardiac arrest may be seen in *cobra* bites. Late occurrence of shock is because of hemolysis, bleeding from internal organs or cardiotoxicity. ECG changes such as: tachycardia, ST-T segment changes, and first degree AV blocks have been described.

Pulmonary: Acute pulmonary edema may occur because of left ventricular failure or may result from extravasation of proteins through damaged alveolar membranes.

Musculoskeletal: Severe localized skin and muscle pain, localized myonecrosis as well as subcutaneous hemorrhage and skin necrosis are common. Severe muscle necrosis may lead to rhabdomyolysis, and myoglobinuria with hyperkalemia. The edema initially is subcutaneous and may progress to involve the entire extremity and sometimes even lead to development of a compartment syndrome in the affected extremity.

Acute renal failure may occur either from hemolysis, rhabdomyolysis, hypotension or DIC or due to direct toxic effect. It may be in form of acute tubular or patchy cortical necrosis, glomerulonephritis, interstitial nephritis or papillary necrosis.

Anaphylaxis and other types of allergic reactions to the snake venom have also been reported in individuals bitten on more than one occasion.

A comparison of clinical syndromes caused by snake-bites commonly seen in India is shown in Table 4.

MANAGEMENT

First Aid and Prehospital Measures

The aim is rapid and safe transport to a place where optimal medical care is available. Get to the nearest hospital immediately.

1. Ensure airway, breathing and intravenous access.
2. Allay anxiety and fear by anxiolytics and reassurance. Analgesics for pain relief may be used.

Table 4 : Comparison of clinical manifestations caused by vipers, Krait and Cobra envenomation

Symptoms and signs	*Viper*	*Krait*	*Cobra*
Pain	+	-	+
Swelling	++ (mins)	-	+ + (hrs)
Vomiting	+	+	+
Painful regional			
Lymphnodes	+	+	+/-
Bleeding fang marks	+	-	-
Nonclotting blood	+	-	-
Hypotension/shock	+	+	+
Neuroparalysis	-	+ +	+
Musculoskeletal	+	-	-
Cardiotoxicity	+	-	+
Renal failure	+ +	-	-

3. Immobilize the bitten part in the same way as a fractured limb. Children can be carried. Use bandages or cloth to hold the splints, not to block the blood supply or apply pressure. Do not apply any compression in the form of tight ligatures.
4. A wide crepe bandage tight enough to obliterate venous return but not arterial pulsations may be applied. It should be loosened intermittently for a few seconds every hour.
5. Local incision, cold compress and use of chemical agents is contraindicated.

II. Identification of Snake

If the snake is available it should be examined to identify and differentiate poisonous from nonpoisonous (Table 5). The ability to identify whether the offending snake is venomous or nonve-nomous is important. This identification process, however, does not have to be made in great detail. There are many pitfalls in the identification process, especially if the clinician is unfamiliar with snakes. In some instances, the head will be mutilated beyond recognition.

History may suggest the type of snake bite. Immediate appearance of important

Table 5: Features that differentiate poisonous from nonpoisonous snakes

	Poisonous snake	*Nonpoisonous snake*
Head		
(i) Scales	Small scales (viper)	Large
(ii) Third labial	Touches eye and nasal shield	Does not touch eye and nasal shield
(iii) Pit	Conspicuous pit between the eye and nostrils (pit viper)	No pit
(iv) fangs	Long, grooved or canalized	Short and solid
BODY		
(i) Belly scales	Large and cover the entire breadth of belly	Small/moderately large and do not cover the entire breadth of belly
(ii) Back scales	Central row of scales on the back are enlarged (Krait)	Scales are not enlarged
TAIL	Compressed/Rattles are present (viper)	Not compressed
BITE	Two fang marks with or without small marks of other teeth	Number of small teeth marks

symptoms and signs suggests a diagnosis of envenomation. Unprovoked, painless bites at night during sleep should raise the suspicion of a krait bite.

Clinicians should be careful when handling these snakes, even when the snake is dead or appears dead, as a dead snake can cause a significant envenomation by means of postmortem reflexes.

A 20 Minute Whole Blood Clotting Test (20 WBCT) has been adopted as a test for coagulopathy. It is simple to carry out but crucially requires a clean, new and dry test tube. A few mL of fresh venous blood is left undisturbed for 20 minutes, and then gently tilted. If the blood is still liquid, it indicates of coagulopathy and confirms that the biting species is Viperine.

III. Hospital Management

1. **Resuscitation:** Airway, breathing, intravenous access, infusion of fluids/ plasma for shock. After establishment of intravenous access, infusion of isotonic crystalloid solutions like Ringer's lactate or normal saline should be considered to combat shock. In severe envenomation albumin or plasma or blood may be infused. Vasopressors like dopamine or dobutamine are used if shock persists or there is severe hypotension.
2. Release the tourniquet, and loosely immobilize and slightly elevate the affected part in a functional position.
3. Cleanse the wound.
4. Give tetanus prophylaxis if it is needed.
5. When the patient is stable, give appropriate analgesic if indicated.
6. Apply a cardiac monitor.
7. Start antivenin therapy (see details below).
8. Shift to intensive care unit for close monitoring.
9. Send laboratory investigations (Table 6): Hemogram, platelet count, cogulation profile, Serum electrolytes (for hyperkalemia) and renal function tests (urea, creatinine) and Electrocardiogram.

Table 6: Essential laboratory data in evaluation and management of poisonous snakebites

- CBC with platelet count
- Urine Analysis
- Blood-chemistry to include blood urea, creatinine, electrolytes, CPK
- PT, PTT
- Serum fibrinogen, fibrin split products
- Blood grouping and cross-matching to hold blood (packed red blood cells)

Grading of Degree of Envenomation (Applicable to Viperine Bites)

Trivial: Signs and symptoms are confined to the local area. There is no localized edema/ pain. No systemic signs and symptoms. No laboratory changes.

Minimal: Signs and symptoms confined to the local area with edema, erythema and pain immediately beyond the area of bite. No systemic signs/symptoms.

Moderate: Signs and symptoms extend beyond the local area with systemic derangements and moderate disturbances of laboratory parameters.

Severe: Local signs and symptoms involve the entire extremity with severe systemic signs and symptoms.

SPECIFIC ANTIVENIN THERAPY

In India, a polyvalent antivenin, active against the four common poisonous snakes in India–cobra, krait, Russel's viper and saw scaled viper (Echis), is available in a lyophilized form. Each vial is reconstituted with 10ml of distilled water. On average potency 1 ml antiserum neutralizes 0.6mg cobra, 0.45mg krait, 0.6 mg Russel's viper and 0.45mg saw scaled viper. A new Fab fragment antivenom (CroFab) for the treatment of crotaline envenomation, the predominant venomous snakebite in the United States is available commercially. It is not effective against King cobra, banded krait and sea-snake.

Indications

It is indicated in all patients who show signs and symptoms of envenomation either local or systemic, and asymptomatic bites occurring indoors and at night as it is highly indicative of krait envenomation. Essentially systemic envenomation will be evident from the 20 Minute Whole Blood Clotting Test, signs of spontaneous bleeding or by visual recognition of neurological impairment such as ptosis. Purely local swelling is not a ground for administering ASV.

Dose and Administration

Symptomatology is not of much help in determining the severity of envenomation as it is too dynamic and constantly evolving. ASV therapy should be individualized. Following is a guideline only;

- Mild local envenomation:20-50 ml of antivenin
- Moderate and severe types: 50-100 ml and 100-150 ml respectively.
- Very severe cases may require a total dose of 250-500 ml. The dose for children is same as is for adults.

The initial dose is 8-10 vials (10 ml each) for both adults and children; it is calculated to neutralize the average dose of venom injected. This ensures that the majority of victims would be covered by the initial dose and keeps the cost of ASV to acceptable levels. A maximum ASV dose of around 25 vials may be used. However, the available data do not suggest any advantage in following a high-dose regime.

Mode of Administration

The total dose should be diluted with 10 ml/kg of distilled water or isotonic saline and infused intravenously at a rate of 4ml/min. The entire dose should be given over 4-6 hours. Adrenaline infusion, antihistamines and corticosteroids should be kept at hand to combat hypersensitivity reaction.

Adverse reactions, either anaphylactoid or pyrogenic, have often been identified as reasons not to administer ASV in smaller local hospitals. The fear of these potentially life threatening reactions has caused reluctance amongst some doctors to treat snakebite. However, if handled early with the primary drug of choice, these reactions are easily surmountable and should not restrict doctors from treating snakebite.

At the first sign of any of the following: urticaria, itching, fever, shaking chills, nausea, vomiting, diarrhea, abdominal cramps, tachycardia, hypotension, bronchospasm and angio-edema, *ASV should be discontinued and 0.01 mg/kg body weight of 1:1000 adrenaline should be given IM.* In addition, to provide protection against anaphylactoid reactions, 0.2 mg/kg of antihistamine and 2 mg/kg of hydrocortisone should be administered intravenously. If after 10 to 15 minutes the patient's condition has not improved or is worsening, a second dose of adrenaline 1:1000 intramuscular is given. This can be repeated for a third and final dose but in the vast majority of reactions, 2 doses of adrenaline will be sufficient. Once the patient has recovered, the ASV can be restarted slowly for 10-15 minutes, keeping the patient under close observation. Then the normal drip rate should be resumed.

ASV test doses have been abandoned. They have no predictive value in anaphylactoid or late serum reactions and may pre-sensitise the patient to the protein.

In anti-hemostatic bites, once the initial dose has been administered over one hour, no further ASV is given for 6 hours. Twenty WBCT test every 6 hours, will determine if additional ASV is required. In the case of neurotoxic bites, once the first dose has been administered, and a Neostigmine test given, the victim is closely monitored. If after 1-2 hours the victim has not improved or has worsened, then a second and final dose should be given.

SUPPORTIVE THERAPY

Local Care

Supportive care includes ***analgesics*** for pain, ***antibiotics*** for infection (cover for anaerobic infection) and ***antitetanus*** prophylaxis. Blisters and superficial necrosis usually heal by themselves. Secondary infection may require antibiotics. Faciotomy is indicated in the anterior tibial compartment syndrome.

Neuroparalytic Symptoms

Anticholinesterases may reverse neurological signs in bites due to cobra. Neostigmine may be started immediately at the first evidence of neuroparalysis. Five intravenous doses of 0.05 mg/kg are administered every 30 minutes initially. The interval between doses is then gradually increased till neurological recovery occurs. Each dose of neostigmine is preceded by intravenous dose of atropine (0.02 mg/kg).

Respiratory muscle paralysis may require mechanical ventilatory support.

Coagulopathy

Administration of antivenin and fresh blood transfusion are the only effective remedies. Role of heparin, epsilon caproic acid and fibrinogen is controversial.

Some Do's and Don'ts

1. Observe the snakebite patient for a minimum of 8 hours.
2. Do not leave the patient unattended.
3. Do not delay immediate or vigorous treatment, if the patient has a moderate or severe envenomation.
4. Do not use of ice or other cold applications. Do not make incisions
5. Do not use steroids as a primary treatment except in severe hypersensitivity reactions.
7. Heparin is generally not recommended for coagulopathies.

PROGNOSIS

A lower body weight increases children's susceptibility to the lethality of the venom. The degree of provocation, number of bites, state of the fangs, number of bites by the snakes in preceding few hours as well as the quantitative and quantitative characters-tics of venom are the major determinants of outcome. The location of the bite is of extreme clinical importance. Incidental injection of venom into an artery or vein greatly enhances the potential for systemic envenomation, commonly resulting in the victim's death. Bites to the head and faces are much more serious than bites sustained on an extremity. Bites on an upper extremity tend to have a worse prognosis than bites on a lower extremity.

In hospitalized children, death occurs in 3-5% patients. The death in viper envenomation occurs because of severe DIC and hemorrhage-internal or from local site, hypotension or pulmonary edema, and in Elapidae bites is due respiratory paralysis.

In the end, it should be understood that many recommended procedures or measures for management of snakebites have not been adequately supported by evidence and are based on consensus. Some aspects of the management are controversial, even among experts. If a treating physician does not have much experience in the management of poisonous snakebites, it is better to seek the advice and protocols of physicians who commonly treat snakebites. The important point is to individualize each victim's treatment strategy.

FURTHER READING

1. Simpson ID. The pediatric management of snakebite the national protocol. Indian Pediatr. 2007;44(3):173-6.
2. Currie BJ. Treatment of snakebite in Australia: the current evidence base and questions requiring collaborative multicentre prospective studies.Toxicon. 2006;48(7):941-56.
3. Nuchprayoon I, Pongpan C, Sripaiboonkij N. The role of prednisolone in reducing limb oedema in children bitten by green pit vipers: a randomized, controlled trial. Ann Trop Med Parasitol 2008; 102(7): 643-9.
4. Chippaux JP, Massougbodji A, Stock RP, Alagon A; Investigators of African Antivipmyn in Benin. Clinical trial of an F(ab')2 polyvalent equine antivenom for African snake bites in Benin.Am J Trop Med Hyg. 2007 77(3):538-46.
5. Kularatne SA, Kumarasiri PV, Pushpakumara SK, *et al.* Routine antibiotic therapy in the management of the local inflammatory swelling in venomous snakebites: results of a placebo-controlled study. Ceylon Med J. 2005;50(4):151-5.
6. Schmidt JM. Antivenom therapy for snakebites in children: is there evidence? Curr Opin Pediatr. 2005;17(2):234-8.
7. Singletary EM, Rochman AS, Bodmer JC, Holstege CP. Envenomations. Med Clin North Am. 2005;89(6):1195-224.
8. Srimannarayana J, Dutta TK, Sahai A, Badrinath S. Rational use of anti-snake venom (ASV): trial of various regimens in hemotoxic snake envenomation.J Assoc Physicians India. 2004;52:788-93.
9. Gold BS, Barish RA, Dart RC.North American snake envenomation: diagnosis, treatment, and management.Emerg Med Clin North Am. 2004 May; 22(2):423-43.

Angela F. Gardner

61 Animal Bites and Injuries

Animal bites have been recognized as a substantial public health problem around the world, disproportionately affecting children.[1-7] Children, perhaps because of their size, kinetic activity level, and lack of caution are more prone to bites than adults. Animal bites may result in infection, disfiguring injury, psychological trauma, and infrequently, death.[8,9,10] The implications for prevention are apparent, and include education for children, parents and pet owners.

EPIDEMIOLOGY

According to the 2007 – 2008 National Pet Owners Survey, approximately 63% of the homes in the United States have a family pet. There are 74.8 million dogs and 88.3 million cats in 71 million households nationwide.[11] An estimated 4.37 million people were bitten by animals annually between 2001 and 2003. Of these, approximately 830,000 required medical attention.[1] This equates to 1.5% of the U.S. population bitten annually, requiring medical attention in 0.3% of the population. Animal bites are a problem world-wide, with dog bites representing the largest portion of injuries requiring medical care.[2-7] Bites from cats represent the second most common source of bites in humans.

Injury rates for dog-bite related injury are highest for children aged 5 to 9 years, and the rate decreases with increasing age.[9] Most bites occur between April and September, with a peak incidence in July. There appears to be an even distribution across the days of the week.[14] Boys are bitten more often than girls in children less than 14 years old. The vast majority of dog bites in children are inflicted by a family dog (30%) or a neighbor's dog (50%).[9] Children less than 6 are most commonly bitten in association with resource (food) guarding, while older children are most commonly bitten in association with territory guarding.[12] According to one report, 75% of all fatal dog bites were inflicted on family members or guests on the family's property.[10]

Adults are most likely to sustain bite injuries to the arm/hand (45.3%), leg/foot (25.8%), and head/neck(22.8%).[9] Children, especially those younger than the age of 4, are most likely to be bitten on the head, neck, or face.[9,13,14] A majority of children sustain bite injuries to one body region only. About 6% have injuries to more than two body areas.[14]

While most bite injuries are treated and released from the emergency department in the United States (98.2%), the number of patients requiring inpatient management is much higher in other countries.[14] This may be in part due to hospitalization of children with deep and/or facial wounds for surgical closure under general anesthesia.[14]

Fatalities from dog bite are relatively rare, but overwhelmingly involve children (70%). Certain breeds of dogs have been associated with human dog-bite related fatalities, mostly Rottweilers (50%) and pit bulls (30%).[15, 16] The authors caution that such studies have limitations, including the inability to correct determine the total number of dogs in a given breed, the popularity of a given breed, and the inability to correctly determine the breed of a mixed-breed dog. Most fatal dog bites involve unrestrained dogs on the owner's property (58%) or unrestrained dogs off the owner's property (24%). Restrained dogs caused the remainder of the fatalities. A single animal per episode caused more than half of the fatal dog bites reported over a twenty-year period. Most fatalities involving more than one dog occurred off the owner's property.[15] Size and propensity for aggression in a given breed may be related to the incidence of human dog bite related fatalities, but many breeds have been associated with fatal attacks, and prevention is needed to decrease the incidence of this tragedy.

MANAGEMENT OF BITE WOUNDS

Diagnosis

A thorough history should be obtained from a reliable source when an animal bites a child. Important aspects of the history include the time since the attack, the nature of the circumstances surrounding the attack, the ownership and medical history of the attacking animal, and the current location of the attacking animal. The child's current medications, allergies, and (tetanus) immunization status should be noted. In addition, it is important to note any underlying conditions that might contribute to the development of infection.

All animal bites should be reported to the proper authorities, using the mechanism appropriate to the facility. In general, domestic pets that have proper and current immunization records can be observed for signs of impending illness. Animals that are unknown (or those whose ownership is unknown) present an increased risk for rabies, especially in an endemic area. Health department and/or animal control authorities should be notified in order to attempt retrieval of the animal, if possible.

Physical Exam

Perform a thorough examination of the wound(s). The location, size, and classification of the wound(s) should be noted. Diagrams or photos are helpful in recording information regarding the wounds. Use descriptive language, such as *avulsion, abrasion, puncture wound,* in describing the injury. Record information regarding the surrounding tissue, including the degree of contamination and the presence of any foreign material in the wound. Note the range of motion of any involved joints or adjacent structures. Carefully document the neurovascular status of the affected area, including pertinent negatives.

In the case of a wound older than a few hours, note the presence of erythema, edema, purulent drainage, or any other finding that may indicate an infection. Explore the wound carefully for the presence of a retained tooth fragment or other foreign body.

Extra care must be taken in the examination of head and face wounds, especially in younger children. A recent Canadian study found that most children (mean age, 7.4) sustained bites of the face (58.5%), followed by an extremity (35.5%).[17]

Younger children sustained more severe bites than older children, often requiring surgical intervention. Similar American studies have correlated an increased likelihood of mortality with a younger age in bite victims.[14,15] In addition, large carnivores may exhibit sufficient crushing force to penetrate the cranium of a child or smaller adult. The result may be a depressed skull fracture, brain laceration, intracranial abscess, or meningitis. Computed tomography (CT) may assist in diagnosing a perforation requiring immediate neurosurgical consultation.

Ancillary Tests

Plain film radiographs should be ordered to exclude foreign bodies in wounds that are in close proximity to a joint and in wounds of the hand(s). Suspected fractures also warrant plain film radiographs.

No blood tests are required to treat dog bites, although laboratory studies may indicated for the evaluation of accompanying trauma.

Routine gram stain and culture are not necessary for wounds that are recent and do not appear to be infected. For wounds that are older than 8 hours and exhibit erythema, warmth, and purulence, aerobic and anaerobic cultures should be obtained. It may be necessary to allow growth of these cultures for up to seven days to allow for the presence of slow-growing pathogens.[18,22] Wounds that fail to respond to antibiotics may also require culture and gram stain.

Treatment

As with all trauma, initial management is based on the ABCs of airway, breathing, and circulation. Following the initial stabilization, attention may be focused on the bite wound(s). The goals of bite wound management are:

1) Prevent infection
2) Minimize disfigurement caused by scarring

PREVENT INFECTION

Early and appropriate treatment of bite wounds decreases the infection rate. Numerous studies show that dog bite wounds treated within eight hours have lower infection rates than do those with treatment delayed by more than eight hours.[18,19] Meticulous wound cleansing, through copious irrigation and careful debridement, is the cornerstone of bite-wound treatment. The wound(s) should be irrigated with sterile normal saline using a system that produces a pressure of five to eight psi, the optimal pressure for mechanical cleansing of bacteria and debris.[18,20,21] A system using a 20 to 35 ml syringe and a 19 or 20 gauge needle of intravenous catheter will produce pressures in the necessary range, and there are commercial wound irrigation systems that will also suffice. The wound should be cleansed thoroughly using the chosen system and devitalized tissue should be carefully removed. Special care must be taken with puncture wounds to insure that irrigation does not inject the tissues with the diluent.

Consultation with the appropriate specialist may be required for extensive, deep, or complicated wounds. Consultation is required for bite wounds involving a joint, the hand(s), or open fractures.

The use of prophylactic antibiotics remains controversial. Fifteen to twenty percent of all animal bite wounds become infected.[21] Crush injuries, hand wounds, and injuries to underlying structures predispose to infection. Immunocompromise or chronic disease may increase the risk of infection. For this reason, most authorities recommend treatment of dog, cat and human bite wounds with prophylactic antibiotics for five to ten days.[18,19,21,22,23]

Pasteurella multocida and *Staphylococcus aureus* occur in 20 to 30 percent of all infected dog bite wounds.[21,22] Other aerobic pathogens include *Streptococcus* species, *Eikenella corrodens, Capnocytophaga canimorsus* and *Corynebacterium* species.[22] Anaerobic organisms implicated in infected dog bite include *Bacteroides fragilis, Veillonella parvula,* and *Fusobacterium* species.

Amoxicillin-clavulanate is the antibiotic of choice for prophylaxis in most animal bites.[21,22,23] Doxycycline, or other tetracyclines, may be used in patients who are allergic to penicillin. However, doxycyline cannot be used in children less than eight years of age or in pregnant women. Erythromycin can be used, but erythromycin, sulfamethoxazole-trimethoprim, cephalexin cefaclor, and dicloxacillin show poor activity against many of the common pathogens found in mammalian bites.[24,25,26] Amoxicillin-clavulanate is suitable for empiric therapy of established infections.

Failure of outpatient therapy may necessitate hospitalization and intravenous antibiotics. Other reasons for hospitalization of children with established dog-bite-wound infections include fever, toxic appearance, rapidly spreading cellulitis, advancement of cellulitis beyond one joint, and involvement of the bone, joint, or tendon. Ticarcillin-clavulanic acid is suitable for intravenous empiric therapy in patients who are not allergic to penicillin. Further therapy should be guided by culture and sensitivity results.

Tetanus Prophylaxis

Appropriate tetanus prophylaxis must be given, based on the child's immunization status. Diptheria-pertussus-tetanus (DPT) vaccine is typically given at two, four and six months of age. A fourth dose is given at 12 to 18 months, at least six months after the last dose. A fifth dose is given at four to six years, followed by a sixth dose at eleven to sixteen. Thereafter, tetanus toxoid with a reduced dose of diphtheria (Td) is given ever ten years, unless the patient sustains a "tetanus-prone" wound, such as an animal bite.

To reduce morbidity secondary to pertussis, the United States approved a tetanus toxoid, reduced diphtheria toxoid and acellular pertussis vaccine (Tdap) in June 2005. The Centers for Disease Control and Prevention now recommend that adults who have not previously received Tdap be given one dose of Tdap in place of the recommended dT should they require tetanus prophylaxis.[27,28] Subsequently, the patient would resume the use of dT for prophylaxis.

Two products were approved for use in children aged 10-18. GlaxoSmithKline's BOOSTRIXâ is indicated for persons 10-18 years of age (www.fda.gov/cber/label/tdapgla050305LB.pdf). Sanofi Pasteru's ADACELÔ is indicated for all persons aged 11-64 (www.fda.gov/cber/label/tape061005LB.pdf). On June 30, 2005, the Advisory Committee on Immunization Practices (ACIP) voted to recommend the routine use of Tdap vaccines in adolescents 11-18 years of age in place of tetanus and diphtheria toxoids (Td) vaccines. (See www.cdc.gov/nip/pr/pr_tdap_jun2005.htm.)

In children who have an unknown or incomplete tetanus immunization series (less than three doses of DTaP), tetanus toxoid should be administered according to age.[27,28]

Children < 7 years: DTaP (pediatric)
Children 7 – 10: Td
Children 11 to adult: Dtap

In addition, all but clean minor wounds require tetanus immune globulin, 250 units administered in the limb contralateral to the toxoid.[27,28]

Children and adolescents who have completed three doses of the tetanus immunization series and who have had a booster within the past 5 years do not require additional tetanus toxoid or tetanus immune globulin, regardless of the severity of the wound.

Children and adolescents who have completed three doses of the tetanus immunization series and who have had a booster within 10 years require tetanus toxoid if the wound is more than clean and minor. There is controversy in the literature regarding the actual existence of "tetanus-prone" wounds, but the Advisory Committee on Immunization Practices divides wounds into "clean and minor" and "major and dirty", with tetanus toxoid required for the "major and dirty" category. Tetanus immune globulin is not required for children who have completed the initial three doses and who have had a booster within 10 years.

Children and adolescents who have completed three doses of the tetanus immunization series and HAVE NOT had a booster within 10 years require intramuscular tetanus toxoid. Those with clean, minor wounds do not require tetanus immune globulin. Major, dirty wounds require tetanus immune globulin, 250 units given by intramuscular injection.

Rabies Prophylaxis

Rabies is the tenth most common cause of death globally.[29] The incidence of rabies in the United States had fallen to approximately one case per year from 1990 to 1999, but 25 cases have been reported since 2000, most attributed to bats.[30] Rabies is found throughout the world, most commonly in temperate or tropical climates. Although in developed countries the source of rabies is rarely domesticated animals, the reverse is true in developing nations. By some estimates most (99%) of the cases of human rabies are the result of dog bites.[31] In Thailand, 90.6% of human rabies infections were attributed to dog bites, followed by 6% from unknown sources and 3.6% from cat attacks. The eradication of human rabies appears to depend on the eradication of stray animals and the implementation of effective post exposure prophylaxis.

Effective post exposure prophylaxis (PEP) depends on identifying a possible exposure to rabies. Animal bites are obvious exposures, depending on the circumstances of the attack. An unprovoked bite from a dog is considered more likely to have been inflicted by a rabid animal than a provoked bite. Nonbite exposure includes the contamination of scratches or abrasions with saliva, cerebrospinal fluid, or brain tissue of an infected animal. The rabies virus does pass through intact mucous membranes, and thus any mucous membrane contact with saliva from a possible rabid animal is considered an exposure.

In areas where rabies is not zoonotic, including much of the United States, a healthy domestic dog or cat that bites a person should be confined and observed for ten days. No one in the United States has died of rabies when the attacking dog or cat has been healthy after 10 days of observation.[33] It should be noted that many states along the U.S. border with Mexico and some areas of south Texas are considered enzootic for canine rabies. In these areas, in most of Asia, and in essentially all of Latin America and Africa, post exposure prophylaxis should be started immediately after a bite by a cat or a dog, but can be terminated if the animal remains healthy after a 10-day observation period. In all areas, an attacking animal should be considered rabid if it escapes and cannot be reliably recovered.

Immediate and thorough cleansing of the wound, as described in the previous section, are essential to reduce the viral inoculum. Experimental studies with various cleansing agents have been conducted, but the best cleansing agent available immediately should be used.

The only rabies immune globulin licensed for use in the United States is human rabies immune globulin (HRIG). It is derived from cold fractionation of plasma from hyperimmunized human donors, and is virtually free of significant side effects.[34] In developing countries, immune serum is often unavailable or very expensive. The immune serum usually available in developing countries is of equine origin (ERIG). The dose of HRIG is 20 IU/kg and the dose of ERIG is 40 IU/kg. Most experts recommend that as much of the dose as possible be given around the wound site. The remainder may be given intramuscularly at a site distant from the site used for the vaccine. Immune globulin should be given as soon as possible after the injury, up to 7 days. The recommended dosage should not be exceeded because it will inhibit the action of the vaccine.

The Essen scheme is currently recommended in the United States for the administration of rabies vaccine. Immunoprophylaxis with the vaccine is recommended to begin as soon as possible after the bite. Because the incubation time for rabies is lengthy, there is no established upper limit for the time elapsed between a possible exposure and administration of the vaccine. The active immunity induced by the administration of the vaccine occurs after the administration of 1.0 ml of vaccine in the deltoid muscle on days 0,3,7,14, and 28.

The rabies vaccines available in the United States are prepared from viruses grown in cell cultures and inactivated by b-propiolactone. HDCV, produced in cultures of human diploid cells, has been available since 1980. Rabies Vaccine Absorbed (RVA), cultured from the cells of rhesus monkeys, was used to vaccinate humans allergic to HDCV, but has been unavailable in the United States since 2006. Purified chick embryo vaccine (PCEV) has been available since 1997. All three preparations are thought to be equally efficacious and safe for post exposure therapy.[34]

Minimize Disfigurement from Scarring

Wound closure following a domestic animal bite remains an area of divisiveness in the medical field. Governing the decision concerning whether to close a wound or not are three factors: cosmetic appearance, function, and risk of infection. Optimal therapy involves prompt treatment to prevent infection, as described above.

Puncture wounds large enough to allow irrigation and drainage of the irrigant without suffusion of the surrounding tissue should be irrigated. Small puncture wounds should be debrided and irrigated as well as possible without damaging the surrounding tissue. In general, unless closure is essential for cosmetic purposes, puncture wounds should be left open.

Wounds of the face and scalp tend to heal rapidly, perhaps due to the generous blood supply, and may be closed primarily. Plastic surgery consultation may be necessary for complex wounds, multiple wounds, or if general anesthesia is required for completion of the procedure.

Bite wounds of the hand have been studied extensively and represent a risk to future function and a high risk of infection. The fascial spaces and tendon sheaths of the hand represent a unique anatomical challenge to proper irrigation and cleansing of wounds in that they communicate and spread bacterial infection through movement of the structure. Specialty consultation should be used liberally in caring for acute bites of the hand. Evidence of established infection is reason for admission and administration of intravenous antibiotics.

Delayed primary closure may be used for puncture wounds, wounds that appear clinically infected, and wounds that are more than 24 hours old. As the scheduling and follow-up required for delayed primary closure are difficult to achieve satisfactorily in the emergency department environment, consultation of the appropriate specialty service may be necessary.

All bite wounds should be immobilized and elevated if possible. Most should be re-examined in 24 to 48 hours.

PREVENTION

Each year the Centers for Disease Control and Prevention sponsors "National Dog Bite Prevention Week." The following is summarized from the material distributed each year.

Before Buying a Dog

- Consult a professional to learn about suitable breeds of dogs for the household.
- Do not bring a dog with a history of aggression into a household with children.
- Delay acquiring a dog if a child is fearful or apprehensive about the dog.
- Spend time with the dog before adopting or buying it.
- Use caution when bringing a dog into the home of an infant or toddler.
- Spay/neuter virtually all dogs. (This reduces aggressive tendencies.)

Teach children to prevent bites:

- Do not approach an unfamiliar dog.
- Do not pet a dog without allowing it to see and sniff you first.
- Never "hug and kiss" a dog. The animal will see this as weakness.
- Remain motionless when approached by a dog. (Be like a tree.)
- If knocked over by a dog, roll into a ball and lie very still. (Be like a log.)
- Do not play with a dog unless supervised by an adult.
- Avoid direct eye contact with a dog.
- Do not disturb a dog that is sleeping, eating, or caring for puppies.
- If bitten, immediately tell an adult.

REFERENCES

1. Gilchrist J, Sacks J J, White D, et al. Dog bites: still a problem? Injury Prevention. 2008;14:296-301.
2. Matter HC. The epidemiology of bite and scratch injuries by vertebrate animals in Switzerland. Eur J Epidemiol. 1998 Jul;14(5):483-490.
3. Ostanello F, Gherardi A, Caprioli A, et al. Incidence of injuries caused by dogs and cats treated in emergency departments in a major Italian city. Emerg Med J. 2005 Apr;22(4):260-262.
4. MacBean CE, Taylor DM, Ashby K. Animal and human bite injuries in Victoria, 1998 – 2004. Med J Aust. 2007 Jan 1;186(1):38-40.
5. Mendez GR, Gomez TM, Somoza AI, et al. Dog bite-related injuries treated in a pediatric surgery department: analysis of 654 cases in 10 years. An Esp Pediatr. 2002 May;56(5):425-429. [Translated from Spanish]
6. Kahn A, Bauche P, Lamoureux J, et al. Child victims of dog bites treated in emergency departments: a prospective survey. Eur J Pediatr. 2003 Apr;162(4):254-258.
7. Fèvre EM, Kaboyo RW, Persson V, et al. The epidemiology of animal bite injuries in Uganda and projections of the burden of rabies. Trop Med Int Health. 2005 Aug;10(8):790-798.
8. Overall KL, Love M. Dog bites to humans: demography, epidemiology, injury, and risk. J Am Vet Med Assoc. 2001;218:1923-1934.
9. CDC. National estimates of nonfatal injuries treated in hospital emergency departments – United States, 2001.MMWR 2003 July;52(26):605-610.
10. Sacks JJ, Sinclair L, Gilchrist J, et al. Breeds of dogs involved in fatal human attacks in the United States between 1997 and 1998. J Am Vet Med Assoc. 2000;217:836-840.
11. American Pet Products Manufacturers Association. 2007/2008 APPMA National Pet Owners Survey. Greenwich, Connecticut: American Pet Products Manufacturers Association, 2008.
12. Reisner IR, Shofer FS, Nance ML. Behavioral assessment of child-directed canine aggression. Inj Prev. 2007 Oct;13(5):348-351.
13. Steele MT, Ma OJ, Nakase J, et al. Epidemiology of animal exposures presenting to emergency departments. Acad Emerge Med. 2007 May;14(5):398-403.

14. Schalamon J, Ainoedhofer H, Singer G, et al. Analysis of dog bites in children who are younger than 17 years. Pediatrics. 2006 Mar;117(3)e374-e379.
15. Sacks JS, Sinclair L, Gilchrist J, et al. Breeds of dogs involved in fatal human attacks in the United States between 1979 and 1998. Vet Med Today: Special Report. JAVMA. 2000 Sept217(6)836-840.
16. Sacks JJ, Lockwood R, Hornreich J, et al. Fatal dog attacks, 1989 – 1994. Pediatrics. 1996;97:891-895.
17. Lang, ME, Klassen T. Dog bites in Canadian children: a five-year review of severity and emergency department management. Can J Emerg Med 2005;7(5):309-314.
18. Goldstein EJ, Richwald GA. Human and animal bite wounds. Am Fam Physician 1987;36:101-109.
19. Goldstein EJ. Infectious complications and therapy of bite wounds. JAPMA 1989;28:329-331.
20. Ball V, Younggren BN. Emergency management of difficult wounds: part I. Emerg Med Clin North Am. 2007;25:101-121.
21. Presutti RJ. Prevention and treatment of dog bites. Am Fam Physician. 2001;63:1567-1572.
22. Lewis KT, Stiles M. Management of cat and dog bites. Am Fam Physician 1995;52:479-85,489-90.
23. Callaham M. Prophylactic antibiotics in common dog bite wounds: A controlled study. Ann Emerg Med 1980;9:410-414.
24. Goldstein EJ, Citron DM. Comparative activities of cefuroxime, amoxicillin-clavulanic acid, ciprofloxacin, enoxacin, and ofloacin against aerobic and anaerobic bacteria isolated from bite wounds. Antimicrob Agents Chemother 1988;32: 1143-1148.
25. Brook I. Microbiology of humand and animal bite wounds in children. Pediatr Infect Dis J 1987;6:29-32.
26. Levin JM, Talan DA. Erythromycin failure with subsequent Pasteurella multocida meningitis and septic arthritis in a cat-bite victim. Ann Emerg Med 1990;19:1458-1461.
27. Centers for Disease Control and Prevention. Preventing tetanus, diphtheria, and pertussis among adolescents: use of tetanus toxoid, reduced diphtheria toxoid and acellular pertussis vaccines: recommendations of the Advisory Committee on Immunization Practices (ACIP). MMWR 2006:55(No.RR-3).
28. Centers for Disease Control and Prevention. General recommendations on immunization: recommendations of the Advisory Committee on Immunization Practices (ACIP). MMWR 2006:55(No.RR-15).
29. Place #94 here.
30. Blanton JD, Hanlon CA, rupprecht CE. Rabies surveillance in the United States during 2006. J Am Vet Med Assoc 2007;231:540-546.
31. Sinclair CL, Zhou C. Descriptive epidemiology of animal bites in Indiana, 1990-92: A rationale for intervention. Public Health Rep 1995;110:64.
32. Schuurman B, van Griethuysen AJ, Marcelis JH, et al. Rat bite fever after a bite froma tame pet rat. Ned Tidjschr Geneeskd 1998;142:2006-2009.
33. Norwood S, McAuley C, Vallina VL, et al. mechanisms and patterns of injuries related to large animals. J Trauma 2000;48:740-744.
34. Bucherl W, Buckley E, Deulofeu V. Venomous animals and their venoms. New York, Academic Press, 1968.

Sunit Singhi

62 Scorpion and Insect Stings

SCORPION STING

Scorpion stings are a major public health problem in many tropical countries. Worldwide, there are about 100,000 cases of scorpion envenomation. For every individual killed by snake envenomation, approximately 10 are killed due to scorpion stings. In India the incidence is higher in Tamil Nadu, Maharashtra, Andhra Pradesh and Bihar. There are 2000 species of scorpions in the world, out of which 50 are poisonous. Almost all of lethal scorpions, except the *Hemiscorpius* species, belong to the scorpion family called the *Buthidae* and live in warm , dry regions. The lethal members of the Buthidae family include the genera of *Buthus, Parabuthus, Mesobuthus, Tityus, Leiurus, Androctonus,* and *Centruroides*. In India there are 86 species, out of which 2 are poisonous;they are *Mesobuthus tamulus* (red scorpion) and *Palamnieus swammerdami*.

Accidental stings are more common during summer months and occurs when scorpions are touched while in their hiding places. Most of the stings occur on the hands and feet.

Pathophysiology

The venom glands of the scorpion are located on the tail lateral to the tip of the stinger. The potency of the venom varies with the species. Venom deposited via the intravenous route can cause symptoms within 5 minutes after the injection. The venom is composed of varying concentrations of neurotoxin, cardiotoxin, nephrotoxin, hemolytic toxin, phosphodiesterases, phospholipases, hyaluronidases, histamine, serotonin, tryptophan, and cytokine releasers. The most potent toxin is the neurotoxin which results in autonomic and neuromuscular overexcitation symptoms, and prevents normal nerve impulse transmissions.

Venom alters voltage dependent ion channels, open presynaptic sodium channels and inhibit calcium dependent potassium channel, which has direct effect on the gating mechanisms of excitable membranes. It results in release of excessive neurotransmitters such as epinephrine, norepinephrine, acetylcholine, glutamate, and aspartate from sympathetic nerve endings and adrenal medulla, causing initially *cholinergic storm* followed by *adrenergic storm.*

Release of catecholamines results in variety of metabolic changes *viz.* glycogenolysis, lipolysis , depletion of tissue glycogen content of atria, ventricles, liver in addition to cardiac sarcolemmal defects, elevation in serum levels of glucose and free fatty acids. Intense vasoconstriction, increased myocardial oxygen demand, results in myocardium ischemia and myocardial toxicity.

In Indian scorpion stings cardiac toxicity is much more pronounced, while neurotoxicity is more common in South Africa and USA. Polypeptides of yellow scorpion (*Buthus cosmobuthus* and *Hemiscorpus*) also cause direct local inflammation, skin necrosis, lymphangitis at the site of sting.

Initiation of systemic inflammatory response, increased levels of various cytokines -interleukin-6, IL-1a and IFN-gamma, NO, alpha-1-antitrypsin – may cause direct tissue injury acute disseminated intravascular coagulation, clotting alterations, acute lung injury and increased capillary permeability.

While adults are stung more often than children, children are more likely to develop a more rapid progression and increased severity of symptoms because of their lower body weight.

Clinical Features

For children presenting with scorpion stings, it is important to ascertain the time of envenomation, nature of the incident, description of the scorpion, local and systemic symptoms. Symptoms may start within 5 minutes. Clinical picture evolves over 30 minutes to six hours.

Severe sharp burning pain (without progression) at the sting site, followed by pruritus, erythema, local tissue swelling, and ascending hyperesthesia, is characteristically seen in Indian subcontinent. The local evidence of a sting may be minimal or absent in as many as 50% of cases of neurotoxic scorpion stings.

Closer proximity of the sting to the head and torso results in a quicker onset of systemic manifestations. They may display disproportionate restlessness, inconsolable crying; uncontrollable jerking of the extremities; and chaotic thrashing, flailing, and writhing combined with contorted facial grimaces.

There are prominent autonomic nervous system signs: sympathetic, parasympathetic or a combination of signs. Symptoms of cholinergic storm, sweating, salivation, vomiting, priapism, fever, shivering, are evident early; between 0-4 hours after sting (can last for 6-13 hours). Manifestations of adrenergic storm, tachycardia, hypertension, myocardial dysfunction , arrhythmias, pulmonary edema, non–cardiogenic pulmonary edema, appear between 4-48 hours. Common signs include mydriasis, nystagmus, hypersalivation, dysphagia, and restlessness. Hypertension is secondary to catecholamine and renin stimulation and can be observed as early as within 5 minutes after the sting; this lasts a few hours. It may be severe enough to cause ventricular failure or hypertensive encephalopathy. Initial hypotension is less common. Hypotension and shock occur because of severe LV dysfunction, or because of exhausted catecholamine stores, or profuse loss of fluids from sweating, vomiting, diarrhea.

The grading of the scorpion envenomations depends on presence and severity of cardiac and neurological signs. The neurologic signs range from local pain or paresthesia at the sting site to cranial nerve and somatic neuromuscular dysfunction. The sensorium initially is normal. Classic rotatory eye movement may result in ptosis and blurred vision. Some patients have mydriasis, tongue fasciculations, dysphagia, dysarthria, and stridor secondary to pharyngeal reflex loss or muscle spasm. Convulsions, cerebral infarcts, aphasia, hemiplegic, cerebral hemorrhage can occur as complications of clotting alterations and disseminated intravascular coagulation.

The mode of death is usually via respiratory failure secondary to anaphylaxis, bronchoconstriction, bronchorrhea, pharyngeal secretions, and/or diaphragmatic paralysis, though venom-induced multiorgan failure plays a large role. Acute pancreatitis has been reported from Trinidad.

Differential Diagnoses include botulism, organophosphate toxicity, myasthenia gravis diphtheria, Guillain-Barré syndrome, neuroleptic overdose and sympathomimetic overdose. **Laboratory investigations** may show evidence of organ dysfunctions. Echocardiography is useful in evaluation of myocardial contractility; diffuse global biventricular hypokinesis with a decreased left and right ventricular ejection fraction. ECG changes are observed in approximately two-third of children in form of sinus tachycardia, QTc prolongation, ST changes, T-wave inversion, ventricular repolarization abnormalities, bundle-branch block and first-degree block.

Treatment

Treatment begins with moving the patient away from the scorpion and stabilizing the patient's airway and vital signs, followed by administration of antivenin and institution of symptomatic and local treatment. Close monitoring is essential for early recognition of circulatory failure.

Local treatment includes use of a negative-pressure extraction device, use of ice bags, analgesics and if needed local infiltration of lignocaine to reduce pain and to slow the absorption of venom via vasoconstriction, immobilization of the affected part below the level of the heart, calming the child. Sedation may be required in some cases to restrain an agitated child. Diazepam is recommended (in concert with GABA open ion channels antagonizes toxin's ability to stimulate specific ion channel). Long-acting sedatives should be avoided.

Establish airway, breathing, and circulation (ie, ABCs) to provide adequate airway, ventilation, and perfusion. Monitor vital signs (eg, pulse oximetry; heart rate, blood pressure, and respiratory rate monitor). Administer oxygen. Administer intravenous fluids to help prevent hypovolemia.

For hyperdynamic cardiovascular changes, administration of a combination of beta-blockers with sympathetic alpha-blockers is most effective in reversing the venom-induced effect. Early use of prazosin (30 microgram/kg/dose) in children with evidence of autonomic storm has proven beneficial; it suppresses sympathetic outflow and activates venom-inhibited potassium channels. It is repeated in the same dose at the end of 3 hours according to clinical response and later every 6 hours till extremities are warm. In case of vomiting it can be administered through nasogastric tube. After giving prazosin, the child should not sit up and the mother is advised not to lift the child to prevent the effects of 'First dose' phenomenon due to prazosin. Prazosin can be given irrespective of the blood pressure provided there is no hypovolemia. It should not be given as prophylaxis in children when pain is the only symptom. Avoid using beta-blockers alone because this leads to an unopposed alpha-adrenergic effect. Also, nitrates can be used for hypertension and myocardial ischemia. In children with bradycardia atropine may be useful.

For hypodynamic cardiac changes, a titrated monitored fluid infusion with afterload reduction helps reduce mortality. A diuretic may be used for pulmonary edema in the absence of hypovolemia, but an afterload reducer, such as prazosin, nifedipine, nitroprusside, hydralazine, or angiotensin-converting enzyme inhibitors, is better. Dobutamine seems to be a better choice than dopamine for the inotropic effect. Dobutamine infusion (5-15 microgram/kg/min) is preferred when no improvement is seen after 4-6 hours. Finally, a pressor such as norepinephrine can be used as a last resort to correct hypotension refractory to fluid therapy.

Role of specific antivenin is not fully established. As the venom reaches target too rapidly, antivenom is useful if administered within 30 minutes of sting. However, routine administration has not offered better outcome, irrespective of clinical severity.

Cortico-steroids are contraindicated; has been shown to enhance the necrotizing effects of excessive catecholamines on myocardium.

Prognosis

Case fatality rate in children due to scorpion sting has declined from 13% to 3% after prazosin was introduced as the first line of management. Poor prognostic factors include age <6 years, delay in initiating prazosin therapy, encephalopathy, pulmonary edema and arrhythmia. Dilated cardiomyopathy has been reported among survivors.

INSECT STING

Allergic reactions to insect stings are common and are often a serious medical problem. Incidence of anaphylaxis to insect stings in the general population over a specified period range form 0.3 to 3%.

Insects that sting are members of the order Hymenoptera of the class insets. 2 major subgroups are: (1) Vespids – yellow jacket, hornet and wasp. (2) Apids – honey bee, brumble bee.

The stinging apparatus in the insects originate in the abdomen of the female insect. It consists of a sac containing venom attached to a barbed stinger. A sting occurs when the sac contracts and venom is deposited into tissue. The stingers of the vespids have few barbs and they can inflict multiple stings unlike the apids who can sting only once.

The allergens in the hornet's venom are phospholipase, hyaluronidase and a protein known as antigen 5.

Local Reactions to Stings

The usual or "normal" reaction to an insect sting is localized pain, swelling, and erythema at the site of the sting. This reaction usually subsides spontaneously within a few hours. Analgesics and cold compresses may only be required.

Within 48 hours of sting the swelling at the sting site extends over a large area and remains so for upto 7 days. This lesion may often be confused with cellulities but infection is never associated with insect sting. It is generally an allergic local reaction to the sting. Treatment includes analgesics and antihistaminics like diphenhydramine. If reaction is very extensive oral steroids may be given for 2-3 days. Topical application of papain may be tried. Tetanus prophylaxis is not required.

Anaphylaxis

Anaphylaxis occurs more often in males than in females. Symptoms usually occur 10-20 mins following a sting but may be delayed for upto 72 hours. One third of patients who have analphylaxis have history of atopic disease. The most common symptoms of anaphylaxis following insect sting are dermal urticaria, flushing and angioedema. Life threatening events like shock, hypotension edema of upper airways and bronchospasm may occur in some cases. IgE antibodies mediate this reaction. The rate of severe reactions to subsequent stings is lower in children than adults and the symptoms during subsequent episodes stimulate those of the initial attack.

Toxic Reactions

Toxic reactions to constituents of venom may occur after many simultaneous stings and has the same clinical features as anaphylaxis.

Unusual Reactions

Rare reports of abnormalities such as vasculitis, nephrosis, neuritis, encephalitis and serum sickness may occur following insect stings. These usually last for days to weeks following the sting.

Therapy of Acute Reaction

If the insect's stinging apparatus if attached to the skin, it should be removed gently taking care not to squeeze the sac which may cause further envenomation. Subcutaneous epinephrine in 1:1000 dilution (0.2 – 0.5 ml) every 20-30 minutes if required. Intravenous epinephrine (1 in 10.000 dilution) may be required rarely if there is profound shock. Depending on the clinical condition child may need intravenous fluids, vasopressors, bronchodilators and oxygen. Airway is to be maintained either by endotracheal intubation of tracheostomy. Upper airway edema may be managed with acrosolized epinephrine and steroids. (methyl prednisolone initially intravenously thereafter oral steroids.) Urticaria and itching may be treated with antihistaminics like diphenhydramine.

Prophylaxis

All children who have once experience anaphylactic reaction to hornet sting and are skin test positive against venom antigen should take prophylaxis. They should be properly clothed with full-sleeved shirts, slacks, pants and shoes. White or dark and drab colored outfit are preferable to bright colored ones. Cosmetics and perfumes, which may attract the insects, should not be worn. Those who are prone to such anaphylactic reactions should carry lifesaving drugs like adrenaline and diphenhydramine alongwith them.

The other mode of prophylaxis is by venom immunotherapy, which is available abroad. It is indicated in all children with moderate to severe anaphylactic reaction and possibly also if one has had either serum sickness or toxic reaction following a sting. It is not indicated in children with normal reaction, large local reaction and mild dermal anaphylactic reaction.

Single or multiple venom immunotherapies can be provided initial dose ranges from 0.01 to 0.1 μg depending on the degree of skin test reaction. Incremental doses of the antigen are to be given either daily or weekly. Maintenance dose is 50-100 μg of single venom or 300 μg of mixed vespid venom. Intervals of dose during maintenance therapy in the 1st year are 4 weeks, 2nd year 6 weeks, and 3rd year 8 weeks. Duration of immunotherapy extends either till the skin test becomes negative or for 3-5 years (Robert E Reisman NEJM 1994, 331 (8) : 523 – 527).

FURTHER READING

1. Mahadevan S. Scorpion sting. Indian Pediatr 2000; 37: 504-513.
2. Sofer S, Guero M. Vasodilators and hypertensive encephalopathy follwoing scorpion envenomation in children. Chest 1990; 97: 118-120.
3. Bawaskar HS, Bawaskar PH. Cardiovascular manifestations of severe scorpion sting in India (Review of 34 children). Ann Trop Pediatr 1991; 11: 381-387.
4. Bawaskar HS, Bawaskar PH. Prazosin for vasodilator treatment of acute pulmonary edema due to scorpion sting. Ann Trop Med Parasitol 1987; 1: 719-723.
5. Elatrous S, Nouria S, Besbes-Ouanes L, Boussarsar M, Boukef R, Marghil S, *et al.* Dobutamine in severe scorpion envenomation. Chest 1999; 116: 748-753.
6. Ismail M. The scorpion envenoming syndrome. Toxicon 1982; 20: 337-344.
7. Freire-maia L, Campos JA. Pathophysiology and treatment of scorpion poisoning. *In:* Ownby CL, Odell GV, editors. Natural Toxins. Pergamon Press Oxford, 1980, p 139-159.
8. Abroug F, Elatrous S, Nouria S, Haguiga , Touzi N, Bouchoucha S, Serotherapy in scorpion envenomation: a randomized controlled trial. Lancet 1999; 354: 906-909.
9. Bawaskar HS, Bawaskar PH. Vasodilators: Scoprion envenoming and the heart (An Indian experience). Toxicon 1994; 32: 1031-1040.
10. Muller GJ. Scorpionism in South Africa. A report

of 42 serious envenomations. South Afr Med J 1993; 83: 405-411.
11. Bawaskar HS, Bawaskar PH. Prazosin in the management of cardiovascular manifestations of scorpion sting. Lancet 1986; 1: 510-511.
12. Bawaskar HS, Bawaskar PH. Management of cardiovascular manifestations of poisoning by the Indian red scorpion (Mesobuthus tamulus). Brit Heart J 1992; 68: 487-480.
13. Gueron M, Adolph RJ, Grupp IL. Hemo-dynamic and myocardial consequences of scorpion venom. Am J Cardiol 1980; 45: 979-986.
14. Das S, Nalini P, Shanti A, Sethuraman KR, Balachander J. Cardiac involvement and scorpion envenomation in children. J Trop Pediatr 1995; 41: 338-340.
15. Dudin AA, Ramband-Cousson A, Thaliji A. Scorpion sting in children in Jerusalem area–A review of 54 cases. Ann Trop Pediatr 1991; 11: 217-223.
16. Amitai Y, Mines Y, Aker M, Goitein K. Scorpion stings in children–A review of 51 cases. Clin Pediatr 1985; 24: 136-140.
17. Abrough F, Ayari M, Nouria S. Assessment of left ventricular function in severe scorpion envenomation–combined hemodynamic and ECHO-doppler study. Inten Care Med 1995; 21: 629-635.
18. Goddard J, deShazo R. Bed bugs (Cimex lectularius) and clinical consequences of their bites. JAMA. 2009 1;301(13):1358-66.
19. King TP, Guralnick M. Hymenoptera allergens. Clin Allergy Immunol. 2008;21:237-49.
20. Finegold I. Issues in stinging insect allergy immunotherapy: a review. Curr Opin Allergy Clin Immunol. 2008;8(4):343-7.
21. Clark S, Camargo CA Jr. Emergency treatment and prevention of insect-sting anaphylaxis. Curr Opin Allergy Clin Immunol. 2006;6(4):279-83.

Sunit Singhi

63 Anaphylaxis

Anaphylaxis is a potentially life-threatening allergic reaction. It most commonly is a IgE mediated reaction. Affected systems include skin (90%), respiratory 0%), gastrointestinal, cardiac, and CNS. Therefore, a patient may have wide range of clinical manifestations (Table 1). Good history and examination is crucial. The common causative agents include food (peanuts and pulses) and drugs penicillin). Very often the etiologic agent may not be evident. Some patients may exhibit a biphasic form or a late phase. The episode appears to get resolved, and then symptoms recur after several hours. It may occur in up to 30%. A severity classification is given in table 2. It can occur despite appropriate treatment; therefore, observe all patients for several hours. Late phase can occur 8-12 hours after the initial attack. There is no reliable predictor of biphasic or protracted anaphylaxis.

CLINICAL PRESENTATION

Onset of symptom is usually within 5-30 minutes of exposure to antigen; however, symptoms may be delayed up to an hour or more. Early administration of intramuscular

Table 1: Sings and symptoms of anaphylaxis

Respiratory	Upper: hoarseness, stridor, oropharyngeal or laryngeal edema, cough, complete obstruction.
	Lower: bronchospasm, tachypnea, cyanosis, use of accessory muscles, respiratory arrest.
Skin	Sensation of warmth, flushing, erythema, general pruritus, urticaria, angioedema.
Gastrointestinal	Nausea, vomiting, crampy abdominal pain, diarrhea.
Cardiovascular	Tachycardia, hypotension, arrhythmias, cardiac arrest.
Neurologic	Dizziness, weakness, syncope, seizures.
Other	Conjuctival injection, lacrimation, sneezing, mouth burning, itch.

Table 2: Grading of systemic reactions due to anaphylaxis

1.	Mild: Onset usually within 2 hours of exposure peripheral tingling, warm sensation followed by fullness of month and throat, nasal congetia periorbital edema, itching, tearing of the eyes and sneezing. Duration upto 2 days.
2.	Moderate: Onset and duration like mild reaction. Above plus broncho-spasm and/or edema of airway and larynx with dyspnea, cough and sneezing, flushing is common. Angioedema, urticaria, nasal and vomiting may occur.
3.	Severe: Onset abrupt, progress rapidly to are within minutes to intense bronchospasm and laryngeal edema; hoarseness, stridor, severe breathlessness and cyanosis, edema and hyper motility cause dysphasia, abdominal cramps, diarrhoea and vomiting. Cardiovascular collapse leads to hypotension, cardiac arrhythmia and shock.

epinephrine is critical. Delayed administration of epinephrine may increase the risk of a biphasic reaction.

ETIOLOGY

Drugs: Antibiotics, chemotherapeutic agents, radiocontrast media, blood products, aspirin, NSAIDs, gamma globulin, insulin, heparin, opiates.

Food: Nuts (peanuts, cashews, almonds, pecans, walnuts), milk, eggs, wheat, fish, seeds (sesame, sunflower, poppy), spices (cinnamon, nutmeg, mustard, saga), fruits (apples, bananas, peaches, oranges), chocolate, potato, corn, additives.

Latex

Venoms: Vasps and bees.

Exercise

Idiopathic

DIFFERENTIAL DIAGNOSIS

- Severe asthma
- Hereditary angioneurotic edema Foreign body aspiration
- Vasovagal response
- Hyperventilation syndrome
- Pheochromocytoma
- Drug overdose

MANAGEMENT

1. Care of ABC-Secure the airway and, give oxygen. If life-threatening airway obstruction occurs, intubate; if unsuccessful, perform cricothyroidotomy.
2. Give epinephrine 1:1,000 (0.1 mg/kg), 0.01 mL/kg up to 0.5 mL intramuscularly; it may be repeated every 15 minutes if necessary. Intramuscular epinephrine injections into the thigh have more rapid absorption and higher levels than IM or subcutaneous injections in the arm. IM route is preferred over subcutaneous because of more rapid absorption.
3. If hypotensive or unresponsive to initial dose: Give epinephrine 1: 10,000 IV at a dose of 0.01 mg/kg (0.1 mL/kg), a bolus of normal saline 20mL/kg, IV, and place the patient in recumbent position with feet elevated. If hypotension persists, administer epinephrine infusion 2-4 mcg/kg/min or dopamine 2 – 10 mcg/kg/min to maintain blood pressure.
4. Diphenhydramine 1-2 mg/kg IM or IV up to 50 mg q 4-6 h.
5. Methylprednisolone 1-2 mg/kg up to 125 mg IV q 4-6 h or prednisone 1-2 mg/kg orally up to 80 mg.
6. Consider ranitidine 1-2 mg/kg IV q 6-8 h for severe reactions.
7. Administer SalbutamoL/albuterol for bronchospasm; inhaled epinephrine for stridor.

8. Monitor vital signs frequently.
9. Observe the patient for at least 6-8 hours and at least 24 hours if severe reaction or history of asthma.

DISCHARGE PATIENT

- Counseling on avoidance of allergen.
- Referral to allergist is indicated for allergy testing.
- Medication: diphenhydramine and short course of steroids.
- Medic-alert bracelet information.

FURTHER READING

- Brown SG, Clinical features and severity grading of anaphylaxis, J. allergy Clin Immunol, 2004: 114(2):371-376.
- Chowdhury BA. Intramuscular versus subcutaneous injection of epinephrine in the treatment of anaphylaxis. J allergy Clin Immunol, 2002;109(4): 720.
- Lieberman P. The diagnosis and management of anaphylaxis. J allergy Clin Immunol. 2005;115(3):584-591.

Brian S. Zachariah

64 Hypothermia

Hypothermia is a condition in which the body's usual mechanisms for temperature regulation are overwhelmed by a cold stressor. It may be classified as accidental or intentional or as primary or secondary. Hypothermia is also classified frequently as mild, moderate or severe depending on the patient's core temperature.

Intentional or therapeutic, hypothermia is a deliberately induced state of altered core body temperature usually used as a neuroprotective measure, for example after cardiac arrest. This is uncommonly used in the pediatric population and will not be discussed further in this chapter. Secondary hypothermia is a lowered core temperature as a result of a medical illness, such as profound hypothyroidism, which lowers the body's temperature set-point. This is also uncommon in the pediatric age group and will likewise not be discussed further. Therefore, the focus of this chapter is accidental, primary hypothermia usually as a result of environmental exposure in an otherwise healthy pediatric patient.

The body loses heat via several mechanisms, the most important of which under dry conditions, is radiation. In the adult and older child this may account for 55 to 65% of total heat loss. This percentage may be even greater in an infant. An infant's exposed head alone may be responsible for upto 50% of body heat loss at an ambient temperature of 9°C (39°F). Conduction is the direct transfer of heat to another object and usually accounts for only 2 to 3% of heat loss in dry conditions. However this may increase 20 to 30 times if the body is submerged in cold water. Convection may also be viewed as the direct transfer of heat, however to the circulating air rather than to another object. It usually accounts for approximately 10% of body heat loss but increases on cold, windy days. Conductive and convective losses are the most common causes of accidental hypothermia.

Evaporation may also be an important source of heat loss, accounting for up to 25% of total heat loss on a cold day. Evaporative heat loss includes insensible water losses from the skin as well as the evaporation of water vapor from the respiratory tract. This can be more significant than is commonly realized. For example, 580 calories are lost for each gram of water which evaporates from the skin or respiratory tract (Edlich).

PATHOPHYSIOLOGY

Hypothermia is also classified as either mild (35 to 33°C), moderate (32 to 29°C), and severe (less than 29°C). The initial response to cold stress is excitatory. The basal metabolic rate increases as does the heart rate, respiratory rate and blood pressure. However, as core temperature reaches approximately 32°C bodily functions begin to slow. Basal metabolic rate drops approximately 10% for each degree centigrade of core temperature decrease and oxygen consumption also decreases (Table 1).

Table 1: Temperature and pathophysiologic correlation

Core Temperature		
°C	°F	**Pathophysiologic Changes**
Mild Hypothermia		
37.6	99.6	Normal rectal temperature
35	95	Excitatory phase: Metabolic rate increases, vasoconstriction, maximal shivering
34	93.2	BP, heart rate, respiratory rate all increase
33	91.4	Confusion, ataxia, slurred speech
Moderate Hypothermia		
32	89.6	Stupor, decreased oxygen consumption
31	87.6	BP, heart rate, respiratory rate all decrease
30	86	Shivering stops
29	85.2	Atrial fibrillation
Severe Hypothermia		
28	82.4	Increased risk of VF. BMR approximately 50%
27	80.6	Unconsciousness
26	78.8	DTRs absent
23	73.4	Pupils fixed and dilated
20	68	Asystole, flat EEG

As core temperature drops below 32° and moderate hypothermia ensues cardiovascular function begins to decline. The electrical conduction system of the heart is affected to a greater degree than is the myocardium itself. Moderate hypothermia is associated with widening of the QRS complex and prolongation of the PR and QT intervals. Bradycardia and atrial arrhythmias are also commonly seen. This bradycardia is due to decreased depolarization of cardiac pacemaker cells and is not vagally mediated. Therefore it may be refractory to standard therapy such as atropine. Osborne or J waves (Figure 1) are often associated with hypothermia but they may be a normal variant and are also seen in other disease conditions such as sepsis and myocardial ischemia as well. Ventricular fibrillation may develop with severe hypothermia as core temperature approaches 29°C (Danzl). Asystole may also be the presenting ECG rhythm, particularly in severe hypothermia with very low (approximately 20 degrees centigrade) core temperatures.

Hypothermia also causes a progressive slowing of nerve conduction (Moss, Patton). With mild hypothermia this may appear as confusion, ataxia, clumsiness and slurred speech. Shivering is also common but begins to stop as core temperature approaches 30°C. Also as moderate hypothermia develops decreased mental status occurs and depressed brain-stem function further depresses heart rate, blood pressure, and respiratory rate. In severe hypothermia reflexes usually disappear around 27°C and unconsciousness usually occurs around 26°C. Pupils become fixed and dilated at approximately 23°C and at the later stages of severe hypothermia the patient frequently appears clinically dead when first encountered by rescuers.

The respiratory system is also affected, particularly in moderate to severe hypother-

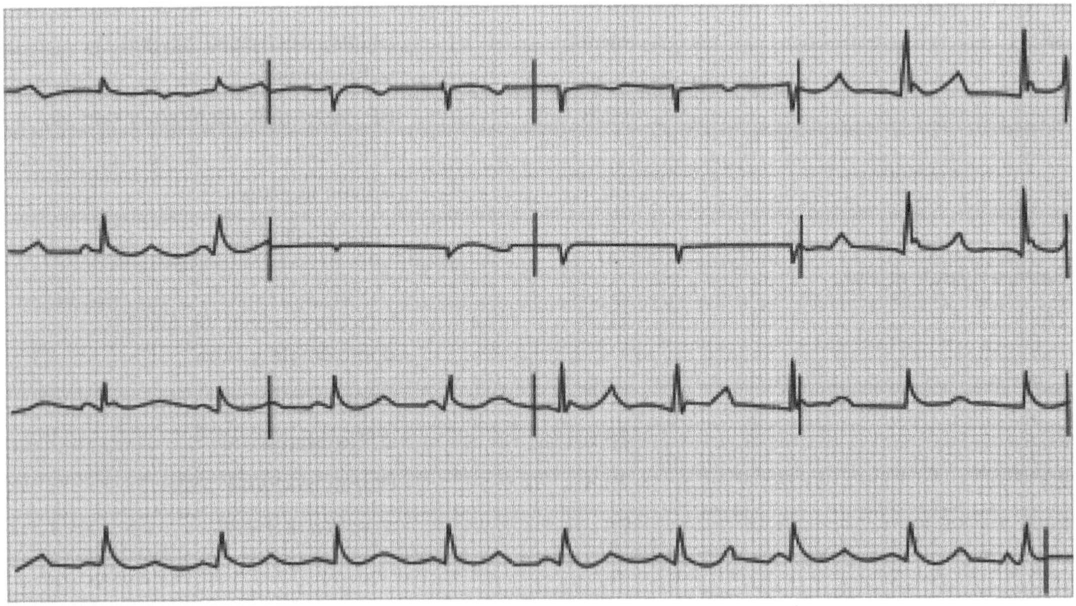

Figure 1

mia. As core temperature falls below 32°C the respiratory rate and minute volume decline. The cough reflex is lost and non-cardiogenic pulmonary edema may occur. Spontaneous respiration ceases in severe hypothermia, usually at a temperature of approximately 24°C.

While cardiovascular and central nervous system effects predominate, hypothermia affects virtually all organ systems and multiple physiological and laboratory abnormalities may be noted. As core temperature decreases gastric dilation and a paralytic ileus may develop, hepatic metabolism decreases and pancreatitis is not uncommon. Also a cold diuresis develops associated with an increased output of dilute urine (Moss). As kidney function decreases nitrogenous waste may accumulate and BUN may rise. Acidosis may also develop as endogenous acids cannot be cleared by the kidney. And the combination of decreased renal and hepatic function may lead to increased concentrations of exogenously administered medications.

The cold diuresis of dilute urine along with interstitial edema results in a decrease in intravascular plasma volume and hemoconcentration. This in turn increases blood viscosity. Cold temperatures also shift the oxyhemoglobin dissociation curve to the left resulting in less oxygen delivery to the tissues. Severe hypothermia may cause prolonged bleeding and elevated coagulation times and even frank DIC may result. Due to hepatic and splenic sequestration, leukocyte and platelet counts may be decreased (Wong).

PREDISPOSING CONDITIONS

Aside from iatrogenic hypothermia in the delivery room or neonatal unit, accidental hypothermia is primarily an environmental disease. Even healthy children exposed to severe cold weather conditions can become hypothermic. Outdoor winter activities and cold-water immersion are frequently associated with hypothermia. However, a child need not be exposed to the external environment to become hypothermic. Inadequate household heating during the cold winter months for example is a common cause for hypothermia in urban areas.

Children in general and neonates in particular are especially likely to develop hypothermia. Neonates, particularly premature infants, lack adequate temperature regulation. Also their large surface area relative to their mass, their paucity of subcutaneous fat, and their inability to shiver make them particularly vulnerable to cold stress. Also premature infants lack adequate brown fat stores and instead tend to conserve heat by vasoconstriction. In turn this vasoconstriction can lead to anaerobic metabolism and acidosis which further reduces their ability to tolerate cold conditions (Fant).

Overall the conditions which predispose a child to hypothermia can be divided into defects of temperature regulation, thermogenesis, and heat conservation. Temperature regulation is controlled by the hypothalamus and may be affected by congenital anomalies as well as by acquired conditions such as central nervous system hemorrhage, meningitis, encephalitis, neoplasms, or kernicterus (Lonning). In addition, medications such as the phenothiazines, tricyclic antidepressants, barbiturates and narcotics can impair thermoregulation as can toxins such as ethanol, carbon monoxide and the organophosphates.

Thermogenesis may be impaired by malnutrition, hypoglycemia, hypothyroidism, hypopituitarism, and hypoadrenalism. Heat conservation may be impaired by loss of intact skin such as occurs with a large burns and exploited dermatoses. In addition, spinal cord injuries and neuromuscular diseases may impair cold perception preventing the patient from seeking shelter or taking other routine measures to prevent heat loss. They may also interfere with the body's natural heat conservation and heat production mechanisms such as vasoconstriction and shivering.

Finally, a variety of conditions such as sepsis (daga), trauma, diabetic ketoacidosis, renal failure, and congenital heart disease are frequently associated with hypothermia.

HISTORY AND PHYSICAL EXAMINATION

Hypothermia may be obvious in the setting of severe environmental exposure however, the presentation may be subtle or even overlooked with exposure to less extreme cold. In fact, mild to moderate hypothermia may present with subtle or misleading symptoms such as confusion, dizziness, chills or dyspnea (Edelstein). Therefore, as usual, history is often the key to making the diagnosis.

In many cases the history must be obtained from the child's parents or companions or the responding medics. Early symptoms of hypothermia may include mood changes, irritability, and poor judgement. Companions may note paradoxical undressing (removing clothing in response to prolonged and severe cold stress), shivering, or rhythmic motions such as rocking. Later in the course of hypothermia the patient may present in coma or cardiac arrest and without an adequate history the precipitating cause may be missed and the appropriate treatment not delivered. A complete history should also include an inquiry about the use of alcohol or illicit drugs as these are commonly associated with hypothermia particularly in older children. Also a past medical history is important as underlying medical conditions frequently lead to or worsen hypothermia.

While a proper history is important, the key to the diagnosis of hypothermia is the rapid determination of core body temperature. In the field this may be difficult, although low-reading glass thermometers are often carried by EMS providers in areas where hypothermia is of particular concern. These thermometers may be used either orally or rectally, but may not accurately reflect core temperature. Once the patient arrives in the emergency department, core temperature is best measured with a low-reading probe placed in the bladder, rectum or esophagus. Even with a temperature probe in place continued caution and diligence is still indicated. Inaccurately low temperatures may be recorded if the rectal probe is lodged in the stool. for example. Probes may also become dislodged and there may be a lag between the probe's reading and the true core temperature during the rewarming process.

Careful assessment and management of the ABC's is indicated. Of note, profound bradycardia and intense vasoconstriction may make a peripheral pulse difficult to detect. In the field a full minute should be taken to assess the presence of a pulse before concluding that none is present. In the emergency department, a Doppler may assist in obtaining both pulse and blood pressure readings. A complete secondary survey (head-to-toe examination) should be performed looking particularly for signs of trauma, complications of hypothermia, and/or signs of any underlying condition which may have caused or worsen the hypothermia. A complete neurological examination is indicated as the degree of neurological impairment correlates closely with the degree of core temperature lowering.

Ancillary Tests

If the patient is hypoxic then a chest x-ray should be obtained. Aspiration pneumonia and noncardiogenic pulmonary edema are often identified. A chest X-ray also may be indicated if trauma is the cause of, or associated with, the hypothermia. Also in patients with trauma or an altered mental status of unknown cause a noncontrast head CT scan and other standard trauma or altered mental status work up may be indicated.

An ECG may show prolonged PR, QRS, and QT intervals or atrial or ventricular arrhythmias as discussed above. Also as previously discussed, J or Osborne waves may be seen and are often proportional to the degree of hypothermia, commonly occurring with temperatures below 30°C. However, Osborne waves are not diagnostic of hypothermia and may occur in other conditions such as cardiac ischemia or CNS lesions and in fact may be a normal variant in some children (Paton).

The main purpose of laboratory tests is to detect either complications of hypothermia or to identify any underlying medical conditions which may contribute to or complicate the diagnosis or alter the treatment plan. Commonly performed tests include a complete blood count, glucose, electrolytes, anticoagulation studies, liver function tests, urinalysis and toxicologic screens. As sepsis is commonly associated with hypothermia, especially in infants, blood cultures and a septic workup may be indicated.

A variety of abnormalities are commonly seen on laboratory studies. Due to cold diuresis, many hypothermic patients are volume contracted and as a result hematocrit levels may be deceptively high. Leukocytes may be elevated with infection or depressed due to hepatic and splenic sequestration. Electrolyte abnormalities are common but they tend to occur in a varied and unpredictable fashion. For example, hyperglycemia may occur with acute hypothermia with impaired insulin function, decreased renal clearance, and reduced hepatic metabolism. On the other hand, hypoglycemia may occur in chronic or secondary hypothermia from malnutrition and depletion of glycogen stores. While other electrolyte changes such as elevated BUN and creatinine may occur in an unpredictable fashion, serum potassium levels may be useful in evaluating prognosis. Elevated potassium levels occur from cellular destruction and a level greater than or equal to 10 mmol/liter is associated with a low likelihood of recovery (Edelstein).

Liver function tests are often elevated and amylase may be elevated if pancreatitis develops secondary to hypothermia. Moderate to severe hypothermia often leads to a disruption in the regulation mechanism and frank DIC may develop. Since most coagulation studies are performed in a laboratory at 37°C, the hypothermic patient may develop a clinically-evident coagulopathy which is not reflected in the deceptively normal laboratory values.

This difference between the patient's core temperature and the temperature at which laboratory studies are performed is also significant in the interpretation of arterial blood gases. Metabolic (lactic) acidosis is common in hypothermia due to shivering, poor tissue perfusion, impaired hepatic metabolism, impaired buffering capacity of cold blood, and reduced renal clearance of lactic acid. PO_2 and PCO_2 levels may also be affected by the balance between the reduced cardiac function (supply) and the reduced metabolic demand seen in hypothermia (Danzl, Pozos). All modern blood gas analyzers warm the sample to 37 degrees C before performing the analysis and because gases are less soluble at lower temperatures many incorrectly believe that arterial blood gases may show oxygen and carbon dioxide levels higher and a pH lower than that found in the patient as the blood is warmed by the machine. However, ABGs obtained on hypothermic patients should not be corrected for temperature and the best approach is to compare uncorrected ABG values with the normal values at 37 degrees C (Edelstein, Delaney).

MANAGEMENT

Hypothermia treatment focuses on preventing further heat loss, supporting the cardiopulmonary system, rewarming the body's core and preventing or correcting complications, most notably ventricular fibrillation or other malignant cardiac rhythms.

Since death may be difficult to determine in the profoundly hypothermic patient, and since good neurologic outcome is possible after prolonged, hypothermic, cardiac arrest, aggressive resuscitation measures are warranted, even in apparently deceased victims, until they have been warmed to above 32 degrees C (Kelly).

Treatment of hypothermia is driven by the severity of the hypothermia, so obtaining a reliable core temperature is a vital early step. An overview of hypothermia treatment is found in Table 2. However, in the field environment, before a core temperature reading can be obtained friends, bystanders or first-responders should begin treatment by preventing further cooling. This can be done by removing wet clothing and replacing it with dry clothing, blankets, or sleeping bags, etc. Conscious patients may be given warm food and drink, but they should rest and not risk further heat loss by continued activity in a cold environment.

Trained rescuers should begin begin rewarming efforts in the field. The one exception is in the case of frostbite where rewarming of the extremity would preclude self-rescue. Chemical heat packs or hot water bottles applied to the axillae, groin and abdomen are a good, field-expedient active external rewarming technique. Care should be taken however to avoid causing burns from overly aggressive active external rewarming.

Patients should always be handled and moved gently to avoid cardiac dysrhythmias. The ABCs should be carefully assessed and managed. Supplemental oxygen should be supplied and the patient intubated if respiratory failure is present. It may be necessary to palpate the pulse for a full minute before deciding that one is absent. If no cardiac monitor is available, the patient is severely hypothermic, and no pulse or other signs of life are apparent, then CPR should be started. However, if a cardiac monitor is available it should be used and CPR withheld even if only a weak pulse or any organized cardiac activity is present.

Table 2: Overview of hypothermia management

Obtain core temperature			
35-33°C (Mild)	32-29°C (Moderate)	< 29°C (Severe)	
Passive Ext. Rewarming Active Ext. Rewarming	Passive Ext. Rewarming (Noninvasive) Active Int. Rewarming Active. Ext. Rewarming	Cardiac Arrest Rhythm Asystole VF	Noncardiac Arrest Rhythm
		CPR	Avoid Compressions
		Defib 2 J/kg (VF)	Active Int. Rewarming- both noninvasive and invasive as appropriate and available
		Intubate Continue CPR	
		Invasive Active Int. Rewarming as available Continue CPR until rewarmed or stable	

While generally ineffective while the patient is still hypothermic, one attempt at defibrillation of ventricular fibrillation (VF) at 2 joules/kilogram should be attempted (Orlowske). CPR should be continued, but further attempts at defibrillation as well as further cardioactive medications should be avoided until the patient arrives at the Emergency Department. Pacing, atropine and lidocaine are all generally ineffective in the hypothermic patient. Bretylium on the other hand has been shown to be effective in both the prophylaxis and treatment of hypothermic VF at an initial dose of 5 mg/kg IV. However, it is no longer widely available.

Care in the ED is very similar to prehospital care although more resources are generally available. If not already done wet clothing should be removed and replaced with warm, dry materials. An accurate core temperature should be obtained as previously discussed. Again careful attention to the ABCs is necessary. Endotracheal intubation, placement of a urinary catheter and IV access should not be delayed but should be performed gently to avoid precipitating a cardiac dysrhythmia. As previously mentioned, bretylium may be the most effective drug to treat cardiac ectopy in hypothermic patients. If available, an initial dose of 5 mg per kilogram IV (repeated at 10 mg per kilogram, as needed) should be administered to treat cardiac dysrhythmias. In fact, the US Wilderness Emergency Medical Services Institute recommends empiric bretylium for all patients with profound hypothermia (Edelstein). Amiodarone should also be considered if the patient remains in VF after rewarming above 30 degrees C.

Normal saline or D5 normal saline are the fluids of choice. Lactated Ringers is not recommended because the hypothermic liver cannot metabolize lactate. Fluids should generally be warmed to between 45 and 65°C. This can be done with a fluid warmer or via storing intravenous fluid bags in a heater. If neither of these are available, intravenous fluids (that do not contain dextrose) can be heated in a microwave oven.

REWARMING TECHNIQUES

Overall, the rewarming techniques used both in the field and in the Emergency Department can be divided into two categories: passive rewarming and active rewarming.

Passive rewarming is used, mostly in the field, in cases of mild hypothermia to prevent further heat loss and allow endogenously produced heat to rewarm the patient. Passive rewarming techniques include removing affected patients from the cold environment and replacing their wet clothing with dry materials.

Active rewarming techniques are utilized in moderate to severe hypothermia when endogenous thermogenesis is inadequate. These can be further divided into active external rewarming and active internal rewarming techniques. Active external rewarming includes techniques such as the use of hot packs, radiant warmers, heated blankets and incubators. These may be appropriate in mild to moderate hypothermia but should be avoided in severe hypothermia as they are often ineffective and may even result in core temperature to drop (the decreasing core temperature after rewarming has started). Not only can this cause a decrease in core temperature but the flow of cold, acidic blood back to the core can precipitate ventricular fibrillation in an already compromised myocardium.

The methods of choice for severe hypothermia instead are the active internal rewarming techniques. Examples include the use of warm IV fluids, warm humidified oxygen, gastric, peritoneal or pleural lavage, mediastinal irrigation, hemodialysis and cardiopulmonary bypass. These techniques result in rewarming rates between 2.5 and 20°C per hour with the more aggressive techniques such as thoracic lavage or cardiopulmonary bypass generally resulting in faster rewarming rates.

Most patients with mild to moderate hypothermia will not require intensive intervention and will recover satisfactorily. However, aggressive treatment even for those patients who are comatose, have nonperfusing rhythms or appear dead is justified in the literature with intact neurological survival even in patients who initially presented with hypothermic cardiac arrest (Edelstein). In such cases the more aggressive active internal rewarming techniques discussed above may be necessary and should be continued until the patient either recovers or remains clinically dead after rewarming.

This may be particularly important in the case of cold or ice-water submersion injuries, especially in children. Children submerged in cold water cool rapidly due to their large surface area and low subcutaneous fat insulation. This rapid cooling is thought to protect cellular function. Therefore, such children should be aggressively treated even if they have been submerged for lengthy periods of time prior to rescue.

Survivors of moderate hypothermia should be admitted to the hospital and victims of severe hypothermia to the ICU. Cardiac and respiratory function should be closely monitored. Hypotension should be treated with IV fluids. Pulmonary edema may develp and should be treated with oxygen, empiric antibiotic coverage for aspiration pneumonia and diuretics, if necessary. Rhabdomyolysis may develop. Frostbite may require surgical exploration or even debridement. Pancreatitis is also not an uncommon complication of hypothermia.

PREVENTION

As is frequently the case, preventing hypothermia is far simpler than than treating it. Children involved in outdoor winter activities should be taught to dress appropriately and to change clothing immediately if it becomes wet. They should also be taught how to recognize the signs of hypothermia and to begin first aid for hypothermia if they recognize them in themselves or their companions.

In other settings, iatrogenic hypothermia is a greater risk. Newborns should be dried and wrapped in blankets immediately after delivery. Their heads should be covered and examinations should be performed under a radiant warmer.

Also, underlying medical conditions that may predispose a child to hypothermia should be identified by their primary care provider and special precautions should be taken to prevent hypothermia in these cases. Also, adequately heated homes and good nutrition help prevent hypothermia and referral to social service agencies may be necessary to ensure these for vulnerable children.

CONCLUSION

Hypothermia is generally an environmental illness and is most common in cold winter months. However, it can occur in temperate climates and warm months as well. Infants and those children with underlying medical conditions are especially at risk for hypothermia both from environmental exposure and otherwise.

An accurate core temperature is key to the diagnosis and treatment of hypothermia. Mild hypothermia can be treated conservatively. Moderate hypothermia may require more involved rewarming techniques. Severe hypothermia should be treated aggressive, usually invasively, even if the child appears clinically dead on initial presentation.

REFERENCES

1. Edlich RF, Chang DE, Birk KA, *et al.* Cold injuries. Compr Ther 1989; 15:13-21.
2. Danzl DF. Accidental hypothermia. In Marx, J et al eds. Rosen's Emergency Medicine: Concepts and Clincal Practice. St. Louis: Mosby, 2005.
3. Moss J. Accidental severe hypothermia. Surg Gynecol Obstet 1986;162:501-513.
4. Patton BC. Accidental hypthothermia. Pharmacol Ther 1983;22:331-377.
5. Wong KC. Physiology and pharmacology of hypothermia. West J Med 1983;138:227-232.
6. Fant M, Cloherty IP. Temperature control. In Cloherty JP, Stark AR, eds. Manual of neonatal care. Boston: Little, Brown, 1985.
7. Lonning PE, Skulberg A, Abyhom F. Accidental hypothermia review of the literature. Acta Anaesthesiol Scan 1986;30:601-613.
8. Daga R, Gorodischer R. Infections in hypothermic infants younger than 3 months old. Am J Dis Child 1984;138:483-485.
9. Edelstein JA, James, L, Silverberg MA, *et al.* Hypothermia. eMedicine, Dec. 2007.
10. Danzl DF, Pozos RD, Auerbach PS, *et al.* Multicenter hypothermia survey. Ann Emerg Med 1987;16:1042-1055.
11. Delaney KA, Howland MA, Vasallo S, *et al.* Assessment of acid-base disturbances in hypothermia and their physiologic consequences. Ann Emerg Med 1989;18:72-82.

- Kelly KJ, Glaeser P, Rice TB *et al.* Profound accidental hypothermia and freeze injury of the extremities in a child. Crit Care Med 1990;18:679-680.
- Orlowske JP. Drowning, near-drowning, and ice-water submersions. Pediatr Clin North Am 1987;34:75-92.

In the previous edition this chapter was written by Steven C. Jackson, MD Staff Emergency Physician Adventist Hospital Portland, Oregon

Yuri Gilhotra and Sonia Singh

65 Heat-induced Illness

Children frequently present to the emergency department because of an abnormally elevated body temperature or hyperthermia. Hyperthermia in the pediatric patient differs physiologically from fever. Fever (rectal temperature greater than or equal to 38 C) is caused by an elevation of body temperature secondary to changes of the thermo-regulatory control center in the hypo-thalamus' Hyperthermia in children, high body temperature not caused by hypo-thalamic thermoregulatory mechanisms, is commonly caused by one of the following:

- Overheating.
- Increased heat production.
- Reduced heat loss.

In the small infant or neonate, overheating is almost always the cause. In children, heat-induced illness is a common cause of non-traumatic death. As children have a greater body surface area relative to mass they are at particular risk of hyper-thermia.

CAUSES

Overheating

This is commonly seen in settings of high ambient temperature and humidity. Children involved with athletic events and other summertime sporting events are at risk particularly during summer months and heat waves. Young children left in locked cars in summer are also vulnerable to heat injury, since the ambient temperature inside the car can reach to 60° C.

Increased Heat Production

Metabolic illness such as hyperthyroidism can cause an increase in heat production. Drugs (anticholinergics, sympathomimetics, aspirin, neuroleptic agents, and selective reuptake inhibitors) as well as seizures are associated with increased heat production.

Decreased Heat Loss

This is commonly seen in disease states such as cystic fibrosis and heart disease. Drugs (phenothiazines, anticholinergics), over-wrapped babies and excessive clothing on hot and humid days can cause a decrease in heat loss.

CLINICAL FEATURES

Heat-related injuries span a wide range of pathological adversities from benign heat cramps to lethal heat stroke. Overheating syndromes represent a continuum of physiological derangement in which cerebral dysfunction is at the extreme end of the spectrum. The spectrum of heat injuries depicts an inability to physiologically react to environmental conditions, insufficient correction of fluid and electrolyte losses, and the result of coming into contact with a host of various heat sources. One must also consider child safety and neglect issues.

Heat Injury

Minor syndromes
- Heat edema
- Prickly Heat
- Heat syncope
- Heat Cramps
- Heat Exhaustion

Major Syndromes
- Heatstroke

The Neonate and Infant

Overheating is the most common cause of hyperthermia in the neonate or infant. It is important to distinguish the healthy overheated infant from the febrile infanf (Table 1)

Table 1: The Overheated and Febrile Infant

Overheated Infant	*Febrile Infant*
High rectal temperature	High rectal temperature
Warm hands and feet	Cool hands and feet
Pink skin	Pale skin
Extended posture	Lethargic
Healthy appearance	Looks unwell
Abdominal temperature exceeds hand temperature by less than 2C	Abdominal temperature exceeds hand temperature by more than 3C

Mild overheating as a result of over-wrapping is generally not dangerous, although there may be an association with apnoeic episodes in premature babier. Significant hyperthermia is dangerous and has been linked with sudden death*-;, particularly in families with a history of malignant hyperthermia.

Heat Edema

This is a self-limited process manifested by mild swelling and tightening of the hands and feet that appears within the first few days of exposure to a hot environment. It is caused by cutaneous vasodilatation and orthostatic pooling of interstitial fluid in the extremities. Usually resolves spontaneously in a few days but can take up to 6 weeks. No special treatment is necessary.

Prickly Heat

This is a pruritic, maculopapular, erythematous rash over clothed areas of the body. Also known as lichen tropicus, miliaria rubra and heat rash. It is caused by acute inflammation of the sweat ducts by blockage of the sweat pores by macerated stratum corneum. Initially itching is the main feature and may respond to antihistamines. The ducts may become secondarily infected with Staphylococcus aureus. Prickly heat can be prevented by wearing clean, light and loose-fitting clothes and avoiding sweat-generating conditions.

Heat Syncope

Heat syncope commonly involves children who have been standing for prolonged periods in hot and humid weather or who have undergone strenuous exertion. It is essentially benign and the mechanism is similar to vasovagal syncope. Treatment consists of placing the patient in the

Trendelenburg position and rehydration with oral or IV isotonic fluids. Hospitalisation is usually not nevessary

Heat Cramps

Heat cramps are severe, painful, involuntary, spasmodic contractions of skeletal muscles, usually those of the calves but may involve the thighs and shoulders. They occur in children who are sweating profusely and replace fluid losses with water or other hypotonic solutions. Cramps may 'occur at the time of exercise or after a latent period of several hours. The exact pathogenesis is unknown but it is generally accepted to be caused by a relative deficiency of sodium, potassium and fluid at the cellular level.

Treatment consists of rest in a cooled environment and fluid and salt replacement, either orally or intravenously with isotonic fluids (0.9% NaCI). Rhabdomyolysis is a rare complication and occurs secondary to protracted and diffuse muscle spasm. Massage and stretching of the involved muscles may be useful for reducing pain and facilitating return of the athlete to the sport or game. Heat cramps can be prevented by maintaining adequate dietary salt intake or drinking commercial electrolyte beverages.

Heat Exhaustion

Heat exhaustion presents in children with vomiting, headache, lethargy, weakness, hyperpyrexia and with a normal menial state. Physiologically it is caused predominantly by water depletion, but in some pediatric patients (e.g. those with cystic fibrosis, in whom greater amounts of salt are lost in their sweat), heat exhaustion can occur predominantly due to salt depletion"

Heat exhaustion is also treated by rest and volume and electrolyte replacement. Generally, these patients do not require hospitalization.

HEATSTROKE

Heat stroke is a medical emergency. The cardinal features of heatstroke are core temperature greater than 40.5C (104.9F) and an altered mental state. Heat stroke can lead to multi-organ failure and is associated with a high mortality rate. Classic pediatric presentations include the adolescent who is staying outdoors in bright sun and exercising vigorously in a hot and humid environment or children who are left in cars in hot weather.

The CNS is especially vulnerable in heatstroke and children may have irritability, confusion, seizures and coma. The cerebellum is highly sensitive to heat, and ataxia can be an early finding. Cerebral edema is quite common and CNS dysfunction is universal at temperatures higher than 42C. Liver injury, renal failure secondary to rhabdomyolysis, non-cardiogenic pulmonary edema, and disseminated intravascular coagulation are all part of the multi-system involvement.

Treatment of Heatstroke

Initial Resuscitation

Initial attention must be paid to the ABCs and children should be moved to the resuscitation room. High flow oxygen, cardiac monitoring, pulse oximetry, intravenous access with intravenous fluid infusions of either normal saline or Ringer's lactate must be started immediately. Core temperature monitoring (rectal probe or oesophageal probe if intubated) and insertion of a foley catheter should occur early. Diagnostic studies looking for end-organ damage include complete blood count, electrolytes, renal function, liver function tests, coagulation profile, creatinine kinase, urinalysis, ECG, chest radiograph. Computed tomography of the head and lumbar puncture may also be indicated as part of the evaluation of altered mental status.

Cooling Techniques

Once initial resuscitation has been instituted, rapid external cooling is the next immediate goal with reduction of the core temperature to 40C (104F). Convection methods (evaporative cooling) are the simplest and fastest non-invasive technique. It involves removing the child's clothing, sponging the skin or spraying tepid water onto the patient and then placing a fan close to the skin. Ice packs can be applies to neck, groin and axillae. Two problems associated with evaporative cooling are shivering which can generate heat, and the inability of cardiac electrodes to adhere to the skin. Shivering is treated with intravenous benzodiazepines and secondarily with phenothiazines. Antipyretics have no role and should be avoided. Immersion cooling where the undressed child is placed in a tub of water covering the trunk and extremities is limited to situations where evaporative cooling is not possible. Problems include displacement of monitoring and temperature probes and the inability to perform defibrillation or resuscitative procedures. In extreme cases more invasive lavage cooling methods may be considered. Gastric lavage is safe in the intubated patient, and peritoneal lavage is an effective rapid cooling technique. In refractory heatstroke cardiopulmonary bypass is an option if available. Complications such as shock, non-cardiogenic pulmonary edema, cerebral edema, consumptive coagulopathy, renal failure and hepatic failure should be treated as outlined in other chapters of this book. The mortality rate for heatstroke is 10%.

MALIGNANT HYPERTHERMIA

This is a complication of some anesthetic agents, and the suspected agent should be stopped immediately, especially if it is an inhalational anaesthetic. Treatment involves the administration of dantrolene, a specific antidote, which inhibits the release of calcium into muscles. Other treatments include hyperventilation with 100% oxygen, bicarbonate, lidocaine to treat arrhythmias, and aggressive cooling of the child. The principles of cooling in malignant hyperthermia are similar to those of heatstroke. The mortality rate for malignant hyperthermia is 7%.

Neuroleptic Malignant Syndrome

Neuroleptic malignant syndrome (NMS) is a rare, life-threatening, idiosyncratic reaction to neuroleptic medications which can cause extreme hyperthermia. Common causative agents include phenothiazenes, thioxanthenes, butyrophenones (especially haloperidol), tricyclic antidepressants, and lithium". Benzodiazepines and chlorpro-mazine are the mainstay of therapy and in severe cases dantrolene may be used. In most patients, symptoms resolve within 24-48 hours after stopping the drug.

PREVENTION

Prevention, particularly in babies and infants, is based on education of new parents about the risks of sun exposure, excess clothing and leaving children in cars, even for brief periods. Sports medicine guidelines regarding older children taking part in sporting activities in hot, humid weather may be useful.

FURTHER READING

1. Behrman RE et al 1996 Textbook of Paediatrics. Saunders, London, 2106.
2. Roberton NRC 1999 Temperature control and its disorders. In: Rennie JM, Roberton NRC (eds). Textbook of Neonatology. Churchill Livingstone, London, 229.
3. Denborough MA, Galloway GJ, Hopkinson KC 1982. Malignant hyperpyrexia and sudden infant death. Lancet Nov 13;2(8307):1068-9.
4. Thompson A 1996 Environmental emergencies. In: Fleisher GR et al (eds) Synopsis of Pediatric Emergency Medicine. Williams and Wilkins, Philadelphia, 452-456.

Banani Poddar

66 Burns and Electrocution

BURNS

Burns in childhood are often accidental and carry a high morbidity and mortality, the latter being more so in the developing world. While in the 1940s only half the patients with burns involving 40% of the body surface area would have survived; today, over 50% of those with burns involving 80% of the body surface survive in developed countries[1]. In children, adolescents and young adults the survival is even higher with over 80% survival with burns involving 90% body surface area. However, specialised burn care facilities are scarce in the developing countries and the mortality and morbidity are higher. The factors, which increase the risk of death, are extremes of age; body surface area burnt exceeding 40% and the presence of inhalational injury[2]. In Indian children, the factors affecting mortality were presence of infection and large surface area burns[3].

Serious burns evolve through a continuum of phases; namely[4]

a) Burn shock, which is fatal to those with large burns and manifests in the first few days,
b) Burn wound sepsis, which manifests in the first few post-injury weeks and is often difficult to treat, and
c) Post burn deformity, which occurs in the survivors as their wounds heal.

Mechanisms of Injury[5]

Scalds: Most of the burns in children below 4 years of age is due to scalds, i.e., due to hot liquids or bath water. These are usually epidermal or superficial dermal burns.

Flame burns: This in common in older children. These tend to be deep dermal or full thickness burns, and often associated inhalational injury.

Contact burns: Contact with a hot substance, e.g., a hot iron, is responsible for this and can occur in smaller children.

Electrical and chemical burns are the least common.

Child abuse accounts for around 5 -10 % of burns in the developed countries. In India, in addition, children are sometimes included in suicidal burns committed by the mother[3].

Physiology of Burn Injury[4, 5]

The three zones of a burn, from the point of maximum injury to the surrounding, are

a) Zone of coagulation, where there is irreversible tissue loss due to coagulation of the proteins.
b) Zone of stasis, where there is decreased

tissue perfusion, but the tissue is potentially salvageable with good resuscitation, and

c) Zone of hyperemia, where there is increased tissue perfusion; this zone usually recovers.

Apart from the above local effects, when the burn area exceeds 20% of the body surface area, cytokines and inflammatory mediators released from the site of injury results in systemic effects. Increased capillary permeability leading to loss of proteins and fluids into the interstitial compartment, peripheral and splanchnic vasoconstriction and decreased myocardial contractility all lead to tissue hypoperfusion. A hypermetabolic response is seen following successful resuscitation along with insulin resistance, protein catabolism and increased gluconeogenesis. To counteract this and to prevent gut mucosal damage due to splanchnic vasoconstriction, early and aggressive enteral nutrition is required. Bronchoconstriction can occur with inhalation injury and ARDS with severe burns. A non-specific down regulation of the immune response is also seen.

Management

First Aid[6]:

First, the burning process should be stopped, if possible, and the patient removed to safety.Clothing can retain heat and should be removed as soon as possible; however, removal of adherent clothing such as synthetic clothing should not be attempted.

Active cooling prevents progression of the wound, if performed within the first 20 minutes of the injury. Immersion or irrigation with tap water for 20 minutes is recommended. Ice cold water should not be used; it may induce intense vasoconstriction. Cooling large areas of skin can lead to hypothermia and should be avoided. Irrigation is also recommended in chemical burns.

Pain is reduced to a large extent by covering the wound, but may require oral non-steroidal anti-inflammatory agents or narcotics for large burns.

The burn should be covered with a clean cotton sheet/cloth or even cling film and then a blanket placed over this to keep the patient warm. It is important to remember that the dressings should not be wrapped around as subsequent edema can lead to constriction. Wet dressings should not be used.

Burns are tetanus-prone wounds. If unimmunized or in doubt, tetanus vaccine should be administered. In case of large or heavily contaminated wounds, passive prophylaxis with immunoglobulin is recommended.

Topical creams applied to the burn wounds at this stage can interfere with subsequent assessment of the depth and extent of the burn and should be avoided.

Minor Burns[3, 6]:

Minor burns are those that are small (<5% body surface area) and superficial and not affecting important areas such as face etc or <1% body surface area if deep. These children are best managed as outpatients.

A complete assessment for depth and extent of burn is made and details of any illness, which could affect the management or outcome, are noted.

Usually a fresh burn wound is sterile; however, it should be cleaned with water and a mild antibacterial substance (or soap) if any visible dirt is present. Small blisters are left as such and large blisters may be de-roofed if they affect the function of the part affected.

Elevation of the affected part to reduce edema is important in the first few days (e.g., in case of facial burns, the child should sleep with the head propped up).

Dressings should be of simple gauze impregnated with sterile petroleum jelly. Topical creams should be applied only after 24 – 48 hours after reassessing the wound.

Dressings are first changed after 24-48 hours and silver sulfadiazine may be used at this time. Various other specialized dressings and topical agents are available, but only add to the cost. Subsequent dressing changes should be at least once in 3 – 5 days and depends on how the healing is progressing. If there is a foul smell, discharge or pain, the dressing should be changed immediately.

Pain relief is important and usually oral non-steroidal anti inflammatory agents suffice. Healing burns are also pruritic and adequate application of moisturiser cream is helpful.

Burn wounds that do not heal in three weeks should be referred to a burn centre.

Referral and Transport Considerations

The following are the patients who should be referred to specialized burn units:

a) Partial thickness burns covering > 10% of body surface area or full thickness burns involving >5% of body surface area
b) Burns involving face, hands, feet, genitalia, perineum and major joints.
c) Chemical burns.
d) Inhalational injury.
e) Any co-morbid condition which could affect the management or prolong recovery.

The important issues to consider during transport of seriously burnt children include control of the airway, appropriate venous access, placement of nasogastric and bladder catheters, maintenance of body temperature and starting intravenous fluids if transport time is expected to be longer than one hour. Proper documentation of the events of the injury apart from drugs administered should accompany the patient.

Major Burns[3, 7-9]

A burn covering body surface area greater than 10% in a child is a major burn. The patient's history should ascertain the type of injury, whether it was in a closed space, the possibilities of other injuries (e.g., following fall from a height) and the nature of the first aid treatment given. Presence of other illnesses or medical conditions should be noted.

Stabilization-ABC and Early Mangement

Any patient with major burns should be initially managed similar to a patient with multiple trauma with special attention given to the airway and breathing.

The airway must be assessed if it is compromised or is at risk of compromise. Aspiration of hot liquids or inhalation of hot gases results in upper airway burns, in which case there will be progressive airway edema. Erythema/edema of the oropharynx on inspection, hoarseness or harsh cough, and the presence of stridor, tachypnea or dyspnoea should be taken as indications for intubation apart from any doubt regarding inhalational injury (see later). Hence, the airway must be secured by endotracheal intubation by an experienced person, in case of any doubt. The tube should be properly secured as re-intubation will be increasingly difficult.

Oxygen administration in high concentration is started in all burn patients. The possible reasons for requiring respiratory support include

a) Deep circumferential burns of the chest, which can limit chest movements.
b) Smoke inhalation leading to inhalational injury.
c) Carbon monoxide poisoning

A reliable vascular access is a must for resuscitation. If venous access cannot be easily obtained, intraosseous access is an acceptable option to begin resuscitation. In case of large injuries, central venous access may be preferred. Till such time as the exact fluid requirement is calculated, 10 – 20 ml/kg/hr of normal saline or Ringer's lactate should be started for any child with >10% burns.

A nasogastric tube is placed simultaneously. This will help in decompressing the stomach and for early aggressive enteral nutrition.

Neurological assessment for any altered sensorium is documented. Hypoxemia or hypovolemia can contribute to the same, as also carbon monoxide poisoning.The patient is exposed and examined thoroughly for the presence of head, chest or abdominal injuries and to assess the extent of the burn injury. While doing so, the child should not be allowed to get hypothermic.

Analgesia is important and intravenous morphine is usually required.

Investigations that need to be done include a blood group and cross match, full blood count, renal function and electrolytes and coagulation profile. In case of respiratory distress, chest x-ray and arterial blood gas is required, in addition to the above.

Secondary Survey

A head-to-toe examination for burn – specific issues is carried out.

Carbon monoxide narcosis is suspected in any patient with burns in an enclosed space. The child would present with altered sensorium with normal pulse oximetry. Levels between 10 – 20 % cause nausea and headache, between 20 – 30 % lead to drowsiness and levels above 40% result in coma and respiratory depression. Arterial blood gas examination reveals metabolic acidosis. Co-oximetry, if available, can diagnose raised carbon monoxide levels. 100% oxygen is used for treatment as this displaces carbon monoxide from bound proteins six times faster than atmospheric oxygen. Mechanical ventilation should be instituted if levels are above 25 – 30%. Hyperbaric oxygen therapy may be helpful in early recovery.

Burns of the eye and external ear are assessed now as facial edema may make it difficult to do so later. Topical creams are applied to the external ear and ophthalmologic consultation sought in case of eye injuries.

Circumferential burns across the chest may need torso escharotomy. Similarly, progressive edema can develop in extremities leading to compartment syndrome. Frequent evaluation is needed and fasciotomy/escharotomy may be required. Coagulation electrocautery should be used for escharotomy to minimize blood loss.

Depth of Burns

Depending on the layers of the skin affected, burns are classified as:

a) Superficial – The epidermis alone is affected. It appears red and moist and when blanched, the refill is brisk.
b) Superficial dermal – The epidermis with the upper layers of the dermis are burnt and blisters are seen. A pale, dry wound is seen which refills slowly on blanching. The above two are very painful when touched.
c) Deep dermal – The burn extends into the deeper layers of the dermis. There is a fixed red colour with no blanching.
d) Full thickness – The burn extends through all the skin layers into the subcutaneous tissue. They are dry, leathery, waxy and hard and do not blanch or bleed.

The first three are referred to as partial thickness burns. Pain is not obvious in the latter two types of burns. Superficial burns heal spontaneously by epithelialisation. Skin adnexa are lesser in number in deep dermal burns and are absent in full thickness burns; hence, healing is associated with contraction and these wounds require surgical intervention.

However, a burn is a dynamic wound and can change with resuscitation; hence it will need to be reassessed frequently later.

Assessment of Burn Area

An accurate estimate of the body surface area burnt is essential as therapy and prognosis depend on this. A fairly accurate estimate is obtained from the Lund and Browder chart (as shown in the Figure), which takes into account the variation in body shape at different ages. The popular 'rule of nines' is inaccurate in children and should not be used.

Erythema should not be included while calculating burn area. In India, pigmented skin makes assessment difficult

Fluid Resuscitation

One of the most important aspects of management of burn management is fluid resuscitation. This is required in burn injuries involving >15% of the body surface area. While good resuscitation maintains tissue perfusion to the zone of stasis and prevents deepening of the burn wound, too much fluid leads to edema and hence tissue hypoxia.

A systemic capillary leak occurs in the first 24 hours after injury. It may be prolonged if there is delay in initiation of resuscitation and in the presence of inhalational injury.

While many formulae predict the volume requirements based on the body surface area involved, it is important to understand that these are only guidelines and continuous monitoring to achieve the resuscitation end points is required. The Parkland formula is used to assess the initial 24 hours fluid requirement (see Table 1), of which half is given in the first 8 hours and the remaining half over the next 16 hours. Crystalloid alone is recommended in the first 24 hours and colloid is administered after this period when the capillary integrity improves. Ringer's lactate alone is adequate for older children but 5% dextrose in addition to this is required in children below 20 kg to prevent hypoglycemia.

The end points of resuscitation are similar to any other shock situation and include

a) Arousable and comfortable child
b) Warm peripheries
c) Systolic blood pressure above the 5th centile for age
d) Pulse rate acceptable for age
e) Urine output 0.5 -1 ml/kg body weight per hour (nil glucose)
f) Base deficit < 2

Table 1: Fluid requirements in children with burns (Parkland formula)

First 24 hours

Children < 20 kg

1. Ringer's lactate: 4 ml/kg /% burn in 24 hours; first half in 8 hours
2. Ringer's lactate with 5% dextrose: Maintenance rate

Children > 20 kg

1. Ringer's lactate: 2-4 ml/kg /% burn in 24 hours

Second 24 hours

Crystalloid: Half of first 24 hours' fluid guided by urine output Colloid (preferably 5% human albumin)

1. 00 - 30 % burns: None
2. 30 – 50 % burns: 0.3 ml/kg /% burn in 24 hours
3. 50 – 70 % burns: 0.4 ml/kg /% burn in 24 hours
4. 70 – 100% burns: 0.5 ml/kg /% burn in 24 hours

Assessment of packed cell volume, serum sodium, base excess and lactate every 4 to six hours should guide further resuscitation.

A central line placement is helpful in patients requiring large volumes of IV fluids (>6 ml /kg / % body surface area). Early administration of colloids may be helpful in these patients. Myocardial dysfunction may be seen in children with large area burns; this may require infusion of β adrenergic agents.

Return of capillary integrity after 18 – 24 hours largely depends on the initial resuscitation. Fluid requirements abruptly decrease after return of capillary integrity; it is important to recognize this and decrease

% Total Body Surface Area Burn
Be clear and accurate, and do not include erythema
(Lund and Browder)

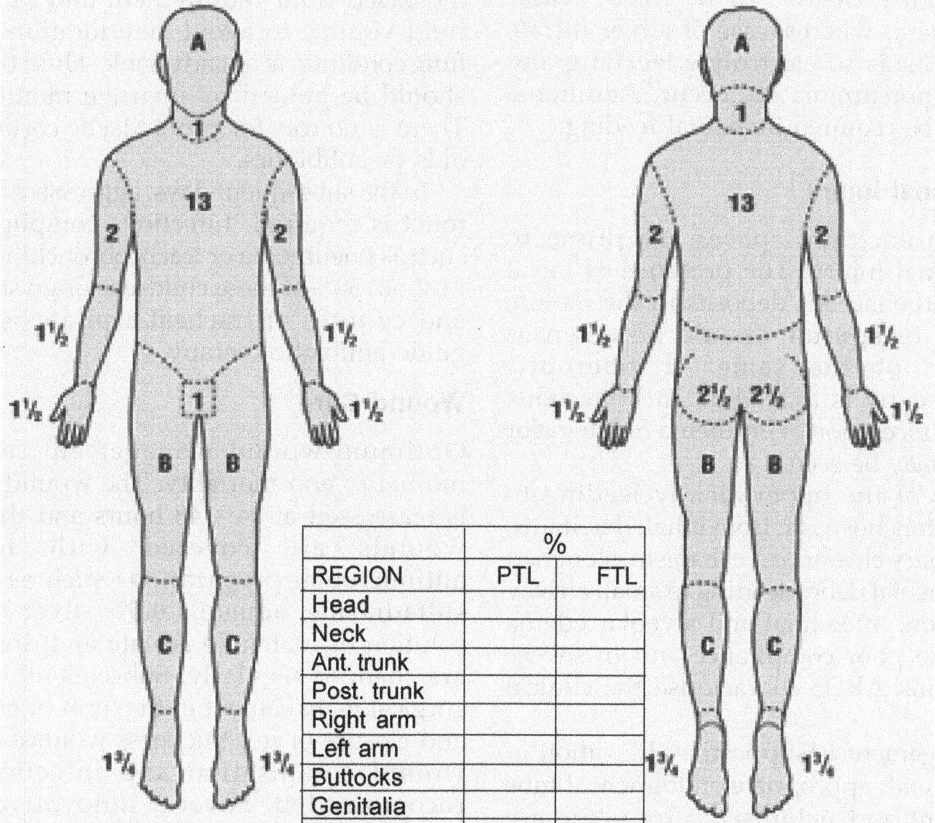

REGION	% PTL	% FTL
Head		
Neck		
Ant. trunk		
Post. trunk		
Right arm		
Left arm		
Buttocks		
Genitalia		
Right leg		
Left leg		
Total burn		

Area	Age 0	1	5	10	15	Adult
A = ½ OF HEAD	9½	8½	6½	5½	4½	3½
B = ½ OF THIGH	2¾	3¼	4	4½	4½	4¾
C = ½ OF ONE LOWER LEG	2½	2½	2¾	3	3¼	3½

Fig. 1: Lund and Browder chart to assess the % of total body surface area burn (reprinted from reference 8 with permission of the publisher)

fluids accordingly. After this point, wound management has an influence on the electrolyte composition of fluids. Use of silver sulfadiazine leads to a free water requirement, whereas use of silver nitrate solution leads to electrolyte leeching and hence hyponatremia can occur. Additional salt may be required in enteral feeding.

Inhalational Injury

Burns in enclosed spaces are prone to inhalational injury. The presence of facial burns, carbonaceous deposits in the mouth, pharynx or sputum should be taken as evidence of the same. If fiberoptic bronchoscopy is available, carbonaceous deposits, ulceration or erythema of the major airways may be seen.

Burns of the upper airway leading to edema, bronchospasm from inhaled irritants, loss of ciliary clearance mechanism, sloughed endobronchial debris leading to small airway obstruction, interstitial and alveolar edema leading to poor compliance and in severe forms frank ARDS characterise the clinical picture.

Management is supportive. Elevation of the head end, appropriate endotracheal tube placement and nebulised adrenaline are effective for upper airway edema. This usually subsides in 2 - 3 days time.

The indications of mechanical ventilation are as in any other hypoxemic respiratory failure. If mechanical ventilation is required, air trapping should be expected. Bronchodilators are liberally used to overcome bronchospasm. Low tidal volume, low respiratory rates and long expiratory times should be ensured to avoid dynamic hyperinflation. Adequate oxygenation should be maintained with minimal iatrogenic lung insult; hence strategies include permissive hypercapnia and keeping the plateau pressures below 30 cm H_2O water. Gas exchange usually worsens 48 – 72 hours after the injury and any urgent surgeries are best completed in this early period.

Inhalational injury is associated with an increased fluid requirement and reducing fluid volume to avoid deterioration of the lung condition is not advisable. Fluid therapy should be guided by invasive monitoring. There is no role for prophylactic corticosteroids or antibiotics.

In the subsequent days, aggressive airway toilet is required. Infectious complications such as pneumonia or tracheobronchitis occur in about 30% of these children. Gram staining and cultures of tracheal aspirates should guide antibiotic therapy.

Wound Care

Optimum wound management reduces morbidity and mortality. The wound depth is reassessed at 24 – 48 hours and then the wounds are covered with topical antimicrobial preparations such as silver sulfadiazine, aqueous 0.5% silver nitrate solution or mafenide acetate and dressings are changed regularly. Subsequently, early surgical management in the form of excision and closure of full thickness wounds before wound colonisation and infection are recommended. Several innovative skin substitutes and better techniques of burn wound excision have substantially improved the outcome.

Maintaining the limbs in the neutral position so as to prevent contractures and early introduction of physiotherapy is important for return to full functional capacity.

Nutrition

A hypermetabolic response is seen following burn injury and this should be countered with an early and aggressive feeding regimen. Enteral feeding should be established around 24 hours after the injury. Tube feeding is recommended if the affected body surface area exceeds 20%. Gastric stasis may occur;

in these cases, nasojejunal feeding should be instituted.

The standard formulae to predict resting energy expenditure are inaccurate in children with extensive burns and hence the total caloric intake should be 1½ times the normal requirement with 2.5 – 3 gm/kg/day of protein. Hypothermia increases the energy requirements and hence should be avoided. Good wound management with surgical excision and closure decreases the caloric requirement.

Liberal use of multivitamins and trace elements is advisable once the caloric intake is satisfactory.

Other Issues

Renal failure in a child with burns early after the injury reflects poor or delayed resuscitation and rarely, myoglobinuria. Later in the course of the injury, sepsis is the leading cause of renal failure. Renal support should be introduced early rather than late so that nutritional support is not curtailed.

Myocardial dysfunction is seen in some children with major burns. Inotropic agents such as dobutamine, which do not cause vasoconstriction, are preferred, provided there is no hypotension.

Infections are responsible for up to 75% of mortality in patients successfully resuscitated.

Differentiating infection from the systemic inflammatory response due to burns can be difficult; similarly, microbial colonisation of the wounds makes wound swab culture a surveillance tool rather than a diagnostic tool. Common organisms include Streptococci, Staphylococci, Pseudomonas, Acinetobacter and Proteus species. Prophylactic antibiotics have no role in the management and short courses of antibiotics with narrow spectrum of activity should be prescribed, when required.

ELECTRICAL INJURIES[5, 10]

Electrical injuries are distinct as in addition to burns sustained, the current passing through the body disturbs the cardiac rhythm and the nervous system. They account for around 2 – 3 % of all burns in children that require emergency management. Most of the electrical injuries in children occur at home. Lightning accounts for some of these injuries and they carry the highest mortality.

Electric current traveling through the body creates an 'entry' point and an 'exit' point. While traveling between these two points, it damages the tissues between these two points by generating heat. A vertical pathway of the electric current is most harmful, affecting all the major organ systems. Hand to hand horizontal path spares the brain but can affect the spinal cord and respiratory muscles. A pathway through the lower part of the body can cause severe local damage but affects no major organ.

The main determinant of the degree of damage is the voltage of the electric current. The duration of contact affects the intensity of energy traveling through the body and hence, the damage. Alternating current (AC) is more damaging than direct current (DC). There is usually a single muscle contraction in DC, which may throw the victim away, whereas tetanic contractions in AC cause a 'locking on' phenomenon. Children are more prone to severe injuries as their skin is thin and offers low resistance. Presence of moisture/wetness also decreases the resistance and increases the intensity of current. Infants and toddlers, who tend to mouth electrical cords suffer severe full thickness burns of the lips, tongue etc for this reason.

a) Low voltage injuries (as with domestic electricity) usually cause superficial burns and may lead to arrhythmias in the form of ventricular fibrillation. Tetanic contractions occur as the current is usually

AC and rhabdomyolysis may be seen. Mortality is usually low.

b) High voltage injuries (>1000 V), on the other hand, lead to deep burns and often extensive tissue damage, blunt injury due to fall, arrhythmias, tetanic contractions of respiratory muscles leading to hypoxia, rhabdomyolysis and carry a moderate mortality.

c) Lightning carries extremely high voltage (in excess of $30x10^6$), though the duration of contact is instantaneous and it is a DC current. Direct CNS injury leading to respiratory arrest, cardiac asystole and blast effect leading to blunt injury culminate in a high mortality.

d) Flash injuries occur when electric current from a high voltage source arcs over the body (or from the source to the person before actually touching the source). High temperatures are generated (5000°C) and severe thermal injuries occur. Also, clothing etc can be set alight causing flame burns.

The morbidity and mortality of electric injuries are on account of the following systemic effects.

Cardiovascular System

Cardiac arrhythmias may be precipitated. Low voltage usually causes ventricular fibrillation, while higher voltages cause cardiac asystole. Due to the inherent automaticity of the heart, spontaneous rhythm can return after the latter. Conduction blocks may also occur. Usually the arrhythmias occur at the time of the injury; delayed ones are rare and are seen in those with pre existing heart disease or if there is direct necrosis of the myocardium.

Vascular injury is seen in the form of medial necrosis with aneurysm formation and rupture. When this occurs in limbs, it can lead to compartment syndrome.

Nervous System

When electric current passes through the brain, the most serious effect is injury to the respiratory control centre leading to respiratory arrest. Acute cranial nerve dysfunction or seizures can occur. Spinal injury or cervical cord transection can occur with hand to hand flow. Tetanic contractions of the respiratory muscles can cause suffocation and anoxia. Traumatic brain and spinal injury can occur secondary to a fall. Autonomic disturbances can also be seen transiently.

Other Effects

Burns of various degrees are seen and often, there is extensive damage in the deeper tissues without the overlying skin being burnt.

The kidneys are not directly affected but may be affected due to anoxia/ischemia. Rhabdomyolysis leading to myoglobinuria can affect the kidneys and precipitate acute renal failure.

The lungs are not directly affected though severe compromise of respiration can occur due to respiratory center injury or tetanic respiratory muscle contraction.

Eye and ear injuries can occur in form of cataracts, rupture of tympanic membranes and hearing deficit. Skeletal injury can occur due to falls.

Management

A child with electrical injuries should be managed as in burns; however, certain unique aspects of management are as below:

1. While giving first aid, the safety of approaching the victim should be kept in mind and either the source of the current should be cut off or properly insulated equipment used. With high voltages, the ground on which the victim is lying can also conduct electricity, especially if it is wet.

2. The extent of cutaneous burns should not be used as a guide to the deeper burns. Similarly, vertebral or other skeletal injuries can occur following violent muscle contractions without any external injury.
3. Fluid resuscitation should be liberal keeping in mind that along with external burns, there is internal visceral injury and rhabdomyolysis. A good vascular access should be established once the airway and breathing are taken care of.
4. Cardiac rhythm disturbances can occur later; hence monitoring should continue for 24 hours if there is no rhythm disturbance initially. Children who have been brought after an electric injury but with no loss of consciousness or burns with normal neurological examination and cardiac rhythm can be safely discharged.

The management of electrical injuries is thus supportive with no specific therapy. Multiorgan failure can develop and needs intensive care management. The prognosis depends on the severity of the initial injury and the subsequent complications.

Prevention

Both thermal and electrical burns are potentially preventable. Perhaps, much more important than management is prevention, especially with regard to children, since most of these injuries occur at home. Safety of electrical appliances should be ensured at all times, which can be implemented through public education and legislation.

REFERENCES

1. Saffle JR. Predicting outcomes of burns. N Engl J Med 1998; 338(6); 387 – 8.
2. Ryan CM, Schoenfeld DA, Thorpe WP, Sheridan RL, Cassem EH, Tompkins RG. Objective estimates of the probability of death from burn injuries. N Engl J Med 1998; 338(6):362-366.
3. Ramakrishnan KM, Sankar J, Venkatraman J. Profile of pediatric burns Indian experience in a tertiary care burn unit. Burns 2005; 31(3): 351 -3.
4. Sheridan RL. Burns. Crit Care Med 2002; 30(11 Suppl): S500-14.
5. Hettiaratchy S, Dziewulski P. ABC of burns-Pathophysiology and types of burns. BMJ 2004; 328: 1427-9.
6. HudspithJ, Rayatt S. ABC of burns-First aid and treatment of minor burns. BMJ 2004; 328: 1487-9.
7. Hettiaratchy S, Papini R. ABC of burns- Initial management of a major burn: I- overview. BMJ 2004; 328:1555-7.
8. Hettiaratchy S, Papini R. ABC of burns- Initial management of a major burn: II- assessment and resuscitation. BMJ 2004; 329: 101-3.
9. Ansermino M, Hemsley C. ABC of burns-Intensive care management and control of infection. BMJ 2004; 329:220-3.
10. Koumborlis AC. Elelctrical injuries. Crit Care Med 2002; 30(11 Suppl): S424-30.

Lokesh Tiwari and Sunit Singhi

67 Near Drowning

Drowning is a leading preventable cause of unintentional morbidity and mortality. Internationally submersion is responsible for approximately 15% of injury deaths in children 1 to 14 years of age. It is a significant cause of disability and death in children younger than 4 years. Near drowning is the clinical syndrome that develops in individuals who survive an immersion episode.

DEFINITIONS

Drowning is a process resulting in primary respiratory impairment from submersion/ immersion in a liquid medium. *Drowning* occurs when submersion results in asphyxia and death at the time or shortly thereafter. If death occurs within 24 hours after submersion, the term *drowning-related death* is used.

Persons who survive for at least 24 hours following submersion, regardless of the duration and extent of recovery, have been termed *near-drowning victims,* but the term near-drowning has now been replaced by *submersion injury* with all of its clinical consequences regardless of outcome.

Wet drowning occurs in 80% to 90% of submersions and refers to events when victims aspirate fluid. After initial laryngospasm abates and the glottis opens, the unconscious victim aspirates water and subsequently develops pulmonary edema.

Dry drowning occurs in 10% to 15% of cases, less common in children. Reflex laryngospasm prevents significant inhalation of immersion fluid; death may occur because of asphyxia. Pulmonary edema in this setting is secondary to fluid extravasated from the intra- to extravascular space in the lung parenchyma secondary to high negative intrathoracic pressures from attempts to inspire on a closed glottis.

The term *secondary drowning* refers to the delayed respiratory distress syndrome (ARDS) after a near drowning episode.

There are certain factors associated with high incidence of drowning (Table 1).

Table 1: Factors Common to Drowning Incidents

Age	Toddlers, teenage boys
Location	Home, swimming pools
Gender	Males predominate in every age group
Drugs	Particularly alcohol
Trauma	Secondary to diving, falls, horseplay

The immediate consequences of immersion are shown in figure 1. initially, immersion induces a voluntary breath holding period (the so called 'diving reflex') this eventually breaks under the intense stimulation of a rising $PaCO_2$, with subsequent inspiration leading to inhalation of immersion fluid. The consequences thereafter depend upon the nature of the fluid (fresh or sea water), and whether reflex laryngospasm prevents significant aspiration ('dry drowning') (Table 2).

TYPE OF ASPIRATED FLUID

Differences between fresh water and sea water drowning are enumerated in Table 2. The extent, to which these changes occur, however, depends on the amount of aspirated fluid.

CLINICAL FEATURES

The features of near drowning include the pathophysiological consequences of the immersion, the nature of the drowning episode, hypothermia and associated problems (e.g. cervical spine or head trauma). These are shown in Table 3.

MANAGEMENT

Because the full extent of CNS injury can not be adequately determined immediately after the rescue, all victims of near drowning should receive aggressive basic and advanced

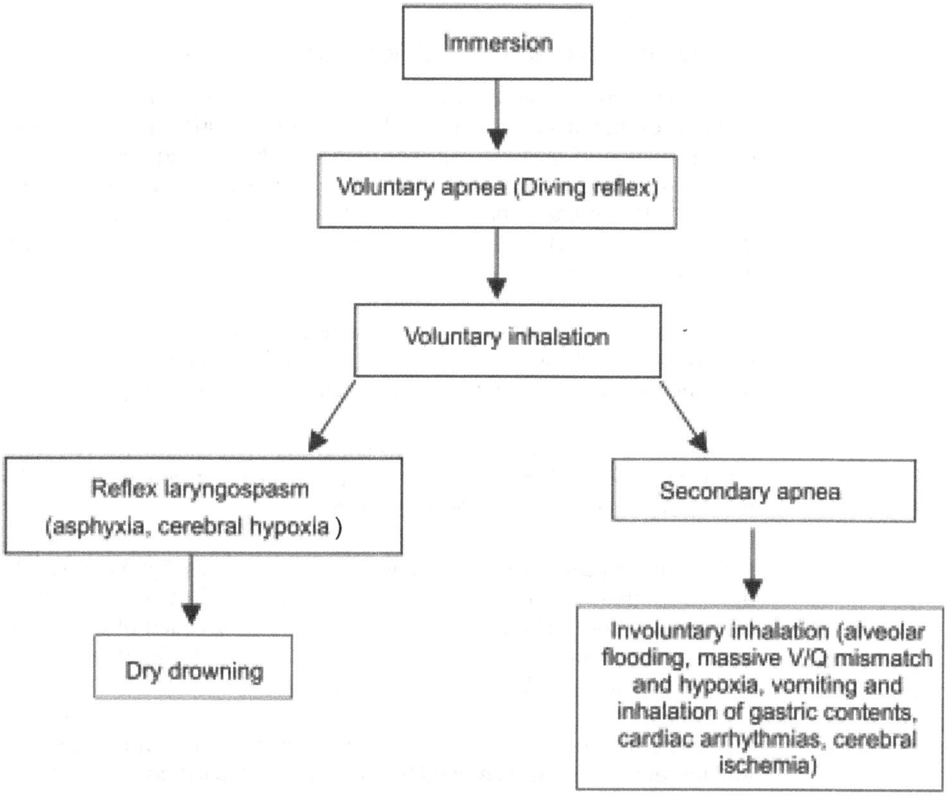

Fig. 1: Consequences of immersion

Table 2: Differences between fresh water and salt water drowning

	Fresh water (hypotonic)	*Salt water (hypertonic)*
Hematocrit	Hemodilution	Hemoconcentration
Intravascular volume	Hypervolemia (transient)	Hypovolemia
Hemolysis & Hb-urea	Present	Absent
Electrolytes disturbance	High K^+, low Na^+ and Ca^{++}	Low K^+, high Na^+ & Ca^{++}
Mechanism	Hypotonic fluid in lungs is drawn into circulaton, in severe cases leading to intravascular hemolysis and hyperkalemia. Decrease in surfactant results in atelectasis, intrapulmonary shunt & pulmonary edema.	Alveoli filled with salt water draw plasma across alveolar-capillary barrier, flooding the alveoli and denaturing surfactant resulting in pulmonary edema & shunt.

Table 3: Consequences of near-drowning

Respiratory	Inhalation of as little as 2.5 ml /kg can cause marked pulmonary insufficiency, features of increased airway resistance, loss of surfactant, alveolar flooding with disruption of alveolar-capillary barrier, reduced lung compliance, intense pulmonary vasoconstriction and severe hypoxemia. ARDS may develop occasionally after an intervening period of recovery. Bacterial pneumonia resulting from aspiration of contaminated water may further contribute to pulmonary insufficiency.
Cardiovascular	ECG may be abnormal, impaired hemodynamic performance because of hypoxia and acidosis, hypothermia, pulmonary and systemic vasoconstriction, and pulmonary edema. Intravascular hemolysis is rarely a problem.
Metabolic	Hypothermia may complicate resuscitation but may also aid survival and neurological recovery. Inhalation of a volume of fluid sufficient to disturb ionic homeostasis is very uncommon in survivors.
Neurological	Initial neurological assessment may be complicated by hypothermia, drug and alcohol abuse, head injury, seizures etc. cerebral edema may develop in response to cerebral ischemia. With improved techniques of cardiopulmonary support, the extent of CNS injury has been the major determinant of survival and neurological morbidity in patients reaching the PICU after near drowning.
Other Organ Systems	Multisystem failure resulting from prolonged ischemic hypoxic state, sepsis, and therapeutic modalities used to manage these children may complicate the clinical course.

life support at the site of the accident and in the emergency department. The success or failure of cardiopulmonary resuscitation (CPR) at the site of the accident often determines the outcome. Asymptomatic victims should be monitored for at least 24 hours for risk of secondary drowning. An outline of management is given in Table 4.

Table 4: Outline of management of a near – drowning victim

First Aid : clear airway, mouth to mouth breathing, keep patient warm.

- Hospitalize all patients for at least 24 hours/ overnight.

In Hospital

- 100% oxygen.
- Nasogastric tube to empty the stomach
- Mechanical ventilation if not breathing,or CO_2 retention
- IPPV with PEEP is (preferred) may be needed for a minimum of 1-2 days.
- Treat shock if present
- Plasma 10ml/kg for fresh water drowning
- Packed cells 10ml/kg for fresh water drowning
- Pulmonary toilet – prevention of aspiration of secretion.
- Aspirated material may precipitate broncho spasm in some. Give Aminophylline/ Corticosteroids.
- Treat acidosis to return pH to $\leq$ 7.10. If reports are not available and child is unresponsive try 1 mmol/kg of $NaHCO_3$.
- Rewarm hypothermic patient 0.5° C/hour
- Antibiotics to treat pulmonary infection
- Seizures—Use diazepam/midazolam
- Care of raised ICP
  a) Mannitol 0.25-0.5 g/kg.
  b) IV dexamethasone 0.1-0.2 mg/kg 6 hourly
  c) IV diuretics frusemide 1 mg/kg
  d) Monitor ICP.

Airway, Breathing and Circulation

Management of the drowning victim's airway and breathing is similar to that recommended for any victim of cardiopulmonary arrest. Attempts to remove water from the breathing passages by any mean other than suction (e.g, abdominal thrusts or the Heimlich maneuver) are unnecessary and potentially dangerous. As with any form of accidental injury, other forms of associated trauma must be considered.

Maintaining adequate airway, breathing and circulatory status should take priority. Electrocardiogram (ECG) monitoring is crucial to detect ventricular dysrhythmias and asystole. Arterial blood gas determination should be performed as hypotension and shock may result from the asphyxial episode and are commonly encountered during the early resuscitation phase. At the same time full blood count, urea, creatinine, electrolytes, clotting studies, urine/plasma for free haemoglobin and chest X ray should be obtained. Head CT cervical spine studies should be asked, if clinically indicated.

Hypothermia

Severe bradycardia and intense vasoconstriction associated with marked hypothermia (< 32°C) may make near – drowning victims appear dead. Resuscitative efforts should be continued, while body temperature is normalized.

Prevent additional evaporative heat loss by removing wet garments and insulating the victim from further environmental exposures. For patients with moderate to severe hypothermia, therapy is determined by the presence or absence of a perfusing rhythm. Management of the patient with moderate to severe hypothermia is as follows:

– Mild (>34°C [>93.2°F]): passive rewarming.
– Moderate (30°C to 34°C [86°F to 93.2°F]): active external rewarming.

- Severe (<30°C [86°F]): active internal rewarming; consider extracorporeal membrane oxygenation.
- Rewarming should proceed slowly; at 0.5°C/hour.

Further Cardiopulmonary Support

Early use of PEEP is effective in reversing hypoxemia. PEEP maintains alveolar stability and alveolar recruitment and increases FRC. PEEP also displaces intra alveolar water into interstitial and perilymphatic spaces resulting into decreased venous admixture and improved compliance. On the other hand excessive amount of PEEP can result in decreased venous return and cardiac output, pulmonary over distension and decreased compliance and barotraumas.

Intravenous access with two large-bore venous catheters or central lines must be established, and infusion of normal saline at a brisk rate should be started. Circulation support should be undertaken with fluids and ionotrops as directed by central venous and pulmonary artery catheterization. Pressor agents, such as dopamine, dobutamine, or epinephrine, may be required to maintain a mean arterial pressure adequate for tissue perfusion, but these should be used only after intravascular volume is restored.

Central Nervous System

The extent of cerebral hypoxia can be quantified by Conn's criteria as category A (awake), category B (blunted consciousness), and category C (comatose). Category C is subclassified into C_1 (decorticate), C_2 (decerebrate), and C_3 (flaccid) as shown in tables. Both the GCS and Conn's classification are helpful in determining management and judging response to therapy and for prognostication.

The best neurologic outcome in near drowning victim requires optimal management of respiration and hemo-dynamics. Maintainance of cerebral perfusion, oxygenation and normocapnia is advised in patients who have suffered a significant cerebral ischemic episode. Head CT may be obtained. It may demonstrate cerebral edema and also exclude focal pathology. Intracranial hypertension caused by cerebral edema should be treated as discussed elsewhere. Moderate hypothermia may afford some cerebral protection. Because glucose is a vital metabolite for the nervous system, fluid management for resuscitation of the CNS should also focus on preventing episodes of hypo or hyperglycemia.

Steroids are not recommended due to side effects like immunosuppression, suppression of fever, and hyperglycemia which may further complicate the clinical picture.

Other Measures

a. Insert nasogastric tube to decompress stomach, which may be distended with swallowed fluid.
b. Acidosis should be corrected with sodium bicarbonate if pH is less than 7.0.
c. Consider broad spectrum antibiotics to treat pulmonary infection.
d. Aspirated material may precipitate bronchospasm in some cases. Consider bronchodilators or corticosteroids in such cases.

OUTCOME

The single most important and prognostically significant consequence of submersion is a decreased oxygen delivery to the tissues. A number of clinical variables determine the magnitude of hypoxia and the subject's ability to withstand it. Factors influencing recovery include

1. Age: younger victims (particularly children) have more potential for good neurological recovery.
2. Type of drowning: Cold immersion and dry drowning have better outcome.
3. Volume of aspirate: >22 ml/kg, invariably fatal.

4. Duration of submersion: >10 minutes associated with poor outcome.
5. The following admission feature predict poor recovery.
a. Need for cardiopulmonary resuscitation (CPR) >25 minutes.
b. Fixed dilated pupils.
c. pH< 7.
d. Absent or abnormal movements 24 hours after injury.

Radiological studies should include a chest radiograph to determine the presence or absence of pneumothorax or pneumomediastinum. Unless head injury is suspected, computed tomography scan of the head is usually not necessary because early findings are often normal even in the face of severe hypoxic damage.

The theory of controlled hyperventilation to a $PaCO_2$ of 30 mm Hg has not been validated scientifically and has even been shown to worsen certain outcomes. It is vital to consider elevation in intracranial pressure when selecting RSI medications. One recommended combination would include premedication with lidocaine, vecuronium and fentanyl, followed by etomidate and succinylcholine for sedation and paralysis.

Table 5: Conn's Criteria

CATEGORY	DESCRIPTION
A	Awake—fully oriented
B	Blunted—arousable; purposeful response to pain
C	Comatose—not arousable; abnormal response to pain
C_1	Flexor response to pain
C_2	Extensor response to pain
C_3	Flaccid
C_4	Arrested

FURTHER READING

1. Idris AH, Berg RA, Bierens J, Bossaert L, Branche CM, Gabrielli A, Graves SA, Handley AJ, Hoelle R, Morley PT, Papa L, Pepe PE, Quan L, Szpilman D, Wigginton JG, Modell JH. Recommended guidelines for uniform reporting of data from drowning: the "Utstein style." *Resuscitation.* 2003;59:45–57.
2. American Heart Association. Standards and guidelines for cardiopulmonary resuscitation and emergency cardiac care. *Circulation* 2005;112;IV-133-IV-135. available at http://circ.ahajournals.org/cgi/content/full/112/24_suppl/IV-133.
3. American Heart Association. Standards and guidelines for cardiopulmonary resuscitation and emergency cardiac care. *Circulation* 2005;112;IV-136-IV-138. Available at http://circ.ahajournals.org/cgi/content/full/112/24_suppl/IV-136.
4. CR: *Environmental emergencies.* In: Fleisher GR, Ludwig S, ed. *Textbook of Emergency Medicine*, 4th ed. Philadelphia: Lippincott Williams & Wilkins; 2000.
5. Mehta SR, Srinivasan KV, Bindra MS, et al: Near drowning in cold water. *J Assoc Phys India* 2000; 48:674-676.
6. Bierens JJ, Knape JT, Gelissen HP: Drowning. *Curr Opin Crit Care* 2002; 8(6):578-586.
7. Burford AE, Ryan LM, Stone BJ, Hirshon JM, Klein BL. Drowning and near-drowning in children and adolescents: a succinct review for emergency physicians and nurses. Pediatr Emerg Care. 2005 Sep;21(9):610-6.
8. Gheen KM. Near-drowning and cold water submersion. Semin Pediatr Surg. 2001 Feb;10(1):26-7.
9. Harries M. Near drowning. BMJ. 2003 Dec 6;327(7427):1336-8.
10. Lord SR, Davis PR. Drowning, near drowning and immersion syndrome .J R Army Med Corps. 2005 Dec;151(4):250-5.
11. Papa L, Hoelle R, Idris A. Systematic review of definitions for drowning incidents. Resuscitation. 2005 Jun;65(3):255-64.
12. Singhi S, Tiwari L. Management of intracranial hyper- tension. Indian J paediatr. 2009;76:519-29.
13. Zuckerman GB, Conway EE Jr. Drowning and near drowning: a pediatric epidemic. Pediatr Ann. 2000 Jun;29(6):360-6.

Lokesh Tiwari and Sunit Singhi

68 Smoke Inhalation Injury

Smoke inhalation and upper airway burns are major concern in victims burnt in enclosed spaces. Airway injury occurs in up to one third of those with major burns, and the risk of concurrent pulmonary damage is directly related to the extent of surface burns present. Smoke inhalation is the primary cause of death in about 60% to 80% of victims of burn injuries. Burn-related death rate is 20% higher in people with combined inhalation injury and cutaneous burns than in those with cutaneous burns alone. Inhalation injury greatly increases the incidence of respiratory failure and acute respiratory distress syndrome. It is also the cause of most early deaths in burn victims.

PATHOPHYSIOLOGY

Smoke inhalation may cause injury in several ways. These include:

1. **Thermal injury**: This is largely restricted to the upper airway due to reflex closure of the glottis and dissipation of thermal energy by the airways. It results in edema of upper airway and large bronchi. Signs of upper airway obstruction- stridor, hoarseness and respiratory difficulty may develop rapidly.
2. **Distal pulmonary damage**: It results from the inhalation of toxic and corrosive chemicals such as hydrochloric acid, phosgene, oxides of sulphur, and nitrogen. In most of the cases, damage to the bronchi and trachea are the result of chemical injury and actual thermal injury to the airway is rare. Activation of inflammatory cascade leads to increased capillary permeability and pulmonary edema. Fluid losses associated with such pulmonary edema may contribute to 'burn shock' syndrome. These patients develop breathing difficulty, wheeze and blackish sputum.
3. **Poisoning** caused by inhalation of toxic products of combustion such as carbon monoxide and cyanide (Discussed under poisoning).

Irritant gases in smoke cause bronchospasm, laryngeal edema, bronchorrhea, ciliary dysfunction, and inspissation of desquamated cells. Circumferential burns can cause extrinsic upper airway occlusion from encircling eschars. The constituents of smoke can destroy surfactant leading to atelectasis, increasing pulmonary vascular resistance, and pulmonary to edema. The risk of pneumonia is high in the presence of atelectasis, bronchorrhea, impairment of mucociliary clearance, and ineffective cough secondary to pain or excessive sedation.

Components of Fire Smoke

The extent of inhalation damage produced depends on ignition source, temperature, concentration and solubility of toxic gases generated. Thus it is important to know source of the fire and combustion products generated when treating a fire victim (Table 1). Fire smoke consists of a variable mixture of thermal loads, gaseous vapours and particulate matter depending on the materials burnt, temperature, rate of combustion, oxygen availability, and ventilation. All components of fire smoke are capable of damaging airway mucosa.

The water solubility of various respiratory irritants determines their site of action (6). Ammonia, hydrogen chloride, sulfur dioxide, and other highly water-soluble compounds typically affect the mucosal surface of the upper airways and produce almost instantaneous pain in the eyes, nostrils, mouth, and pharynx. Less water-soluble agents, such as chlorine, nitrogen oxides, and phosgene, affect the distal airways. Because these agents are not as irritating to the upper airways, exposure is less likely to be perceived and, in turn, to provoke escape responses, thereby leading to greater exposure of lung parenchyma.

Asphyxiants are gases that physically displace oxygen from the environment. Simple asphyxiants, such as nitrogen, carbon dioxide, and methane, produce hypoxia by lowering the ambient oxygen tension. As ambient oxygen concentrations fall to 10%, victims may complain of dizziness, dyspnea, and tachypnea. As levels fall to about 7%, mental impairment with stupor can occur. Levels below 5% are incompatible with life. Chemical asphyxiants, such as carbon monoxide and hydrogen cyanide, directly interfere with the delivery and utilization of

Table 1: Components of fire smoke

By-products of combustion	*Gases found in fire smoke*
Burning wood	**Irritants**
Acetic acid	Acrolein
Alcohols	Aldehydes
Aldehydes	Ammonia
Carbon dioxide	Chlorine
Carbon monoxide	Hydrogen chloride
Ketones	Isocyanides
Methane	Nitrogen oxide
Tars	Phosgene
Burning cotton or wool	Sulfur dioxide
Carbon monoxide	**Asphyxiants**
Hydrogen cyanide	Carbon dioxide
Ammonia	Methane
Sulphide	Nitrogen
Burning plastics	Carbon monoxide
Carbon monoxide	Hydrogen cyanide
Hydrochloric acid	
Phosgene	

oxygen. Anemic hypoxia caused by a diminished erythrocyte oxygen-carrying capacity can develop following carbon monoxide exposure. Hydrogen cyanide disrupts the cytochrome oxidase enzymes of the electron transport chain, resulting in histotoxic hypoxia.

DIAGNOSIS

Smoke inhalation injury should be suspected in fire victims trapped in a confined space or who lost consciousness during a fire. Inhalation injury is likely in the presence of facial and upper cervical burns, singed eyebrows and nasal vibrissae, and victims having respiratory signs like bronchial breath sounds, wheezing, cyanosis, and carbonaceous sputum.

The chest x-ray may be normal in the acute period, and therefore often unhelpful in first 24 hours. Chest X ray taken after 24 to 36 hours may show patchy atelectasis to diffuse interstitial and alveolar involvement. A xenon 133 ventilation-perfusion lung scan may reveal nonhomogeneous uptake and can be an accurate means of detecting lower airway damage. CT chest is good modality for detecting delayed respiratory sequelae, like bronchiectasis, bronchiolitis obliterans, or pulmonary fibrosis.

Bronchoscopy is considered the "gold standard" for early evaluation of upper airway injury, but the best results are obtained within the first 24 hours. Bronchoscopy can also be used to detect late pulmonary sequelae.

Pulmonary function testing can confirm obstructive or restrictive ventilatory defects. In ventilated patients deformities in flow-volume curves can indicate the presence of obstruction in the upper airways. Hypoxemia and hypocarbia occurs in most smoke inhalation patients, but hypercarbia can occur in patients with severe airway obstruction or extensive alveolar injury. An increased mixed venous PO2 and a decreased difference in arteriovenous oxygen content suggest concurrent carbon monoxide and hydrogen cyanide poisoning.

Other diagnostic methods include bronchoalveolar lavage, showing an increased number of polymorphonuclear cells and alveolar macrophages, and transbronchial biopsy, which can be used to diagnose bronchiolitis obliterans and interstitial fibrosis.

MANAGEMENT

Thermal Injury to the Airways

Airway obstruction can progress very rapidly, but the onset may be delayed for up to 24 hours following injury. All such patients should therefore be monitored and immediately intubated if signs of airway obstruction appear. Other indications for intubation are: Facial burns with depressed conscious level or with circumferential neck burns, full-thickness burns to nose and lips, pharyngeal edema.

There is no place for conservative management in such circumstances; it is better to intubate early than to delay and face complete airway obstruction. Endotracheal intubation is likely to be impossible if there is complete airway obstruction. In such patients an emergency tracheostomy is indicated. The procedure may be difficult in the presence of cervical burns.

Once the airway is intubated, the extent of the thermal injury to the lower respiratory tract should be defined by fiber-optic bronchoscopy. Airway edema is usually maximal 24 hours post burn, and resolves after 4-5 days. Steroids are not recommended (8). Inhaled bronchodilators may be helpful in reducing bronchospasm, and humidification can relieve excessive airway drying or mucous plugging.

Distal Pulmonary Damage and Respiratory Failure

Maintenance of airway patency, adequate oxygenation and ventilation, aggressive pulmonary toilet, and stabilization of hemodynamic status are the cornerstones of therapy. Maintenance of optimal fluid status is essential. Patients with concurrent surface burns and inhalation injury require 2 mL per % burns per kg more fluid than those with cutaneous burns alone to support adequate cardiac and urine output.

Respiratory failure and the need for mechanical ventilation should be assessed and managed in the usual fashion. Carbon monoxide poisoning complicates the assessment of oxygenation). Defects in gas exchange may be severe, particularly if ARDS develops, and a lung protective strategy utilizing low tidal ventilation should be instituted. Prophylactic antibiotics have no value in this chemical pneumonitis, and the subsequent burn management and treatment of eventual bacterial pneumonia can be made more difficult by the development of resistant organisms if antibiotics are used early.

CARBON MONOXIDE (CO) POISONING

CO interferes with tissue oxygenation in several ways: it binds avidly to hemoglobin prevents oxygen carriage; it promotes a left shift of the oxyhemoglobin dissociation curve, making hemoglobin less likely to give up oxygen to the tissues; and it binds to other heme proteins such as the cytochrome oxidases and impairs oxidative processes at the mitochondrial level. It is this, rather than binding to hemoglobin (Hb), which is principally responsible for the toxic effects of CO.

The clinical features of CO poisoning include nausea and vomiting, headache, hyperventilation, hypotension, increased muscle tone, and coma. Classically patients appear with cherry-pink skin, although cyanosis is more common. Pulse oximeters over-read because they are unable to distinguish HbCO from HbO_2. Arterial blood gases and co-oximetry reveals the true picture of a normal PaO_2, a low SpO_2, and a high HbCO level. HbCO levels of 20% suggest a significant injury, whilst levels of 60% are life-threatening.

Treatment is largely supportive. Specific measures include oxygen therapy at highest concentration available. Treatment with high inspired oxygen concentrations promotes the displacement of CO from heme-binding sites. The half-life of HbCO is brought down to 60 min from 240 min at room air with inspired oxygen concentration of 100%.

Intubation and ventilation with 100% oxygen may be appropriate. Clearance from tissue binding sites is slower than from hemoglobin, and therapy is therefore maintained until the systemic consequences of poisoning (acidosis, coma, etc.) resolve.

Hyperbaric oxygen therapy for 1-2 hours at 3 times atmospheric pressure (repeated after 24 hours) is more effective than normobaric oxygen therapy, and reduce long-term neurological sequelae. Although its limited access restricts its usefulness somewhat, transfer to the nearest hyperbaric chamber should be considered if patient fails to respond to conventional therapy, is comatose or has high HbCO levels.

Dantrolene (1mg/kg) can be used to reduce oxygen demand.

CYANIDE POISONING

Combustion of synthetic fabrics and furnishings generates cyanide and other toxic products. Any patient with evidence of inhalational injury should be treated for cyanide poisoning with 10mL 3% sodium nitrite over 3 minutes followed by 25 mL 50% sodium thiosulphate over 10 minutes.

FURTHER READING

1. Alarie Y. Toxicity of fire smoke. Crit Rev Toxicol. 2002;32(4):259-89.
2. American Burn Association. Inhalation injury: diagnosis. J Am Coll Surg. 2003;196(2):307-12.
3. Baud FJ. Cyanide: critical issues in diagnosis and treatment. Hum Exp Toxicol. 2007 Mar;26(3):191-201.
4. Enkhbaatar P, Traber DL. Pathophysiology of acute lung injury in combined burn and smoke inhalation injury. Clin Sci (Lond). 2004;107(2):137-43.
5. Lee AS, Mellins RB. Lung injury from smoke inhalation. Paediatr Respir Rev. 2006;7(2):123-8.
6. Milcak RP, Suman OE, Herndon DN. Respiratory management of inhalation injury. Burns. 2007;33(1):2-13.
7. Miller K, Chang A. Acute inhalation injury. Emerg Med Clin North Am. 2003;21(2):533-57.
8. Murakami K, Traber DL. Pathophysiological basis of smoke inhalation injury. News Physiol Sci. 2003;18:125-9.
9. Pham TN, Gibran NS. Thermal and electrical injury. Surg Clin North Am. 2007;87(1):185-206.
10. Prockop LD, Chichkova RI. Carbon monoxide intoxication: an updated review. J Neurol Sci. 2007;262(1-2):122-30.
11. Sicoutris CP, Holmes JH. Fire and smoke injuries. Crit Care Nurs Clin North Am. 2006;18(3):403-17.
12. Stoller KP. Hyperbaric oxygen and carbon monoxide poisoning: a critical review. Neurol Res. 2007;29(2):146-55.
13. Weaver LK. Clinical practice. Carbon monoxide poisoning. N Engl J Med. 2009 19;360(12):1217-25

Bhavneet Bharti, MD

69 Malnutrition Related Emergencies

Medical emergencies in children are often challenging and frightening. This fact assumes much greater importance if such emergencies are confronted in a child with underlying malnutrition, the latter metamorphosing common illnesses like respiratory infections, measles, diarrhea etc. into life threatening emergencies (only under-nutrition is being considered for the purpose of this article). Presence of severe malnutrition is well known reason for exponential increase in the risk of morbidity and mortality potential of emergency illnesses in such children. In fact, pediatric emergencies and their management in severely malnourished children need to be viewed differently by mainly following perspectives: 1) Malnutrition, either primary or secondary, provides a very vulnerable immunological milieu for infective illnesses in emergency setting; 2) Clinical presentation may be deceptively milder and not-so explosive, yet sinister in severely malnourished children; 3) Many of classic signs and symptoms of many emergency illnesses can be masked by underlying malnutrition in an affected child and such diseases may masquerade as nonspecific or vague symptoms. 4) Management of emergency illnesses in severely malnourished children necessitates proactive as well as preemptive approach to forestall and mitigate any impending disastrous outcome.

The high mortality rates, with death commonly occurring during the first 48 hours after hospital admission in severely malnourished children had often been attributed to faulty case management protocol. A manual by WHO for the senior health workers and physicians clearly delineates and streamlines the standard management protocol in such settings. The focus of this chapter is on common emergencies observed within the first 48 hours of hospitalization in severely malnourished children. Nutritional issues, although most important, are not within the purview of this present article.

Classification of emergencies in malnourished children:

Emergencies archetypal of malnourished children: A) Hypoglycemia B) Hypothermia C) Hypokalemia D) Anemia E) Fluid overload

Emergencies exacerbated in malnourished children: A) Diarrhea with dehydration B) Infections C) Sepsis with septic shock and metabolic acidosis (Figure 1).

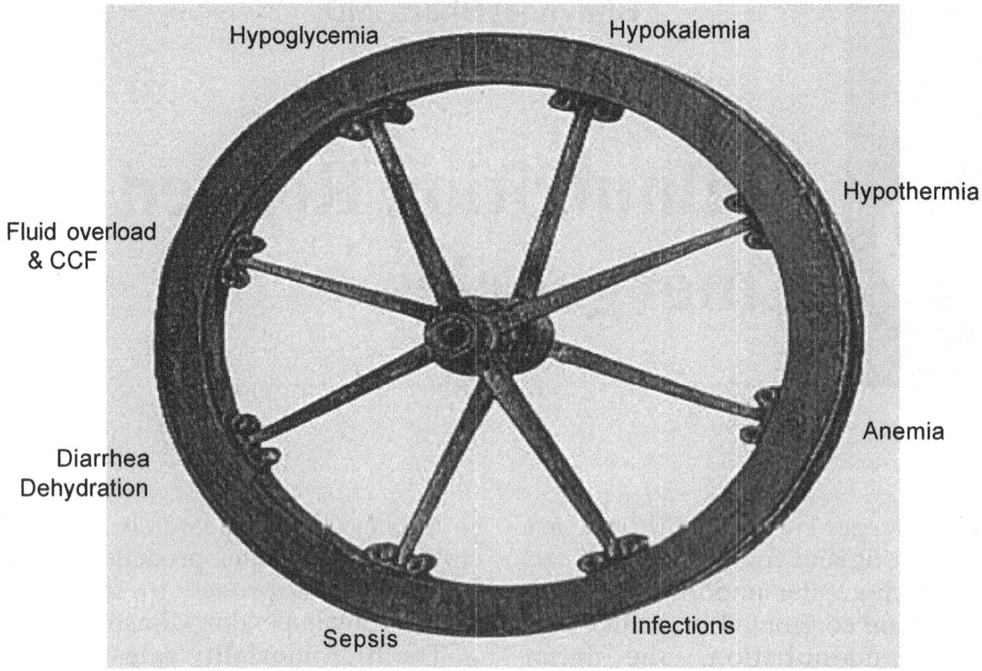

Fig. 1: Wheel of Severe Malnutrition depicting various emergencies

HYPOGLYCEMIA

Hypoglycemia is one of common metabolic emergencies seen in malnourished children. It is imperative to recognize it at the earliest, as it is known to be associated with neurological damage and high fatality. Signs of hypoglycemia include hypothermia, lethargy, limpness and alteration of sensorium. Malnourished children usually do not show signs of sweating or pallor, characteristic features of hypoglycemia, which are seen, in well-nourished children. Drowsiness, apneic spells and convulsions are other life threatening danger signs. Concomitant infections, inadequate feeding in the recent past, delay in presentation to hospital, use of potentially toxic herbal preparations, and the lack of diagnostic facilities may aggravate hypoglycemia. Importantly, hypoglycemia is amenable to inexpensive and widely available treatment.

Hypoglycemia is defined as blood glucose of less than 54 mg/dl. To prevent hypoglycemia it is important to ensure that any malnourished child is fed at 2-3 hourly intervals all through the day and night.

Treatment should be started immediately on clinical suspicion, even in the absence of laboratory confirmation of the diagnosis. If the child is conscious, (s)he should be given 50ml of 10% glucose (or 5 g table sugar dissolved in 50ml water) orally. If the child has altered sensorium or is having seizures, 5 ml/kg of 10% glucose or 2ml/kg of 25% glucose is administered intravenously, followed by 50 ml of 10% glucose by nasogastric tube. In case of difficult intravenous access, the nasogastric dose can precede the intravenous correction. Oral or nasogastric feeds should be started with the improvement in sensorium to prevent future recurrences.

Table 1: Laboratory Tests to be considered in Emergency

Test	*Interpretation and Significance*
Tests that may be useful	
Blood glucose	<54 mg/dl indicative of hypoglycemia
Microscopic examination of blood smear	For presence of malarial parasite
Hemoglobin or PCV	Hemoglobin< 4 g/dl or PCV< 12% indicative of very severe anemia
Examination and culture of urine	Bacteriuria or >10 leukocytes/hpf indicative of infection
Chest X Ray	1. Pneumonia: Malnourished children show less opacities in the lungs 2. Vascular engorgement and cardiomegaly may indicate heart failure 3. X ray may also show features of rickets
Tests that are of little value	
Serum proteins	Only guides the prognosis
Tests for HIV	Should not be done routinely and never without prior counseling
Serum electrolytes	May be helpful in monitoring

Adapted from WHO Manual for the management of severe malnutrition. (Ref 2)

In view of close involvement of hypoglycemia with systemic infections, it is recommended that all such children be started on broad-spectrum antibiotics, as hypoglycemia may be one of the manifestations of sepsis in malnourished children.

HYPOTHERMIA

Hypothermia in a malnourished child is defined as core or rectal temperature < 35.5°C or axillary temperature <35 °C. Marasmic children especially younger infants and those with large areas of denuded skin or serious infections are extremely vulnerable to hypothermia. It is usually as a consequence of reduction in the metabolic rate i.e., in heat production. As a result, the child with severe malnutrition has difficulty in regulating body temperature and follows the ambient temperature closely. It is for this reason that malnourished children are prone for early morning hypothermia and consequent mortality. Hypothermia could be a manifestation of infection, similar to the neonatal responses and warrants the use of broad-spectrum antibiotics. Often hypothermia and hypoglycemia coexist in such children. It is important for the physicians to treat hypothermia with utmost care as use of various warming devices such as hot water bottles, heaters, blowers etc can result in severe thermal injuries. Kangaroo method (the child is placed in skin to skin contact with the mother and both covered well) is an innovative method to manage hypothermia in low birth weight babies; but the principle can be easily extrapolated for malnourished children with no risk of thermal accidents. No external warming device is safe in the absence of close monitoring and supervision. Ideally, it would be appropriate to have regulated room temperature using central air conditioning and using appropriate clothing. Pre warmed fluids could be useful adjunct in children receiving parenteral fluids. Last but not the least, one must ensure that the place where the child is nursed is free from draughts.

HYPOKALEMIA

Severely malnourished children have depleted body stores of potassium, even though it may not manifest in the laboratory values. Severity of malnutrition has been observed to have a significant correlation with the degree of hypokalemia. All hospitalized malnourished children must receive oral potassium supplement in a dose of 4 mmol/kg for a period of 5 days. Potassium containing infusions are usually not necessary in children who do not have significant diarrhea or vomiting. If a child has severe dehydration requiring intravenous fluids or has a very high purge rate that cannot be managed by ORS, then potassium is to be added to the fluids in the following manner: (i) if serum potassium < 2mmol/L, add 40mml/L of KCl; and (ii) if serum potassium is between 2 and 2.5mmol/L, add 30mmol/L of KCl.

Malnourished children with diarrheal losses are also prone to develop neuromuscular weakness and at times, it may be one of the presenting features to Emergency room. The exact mechanism whereby hypokalemia causes muscle weakness is still not known, but it has been shown to change resting membrane potential, limit increase in blood flow in exercising muscles and causes a reduction in muscle glycogen content of experimental animals. The commonest neuromuscular manifestation of hypokalemia is neck flop which is more frequently noticed by mothers. Other manifestations included weakness of trunk and limb muscles, abdominal distension and absent/sluggish bowel sounds. Weakness of limb muscles range from inability to move against resistance to flaccid paralysis. Respiratory muscle involvement and Phantom hernias has also been occasionally reported. These signs usually respond to parenteral potassium supplementations.

SEVERE ANEMIA

Mild to moderate anemia is almost always present in children who are malnourished. However treatment with oral supplements is better deferred as free iron promotes oxidative damage to cell membranes and promote the growth of some pathogens. Studies have shown that giving iron from the time of admission increases mortality in malnourished children.

However, in cases of severe anemia (Hb<4.0 g/dl) a blood transfusion is indicated to avoid heart failure. Such children are given 10 ml/kg of packed cells or whole blood over 3 hours. In patients with impending heart failure, partial exchange transfusion may be preferred.

CONGESTIVE CARDIAC FAILURE & FLUID OVERLOAD

The impaired cardiac function in malnourished children may lead to congestive cardiac failure in case of over hydration or sodium overload. Severe anemia may be one of the contributory factors. The first sign of congestive cardiac failure usually is fast breathing which may be difficult to differentiate from respiratory tract infections and septic shock, both of which may manifest with similar signs. It should be noted that the latter two usually occur within the first 48 hours after presentation and cardiac failure usually presents later. It requires the use of diuretics such as frusemide (1mg/kg) and judicious use of fluids and dobutamine. Cautious use of digoxin is advocated only in presence of firm diagnosis of congestive cardiac failure and hypokalemia corrected or improved.

DIARRHEA AND DEHYDRATION

Diarrhea with accompanying dyselectrolytemia is common emergency in severely malnourished children. Assessment of dehydration in a case of malnutrition could be challenging. Many of the signs that are normally used to assess dehydration in well-nourished child could be unreliable:

(i) The absence of subcutaneous fat and supporting tissue make the skin thin, loose and less elastic thereby overestimating dehydration.
(ii) Edema, on the other hand may mask the diminished skin turgor in children with Kwashiorkar.
(iii) The salivary and lacrimal glands are atrophied in malnutrition, so the children have dry oral mucosa and lack of tears.
(iv) Apathy and irritability may be part of the nutritional deficiencies rather than manifestations of dehydration.

Thus it becomes difficult to detect dehydration reliably and to determine its severity. Moreover, many signs of dehydration may also be seen in septic shock. Hence it often becomes necessary to treat some children for both.

The signs of dehydration that remain reliable in malnourished children are: (i) History of diarrhea; (ii) Excessive thirst; (iii) Sunken eyes; (iv) Weak or absent peripheral pulses; (v) Cool extremities; and (vi) Decreased urine output.

Clinical signs, which are helpful to distinguish between dehydration and septic shock, are enumerated in Table 2.

As far as treatment is concerned, oral route is the preferred route for rehydration until and unless there are any contraindications for the oral use such as cases of severe dehydration, circulatory collapse or shock. Serum sodium levels may be reduced in malnourished children but the total body and cellular sodium may be normal or increased. These children are more prone

Table 2 : Clinical signs of dehydration and septic shock in a malnourished child

Clinical Sign	*Some dehydration*	*Severe dehydration*	*Incipient septic shock*	*Developed septic shock*
Watery diarrhea	Yes	Yes	Yes or no	Yes or no
Thirst	Drinks eagerly	Drinks poorly	No	No
Hypothermia	No	No	Yes or no	Yes or no
Sunken eyes	Yes	Yes	No	No
Weak or absent radial pulse	No	Yes	Yes	Yes
Cold hands and feet	No	Yes	Yes	Yes
Urine flow	Yes	No	Yes	No
Mental state	Restless or irritable	Lethargic, comatose	Apathetic	Lethargic
Hypoglycemia	Sometimes	Sometimes	Sometimes	Sometimes

Adapted from WHO Manual for the management of severe malnutrition (Ref 2).

to develop fluid overload and heart failure. Therefore rehydration is performed slowly .The malnourished children have low potassium values and may have abnormally high sodium levels. Therefore in place of standard ORS solution, WHO recommends the use of a special rehydration solution for the malnourished (ReSoMal). The composition of this solution is given in Table 3. ReSoMal is not available commercially in India, however it can be made from the standard WHO-ORS solution by diluting it in 2 litres of water (instead of 1 litre), adding 50 g of sucrose (25g/l) and 40 ml of mineral mix. The composition of the mineral mix is given in Table 4. Attempts are being made in India to make mineral mix available commercially. Approximately 70 to 100 ml/kg body weight of this solution is given over 12 hours to restore hydration in the following manner: (i) 5 ml/kg every 30 min for the first 2 hours orally or by NG tube; and (ii) 5-10 ml/kg/hour thereafter. The child must be monitored closely for signs of under- and over-hydration and fluid therapy tailored accordingly. Rehydration is indicated by passage of urine and subsidence of thirst.

Table 3: Composition of oral rehydration salt solution for severely malnourished children (ReSoMal)

Component	*Concentration (mmol/l)*
Glucose	125
Sodium	45
Potassium	40
Chloride	70
Citrate	7
Magnesium	3
Zinc	0.3
Copper	0.045
Osmolarity	300

Adapted from WHO Manual for the management of severe malnutrition.(Ref 2)

Table 4: Composition of mineral mix solution

Substance	*Amount*
Potassium chloride	89.5g
Tripotassium citrate	32.4 g
Magnesium chloride	30.5 g
Zinc acetate	3.3 g
Copper sulfate	0.56 g
Sodium selenate	10 mg
Potassium iodide	5 mg
Water	1000 ml

Adapted from WHO Manual for the management of severe malnutrition. (Ref 2)

In order to maintain hydration, children under 2 years of age are given 50-100 ml of ORS after each loose stool; older children should be given 100-200 ml for every loose stool.

Intravenous fluids are indicated only in the presence of severe dehydration and shock. Various fluids used include the following:

1. Half strength Darrow's solution with 5% dextrose
2. Half strength Ringer's Lactate solution with 5% dextrose
3. N/2 saline with 5% glucose/dextrose

The fluid is administered in the following manner: (i) 15 ml/kg is to be given over one hour (ii) Start ReSoMal/ORS simultaneously through NG tube at 10 ml/kg/hour; (iii) Reassess after one hour and repeat the intravenous fluids in case of no improvement; (iv) Switch to ReSoMal/ORS (10 ml/kg/hour) for the next 10 hours; and (v) If the child fails to improve despite intravenous fluid therapy, treat the child as septic shock.

Early administration of oral fluids and feeds is beneficial in malnourished children.

INFECTIONS

Bacterial and viral infections are common in severely malnourished children. Bacterial infections such as pneumonia, diarrhea and urinary tract infection are common. While majority of infections are bacterial, viral infections like measles and chicken pox can be lethal. A high index of suspicion is required for the malnourished children as signs of infection are usually absent in them due to of poor inflammatory response. Prompt and effective treatment of bacterial infections helps in significant reduction in mortality and improvement in nutritional response to feeding. Empirical broad-spectrum anti-microbials are recommended to all malnourished children requiring hospitali-zation. Choice of antibiotics will depend upon on the local susceptibility pattern, cost and availability of the drugs.

In endemic areas, malaria must be ruled out by examination of the peripheral smear. Rapid diagnostic test for malaria may also be useful diagnostic adjuncts if available. Children with malaria may have overlapping clinical signs such as diarrhea.

Septic Shock

Dehydration and septic shock are difficult to discriminate in children with severe malnutrition, as signs of hypovolemia are present in both. Many cases of sepsis have history of diarrhea and dehydration, adding to the diagnostic problem. The signs that may be helpful in differentiating the two are shown in Table 2.

All children with incipient or developed septic shock should be immediately started on broad-spectrum antibiotics. Hypothermia and hypoglycemia must be managed as per protocol. Children with incipient shock are started on early nasogastric feeds.

The treatment protocol for developed septic shock as per WHO is given below:

1. The goal of first hour is to start immediate volume replacement. Recommended fluids are given at the rate of 15 ml/kg/hour, with extreme care to avoid over-hydration and congestive heart failure. If facilities are available, central venous lines could be used to monitor fluids in the facility-based settings especially where the expertise is available.
2. If the child fails to show improvement after one hour of therapy or develops features of congestive cardiac failure, blood or plasma transfusion (10 ml/kg over 3 hours) could be considered depending upon the availability. Monitoring of the fluids given must be done strictly. On earliest features of congestive heart failure development, the rate of transfusion should be slowed and diuretic be used.
3. In cases of septic shock that do not respond to intravenous fluid resuscitation and cannot maintain normal blood pressure on fluid therapy alone, intravenous vasoactive agents such as dopamine and dobutamine should be used. If the shock remains refractory to this therapy, intravenous infusion of epinephrine or norepinephrine, with or without sodium nitroprusside for reduction of afterload should be considered.

METABOLIC ACIDOSIS

Acidosis usually accompanies dehydration, and appropriate correction of dehydration corrects the acidosis as well. It may, however, represent tissue hypoxia due to impaired perfusion in children with septic shock. There is controversial role of bicarbonate in children with persistent clinical features of acidosis (i.e., rapid and deep breathing) after adequate rehydration. The cut off value for the use of bicarbonate therapy could be taken as pH of 6.9 as this degree of acidosis may result in impaired myocardial function.

NURSING NEEDS

Emergency rooms in resource poor settings are often crowded with many children sharing cots and further predisposing to nosocomial infections. Malnourished children are very vulnerable to cross infections because their immune functions are impaired; therefore, good ward hygiene is of utmost importance. The place offered for nursing of these children should be free of draughts to prevent hypothermia. Reverse isolation could be considered as a measure to prevent nosocomial infections if it is available. Bathing should essentially be postponed and if sponging is done, immediate drying is recommended to prevent hypothermia

Finally, one must realize that children who are severely malnourished are likely to have suffered substantial nutrient deficits by the time they arrive at the hospital because of recurrent or persistent episodes of diarrhea or infections. It is therefore imperative to regard severe mal-nutrition as a state of multiple micronutrient deficiencies and to provide vitamins and minerals (twice the recommended dietary allowances) to correct deficiencies. If managed appropriately, the metabolic apparatus will be in working order again, and then it will be safe to move ahead and promote rapid catch-up growth by feeding of high-energy, high-protein diets after the initial acute management of emergencies.

To conclude, it must be reiterated that severely malnourished children die in the hospital of four main causes: hypoglycemia, hypothermia, cardiac failure from over-hydration and electrolyte imbalance, and infection (the infection often being missed completely or treatment being delayed). Differential mortality across various treating units could be attributed to the extent of remedial as well as preventive efforts practiced by their healthcare providers. In short, phrase " forewarned is forearmed" can aptly illustrate the key theme of management of pediatric emergencies in malnourished children and it is absolutely imperative that we must optimize our preventive programmes and encourage community based therapeutic interventions to identify the high risk children and prevent hospital admissions of these severely malnourished children.

FURTHER READING

1. Schofield C, Ashworth A. Why have mortality rates for severe malnutrition remained so high? Bull WHO 1996; 74: 223-229.
2. World Health Organization. Management of severe malnutrition: a manual for physicians and other senior health workers; Geneva, 1999.
3. World Health Organization. Management of the child with a serious infection or severe malnutrition. Guidelines for care at the first-referral level in developing countries. Geneva: WHO, 2000.
4. Ahmed T, Begum B, Badiuzzaman, Ali M, Fuch G. Management of severe malnutrition and diarrhea. Indian J Pediatr 2001; 68: 45-51.
5. Ahmed T , Ali M, Ullah MM, Choudhary IA, Haque ME, Salam MA etal. Mortality in severely malnourished children with diarrhea and use of standardized management protocol. Lancet 1999;353:1919-1922.
6. Rice AL, Sacco L, Hyder A, Black RE. Malnutrition as an underlying cause of childhood deaths associated with infectious diseases in developing countries. Bull World Health Organ 2000; 78: 1207-122.
7. Cavalcante AAM, Pinheiro LMP, Monte C, Guimaraes ARP, Ashworth A. Treatment of malnutrition in Brazil: simple solutions to common problems. Trop Doctor 1998; 28: 95-97
8. Wharton BA, Howells GR, McCance RA. Cardiac failure in kwashiorkor. *Lancet* 1967; ii: 384-387.
9. Bennish ML, Azad AK, Rahman O, Phillips RE. Hypoglycaemia during diarrhoea in childhood. Prevalence, pathophysiology, and outcome. N Engl J Med 1990; 322: 1357-1363.
10. Berkowitz FE. Infections in children with severe protein-energy malnutrition. Pediatr Infect Dis J 1992; 11: 750-759.
11. Manary MJ, Brewster DR. Potassium supplementation in kwashiorkor. J Pediatr Gastroenterol Nutr 1997; 24: 194-201.
12. Chhabra A, Patwari AK,AnejaS,Chandra J, Anand VK, Ahluwalia TP. Neuromuscular manifestations of Diarrhea related hypokalemia. Indian Pediatrics 1995;32:409-15.
13. Ashworth A. Treatment of severe malnutrition .J Pediatr Gastroenterol Nutr 2001; 32: 516-18.

George L. Foltin, Lou E. Romig and Glenda H. Grawe

70 Prehospital Emergency Medical Services

Physicians need to have an understanding of the structure and function of the emergency medical service (EMS) system that cares for their patients and to assure that the care delivered is appropriate for children. EMS is not restricted to the on scene care and transport of a patient, but encompasses the entire spectrum of emergency care (Figure 1). Knowledge of the development of EMS, US public policy and regulation of EMS, types of EMS systems, how EMS systems function, supervision, training and education of EMS providers and the unique environment that they function in are vital to this understanding. Within each of these keep in mind the challenge to integrate specific needs of pediatric patients.

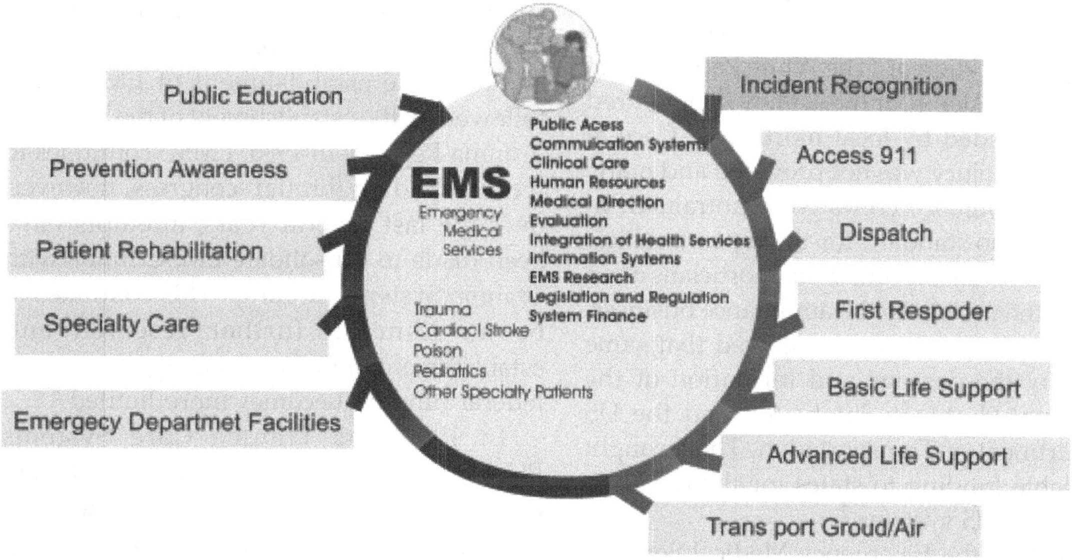

Fig. 1: Spectrum of EMS[1]

DEVELOPMENT OF EMS

EMS has been present since ancient times. There are records from ancient Egypt as well as the New Testament that describe rendering of care to the acutely injured person. EMS as we think of it today, closely parallels the development of battlefield medicine. The initial concepts of triage and battlefield treatment date to the Napoleonic Wars and Clara Barton's work in the civil war is credited with development of triage and treatment methods in the US. It was not until the Korean and Vietnam Wars that the US became adept at providing front line care to soldiers that significantly improved survival of wounded soldiers.

During the Vietnam War, The National Academy of Sciences, National Resource Council, published a report titled "Accidental Death and Disability: The Neglected Disease in Modern Society". This document, later to be called "The White Paper" highlighted the plight of the acutely injured person, and recommendations were made for development of EMS systems. Prior to 1966, the year of the publication of "The White Paper", most transport systems for the acutely ill or injured were provided by local morticians. Care at the site of injury was not provided and many of the ambulance crews were untrained. In addition, no standard for the type of vehicle used was available, thus why morticians often found themselves in the ambulance business. Recommendations were followed that same year by the passage and formation of the National Highway Safety Act and the US Department of Transportation. This brought available funding to states for the development of EMS systems.[2]

In 1973, the Emergency Medical Services Act, created an agency within the Department of Health, Education and Welfare that identified 15 components of EMS systems, unfortunately of these components financial feasibility and medical direction were not present (Table 1). The idea of regionalization of care and the creation of trauma systems was also part of this act. Funding for development of EMS systems continued to be accessible until 1981 when the Omnibus Budget Reconciliation Act changed the allocation of funding to block grants to states that were to address health issues that also encompassed EMS. Unfortunately as a result of the change in funding distribution many programs did not continue or finish developing.

In the 1980's the American Academy of Pediatrics under the direction of Dr. Calvin Sia brought to the forefront the poor outcomes for emergently ill and injured children, which was followed by legislation which created Emergency Medical Services for Children (EMSC) in 1984 under the US Department of Health and Human Resources. This important piece of legislation was to support the development of emergency care for pediatric patients through the continuum of EMS. The establishment of EMSC was followed by the establishment of the Pediatric Trauma Registry in 1985. EMSC continues to receive funding through congress, however; over the last several years, attempts have been made to consolidate EMSC funds with Trauma Systems funding. This continues to be an issue in further research and establishment of pediatric emergency care as federal funding becomes more limited.[3]

In 1990, the Trauma Care Systems Planning and Development Act was created to provide continued development of regionalized trauma care; however, funding has been intermittent and contributed to the delay of a regionalized trauma system.[4]

What legislation has accomplished over the last 40 years is guidelines and funding to continue the development of EMS. Several foundations and organizations have participated in developing a series of "agendas" to guide ongoing development and improvement in EMS systems. These are listed in Table 2 and are the assets targeted for EMS. In 2007, EMS interests were solidified in the Federal Interagency Committee on Emergency Medical Services (FICEMS) to help focus on the "EMS Agenda of the Future" and consolidate the many involved agencies that control EMS funding. Continued awareness of legislation and funding allocation is crucial to the continued development of quality of prehospital care of emergently ill or injured children.[5]

Table 1: Emergency Medical Services System Act of 1973: 15 Components of EMS Systems

- Manpower
- Training
- Communications
- Transportation
- Facilities
- Critical care units
- Public safety agencies
- Consumer participation
- Access to care
- Patient transfer
- Coordinated patient record keeping
- Public information and education
- Review and evaluation
- Disaster plan
- Mutual aid

Table 2: EMS agenda for the future: Systems attributes

- Integration of Health Services
- EMS Research
- Legislation and Regulation
- System Finance
- Human Resources
- Medical Direction
- Education Systems
- Public Education
- Prevention
- Public Access
- Communication Systems
- Clinical Care
- Information Systems
- Evaluation

US Public Policy: How EMS is Regulated

The regulation and administration of EMS systems was delineated 1988 by the Statewide EMS Technical Assessment Program administered by NHTSA. This guides the way EMS systems are established within states.[6] These system elements include regulation and policy that governs each state's EMS system and designates leadership and local authority. For each state there is an acting EMS State Director. This person is appointed by the Governor in most states and acts as the administrative lead for coordination of EMS activities and allocation of funds. Resource allocation and the concept of mutual aid is guided by the state and often integrated into disaster management planning. States are the licensing board for not only personnel but of transportation vehicles utilized by EMS. Communication and coordination along with dissemination of public education and information are initiated at a state level with local system control and integration. Many of the state administrative roles are duplicated at the regional and local levels and have the added role of maintaining operational as well as administrative standards. Medical direction and quality improvement are often controlled at local system level; some rural areas may combine resources and use regional medical direction and quality improvement measures.

Types of EMS Systems

All EMS systems involve the citizens of the community. One of the general goals of all systems is bystander response. In some rural areas, all of the prehospital care is provided by trained local volunteer providers. Many city municipalities have EMS combined with fire or police, fewer have stand alone EMS. Most municipalities train all fire and police as first responders. Other systems rely on hospital based services, although rare. Many areas contract services to private providers for EMS coverage.

How EMS Systems Function

Access and System Entry

Patient and citizen education including

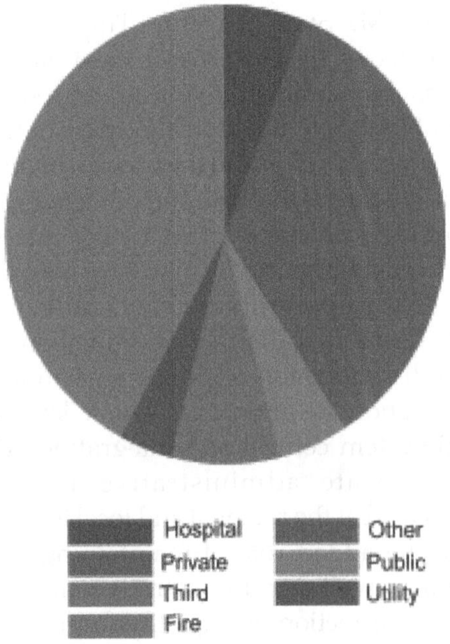

Fig. 2: Service Types

prevention, bystander cardiopulmonary resuscitation (CPR) training and the 911 system all are methods or system access and entry. Simply by improving the use of seat belts and car seats through clinics held at fire stations constitutes access to the system and has been an invaluable tool to improve car restraint use and reduce vehicular injury, especially in the pediatric age group. Bystander CPR is the earliest entry level into the system for emergent arrest and has proven to be of benefit in cities with higher levels of lay CPR education rates. Many cities across the United States participate in the 911 system which was first suggested by "The White Paper" in 1966. In more urbanized areas, "enhanced 911" provides the physical location of the call and improves response to emergency events. There are still rural areas that do not have 911 access points, but that is rapidly becoming less frequent. Enhanced 911 has been difficult to integrate in these rural areas and only through community effort has this been successful. Another difficulty is with cellular and internet based phones that are not integrated into the enhanced 911 systems. Finally, new automated crash notification or "ACN" devices installed in some newer cars make real time notification of accidents a new technology that may further reduce time to incident notification.

Prehospital Care

Prehospital care begins with telephone triage, emergency medical dispatch and pre-arrival instructions. In addition, first response by bystanders, police and fire. Arrival and treatment by BLS and ALS units is the second step to prehospital care followed by transport by EMTs and/or paramedics to a hospital or other destination. Triage decisions for specialty referrals such as trauma centers are made on scene as directed by local protocols.

Transport

Transport decisions are based on local protocol determinations. For pediatric patients, those who are critically ill or injured, they should be taken to the closest designated pediatric trauma center or designated pediatric care facility. This can be an issue for rural systems that do not have specialized care, but the awareness of which facility is best capable to handle the pediatric patient is vital.

In-hospital Emergency Care

Resuscitation, stabilization and admission or transfer to a higher level of care.

Definitive Care

Definitive care is the acute care of the emergent illness or injury by surgery or intensive care.

Rehabilitation

Rehabilitation begins the moment the patient enters the system. The goal of EMS is treatment of the acutely injured with return to society. Rehabilitation is a crucial component to ensure a favorable outcome.

Education, Training and Supervision of EMS Personnel

Education and Training

As an introduction to this section a definition of what type of personnel work within EMS is not only helpful but crucial when working in emergency medicine. Below are listed the different types of EMS personnel with level of training and responsibility.

First Responder: Has completed 40-60 hours of training and provides lifesaving skills, such as CPR, and other basic interventions requiring minimal equipment until other rescuers arrive.[8]

Emergency Medical Technician-B (EMT): Often referred to as "EMT" or a "basic", trained in emergency medical care and transport of ill and injured patients. Functions under medical direction and requires licensure after completion of an accredited EMT course with a minimum of 110 hours of coursework (to include 2 hours anatomy and physiology, 1 hour pharmacology) by a state accredited training program. Coursework is based on the National Standard Curriculum developed by NHTSA and includes 8 modules, one of which focuses exclusively on infants and children. EMT are certified through the state that they practice, but are also encouraged (if not required) to pass the "National Registry EMT" exam at the completion of their training. Most medical directors require further training within the system with a final verification of skills before they begin their position. EMT-Bs are required to complete 48 hours per year or continuing education or complete a 24 hour refresher course to maintain their certification.[9]

Emergency Medical Technician-I: EMT-B providers who have completed additional training at the discretion of their medical director and may perform more advanced care such as IV therapy. EMT-I often complete 200 or more hours of training and have the same continuing education requirements as EMT-Bs.[10]

Emergency Medical Technician-P: "paramedic" highest level of prehospital provider, trained at advanced levels of resuscitation which may include advanced airway management as the discretion of the medical director. Paramedic education requires completion of EMT-B curriculum and approximately 1200 hours of instruction time. Many programs combine resources with colleges to offer paramedic training that has an associate degree granted with it. Of the 1200 hours of training as directed by the NHTSA National Standard Curriculum the average time dedicated to pediatric didactic and practicum experience averages 70-80 hours and varies from course to course. As with EMT-B, all paramedic training courses must be certified by the state EMS office and paramedics are often required to pass a skills test with the medical director of the employing service before beginning job duties. Paramedics are also required to maintain continuing education requirements of at least 48 hours per year to remain eligible for certification.[11]

Emergency Medical Dispatcher: Coordinates telephone and triage with dispatch of appropriate resources to emergency scene and often provides pre arrival instructions. These courses are coordinated by the medical director and the state EMS office. Training is based upon the NHTSA EMD training guidelines.[12]

Medical Director: Trained licensed physician, meeting all requirements and holding licensure in the state in which the service is located and provides service. Additional formal fellowship training is available in EMS and in the future is anticipated to be recognized as a unique specialty by the American Board of Emergency Medicine (ABEM). Most medical directors have a background in either emergency medicine or family medicine. Few medical directors are pediatricians.

Supervision

Prehospital EMS personnel function under a medical director. A medical director is responsible for the performance and decisions of these providers. Most medical directors are practising emergency physicians or in rural areas may have a family medicine practice. Few services large EMS services, such as Houston Fire Department and Cincinnati Fire Department have assistant medical directors that are pediatric emergency medicine physicians.

The medical director develops the protocols within which the providers may practice. Many systems use a system of complaint based algorithom to direct pre-hospital care based on patient assessment. The provider can carry out those tasks, such as giving an initial bolus of normal saline to a tachycardic child with fever and delayed capillary refill, based on the set of protocols that they have. It has only been within the last several years that EMS systems have recognized the need for pediatric specific protocols. EMSC, Minnesota chapter has placed prehospital pediatric advanced life support protocols on the internet for use by systems to help to improve the focus of pediatrics in protocol development which can be accessed at:

http://www.emscmn.org/HealthcareProfessionals/PediatricALSGuidelines.pdf

Medical directors are active in the education and training of EMS personnel and play a part in job description, position requirements as well as equipment selection. One of the most important aspects of a medical director's role is in quality improvement to insure prehospital practices are safe, follow current standards of care and quality patient care. Finally, medical directors serve as a link to other systems including the hospital that are integral in the EMS system as a whole.

Prehospital Environment

Epidemiology

Children comprise approximately 30 percent of all patients who use emergency department facilities. In the prehospital setting, EMS systems report that from 3 percent to 5 percent of ambulance runs are for children under 12 years of age. In systems that consider patients to be pediatric upto 18 years of age, the number jumps to as high as 10 percent.[13,14,15,16]

Problems that result in requests for ambulance usage are evenly divided between medical and trauma in most systems that have reported pediatric epidemiology. The distribution of pediatric calls is also different within age groups as an example; the majority of ambulance calls for children over the age of 2 are for trauma. Vehicular injuries (including passenger and pedestrian- and bicycle-struck incidents) are the most common followed by falls and burns.[17] The medical problems encountered by prehospital care providers in their pediatric patients are different than those encountered in adults. Cardiac-related problems are quite rare in children. Seizures, fever, respiratory distress, near drowning, and poisonings are conditions the prehospital care providers will encounter (Table 3).[14,16]

The number of pediatric patients a prehospital provider encounters yearly depends on the call volume of the EMS system and the demographics of the polulation served. Even prehospital providers who work in an urban setting may not handle more than two pediatric patients a week. The rural provider may receive a pediatric call as seldom as once a month. Overall, less than five percent of children transported by ambulance will have a life-threatening problem and less than one percent will be in full cardiopulmonary arrest.[17,18]

Table 3: Common pediatric prehospital emergencies

Respiratory distress	*Status epilepticus*
Airway trauma	
Head injury with apnea	*Near drowning*
Upper airway obstruction	*Poisoning*
Lower airway disease	Sudden infant death syndrome
Unconscious	*Child abuse*
Shock states	
Dehydration	
Sepsis	
Hemorrhage	

On the other hand, a significant proportion of children transported by ambulance have potentially serious illnesses or injuries. A study at a Midwestern pediatric tertiary center demonstrated an eight-fold higher admission rate for children brought by ambulance as opposed to those arriving by other means. Of these 1 percent died in the emergency department and 14.4 percent required immediate operative or intensive care.[15] Another study performed at a tertiary referral center in New York City demonstrated a five-fold admission rate for children who arrived by ambulance as opposed to those arriving by other means, and 36 percent of these patients required an advanced life support (ALS) decision in the prehospital setting.[18]

The low encounter rate by prehospital providers to sick children results in problems for both emergency medical technicians (EMTs) and paramedics: (1) Hands on experience may be difficult to obtain; (2) skills that have been acquired for handling pediatric patients might deteriorate; and (3) there may be lack of confidence in ability to assess and treat a sick child.

Many courses have been developed nationwide for both initial training and continuing medical education (CME) for prehospital providers at all levels. The American Heart Association/American Academy of Pediatrics, Pediatric Advanced Life Support (PALS) course has been successfully adapted for EMS providers in a number of centers.[19] The issue of lack of formalized focused pediatric training has been addressed by the American Academy of Pediatrics with the development of Pediatric Emergency Care for the Prehospital Provider (PEPP). This extensive modular based course was recently revised and provides a template for the approach and evaluation of the pediatric patient. Fundamental to its basis is the pediatric assessment triangle or "PAT". It emphasizes the importance of recognition of three vital components of the pediatric exam that do require minimal intervention including general appearance, work of breathing, and circulation to the skin.[20] More EMS systems are using the PEPP based format to teach paramedic and EMT personnel pediatric assessment and treatment skills. The national Department of Transportation (DOT) guidelines for initial EMT and paramedic training, have recently been rewritten, and involved input specifically from pediatric emergency medicine providers that will further expand training requirements in pediatrics.[21]

Some special considerations are airway/breathing, spinal immobilization, and circulatory and neurological compromise as is discussed in the next four sections.

Airway/Breathing

As formal pediatric EMS education becomes more accessible, prehospital personnel (both BLS and ALS) are being made aware of the vital role of adequate airway and ventilatory management in the child. Much controversy exists over the best prehospital airway management plan in both pediatrics and adult EMS systems. Intubation skills are taught to EMTs and is part of the NREMT exam. However; at the discretion of the medical director of the system some EMS systems do not allow intubation of any patients, others allow adult but not pediatric intubation and others allow intubation of all ages. In 2000, Dr Mary Gausche-Hill published a study that further question the use of endotracheal intubation in the prehospital pediatric respiratory arrest victim, showing no difference in outcome in patients who were intubated than those who received bag valve mask ventilation that has further continued the debate of the safety of prehospital pediatric intubation and cost to maintain these advanced skills.[22] Ongoing field evaluations of alternative airway adjuncts continues in this area that include the laryngeal mask airway (LMA), but as of yet the only device consistently recommended across all services in bag valve mask for airway support.

Although training in advanced airway and ventilatory skills is now available and emphasized, current educational programs are also emphasizing the basics. Paramedics are being taught to be aggressive but also to recognize when aggressive invasive techniques are not indicated. Children will often respond well to meticulous noninvasive intervention such as airway positioning, suctioning, and high-flow oxygen. Paramedics are learning that they may best serve the patient by settling for an adequate airway, rather than the definitive one. They are extending their understanding to encompass optimal airway management instead of merely immediate management. The well-trained medic recognizes that the rapid transport of a head-injured child undergoing good bag-valve-mask hyperventilation may represent better overall care than transport delayed for a potentially traumatic field intubation of the same trismic, combative patient. This approach serves as an example that prehospital personnel are capable of learning to recognize the fine lines between conservative management, aggressive intervention, and over treatment in the pediatric EMS patient.

Spinal Immobilization

Spinal immobilization is a skill that all prehospital providers routinely provide to the adult patient but that they sometimes find difficult for the child. Faced with a multi victim auto crash, limited equipment, and a combative child with an obvious head injury, it may be difficult to immobilize a squirming child with only a Kendricks extrication device (KED) board, towel rolls, and tape and with no cervical collar. The indications to initiate spinal precautions for both children and adults are intuitively clear although they are little substantiated by research. Along with kinematic, physiological indications and medicolegal considerations, judgement must often be incorporated into the decision-making process. Medics should be allowed the opportunity to practice immobilizing infant mannequins to a back board, and key scenarios should be discussed. For example when faced with a scared, combative 18-month-old with no obvious injuries who just fell off a bed onto a hardwood floor and when knowing that the fight to immobilize the child may worsen any injuries, the paramedic's judgement may lead to transporting the child in a regulation care seat with a parent. On the other hand, severely injured small children should not be hand-carried but rather should be afforded the same rigorous immobilization as the adult passengers in the same vehicle crash would probably receive.

Circulatory Compromise

Paramedics are taught to use the pediatric assessment triangle to aid decision making to circulatory status such as mental status changes, heart rate, capillary refill, and pulse character rather than blood pressure measurements. After determining the patient's status, they must decide if and how they should intervene in the short time they have.

The concept of *prophylactic Ns* is being discouraged for nontraumatized children, recognizing that the stress of IV insertion may compromise the patient's condition. Most of the pediatric medications available to EMTs can be given by inhalant, intranasal, subcutaneous, rectal, or endotracheal routes. Rural versus urban considerations play an important role in deciding the need for vascular access also.

Rapid vascular access for severely ill and injured children has long been a point of frustration for prehospital personnel. IV access in a sick and dehydrated child is challenging in even the best environment, but in a prehospital setting this can pose even more problems. Intraosseous access is now widely accepted across the United States for pediatric patients as an acceptable method for obtaining vascular access when intravenous access is not possible. Studies have demonstrated paramedic intraosseous success rates of 80 percent, 85 percent, and 94 percent, respectively. [23,24,25]

Neurological Compromise

Pre hospital personnel often have difficulty evaluating the mental status of a child. The subtle early changes in mental status exhibited by children are often difficult to pick up, especially in situations where the child has valid psychological reasons to be scared, agitated, or irritable. Furthermore, the preverbal child cannot be examined using the customary adult mental status examination. As they are in regard to adults, the use of nonprecise terms such as *obtunded, comatose,* and *unresponsive* are open to interpretation and should not be used when communicating with medical control. Glasgow Coma Scale (GCS) scores cannot be applied to young children and the pediatric adaptations of the scores have not been validated.

Many EMS systems are use the AVPU (alert, responsive to voice, responsive to pain, or unresponsive) system for radio or phone reports, which can easily be applied to children. The advantages of this system are that it is quick, easy to assess in all age groups, and involves no math. It can be used for serial evaluations since each category represents a theoretical increment in cortical function. The GCS score, however, still has its place and may be required on EMS report forms.

Seizures are a very common chief complaint among pediatric EMS patients and are frightening to both parents and field personnel. Paramedics are restricted in their choices of therapy to a variety of benzodiazepines. These medications can be given IM, IV, rectally or intranasal. The pediatric patient is most likely to have had a febrile seizure, very commonly the patient will no longer be actively seizing. Paramedics must be taught that under no circumstances should they deliver an anticonvulsant to a patient who is not actively seizing. In addition, since the most common reason for respiratory depression in a child with status epilepticus is secondary to administration of a benzodiazepine, prehospital personnel must be trained and ready to manage the airway. Both paramedics and EMTs need to be taught that maintenance of a patent airway with sound BLS technique alone will result in a good outcome for the seizing pediatric patient. Furthermore the most harmful etiologies for reversible seizures are hypoglycemia, hypoxia and poisonings.

THE HOSPITAL SETTING

All pediatric care is not equal. A facility that provides excellent care for adults may not be able to provide the same level of care for children. Many parts of the country do not have criteria for triage of sick, non-traumatized children. Facilities that excel in pediatric care are in place, but prehospital personnel may have to transport medical patients to the nearest facility. Systems loosely based on the trauma system concept are slowly being developed for pediatric medical patients. The prototype is a system developed in California.[26] In this voluntary system, emergency department's criteria for staffing, educational, and equipment guidelines are outlined in order to be designated as *emergency department approved for pediatrics* (EDAP). These facilities act as primary receiving centers for pediatric patients.

Patients may be transported directly or by transfer to a higher level of care, a pediatric critical care center (PCCC). These centers are also designated according to guidelines.

WEB RESOURCES

http://www.nhtsa.dot.gov/ems/
National Highway Traffic and Safety Administration
http://www.naemsp.org/
National Association of EMS Physicians
http://www.nremt.org/
National Registry of Emergency Medical Technicians
http://bolivia.hrsa.gov/emsc/
Emergency Medical Services for Children
http://www.peppsite.com/
PEPP education website
http://www.acep.org/
American College of Physicians
http://www.aap.org/
American Academy of Pediatrics

REFERENCES

1. National Highway Traffic Safety Administration, "Emergency Medical Services 24/7 Care-Everywhere"
2. National Academy of Sciences, National Research Council: Accidental Death and Disability: The Neglected Disease of Modern Society. Washington D.C.: National Academy Press, 1966.
3. Public Health Service Act, Section 1910, Emergency Medical Services for Children, US Department of Health and Human Services, Health Resources and Services Administration, Maternal and Child Health Bureau, and the Department of Transportation, National Highway Traffic Safety Administration, Office of Traffic Injury Control Programs, 1984.
4. Trauma Care Systems Training and Development Act of 1990: Public Law 101-590. Washington, D.C.: 1990.
5. National Highway Traffic Safety Administration: EMS Agenda for the Future. Washington, D.C.: U.S. Department of Transportation.
6. National Highway Traffic Safety Administration: Statewide Technical Assessment Program. Washington D.C.: US Department of Transportation, 1988.
7. Williams, D 2004 JEMS 200 City Survey, A snapshot of facts and trends to create benchmarks for your service JEMS 30(2)42-60, 2005.
8. National Highway Traffic and Safety Administration, First Responder: National Standard Curriculum, Washington D.C.: US Department of Transportation, 1995.
9. National Highway and Traffic Safety Administration, Emergency Medical Technician: National Standard Curriculum, Washington D.C.: US Department of Transportation, 1996.
10. National Highway and Traffic Safety Administration, Emergency Medical Technician - Intermediate: National Standard Curriculum, Washington D.C.: US Department of Transportation, 1998.
11. National Highway and Traffic Safety Association, Emergency Medical Technician Paramedic: National Standard Curriculum, Washington D.C.: US Department of Transportation, 1998.
12. National Highway and Safety Administration, Emergency Medical Dispatch. National Curriculum, Washington D.C.: US Department of Transportation, 1996.
13. Tsai A, Kallsen G. Epidemiology of pediatric prehospital care. Ann Emerg Med 1987;16:284-292.
14. Johnston C, King W. Pediatric prehospital care in a southern regional emergency medical service system. Southern Medical Journal 1988;81(12):1473-1476.
15. Romig L. EMS utilization by the pediatric patient population of a midwestern metropolitan area. Ped Emerg Care (abs) 1988;4(4):297.
16. Seidel J, Hornbein M, Yoshiyama K, et a1. Emergency medical services and the pediatric patient: Are the needs being met? Pediatrics 1984;73:769-772.
17. Seidel JS. EMS-C in urban and rural areas: The California experience. In Haller JA Jr, ed. Emergency medical services for children, Report of the ninety-seventh Ross conference on pediatric research, Columbia, Ohio, Ross Laboratories 1989;22-30.

18. Pon S, Foltin G, Tunik M, *et al.* Utilization of prehospital care by pediatric patients in New York City. Ped Emerg Care (abs) 1989;5(4):286.
19. Romig L. A prehospital modification of the AHA Pediatric Advanced Life Support course. Ped Emerg Care (abs) 1989;5(4):286.
20. American Academy of Pediatrics, Pediatric Education for the Prehospital Provider, 2nd Ed Jones and Bartlett Publishers, Sudbury MA 2005.
21. National Highway Traffic and Safety Administration, National EMS Core Content, Washington D.C.: US Department of Transportation, 2005.
22. Gausche M, Lewis RJ, Stratton SJ *et al,* Effect of Out-of-Hospital Pediatric Endotracheal Intubation on Survival and Neurological Outcome, A Controlled Clinical Trial. JAMA 2000(283); 783-790, 2000.
23. Smith R, Keseg D, Manley L, *et al,* Intraosseous infusions by prehospital personnel in critically ill pediatric patients. Ann Emerg Med 1988; 17(5):491-494.
24. Miner W, Corneli H, Bolte R, *et al.* Prehospital use of intraosseous infusion by paramedics. Pediatric Emergency Care 1989;5(1):5-7.
25. Seigler R, Tecklenburg F, Shealy R. Prehospital intraosseous infusion by emergency medical services personnel: A prospective study. Pediatrics 1989;84(1): 173-177.
26. Los Angeles Pediatric Society. The emergency department approved for pediatrics (EDAP), pediatric critical care center (PCCC) information manual. Los Angeles: Los Angeles Pediatric Society, American Academy of Pediatrics, and Los Angeles County Department of Health Services, 1984.

Sunit Singhi and Bhavneet Bharti

71 Setting Up A Pediatric Emergency Unit

Emergency is defined by WHO as a condition determined clinically or considered (perceived) by the patient or his caretakers as requiring urgent medical services, failing which it could result in loss of limb or life. However, studies have shown that 20 -60 % of all patients presenting to the emergency departments have urgent yet simple and uncomplicated problems that can be cared for quickly and efficiently [1]. The role of an emergency room in the management of pediatric emergencies is to distinguish the child in need of emergency or urgent care from the large numbers of less serious presentations, to provide an area where they can receive effective care. Smaller family norms and rise in literacy are responsible for increasing use of the emergency department (ED). An additional reason for increasing use of ED of a government hospital such as ours may also be availability of no or low cost quality services to patients from lower socio-economic strata, which constitute a major proportion of our population.

In the beginning of the twentieth century, every hospital had an "accident room" which was used for treatment of patients injured in accidents. By 1960's these rooms gradually evolved into "walk in medical clinics" and even patients with medical problems started utilizing them. In 1961, the Platt Committee in UK recommended the name "Accident and Emergency "after which this discipline made rapid progress to gain a status of a full fledged department of all developed countries. However, Pediatric Emergency as a separate specialty was first formulated and developed in United States in 1970[2]. The access to emergency services in India is far from satisfactory and the development of emergency medicine is in its inceptional stages[3,4]. While organization of pediatric emergency services at the national level is beyond the scope of this chapter, all pediatricians have a role to play in the development of emergency services in their hospital. In the public sector often due to limited resources there is a common emergency care area for adults and children. However the emergency care needs of children differ from those of adults, hence planning of an Emergency Unit should address these differences. A unit dedicated exclusively to children would be ideal. A great deal of planning and preparation is required in setting up this sensitive area of the hospital.

ESSENTIAL INPUTS IN PLANNING

The characteristics of population in catchment area determine the provision type and volume of services. Poor and socioeconomically deprived areas place a higher demand on all services than do more affluent areas. One of the debates of recent times is up to which age should we treat children in a pediatric facility. Local policy and practice will determine this issue, but it is important to address this issue and decision be made in the beginning. The needs of the adolescent population are different to those of the infant and toddler. New pathologies start to emerge, which necessitate a different way of thinking. Sociocultural factors, customs and local beliefs of the population should be given due consideration while planning the emergency services. Failure to address these issues will lead to bed blocking, uneven staffing and frustration.

Knowledge of the spectrum of the diseases along with seasonal and temporal variations is an essential input in planning the services. The spectrum of pediatric emergencies as seen in our hospital is given in the Table 1. Integrated management of Childhood illnesses (IMCI) developed by WHO, however, focuses on five major causes of death in childhood: diarrhea, pneumonia, malaria, measles, and malnutrition. It has been recognized that implementing IMCI guidelines implies referring up to 20% of the patients. It is these children who are severely ill and at the highest risk of death. In our experience, the comparative disease burden of pediatric emergencies in a Community vs. Tertiary care hospital is shown in the Table 2. Diarrheal and Acute Respiratory infections were the frequent causes of morbidity at both the places. Neonates formed a significant proportion of patients in both the hospitals. The common neonatal problems included birth asphyxia, sepsis and prematurity with its complications. The peak numbers of emergency visits in both the hospitals were reached in the months of July-August. However peak of respiratory cases was seen in winters. These seasonal variations have important implications for optimizing the allocation of resources according to the seasonal variation in disease frequency.

The severity of the disease presentations at admission further provide the input for planning the resuscitative measures and equipment required .In a study done in our institute on nearly 2000 children below 5 years, 25% of the children required resuscitation in one form or other. Frequencies of various resuscitation measures in three different age groups are given in the Figure 1. Assessing the outcomes of acutely ill patients, that is identification of the risk factors for mortality would further help in resource allocation in the vulnerable section of the patients. Hence, an effective emergency care system is essentially a system of care with linked and interdependent components: prehospital care (including transportation) and care at hospital.

Location of the Pediatric Emergency Department

The emergency department (ED) should be located on the ground floor, with direct access from the main road with ample space

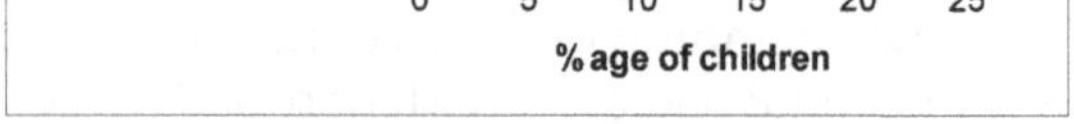

Fig.1: Frequencies of various resuscitative measures in children presenting to Pediatric ED

Table 1: Distribution of 43,800 patients attending pediatric emergency (PGIMER) between 1995-2000, with respect to major diagnosis

Major Illnesses	No.of patients (percentage of total)
Gastrointestinal	**10173(23.3%)**
Diarrhoea	7724
Intestinal obstruction	536
Acute liver failure	496
Others	1387
Respiratory	**10269(23.44%)**
Upper respiratory infection (URI)	3183
Pneumonia	2695
Asthma	2302
Others	2089
Central Nervous System	**7038(16.07%)**
Seizures	3096
Meningitis (bacterial, aseptic)	1222
Encephalitis	669
Others	2051
Neonatal illnesses	**6830(15.59%)**
Suspected sepsis	1657
Jaundice	1577
Birth Asphyxia	951
Others	2645
Systemic infections	**2849(6.73%)**
Septicemia	1126
Malaria	822
Enteric Fever	493
Others	408
Cardiac	**2070 (4.9%)**
Acyanotic heart disease	960
Congenital cyanotic heart disease	863
Others	247
Hematological	**2034(4.8%)**
Renal	**1996 (4.3%)**
Poisoning	**253 (0.58%)**

(Adapted from - Singhi S et al, J Trop Pediatr 2003; 49:207-11, reference 7)

Table 2: Important Causes of Morbidity in patients attending Pediatric emergency service: *Comparison of a tertiary care hospital vs a community hospital .*

Type of Morbidity	Number of Patients (%) seen at	
	Community Hospital, Naraingarh%	Tertiary Care Hospital, PGIMER (%)
Total	596	8301
GIT	249(41)	1713(21)
Diarrhea	228	1175
With no dehydration	151	823
With some dehydration	77	352
Hepatitis	3	96
Abdominal pain	11	129
ARI	108(18)	2003(24)
Pneumonia	87	494
URI	11	703
Asthma	4	468
Foreign body	Nil	53
Neonates	69(11)	1360(16)
Neonatal sepsis	65	408
Neonatal jaundice	4	402
CNS	35(6)	1374(17)
Seizures generalized	17	195
Febrile seizures	3	64
Focal Seizure	NA	325
Hematological	5(1)	223(3)
Sepsis	13(2)	80(1)
Fever without focus	60(10)	31(<1)
Poisoning	5(1)	184(2.3)

(From: Singhi S, Gupta G, Jain V. Comparison of pediatric emergency patients in a tertiary care hospital vs a community hospital. Indian Pediatrics. 2004;41:67-72.)

for ambulance and parking. A covered porch with enough space for the vehicle and the patients to alight at the entrance is important. Proper sign postings should be there and it should be easily located. Though it should be physically separate from other areas in the hospital; it should be easily accessible from the intensive care unit (ICU), blood bank, laboratory, operation theatre (OT) and mortuary. Having ICU and OTs adjacent to the emergency room will have a benefit in allowing rapid transfer of critically ill children to a place of definitive care. Proximity also allows more frequent meeting and informal collaboration, which can help to build teamwork. The radiology service must be close to all emergency services. At the very least, standard X-ray units should be sited or planned close to the emergency. Computerized tomography, ultrasound or magnetic resonance imaging may be necessary for evaluation of sick children and these facilities should be accessible from the emergency. This will facilitate prompt care of the ill child in a facility close to an area where maximal resuscitation expertise is available. The ED should be close to admission, medical records and cashier's booth. Wherever possible admitting function, cashiering, and registration of new patients and creation of their medical record should be done in the ED. Within the treatment setting, distraction therapy can be employed. Familiar cartoon characters on the walls, toys and a friendly relaxed atmosphere can all help diagnosis and treatment[5].

SPACE REQUIREMENTS

It is a frequent misconception among lay planners to think that pediatric facilities need to be smaller than adult facilities because children are smaller than adults. What is forgotten that staff working in both areas is the same shape and size. In addition children in our country are often accompanied by parents and several family members, making if anything the needs of children, in terms of space, greater. Total space requirement depends upon the number of patients attending in a day, the size and the type of hospital and the type of diagnostic and therapeutic facilities available. Simply stated, a daily census of 50 children requires 500 square meters area. To this another 50% should be added to prevent overcrowding. Patient loads generally show an upward trend in this department, hence it is better to plan for over usage than under usage and be prepared for increase overload. Nonetheless, the emergency departments should always have a provision to cater to a major disaster involving many children[5,6].

Architectural Design

It is important to remember the principle "design follows function" in planning the ED. Basically, there are only a few type of designs in the construction of an emergency department: the core type, the arena type and the corridor type. The core design is one in which the treatment spaces are situated around a central point in which emergency department personnel work. Ideally there is a corridor outside the treatment areas from which the patients enter the cubicles. Visitors, ancillary personnel use the corridor outside the core and the support rooms are along the periphery of corridor. This plan or its modifications leaves the greatest freedom for emergency personnel. The arena type is essentially a core plan without the periphery corridor and is good for smaller emergency departments. Many steps are saved since the work centre is almost in the middle.

Corridor plan is desirable if there is separation of various services .In general, accident and emergency units prefer this plan as each speciality can be provided separate space. The design should be such that there is minimum criss- crossing of patient traffic and privacy is maintained while treating. The rooms should be spacious and the joining corridors at least 3 meters in width. Doorways should be so designed as to follow unhindered passage of trolleys. Floor should be nonslippery and wall colors of light shade. We in our ED follow the modified core design with many smaller areas, cubicles and rooms along the corridor (Figure 2).

Physical Facilities and Layout

Facilities in the emergency are broadly classified under two categories: administrative and public facilities and the clinical facilities. Administrative and public areas include reception and public waiting area, space /room for the staff, ambulance driver and attendant. Reception control is required for the observation and control of access to the treatment area and preferably registration. It should be well equipped with communication including inter communication system. There should be some space

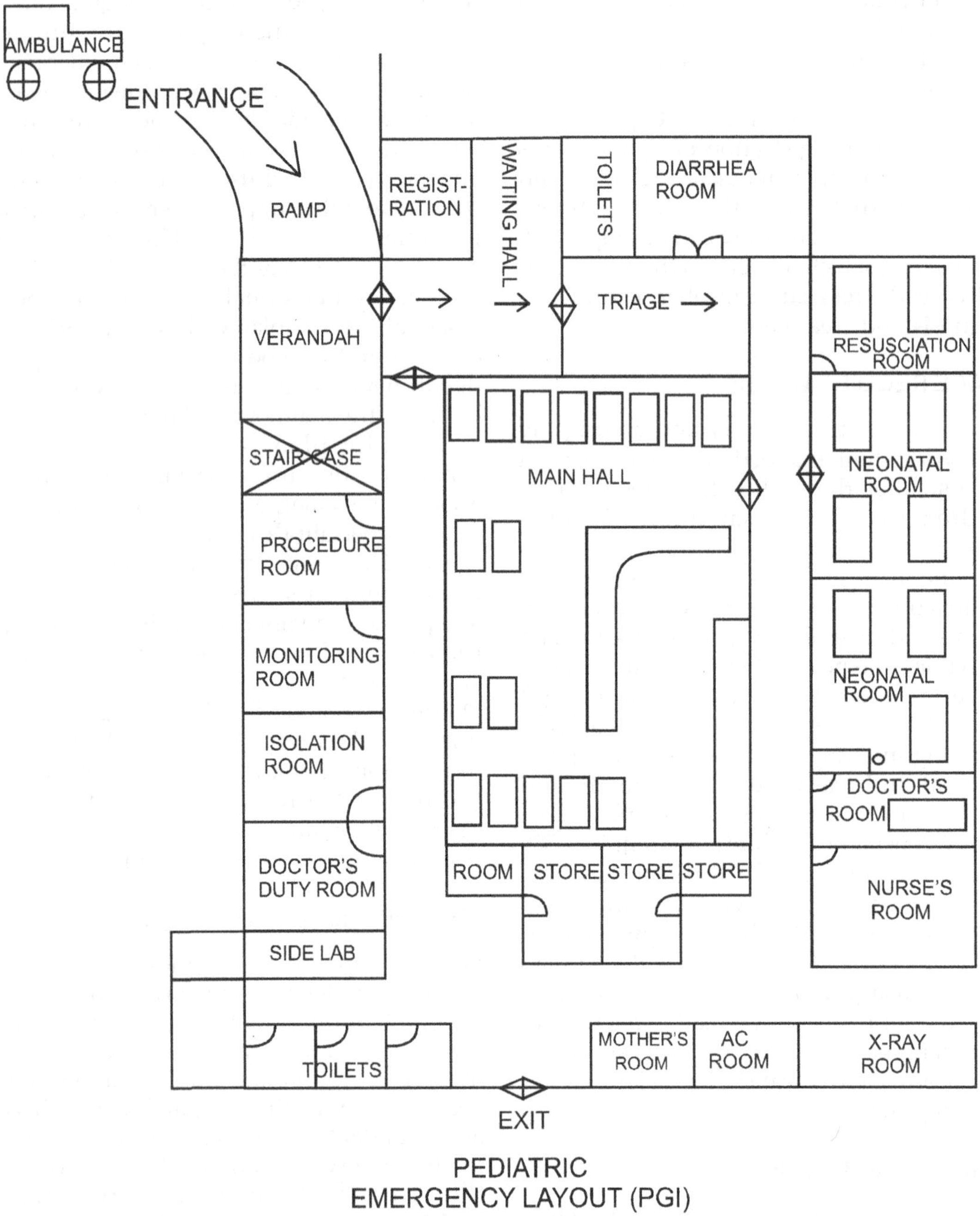

Fig. 2: Pediatric Emergency Layout (PGL)

earmarked for the stretchers and wheel chairs adjacent to the entrance. Public waiting area should have toilet facilities, water coolers, public telephones, facility for charging the mobile phones, snack bar and a vending machine. Separate waiting area for the relaxation of the mothers and other attendants should be available. A cloakroom can ensure safe custody of the attendant's luggage. There should be separate rooms for the various staff working in the emergency including the doctors, nurses and the paramedical staff[5].

Clinical facilities should include two distinct areas after the initial triage and resuscitation: Monitoring and treatment area for the critically ill children and Observation area where sick children are observed for short duration. The monitoring area require intensive monitoring facilities such as in PICUs with individual patient rooms allowing at least 225 ft^2 per patient. Electrical power, oxygen, medical compressed air, and vacuum outlets should be sufficient in number to supply all necessary equipments. In most cases, 12 or more electrical outlets and a minimum of 2 compressed air outlets, 2 oxygen outlets, and 2 vacuum outlets will be necessary per bed space. Reserve emergency power and gas supply (oxygen, compressed air) are essential. Screens or curtains must be provided to ensure patient privacy. Procedure/treatment area for both minor and major procedures should be separately earmarked We in our emergency have two monitoring beds and separate areas for the neonates and for children with diarrhea, as they constitute nearly 16% and 23% of our patients respectively[7]. There is separate isolation room for children with communicable diseases. Floor plan of Pediatric Emergency Department at PGIMER is shown in Figure 2.

PERSONNEL

Staffing an Emergency has always been a challenge to the hospital administrators. Fluctuating patient volumes and acuity prohibit the accurate assignment of the staff to the workload. Ideally pediatricians with skills, knowledge and commitment to care for critically ill children should be present 24 hours per day, 7days per week. However in small emergency rooms providing a basic facility, a trained assistant or a resident can supplement the work of a Pediatrician who is promptly available for supervision and provide directions to the staff.

Nurses are the most important personnel in an ED. To help determine the nurse staffing, workforce measures such as hours per patient visit and nurse to patient ratios have generated considerable debate. The hours per patient visit method for calculating staffing is based on the historic benchmark data. The limitation of this method is that it considers patient volume and available nursing hours without consideration of factors such as patient acuity, length of stay and the nursing interventions and activities. There are others who propose using nurse to patient specific ratios such as in ICU's. A critical limitation in use of ratios is that ratios do not account the variability found in institutions, available internal and external resources (e.g. inpatient beds, equipment, other staff) individual and aggregate patient needs (e.g. volume, intensity, demographics, length of stay) and the nursing expertise required by the patient population. The use of ratios have been challenged because the mandated staffing may be interpreted by the institutions as the maximum required staffing, when in fact it is the minimum mandated staffing standard. Further ratios may lead to minimum safe staffing and patient care instead of best practice staffing and care[8].

To identify safe, effective and realistic best practice staffing in emergency, six key factors have been identified in the projection of staffing requirements which include patient census, patient acuity, patient length of stay, nursing time for nursing interventions, activities by patient acuity, and skill mix for providing patient care based on nursing intervention that can be delegated to an attendant and an adjustment factor for the non patient care time. Continued research is needed to determine patient, nurse, doctors and organizational outcomes in relation to predicted staffing .We have an exclusive pediatric ED which is a part of 180 bedded Advanced Pediatrics Centre providing training to residents in pediatrics and its subspecialties. The centre is a part of 1500 bedded multispeciality and postgraduate teaching and research institute .It has a patient load of nearly 12000 per year and is manned round the clock by four residents (trainees in Pediatrics), a senior resident (a trained pediatrician with postgraduate qualification) and trained nursing and paramedical staff. A consultant supervises patient care round the clock and a senior consultant supervises the overall functioning of the department.

The activities improving the initial emergency management of severely ill children has received substantial attention and resources in developed countries whereas many clinicians have been prepared to deliver rapidly standardized emergency management by undertaking training courses such as the Advanced pediatric life support and PALS and several nursing and paramedic pediatric emergency curricula. Our endeavor should be to train all the physicians and nurses involved directly in care of sick children in pediatric advanced life support (PALS) course followed by recertification at regular intervals. In academic institutions, new residents doctors are frequently replacing the trained residents in order to provide 24-hour facilities. Hence, ongoing training and teaching should be an inherent part of this department.

EQUIPMENTS AND SUPPLIES

Equipments and supplies in the ED can be divided into three categories

General medical supplies – These are supplies that are generally disposable and used as they come from the manufacturer. These supplies may be stored in the ED or in the queue (outside the ED)

Reprocessed items – These items are reused and must be sent elsewhere in the hospital for reprocessing. These include linen, cut down sets, tracheostomy sets, respiratory equipment etc.

Support items – These include operational supplies such as appropriate forms, paper, clips etc.

The suggested equipments, instruments and supplies are listed in the Table 3. Each of these items should be located in or immediately available to the area noted. This list does not include routine medical/surgical supplies such as adhesive bandages, gauze pads and suture material nor does it include routine office items. A wall mounted oxygen and suction facility is a must for the ED's catering to larger workloads. There should be provision of adequate lighting supplemented by procedure lights especially in the procedure rooms.

Maintenance of equipment is a common problem in ED. Common complaints about missing and nonfunctional equipment is a symptom of fragmented maintenance system and lack of accountability for documenting, responding to and following up on maintenance needs. To circumvent this problem maintenance of equipment in emergency should be inventoried and handled on preventive maintenance basis [9].

Table 3: Suggested equipment and supplies for EDs

General requirements	*Airway & Breathing needs*
Cardiac monitors with defibrillator Temporary external pacemaker EKG monitor and machine Pulse oximeter End tidal CO2 detector Heating source Thermometers Weighing machines (adult and infant) Tape measure, Broselow's tape Sphygmomanometer with BP cuffs all sizes Ophthalmoscope/Otoscope Radiograph view Box IV Poles Pediatric restraining devices Biohazard disposal receptacles, including for sharps Garbage receptacles for non-contaminated materials Intradepartmental staff communication system: pagers and mobile phones **Fracture management equipment** Spinal immobilization board Splints Semi rigid neck collars	Suction devices and catheters 6-14 Oral, nasal and nasopharyngeal airways Clear oxygen masks, standard and non breathing Bag-valve- mask respirator (pediatric and infant size) Laryngoscopes, straight and curved, and stylets Endotracheal tubes, sizes 2.5-8.0 Magill forceps Tracheostomy kit Cricothyroidotomy kit **Circulation needs** IV catheters, sets, tubings, poles Butterfly needles Intraosseous needles Infusion pumps and tubing Central venous catheter setups with CVP monitoring equipment Pericacrdiocentesis instruments **Special Pediatric trays** Lumbar puncture Venous cut down Tube thoracostomy with und water seal New Born Kit (Umbilical vessel cannulation supplies) CPAP set Urinary catheter (Sizes 5-12)

Drugs

It is essential that the drugs required for emergency treatment are immediately available without requiring parental purchase.

FUNCTIONAL REQUIREMENTS

Triage

Triage is a brief clinical assessment that determines the time and sequence in which patients should be seen in the ED or, if in the field, the speed of transport and choice of hospital destination. These decisions generally are based on a short evaluation of the patient and an assessment of vital signs. The patient's overall appearance, history of illness and/or injury, and mental status also are important in the triage decision. The assessment is attempted within 15-20 seconds using the PALS guidelines; it is done by the junior resident in our set up. Correct triage depends upon the experience of the triage staff and adherence to objective directions. Subconscious pressures to under-triage (i.e. allocate to a less urgent category) occur when the department is busy and vice versa when the department is quiet. Children presenting as cardiopulmonary failure or cardiac arrest need to be seen, assessed and treated on arrival by the most experienced staff available. Delay in the treatment should be minimal in children presenting as shock or respiratory distress. Triaging gets priority over registration in Emergency. The children who are stable at presentation can wait for treatment. One should remember that triage is a dynamic process. Once the child is placed in a particular category, he should be regularly reassessed to determine if he needs to be moved up or down a category. Parents are usually concerned for their child when they present in Emergency and if they see other children being attended first on the basis of emergency or priority signs. Communication and explanation of the triage system are therefore needed. The initial triage of sick children arriving at hospitals in developing countries is often deficient, with severely ill children experiencing delays in the institution of life saving emergency[6,10].

In recent years, two initiatives have come together in an attempt to improve the emergency management of children in the hospital. Simplified guidelines for emergency triage assessment and treatment (ETAT) in developing countries were developed by the WHO IMCI Referral Care Project and piloted in Brazil and Malawi with good triage results when compared to decisions made by the Advanced Pediatric Life Support (APLS) trained staff. In a study from large volume Pediatric ED from Chennai central-peripheral temperature gap and respiratory failure requiring ventilation were found to be major risk factors for mortality in the children aged >1year.Among the post neonatal group, poor pulse volume and respiratory failure were strong risk factors. Given these results, perhaps the clinical features of circulatory and respiratory failure at presentation as proposed in PALS, APLS and ETAT guidelines are important for triage decisions even in the under resourced ED's of the developing countries (Figure 3).

Components of Model Case Sheet

Initial cardiopulmonary assessment using triage form is the first step in the Emergency followed by noting of the demographics and the reporting date and time. In ED's with heavy emergency loads, comprehensive history and examination may be almost impossible. Depending upon the time available, problem focused, expanded problem focused, detailed or a comprehensive history or examination are undertaken. Proper documentation serves two distinct purposes; clinical necessity and the legal necessity especially because of the increasing malpractice claims. Medical records of the admitted patients are preserved for at least two years and longer for the medico- legal cases such as child abuse. Physicians and nurses must be conversant with consumer protection forums and the Consumer Protection Act, and liability suits arising out of malpractice or negligence, and aware of ways of protecting themselves and hospital legally. Good medical and administrative practices including maintenance of well-documented medical records are a good legal protection.

If the resources permit, computer with internet facilities and networking can further help the pediatrician meet expectation of parents who think that their emergency physician is providing the best and latest in medical knowledge.

Admission and Transfer Criteria

Because hospitals vary significantly in their resources for providing pediatric care, there is no single set of criteria for admission and transfer of pediatric patients that has universal applicability. Each institution must assess its own capabilities and limitations in light of its mission and then formulate guidelines. Once guidelines for transfer of patients have been established, those for admission become less difficult to define. This challenging process requires input from all members of the health care team, including hospital administration. The goal is to ensure that each patient in the facility receives the optimal care that is most appropriate for his or her medical and psychosocial needs. We

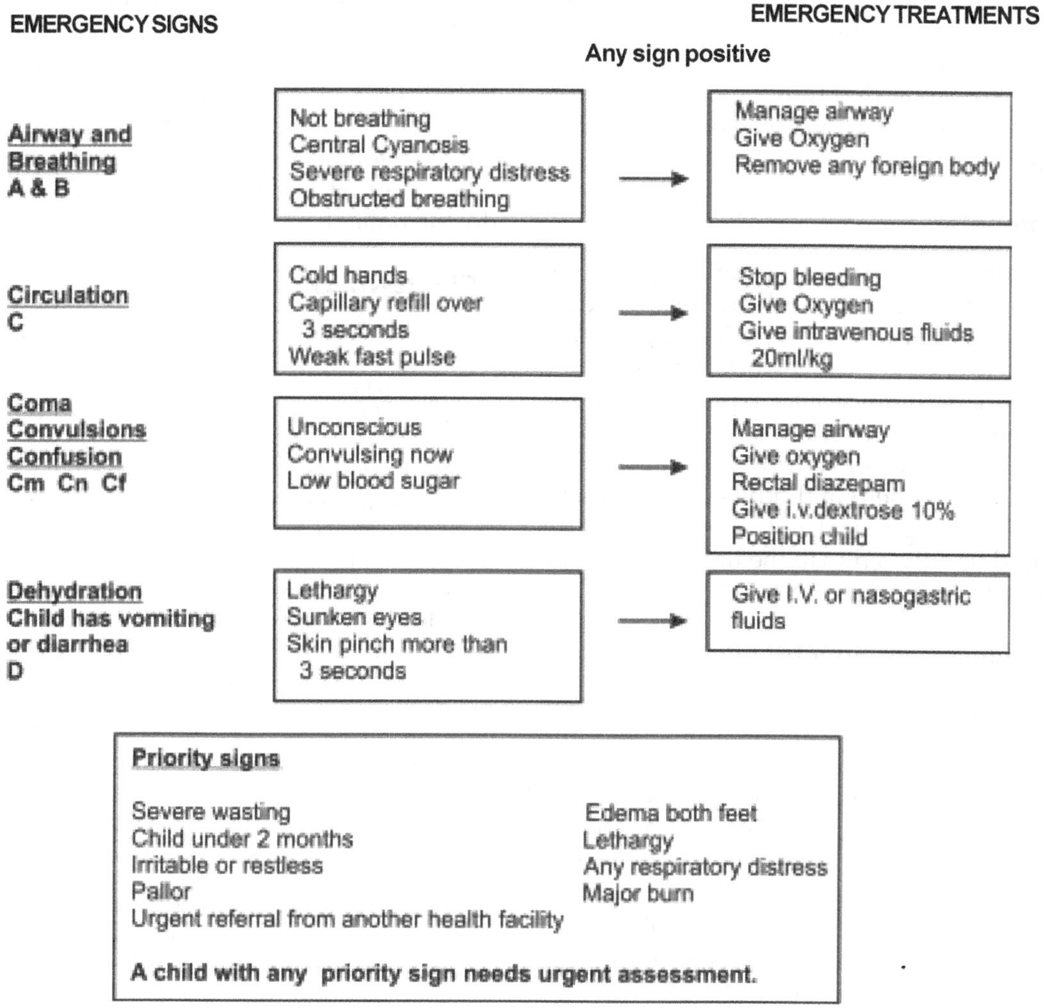

Fig. 3 : Emergency signs (ETAT guidelines)

in our hospital admit all children where the anticipated duration of the stay is more than six hours. An attempt is made to transfer all critically sick children to the Pediatric ICU soon after stabilization and other stable children to their respective units within 24 hours of their arrival.

Protocols

The management of common pediatric emergencies should follow set practices determined prior to child attending the ED. These will give a framework for junior and inexperienced physicians to practice safe and immediate care. Within this framework there should be supervision of experienced physicians to help and advise with difficult cases. As a general rule these protocols should be adhered to in the first instance and only varied by senior advise.

Administrative Functioning

In a tertiary care hospital the junior resident is the primary physician for triage and subsequent assessment and management. The more senior doctor (Senior resident) is consulted for procedures, excessive workload and for stabilization and resuscitation. It is desirable to discuss all problem cases with the Consultant of the unit. The Director or the In charge assumes the overall responsibility of the functioning of the unit.

Audit and Research

Practice review is an important part of the emergency care. The continued questioning of current practice by audit and research is vital to the planning and development of the speciality; without it we cannot hope improvement in the service provided[6].

CONCLUSIONS

Although emergency units in the hospitals vary in shape, size and technology similarities in responsibilities exist. The primary responsibility is to provide quality health care to the communities served. However, in our efforts to provide the efficient technology based, cost effective services to pediatric emergency patients, we must not forget the "human touch". It is the lack of compassionate care that leads to dissatisfaction in the doctor patient relationship [11].

REFERENCES

1. Mayer T, Cates R. Customer service-survival skills. Emergency Physicians of North Virginia.Ltd:2002.
   Available at :wysiwyg:44http:129.174.192.191/jRing/survival skills.htm.
2. Pena ME, Synder BL.Pediatric Emergency medicine.The history of growing discipline. Emerg Med Clin North Am. 1995; 13:235-53.
3. Posaw LL, Agarwal P,Berntein SL.Emergency medicine in New Delhi area,India. Annals Emerg Med 1998;32:609-15.
4. AlagappanK, Cherukuri K, Narang V, KwiatkowskiT, Rajagopalan A.Early development of emergency medicine in Chennai, India. Annals Emer Med 1998;32:604-8.
5. Kunders GD,Gopinath S ,Katakam. Emergency services.In Hospitals Planning,Design and Management.Eds Kunders GD,Gopinath S, Katakam. New Delhi,Tata McGraw-Hill;1998. p.140-5.
6. BeattieTF, Hendry GM, Hewson GC.The Child and the Accident and Emergency Department. In :Pediatric Emergencies.London :Mosby Wolfe;2005 .p. 1-10.
7. Singh S, Jain V, Gupta G. Pediatric Emergencies at Tertiary Care Hospital in India. J Trop Pediatr.2003;49:207-11.
8. Almeida SL. Nursing perspectives on the emergency department. Emerg Med Clin North Am. 2004;22:117-29.
9. Williams M. Materials management and logistics in the emergency department. Emerg Med Clin North Am. 2004;22:195-215.
10. Sandy G, Tamburlini G, Molyneux E,Whitesell P,Campbell H. Arch Dis Child 1999;81:473-7.
11. Chugh K. Organization of Pediatric Emergency Services. In: Principles of Pediatric and Neonatal Emergencies. Eds. Sachdev HPS, Choudhry P,

Bagga A, Chugh K, Ramji S, Puri RK, New Delhi: Jaypee; 2004.p13-19.

12. Singhi S, Gupta G, Jain V. Comparison of pediatric emergency patients in a tertiary care hospital vs a community hospital. Indian Pediatrics 2004; 41:67-72.
13. Integrated Management of Childhood Illness: a WHO/UNICEF Initiative. Bul World health Organ 1997:75(Suppl 1).
14. Robertson A, Molyneux E. Triage in the developing world-can it be done? Arch Dis Child 2001;85:208-13.
15. Simkiss D.Emergency Pediatric Care. J Trop Pediatr 2005; 51:263-4.
16. Santhanam I, Pai M, Kasturi K, Radhamani M.Mortality after admission in the pediatric emergency department:A prospective study from a referral children's hospital in southern India. Pediatr Crit Care Med 2002 ; 3:358-63.
17. Mahawar P, (Guides Singhi S, .Correlation of determinants of hypoxia and resuscitation adequacy in children ≤ 5 years in pediatric emergencies. Thesis, submitted to PGIMER for MD(Pediatrics) 2003.

Index

B

C

O

P

R